Cardiac Imaging in Structural Heart Disease Interventions

Anita M. Kelsey
Sreek Vemulapalli • Anita Sadeghpour
Editors

Cardiac Imaging in Structural Heart Disease Interventions

A Textbook for the Heart Team

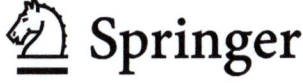

Editors
Anita M. Kelsey
Division of Cardiology
Duke University Medical Center
Durham, NC, USA

Sreek Vemulapalli
Duke University Hospital
Durham, NC, USA

Anita Sadeghpour
MedStar Health Research Institute and
Georgetown University
Washington, DC, DC, USA

ISBN 978-3-031-50742-7   ISBN 978-3-031-50740-3   (eBook)
https://doi.org/10.1007/978-3-031-50740-3

© The Editor(s) (if applicable) and The Author(s), under exclusive license to Springer Nature Switzerland AG 2024

This work is subject to copyright. All rights are solely and exclusively licensed by the Publisher, whether the whole or part of the material is concerned, specifically the rights of translation, reprinting, reuse of illustrations, recitation, broadcasting, reproduction on microfilms or in any other physical way, and transmission or information storage and retrieval, electronic adaptation, computer software, or by similar or dissimilar methodology now known or hereafter developed.
The use of general descriptive names, registered names, trademarks, service marks, etc. in this publication does not imply, even in the absence of a specific statement, that such names are exempt from the relevant protective laws and regulations and therefore free for general use.
The publisher, the authors, and the editors are safe to assume that the advice and information in this book are believed to be true and accurate at the date of publication. Neither the publisher nor the authors or the editors give a warranty, expressed or implied, with respect to the material contained herein or for any errors or omissions that may have been made. The publisher remains neutral with regard to jurisdictional claims in published maps and institutional affiliations.

This Springer imprint is published by the registered company Springer Nature Switzerland AG
The registered company address is: Gewerbestrasse 11, 6330 Cham, Switzerland
If disposing of this product, please recycle the paper.

Your bonus with the purchase of this book

With the purchase of this book, you can use our "SN Flashcards" app to access questions free of charge in order to test your learning and check your understanding of the contents of the book
To use the app, please follow the instructions below:

1. Go to **https://flashcards.springernature.com/login**
2. Create an user account by entering your e-mail adress and assiging a password.
3. Use the link provided in one of the first chapters to access your SN Flashcards set.

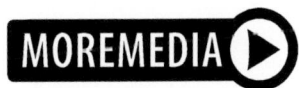

Your personal SN Flashcards link is provided in one of the first chapters.

If the link is missing or does not work, please send an e-mail with the subject "**SN Flashcards** " and the book title to **customerservice@springernature.com**

To my daughter, Michelle, the new cardiologist, for inspiration, to my Pete, for love, to my parents and role models, Margaret and Walter, and to George, where it all began.
Anita McIlveen Kelsey

To my daughter, Ariana, the light of my life and my parents for their love and support.
Anita Sadeghpour

To my daughters, Isabel and Stella, who are my sunshine and hope, my wife Lynn, with whom I have been blessed to walk through life, and my parents, whom I admire more and more with every day I get older.
Sreek Vemulapalli

Foreword

In my many years in cardiovascular medicine, I have seen how critically important education and team care are to realizing the promise of our rapidly advancing technologies and practices, and how hard it can be to deliver needed content in meaningful and accessible ways to the right audiences. Multidisciplinary topics or aspects of medicine requiring team care are a particularly challenging area as expertise is often siloed, yet team members need to be familiar with their colleagues' expertise to provide the most effective and collaborative care. Structural heart interventions are a perfect example of this: structural heart experts, proceduralists, imagers, intensivists are collectively essential to optimal patient care. I recognized this at the beginning of the structural heart intervention boom in the mid-2000s, as the imaging lead investigator in the first randomized trials leading to the initial approvals of two of the most important structural heart device advances: transcatheter heart valves, in the aptly named PARTNER trials using balloon inflatable valves, and the PROTECT and PREVAIL left atrial appendage occlusion trials. In both sets of landmark trials, the imaging teams provided important and powerful input into patient selection, procedural conduct, and long-term success. In turn, the trials provided an indispensable learning environment for imagers (as well as implanters) as we adapted old techniques and learned new ones to better support the heart team and our patients. Some of these insights are still state of the art; for others, these early innovations were foundational as imaging capabilities and skills have advanced to keep pace with rapidly evolving technologies and techniques.

Since then, the need for cross-specialty education in structural heart disease has only grown with the tremendous growth and diversity of procedures and capabilities. In writing *Cardiac Imaging in Structural Heart Disease Interventions: A Textbook for the Heart Team*, long-term esteemed colleagues Drs Kelsey, Vemulapalli, and Sadeghpour have identified a critical gap in educational materials targeting those who may not otherwise be exposed to imaging content but whose daily work would benefit immensely from more in-depth knowledge. By mixing together case studies, highlighting key points, providing summary tables and carefully targeted figures, and ending with board type questions, the authors have made the content highly accessible to those with different learning styles or needs.

This book is set apart and elevated by the decades of experience as imagers and educators of each of the editors and authors. Suitable for trainees and non-imaging experts as well as imagers, this is a book to read through to learn about the state of the art, turning often to the marvelous images and figures in the text and online. In this sense, it is a book about the past and the present. However, it is also a book about the future. It is a reference text to keep handy for years to access a table or figure to shed light on a specific issue, or to flip through to answer a specific question. Most importantly, it is a foundation and inspiration to ongoing advances in imaging and in structural heart disease.

Duke Clinical Research Institute Pamela S. Douglas
Durham, NC, USA
Duke University School of Medicine
Durham, NC, USA

Preface

Structural heart interventions require a team of medical professionals, excellent communication, and detailed cardiac imaging for successful, safe performance of these complex procedures. To facilitate effective communication and successful procedures, a clear understanding of the value of cardiac imaging is required by all members of the multidisciplinary team including cardiothoracic and vascular surgeons, interventional and noninvasive cardiologists, cardiac anesthesiologist, research and clinical nurses, sonographers, cardiovascular/OR technicians, and cardiology/cardiac surgery/cardiac anesthesia fellows. While each brings valuable skills to the team, a shared understanding of the importance and role of imaging is critical to the optimal teamwork and communication necessary for the success of these interventions.

While many great textbooks have addressed different aspects of structural heart disease interventions, few focus on the integration of cardiac imaging; and if cardiac imaging is the focus, the text is directed towards cardiac imagers. We have written this textbook with several features leveraging the tenets of adult learning to provide digestible information accessible to all heart team members:

- Clearly stated learning objectives for each chapter
- Case-based format with emphasis on images and multi-media
- Special emphasis on cardiac imaging within the preprocedural, intraprocedural, and postprocedural heart team discussions
- Comparisons of the additive value of multi-modality cardiovascular imaging
- Imaging pearls for non-imagers
- Key points about the value of each imaging modality and complexities at each stage of the interventional procedure.
- Board-style questions with explanations

We are deeply indebted to the many authors who have contributed their expertise and invaluable perspective in the chapters of this textbook. They have given you, the structural heart team members, a wealth of cardiac imaging insights acquired over many years of experience in the growing field of structural heart interventions.

We hope that you will find this textbook a valuable resource for your structural heart team, offering insights and clinical pearls that will prove instrumental in your team's success in providing these procedures for your cardiac patients.

Durham, NC, USA   Anita M. Kelsey
Durham, NC, USA   Sreek Vemulapalli
Washington, DC, USA   Anita Sadeghpour

Acknowledgments

This textbook would not have been possible without the expertise and effort of many people. We appreciate Pam Douglas who introduced these editors, igniting the creative energies to commence this work. We are indebted to our esteemed contributors who have provided in these pages the culmination of many years of experience in the art of multimodality imaging for structural heart disease interventions. We are also grateful to the Duke Cardiac Diagnostic Unit sonographers who assisted in image acquisition and editing, enhancing the value of this resource for the heart team including Ashlee Davis, Danny Rivera, Andrew Monteagudo, Rachel O'brien, Batina Kight, Carter Davis, and Jayne Leypoldt.

Finally, we would like to recognize friends at Springer Nature, for their unwavering morale and technical support throughout the project, Grant Weston, Hemalatha Gunasekaran, and Emily Wong.

Contents

Part I Cardiac Imaging and Percutaneous Therapeutic Intervention in Valvular Heart Diseases

Transcatheter Aortic Valve Replacement 3
Kavishka Sewnarain, Zain Ally, and Jonathon A. Leipsic

Multimodality Imaging of Mitral Valve Diseases: TEER, Valve in Valve, and Beyond 69
Taimur Safder, Gloria Ayuba, and Vera H. Rigolin

Multimodality Imaging of Tricuspid Valve Disease at the Dawn of Transcatheter Intervention 119
Susheel Kodali and Vratika Agarwal

Multimodality Imaging of Right Ventricular Outflow Tract Disease in Adults with Congenital Heart Disease 137
Toi Spates and Richard A. Krasuski

Pre- and Intraprocedural Imaging Considerations in Paravalvular Leak Closure 155
Adriana Postolache, Simona Sperlongano, Mathieu Lempereur, Raluca Dulgheru, François Damas, Nils Demarneffe, and Patrizio Lancellotti

Part II Percutaneous Therapeutic Intervention in Non-valvular, Non-congenital Structural Heart Diseases

Left Atrial Appendage Closure Periprocedural Imaging 177
Mesfer Alfadhel and Jacqueline Saw

Alcohol Septal Ablation in the Management of Hypertrophic Obstructive Cardiomyopathy (HOCM) 195
Daniel B. Loriaux, Andrew Wang, and Todd L. Kiefer

Percutaneous Closure of Post-myocardial Infarction Ventricular Septal Rupture 229
Jessica Raviv and Barry Love

Part III Interventions in Heart Failure

Interatrial Shunt Devices 245
Taimur Safder, Sanjiv Shah, and Akhil Narang

Part IV Percutaneous Therapeutic Intervention in Adult Congenital Heart Diseases

Patent Foramen Ovale and Atrial Septal Defect 263
Aken Desai, Edward Gill, and John Carroll

Percutaneous Ventricular Septal Defect Closure 283
Kamel Shibbani, Karim A. Diab, Damien Kenny, and Ziyad M. Hijazi

Coronary Cameral Fistula Closure 295
Anita Sadeghpour, Ata Firouzi, and Zahra Hosseini

Transcatheter Closure of Ruptured Sinus of Valsalva 309
Y. Hejazi, Z. M. Hijazi, and A. Sadeghpour

Transcatheter Approach to Coarctation of Aorta and Isolated Interrupted Aortic Arch in Adults 327
Ata Firouzi, Anita Sadeghpour, and Zahra Hosseini

Percutaneous Closure of Patent Ductus Arteriosus 343
Lourdes Prieto and Daniel Duarte

Index 357

Part I

Cardiac Imaging and Percutaneous Therapeutic Intervention in Valvular Heart Diseases

Transcatheter Aortic Valve Replacement

Kavishka Sewnarain, Zain Ally, and Jonathon A. Leipsic

Abstract

Aortic stenosis (AS) is the second most common form of valvular heart disease in the western world with bicuspid aortic valve being the second most common congenital cardiac anomaly, after patent foramen ovale. Isolated aortic regurgitation (AR) is less common than symptomatic AS. Imaging plays a significant role in diagnosis, procedural planning and intraprocedural management in these patients. Management can be either conservative or include valve replacement with either transcatheter or surgical options for symptomatic patients with severe disease. This chapter explores the indications and important imaging features in diagnosis, pre-procedural planning and management. The heart team discussion highlights the multifactorial approach optimizing device choice, aortic root features, chosen access route and the prediction and prevention of complications as well as Food and Drug Administration approval of Transcatheter Aortic Valve Replacement (TAVR) in low-risk patients and Valve in Valve procedures. There is a resurgence in balloon valvuloplasty which is indicated as a bridge to more definitive TAVR and Surgical Aortic Valve Replacement (SAVR) and is now also increasingly utilised in valve orifice dilatation pre and post Transcatheter heart Valve (THV) deployment. Post procedural patient follow-up and imaging is discussed and is aimed at confirmation of procedural success as well as identification of procedural complications and guidance of further clinical decision making.

Keywords

Aortic stenosis · Acquired aortic valve disease · Bicuspid aortic valve · Aortic regurgitation · Transcatheter aortic valve replacement · Transcatheter heart valve · Hypoattenuating leaflet thickening (HALT) · Paravalvular regurgitation · Coronary obstruction · Valve in valve · Balloon valvuloplasty · Echocardiography · Cardiac imaging · Elevated gradients

Supplementary Information The online version contains supplementary material available at https://doi.org/10.1007/978-3-031-50740-3_1.

K. Sewnarain · Z. Ally · J. A. Leipsic (✉)
Department of Radiology, Advanced Cardiovascular Imaging, St. Paul's Hospital, University of British Columbia, Vancouver, BC, Canada
e-mail: jleipsic@providencehealth.bc.ca

Test your learning and check your understanding of this book's contents: use the "Springer Nature Flashcards" app to access questions.

To use the app, please follow the instructions below:
1. Go to https://flashcards.springernature.com/login
2. Create a user account by entering your e-mail address and assigning a password.
3. Use the following link to access your SN Flashcards set: ▶ https://sn.pub/ambACS

If the link is missing or does not work, please send an e-mail with the subject "SN Flashcards" and the book title to customerservice@springernature.com.

Learning Objectives

1. Describe how to diagnose aortic stenosis and use imaging to guide management choices.
2. Describe how to identify bicuspid aortic valve disease and the indications for valve replacement.
3. Describe how to identify aortic regurgitation and recognize the indications for valve replacement.
4. Describe the strengths and weaknesses of available preprocedural imaging modalities and their interpretation in aortic valve disease.
5. Describe how to assess potential TAVR complications through imaging.
6. Describe the role of imaging in balloon valvuloplasty and valve in valve procedures.

Aortic Stenosis

Case Study

A 75-year-old male patient with a history of prior percutaneous coronary intervention (PCI) and coronary artery bypass graft (CABG) presented with chest pain and progressive dyspnea on exertion. He experiences palpitations and dizziness but no syncopal episodes. On physical examination, auscultation revealed a Grade 2/6 systolic ejection murmur at the base radiating to the neck and cardiac apex. Distal pulses were feeble but palpable. ECG did not show an old infarct nor other abnormalities.

Background and Definitions

Aortic Stenosis Definition and Classification

Aortic stenosis (AS) is the second most common cause of valvular heart disease in the western world with the primary pathogenesis shifting from rheumatic to degenerative valve disease in modern times [1]. Patients at higher risk for AS include those with congenital (bicuspid, unicuspid) heart valve variants [2] and comorbidities resulting in abnormal calcium metabolism [3].

Patient risk profile and histopathological leaflet findings in AS are similar to that of coronary atherosclerotic disease, with an inflammatory component, commonly progressing to leaflet calcification and immobility [1]. This results in insidious deterioration in left ventricular outflow with subsequent myocardial hypertrophy, systolic and potentially diastolic dysfunction with resultant heart failure [3]. There is a latent period with symptoms generally only becoming significant with the onset of severe stenosis [3]. Classic symptoms include angina, heart failure or syncope but the elderly may only present with exercise intolerance [1, 3]. Classic clinical signs include a parvus-tardus carotid pulse, a holo/mid/late systolic murmur maximal at the second intercostal space radiating to the carotid vessels and less often to the apex [3].

Imaging plays a central role in the diagnosis, severity grading, procedural planning, and follow up of the patient with AS. The mainstay of imaging in AS is echocardiography (Transthoracic echocardiography (TTE) or Transesophageal echocardiography (TEE)), cardiac catheterization and computed tomography (CT), supplemented by Magnetic Resonance Imaging (MRI) in specific scenarios. Intraprocedural imaging is accomplished with fluoroscopy with or without echocardiography.

Management options are divided into watchful waiting, medical treatment and valve replacement, either via percutaneous or surgical intervention [3]. Watchful waiting is an option in patients with severe stenosis who are truly asymptomatic, with care paid to ensure that symptoms are not erroneously attributed to "aging" [3]. Since onset of symptoms may be sudden, close monitoring is essential with 6–12 months serial echocardiograms [4]. Patients with a velocity of >5 m/s or an increase of >0.3 m/s/year have a strong predilection to valve replacement within 2 years [3] and as a result in patients with very severe AS (defined as an aortic velocity of ≥5 m/s and low surgical risk), AVR is reasonable [4]. Severe AS should be actively excluded in patients with suspected moderate stenosis and low flow low gradient [3]. Follow up echocardiograms should be performed every 12–24 months in moderate stenosis, 3–5 years in mild stenosis or at the onset of new symptoms or clinical findings [3].

Diagnosis and Pre-procedural Evaluation

Echocardiography

Transthoracic echocardiography (TTE) plays an essential role in the non-invasive diagnosis of AS by defining valve morphology and sclerosis and assessing the severity of stenosis and its impact on left ventricular function and remodeling [5]. Severity can be graded as mild, moderate or severe and additionally categorized as having reduced or preserved function with normal or low cardiac outflow [5].

Given the patient's history of coronary artery disease, presenting symptoms, and physical exam findings, diagnoses of progressive coronary artery disease, as well as aortic stenosis were considered. Based on this differential diagnosis, the first step of further diagnostic testing was to obtain a transthoracic echocardiogram, primarily to assess biventricular function and also to evaluate the aortic valve. The echocardiogram revealed severely thickened aortic valve leaflets with severely restricted leaflet motion (Videos 1 and 2). After assessment of the aortic spectral Doppler from multiple echo windows and with multiple sonographers when available [6], the aortic valve Vmax was 3.7 m/s with a mean gradient of 30 mmHg (Fig. 1) [6]. The aortic valve area (AVA) was calculated from the continuity equation at 1.0 cm^2 with an AVA index of 0.5 cm^2/m^2. The stroke volume was calculated at 86 mL with an indexed value of 43 mL/m^2. There was moderate posterior mitral annular calcification and mild central mitral regurgitation. The LVEF was estimated at 60% with the ratio of left ventricular wall thickness to cavity dimension suggestive of left ventricular concentric remodeling (Video 3).

This patient's echocardiographic values demonstrate discrepancy between the observed gradients (which would be classified as moderate) and the calculated AVA and indexed AVA, which would be classified as severe). This AVA–gradi-

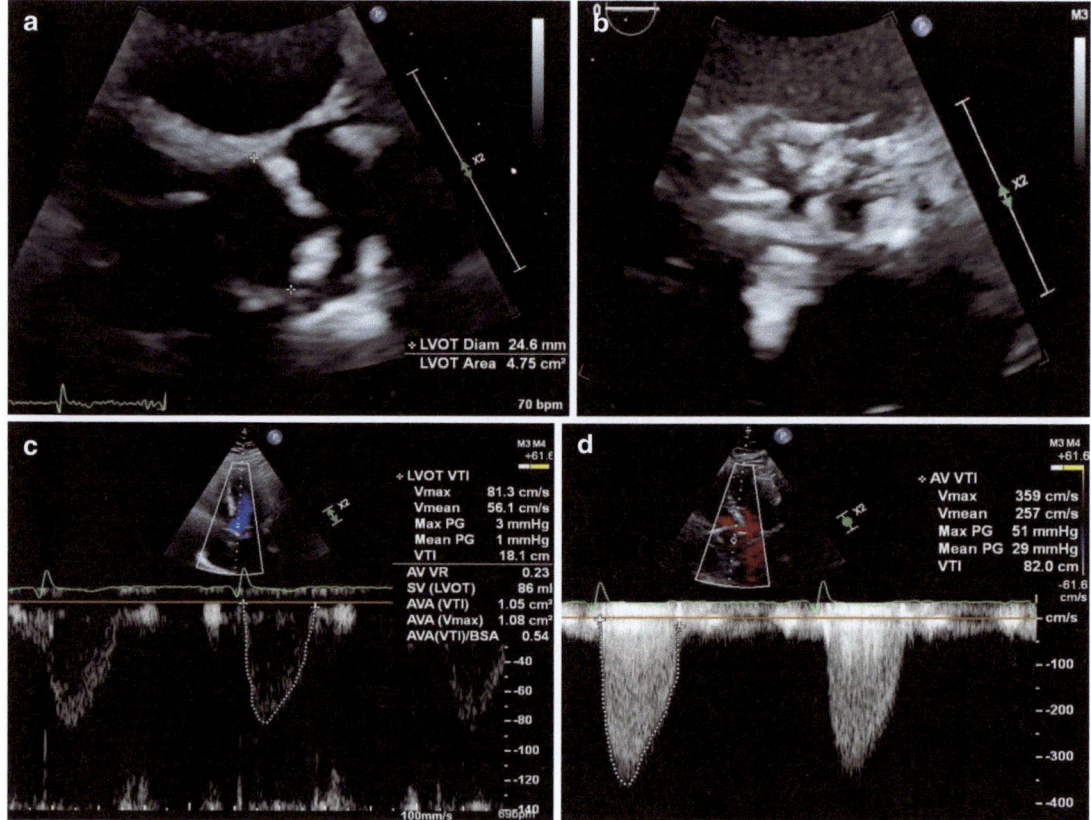

Fig. 1 2D trans thoracic echocardiogram of the aortic valve (**a**) Parasternal long axis zoomed 2D view with a LVOT diameter of 24.6 mm (measured inner edge to inner edge) and thickened coronary leaflets. (**b**) Parasternal short axis demonstrating tricuspid aortic valve with thickened leaflets. (**c**) Pulsed wave doppler of the LVOT with a VTI of 18.1 cm. (**d**) Continuous wave doppler across the aortic valve with a VTI of 82 cm. The mean transvalvular valve gradient was 29 mmHg and the peak transvalvular gradient was 51 mmHg. AVA was calculated at 1 cm^2

ent discordance is a clinically common scenario and the first step is to confirm the accuracy of the echo measurements and calculations, especially the LVOT diameter. The LVOT diameter should be measured in a zoomed image of the LVOT taken from the parasternal long axis view during mid systole from the inner edge to the inner edge. Errors in the measurement are squared as part of the calculation of the AVA, the indexed AVA, and the stroke volume index are the most common source of inaccuracy in AS grading. To confirm the accuracy of the LVOT diameter measurement, the observed value can be compared against the predicted LVOT diameter, calculated as (5.7 × body surface area) + 12.1 where discrepancies of >2 mm suggest inaccurate LVOT diameter measurement [7].

Once the accuracy of the echo measurements is confirmed, further imaging will be needed to confirm the diagnosis of severe AS (Fig. 2) In this case, given that the patient had a normal EF and a normal stroke volume index, to confirm the presumptive diagnosis of normal flow, low-gradient AS, the patient underwent non-contrast and contrast multi-detector CT, both for the purposes of obtaining an aortic valve calcium score [8] as well as potential procedural planning.

Computed Tomography

CT may be used to determine the aortic valve calcium score when there is discordance between echocardiographic findings (i.e. low flow, low gradient and normal flow, low gradient) [9] and aortic valve area in patients with clinical evi-

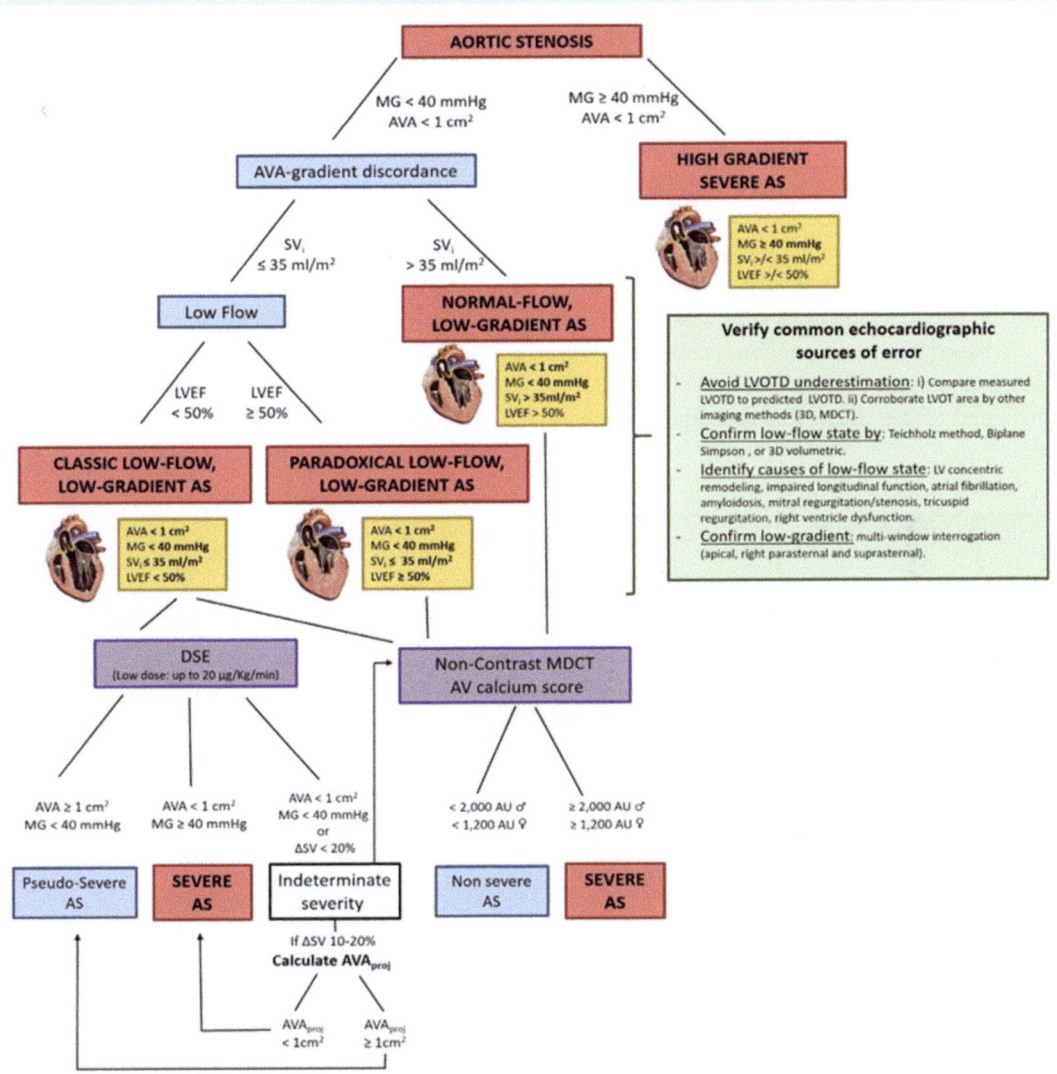

Fig. 2 Algorithm for assessing AS severity in different flow-gradient scenarios. *AS* aortic stenosis; *AU* agatston units; *AV* aortic valve; *AVA* aortic valve area; *AVA$_{proj}$* projected aortic valve area; *DSE* dobutamine stress echocardiography; *LV* left ventricular; *LVEF* left ventricular ejection fraction; *LVOT* left ventricular outflow tract; *LVOTD* left ventricular outflow tract diameter; *MDCT* multidetector computed tomography; *MG* mean transvalvular gradient; *SV* stroke volume; *SV$_i$* indexed stroke volume; *ΔSV* change in stroke volume; *3D* 3-dimensional. Reprinted from JACC Case Reports, Vol 4/3, Iria Silva, Erwan Salaun, Nancy Côté, Philippe Pibarot, Confirmation of Aortic Stenosis Severity in Case of Discordance Between Aortic Valve Area and Gradient, 170–177, Copyright 2022, with permission from Elsevier

dence of severe stenosis [10]. CT leaflet calcium score does not account for pathological leaflets with fibrotic rather than calcific thickening [10] and should be considered especially when evaluating female patients. The presence of a low aortic valve calcium score and echocardiographic significant AS should not preclude TAVR with balloon expandable (BE) devices as these have demonstrated high device success and lower paravalvular regurgitation (PVR) rates in comparison to patients with high valve calcium scores [9]. CT based threshold are gender specific, with stenosis classified as severe when >1300 AU in women and >2000 AU (arbitrary value) in males [10].

The patient's aortic valve was tricuspid and symmetrically calcified with no adverse root features. The calcium score was >2000 Agatston units, consistent with severe AS. Additionally, the systolic annular area was 383 mm², with a perimeter of 69 mm and diameter of 22 mm. There was no annular or LVOT calcification. The distance of the left main and right coronary ostia to the annular plane was measured at 13 mm and 18 mm respectively. The average dimension of the Sinus of Valsalva (SoV) (calculated by averaging the distances measured from cusp to commissure), was 32 mm and the STJ was measured at 27 mm (Fig. 3). Predicted CT derived fluoroscopic projections were cusp overlap view of

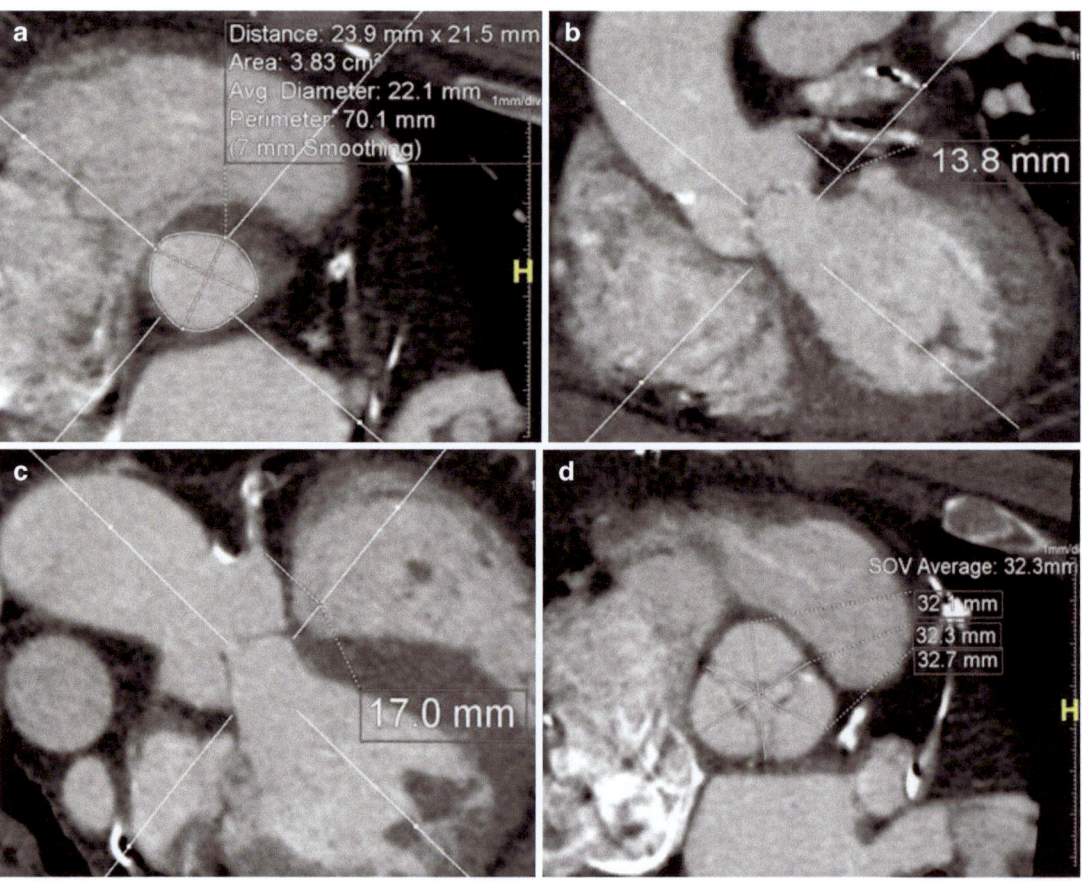

Fig. 3 Post contrast pre TAVR CT imaging. (**a**) Annular area of 383 mm² and perimeter of 70 mm. Measurement taken in the derived annular plane in the systolic phase of the cardiac cycle. (**b**) Left main coronary height of 13.8 mm and (**c**) right coronary height of 17 mm from the annular plane suggests low risk for coronary obstruction. (**d**) The sinuses of Valsalva measured from cusp to commissure and the three measurements averaged to give a SOV average dimensions of 32 mm. This suggests a capacious SOV signifying a low risk for coronary artery obstruction

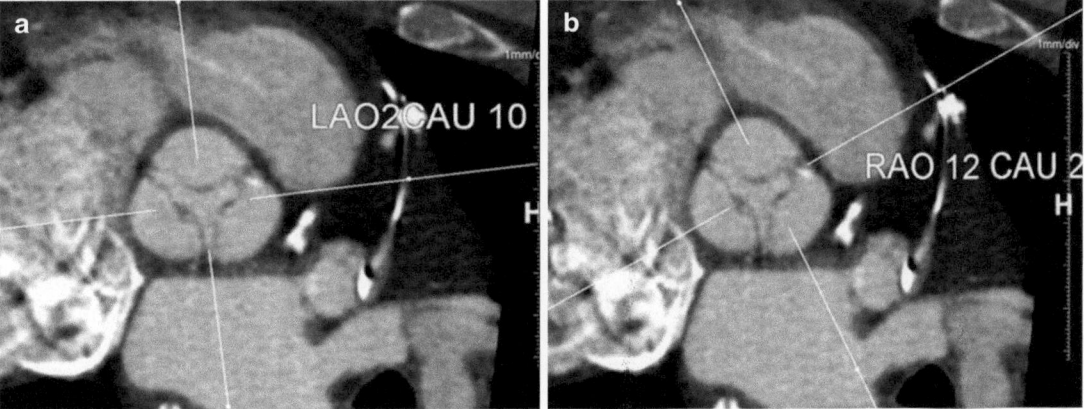

Fig. 4 CT derived projection angles to guide fluoroscopic procedure and obtain a plane orthogonal to the annulus (**a**) right cusp centered view and (**b**) overlap view

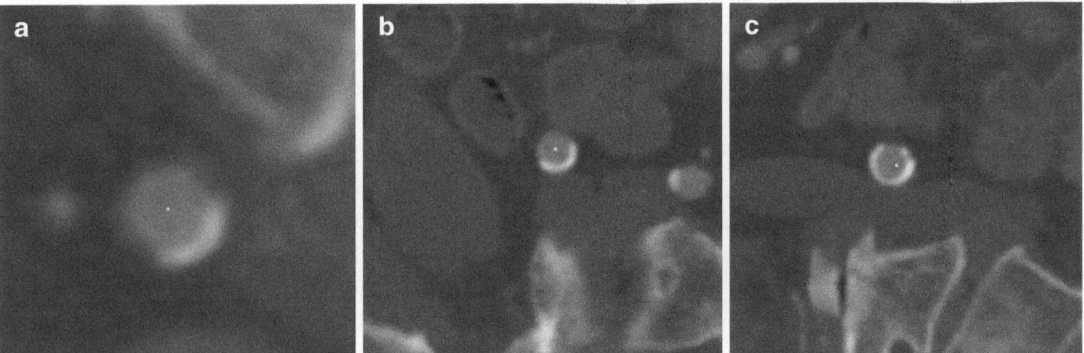

Fig. 5 Short axis images of vascular access of the iliofemoral vessels. Images assessed for degree of calcification. (**a**) Mild crescentic non protruding calcification. (**b**) Horseshoe calcification. (**c**) Near circumferential calcification

RAO 10 CAU 22 and a right cusp centered view could be achieved at RAO12 CAU2 (Fig. 4).

The were no imaging features prohibitive of bifemoral vascular access. There was mild tortuosity and calcific atherosclerotic plaque with minimal luminal diameters of 6 mm in the external iliac arteries on each side (Fig. 5). The ascending aorta had no calcific atherosclerotic plaque. The aortic arch, descending thoracic and abdominal aorta had coalescing non protruding atherosclerotic changes. There was no significant vascular tortuosity (Fig. 6).

Cardiac Catheterization

Preprocedural cardiac and coronary catheterization is performed to determine the presence and severity of coronary atherosclerotic disease and feasibility of future coronary access post TAVR [11]. Cautious attempts at crossing the aortic valve at time of pre procedural angiogram predicts ease of successful negotiation of the valve during the TAVR procedure (however an unsuccessful attempt does not preclude TAVR) followed by LV catheterization to determine, trans aortic pressure gradient, annulus area and the severity of aortic stenosis especially in the setting of discrepant echocardiography results [11] or discordant clinical and non-invasive imaging findings [4]. Assessment of pulmonary artery pressures, pulmonary vascular resistance and cardiac output may also be obtained during right heart catheterization [11]. Access route feasibility for TAVR may also be assessed via aortography and pigtail catheterization [8, 11]. It allows for determination

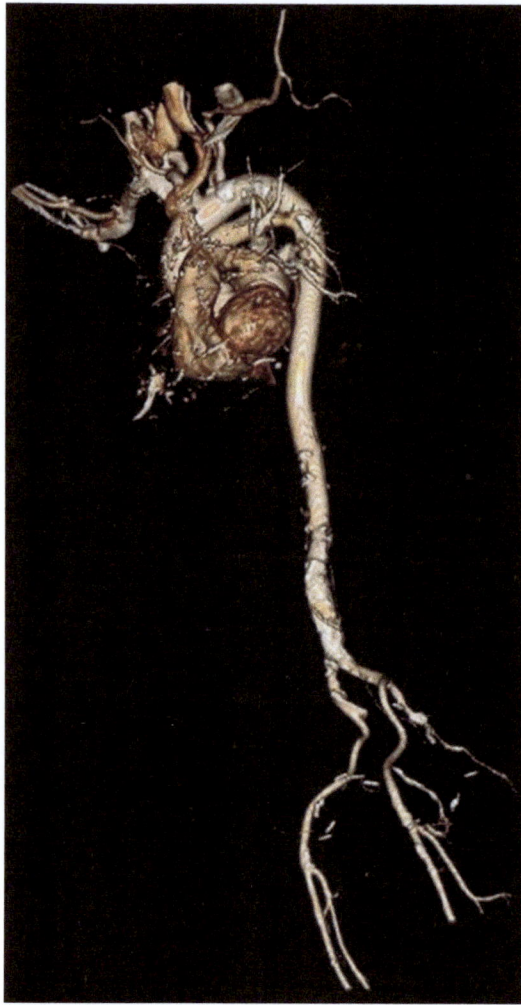

Fig. 6 3D Volume rendered image assessing tortuosity of the vessels being considered for access. Mild tortuosity of iliofemoral vessels

of tortuosity, degree of calcification and luminal caliber [11] however assessment of the latter two is limited [12]. Angiography also allows for assessment of vessel movement with reduced motion implying a more rigid and calcified artery [13]. Accurate assessment of luminal dimension is however limited by lack of orthogonal images in the acquired 2D planar views [8].

The present patient's coronary angiogram demonstrated patent grafts with significant native vessel disease. Aortic root had no dissection, dilatation, or severe calcification. Right heart catheterization had normal pulmonary arterial and right atrial pressures. Cardiac output and Cardiac Index where normal at 3.77 L/min and 1.93 L/min/m^2 respectively (Fig. 7; Video 4). *Right and left iliofemoral arteries were feasible for transfemoral (TF) TAVR without severe stenosis, tortuosity or significant calcification* (Fig. 8; Video 5).

Although not required in our patient, CMR and Nuclear Medicine are further tools in the diagnostic arsenal. CMR provides additional benefit in patients with iodine contrast allergies and impaired renal function [11]. Non contrast CMR was found to be equitable to CT and 2D echo in annular measurement, and further information in the form of biventricular function, severity and presence of AS, aortic regurgitation (AR) or mixed lesions and determination of a physiological orifice area [11]. Detection of mid wall fibrosis by late gadolinium sequences portends left ventricular decompensation and mortality [14]. Calcium however limits assessment of vascular access and aortic root especially in non-contrast studies [11].

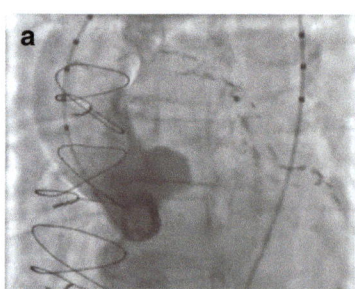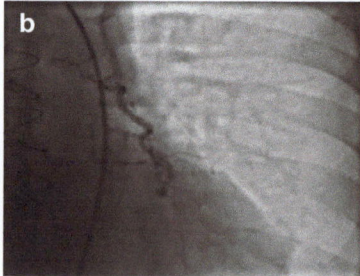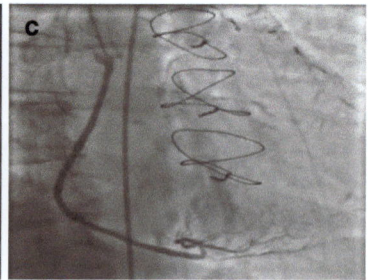

Fig. 7 Angiographic assessment of the aortic root and coronary vessels. (**a**) Non dilated aortic root without severe calcification. Evidence of prior CABG. (**b**) LIMA to LAD and SVG to PDA were patent. (**c**) Patent graft to the right coronary artery

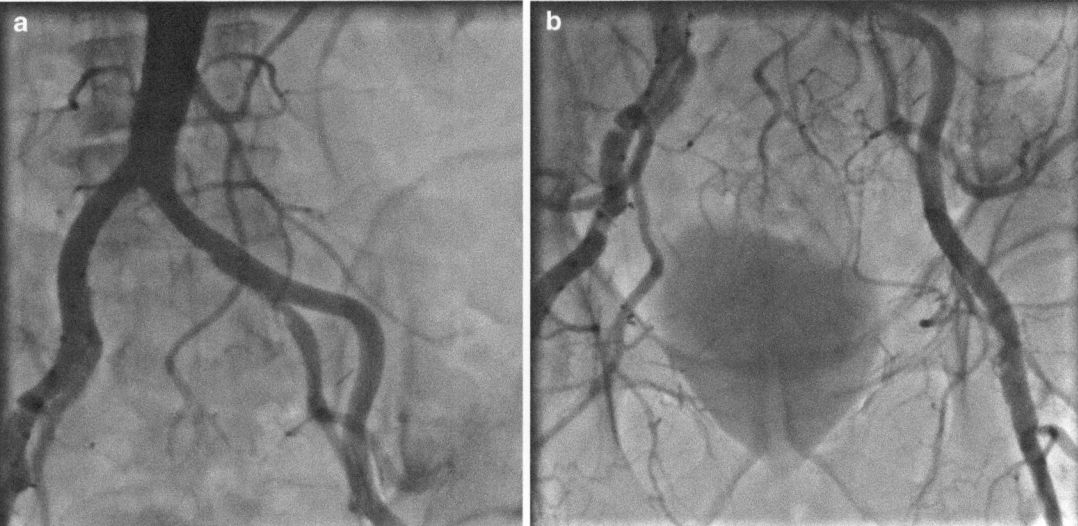

Fig. 8 Aorto femoral access was feasible with no significant stenosis or tortuosity. Mild calcific plaque in the aorta and both iliofemoral vessels

Differential Diagnosis

Prior to testing, the patient's signs and symptoms were most consistent with a differential diagnosis of progressive coronary artery disease and/or aortic stenosis. The patient's echocardiogram, cardiac catheterization, and cardiovascular CT are most consistent with severe, symptomatic AS as the cause of the patient's symptoms. Based on this diagnosis, evaluation for AVR is warranted.

Heart Team Approach and Discussion

Given that the diagnosis of severe, symptomatic AS has been made and a decision to evaluate for the suitability of AVR has been made, the next decision to be undertaken is TAVR vs. SAVR. On the strength of a series of clinical trials of encompassing both the Edwards Sapien and Medtronic CoreValve TAVR platforms, TAVR has been approved by Food and Drug Administration for use in patients at low through high risk of death or major complications during open-heart surgery. As a result, shared decision-making between TAVR and SAVR is often based on anatomy, patient preference, and other considerations.

Decision Between SAVR and TAVR

Valve replacement treatment options include SAVR (bioprosthetic or mechanical) or TAVR.

In patients less than 65 years of age with no high risk or prohibitive features for surgery and with a life expectancy of greater than 20 years, SAVR is the preferred option, mainly due to insufficient data on long term durability of TAVR valves versus SAVR [4]. In patients with SAVR the decision for a mechanical versus a bioprosthetic valve depends on patient preference, potential future childbearing, age of the patient, feasibility of long term anticoagulation use, and a balance between a combination of valve hemodynamic requirements, valve durability and predicted future surgical risk profile [4]. Patients between 65 and 80 years with no contraindication to either SAVR or TAVR may receive either procedure [4]. Patients over 80 years or patients with less than 10 years predicted survival, TAVR is preferred provided there are no contraindications [4]. In addition TAVR is preferred in patients of all ages in whom SAVR is high risk or prohibitive and predicted post TAVR survival is greater than a year with a reasonable quality of life [4].

Cardiac features detectable on imaging that can favor SAVR include suboptimal annular and aortic root findings as listed in Table 1 below,

Table 1 Imaging parameters, their significance in TAVR suitability, and reference values

	Reference values	Significance	Key points
Annulus (measured at blood tissue interface contouring through calcification as if not present [15])		Area and perimeter used for valve sizing and referenced with manufacturer sizing charts	– Smaller annular dimensions acquired by 2D TEE than 3D TEE which in turn were smaller than those acquired by CT [16]. – Should be measured at the largest dimension, usually 20% R-R interval [16] usually at end systole (i.e. the last phase before the mitral valve opens). – Annulus is predominantly ellipsoid in diastole, approximates a circular shape with a larger area, perimeter and short axis diameters in systole [16]. – Occasionally, in the presence of a hypertrophied septum annulus may be smaller in systole due to protrusion of basal septum into the annulus and left ventricular outflow tract (LVOT) [17], an appearance referred to as inverse dynamism
Sinus of Valsalva dimensions (measured cusp to commissure in widest dimension parallel to annulus) [15]	<30 mm [15]	<30 mm predicts risk of coronary artery occlusion [15]	– Risk of coronary occlusion depends on a combination of sinus of Valsalva (SoV) dimension, coronary artery heights, leaflet heights, aortic root dimensions, annular dimension and the choice of prosthetic valve [15]
Coronary to ostial heights	12 mm	Less than 12 mm is at high risk for occlusion [15]	– An accessory coronary artery and separate ostia of the conal artery, left circumflex (LCX) or left anterior descending (LAD) should be identified if present and assessed for risk of occlusion [15]. – Ostial location within the sinus varies with varying proximity to the sinotubular junction (STJ), annulus and commissures [18]. – A low coronary ostial height (less than 12 mm) should be considered in combination with SOV diameter, THV size, annular and root dimensions [17]
LVOT	Access for calcification, sub valvular membrane, septal hypertrophy [19]	There is increasing risk of rupture with increasing severity of calcification [19]	
STJ height (shortest distance between the annular plane and the lowest STJ level) STJ diameter (widest and orthogonal dimensions at the STJ plane)		A STJ height and diameter less than the prosthetic valve places the STJ at risk of injury, of particular importance in the use of balloon expandable valves [15]. Calcification at the STJ may limit balloon and device expansion with risk of device migration [12]	– A STJ height less than the height of the prosthetic valve, implies extension of the valve beyond the STJ and into the proximal ascending aorta [15]

Table 1 (continued)

	Reference values	Significance	Key points
Aortic angulation (angle between the horizontal plane and annular plane of the aortic valve) [20, 21]	48°	Reduced immediate procedural success, with increased risk of device migration, increased requirements for a second valve and balloon dilation, increased fluoroscopy time and post procedural paravalvular leak (PVL) in patients with an aortic angle of ≥48° [21]	– No statistically significant effect of aortic angle on outcomes with new generation valves i.e. self-expandable or balloon expandable [20, 22]
Landing zone calcification		Landing zone calcification, and lack their off, plays an important role in device anchorage [9] however adverse outcomes from annular and sub annular calcification include PVL, conduction abnormalities and annular rupture [15]	– Subjective assessment of number of calcified foci and extent in radial, inferior and circumferential directions and described as mild, moderate or severe. Location to the aortic leaflets and morphology of the calcium namely crescentic/flat or protruding should also be accessed [15]
Ascending aorta		Larger aortic diameters are more commonly present in bicuspid valve morphology, advanced age and female gender (when indexed to BSA) [23]. Ascending aortic calcification	Concerns in the setting of AS and TAVR include progressive dilation, aortic dissection [24], rupture [24], PVL [25] and an increase in all-cause mortality at 2 years [25]. Measurement techniques vary from inner wall to inner wall, outer wall to outer wall and leading edge to leading edge. 2D leading edge to leading edge measurements were found to corelate best with inner wall to inner wall dimensions on CT and MRI [26]. Ascending aorta calcification (porcelain aorta) favors TAVR over SAVR [4]

severe primary mitral regurgitation, dilation of the aortic root and ascending aorta, septal hypertrophy, coronary artery disease requiring CABG, whereas a porcelain aorta favors TAVR [4].

Preprocedural CT provides important information on access feasibility, potential fluoroscopic projections of the aortic root, annular sizing, aortic leaflet and root calcification, risk of coronary obstruction and identifying high risk features for complications [11]. Complementing anatomical coronary assessment, physiological assessment with fractional flow reserve derived from CT is safe and feasible with an acceptable diagnostic accuracy in patients with AS [27]. Importantly, CTA can also be used to provide information regarding vascular dimensions, calcification, tortuosity, all of which are important to determine the optimal vascular access point for a transcatheter intervention (Fig. 9).

Access for TAVR

The advent of pre procedural screening has reduced the incidence of major vascular complications, now occurring in 4–5% of procedures [15]. Improvements in sheath size has reduced the lumen size at which safe access can be achieved however pre-procedural vascular imaging, usually by CTA, is recommended to alert the heart team to precarious anatomy and pre-existing vasculopathy [15].

Trans femoral (TF) access is preferred [28] and demonstrates the lowest complication rate [29]. In the event that TF access is not possible, alternate workable access routes include trans subclavian, trans aortic, trans apical, trans carotid, trans caval and antegrade aortic approaches [28]. Trans aortic and trans apical approaches where initially preferred alternative access routes but following relative inferior outcomes in ran-

From the conventional MPR imaging, the optimal phase with the least motion and widest annular orifice is chosen. Following double oblique manipulation to obtain en face views of the aortic valve, the annular plane is derived from aligning the insertion points(B) of the cusps. The annular area and perimeter (A) are measured optimally using the spline contour with the margins at the interface between the walls of the annulus and the opacified lumen.	
The height of the right (C) and left main (D) coronary arteries are obtained by a vertical perpendicular measurement from the inferior margin of the ostium, of each vessel, to the annular plane.	
The STJ diameter is acquired by perpendicular axial dimensions at the level of the STJ (E). The STJ height is is the lowest vertical perpendicular height of the STJ to the annulus (F).	
The sinus of Valsalva is an averaged dimension of the three cusp to commissure distances (G) in a plane parallel to the annulus at which the sinus is at its widest.	

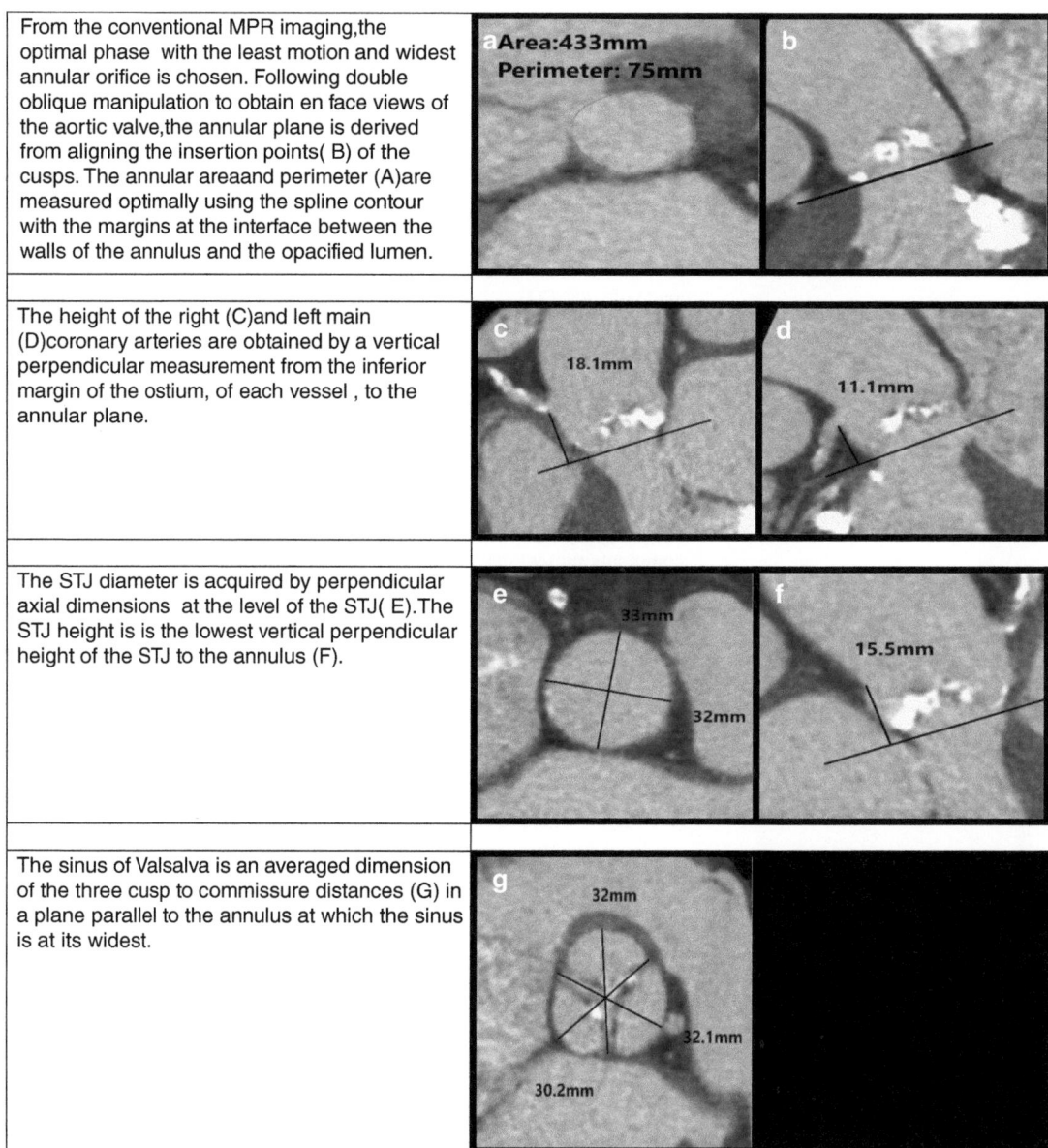

Fig. 9 Aortic annulus measurement by cardiac CT

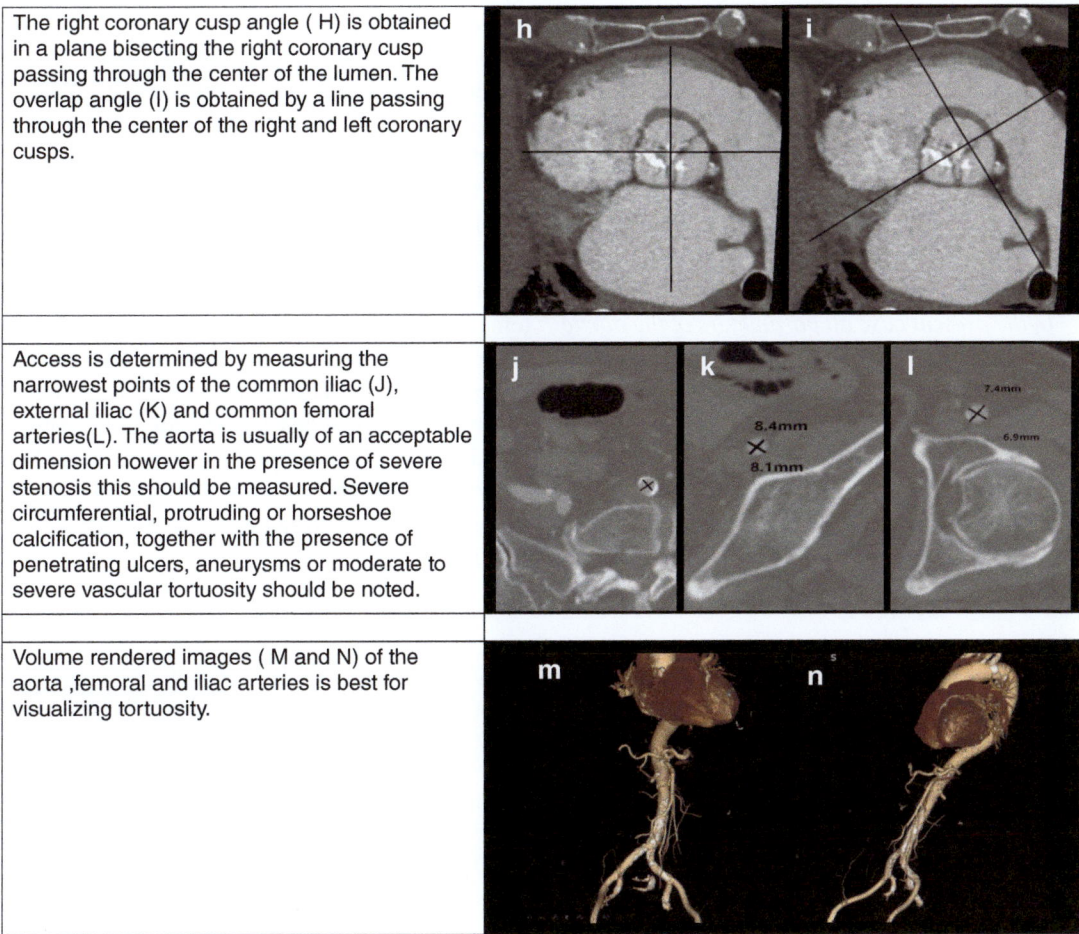

Fig. 9 (continued)

domised studies comparing SAVR to TAVR [29], these are usually reserved for when all other approaches are unsafe or not possible [11]. Mortality rates measured at 1 and 2 years post procedure are similar in the TF and trans subclavian/axillary route, however mortality rates are significantly increased at both time frames in trans aortic and trans apical access [30]. Use of an alternate access is limited by institutional and provider expertise [28].

CT is the preferred modality in preprocedural vascular assessment and has led to a decrease in major and minor complications [11]. Information on calcification, tortuosity, luminal dimension, the presence of aneurysms, vascular dissection and atheroma (which poses a risk for embolization) can be easily ascertained [8]. Comprehensive assessment includes analysis of 3D volume rendered images, curved multiplanar reconstruction and maximum intensity projections [31]. The minimal luminal diameter may be underestimated due to blooming artefact from calcium and overestimation of stenosis as a result of partial volume averaging [13].

Magnetic Resonance Imaging

Gadolinium MRI is comparable to CTA when assessing vessel diameter and angulation [32]. There is however reduced sensitivity in calcified vessels [32] and its use is limited in patients with renal impairment [11]. Ferumoxtyol contrast enhanced MRI provides a reasonable alternative in the setting of renal dysfunction, limiting effects from flow and motion when compared to a non-contrast MRI but extent of calcification may still be underestimated [33]. It is safe and diagnostic at both 1.5 T and 3 T [33]. Non-contrast cardiac MRI for pre-procedure AVR evaluation remains under investigation, however, Pamminger et al. demonstrated strong correlation for luminal dimension and tortuosity determination between non contrast quiescent interval single shot MRI (QISS) and contrast CT angiography, however QISS lacked visualisation of calcified plaque burden [34].

In the present case all parameters of the aortic root are normal with low risk of complications. In addition, the patient has a stent and a saphenous vein to posterior descending artery, left internal mammary to left anterior descending artery and venous to circumflex artery grafts with low risk of coronary obstruction. Additionally, there were no significant contraindications to transfemoral access and TF TAVR.

Valve Choice

Choice for the patient: A 23 mm Sapien Ultra.

The devices currently approved for TAVR in the United States include the Edwards SAPIEN and the Core Valve platforms [35]. The frequency at which the valves are used depends on the familiarity of the operators with the device as well as the patients anatomic and clinical suitability [36]. There are multiple other TAVR systems approved in Europe and there will soon be other TAVR systems available in the United States as well. The principles for choosing between these systems for an individual patient will likely remain similar to what is described above with patient anatomy and operator familiarity with TAVR systems likely remaining the driving factors.

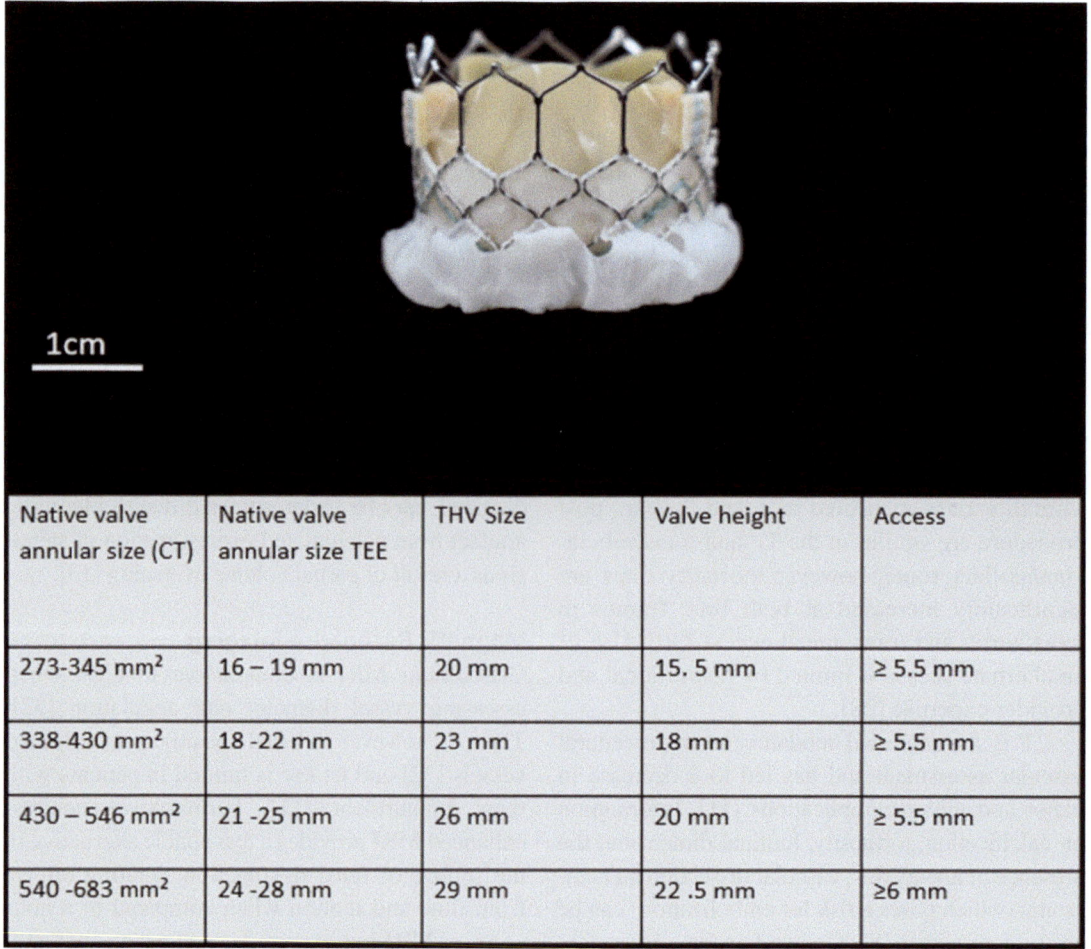

Native valve annular size (CT)	Native valve annular size TEE	THV Size	Valve height	Access
273-345 mm²	16 – 19 mm	20 mm	15. 5 mm	≥ 5.5 mm
338-430 mm²	18 -22 mm	23 mm	18 mm	≥ 5.5 mm
430 – 546 mm²	21 -25 mm	26 mm	20 mm	≥ 5.5 mm
540 -683 mm²	24 -28 mm	29 mm	22 .5 mm	≥6 mm

Fig. 10 Adapted from manufacturer instruction document

Sapien 3 Valve (Fig. 10)

Sapien 3 (S3) is a balloon expandable THV designed to improve positioning, increase paravalvular sealing and decrease vascular complications [37]. The S3-THV has a frame geometry that allows for lower delivery profiles and has higher radial strength when compared to its predecessors thus allowing improved maintenance of circularity after it has been deployed [38]. Available sizes include 20 mm, 23 mm, 26 mm, and 29 mm [39]. The 14F and 16F sheaths used with the S3-THV reduces vascular profile requirements thus allowing more patients to undergo transfemoral TAVI without significant access site bleeding or vascular complications [38].

Evolut Pro and Evolut R (Figs. 11 and 12)

Currently available in four sizes: 23, 26, 29, and 34 mm allowing for treatment in an annulus with a perimeter of 56.5–94.2 mm [39]. The Evolut R is a tricuspid self-expandable valve with high radial force in the lower part of the device facilitating self-expansion [39]. The valve can be recaptured and repositioned and has a 13 mm pericardial skirt at the inflow providing additional seal against PVR [39]. Vessel caliber requirements for access are ≥5 mm for 23 mm, 26 mm, 29 mm and ≥5.5 mm for 34 mm devices [39].

Specific Considerations in the Suitability for TAVR and Valve Choice

Severe left ventricular outflow tract and annular calcification: There is an increased risk of PVL and annular rupture associated with increased LVOT and annular calcification [40]. Annular rupture is most frequent during deployment of a balloon expandable valve or during post dilatation in the setting of PVL [40]. To reduce annular

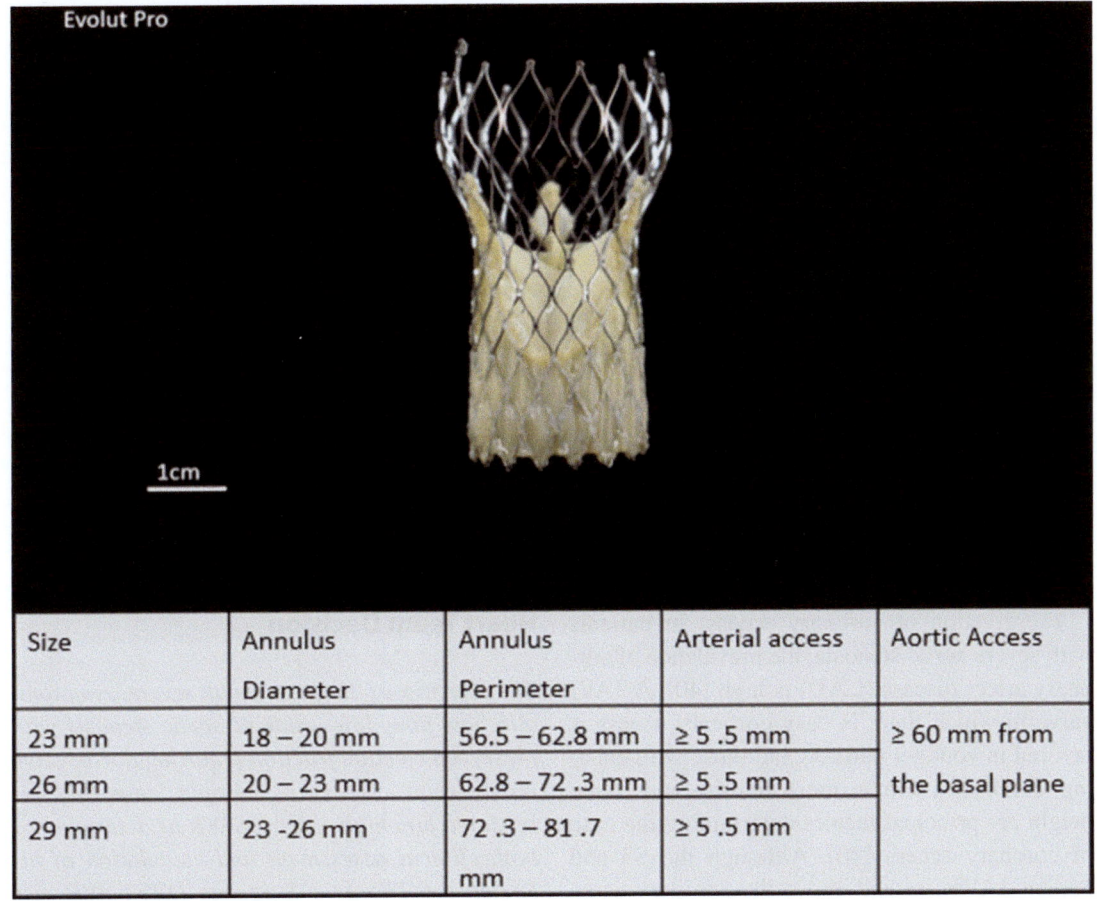

Size	Annulus Diameter	Annulus Perimeter	Arterial access	Aortic Access
23 mm	18 – 20 mm	56.5 – 62.8 mm	≥ 5 .5 mm	≥ 60 mm from the basal plane
26 mm	20 – 23 mm	62.8 – 72 .3 mm	≥ 5 .5 mm	
29 mm	23 -26 mm	72 .3 – 81 .7 mm	≥ 5 .5 mm	

Fig. 11 Adapted from manufacturer instruction document

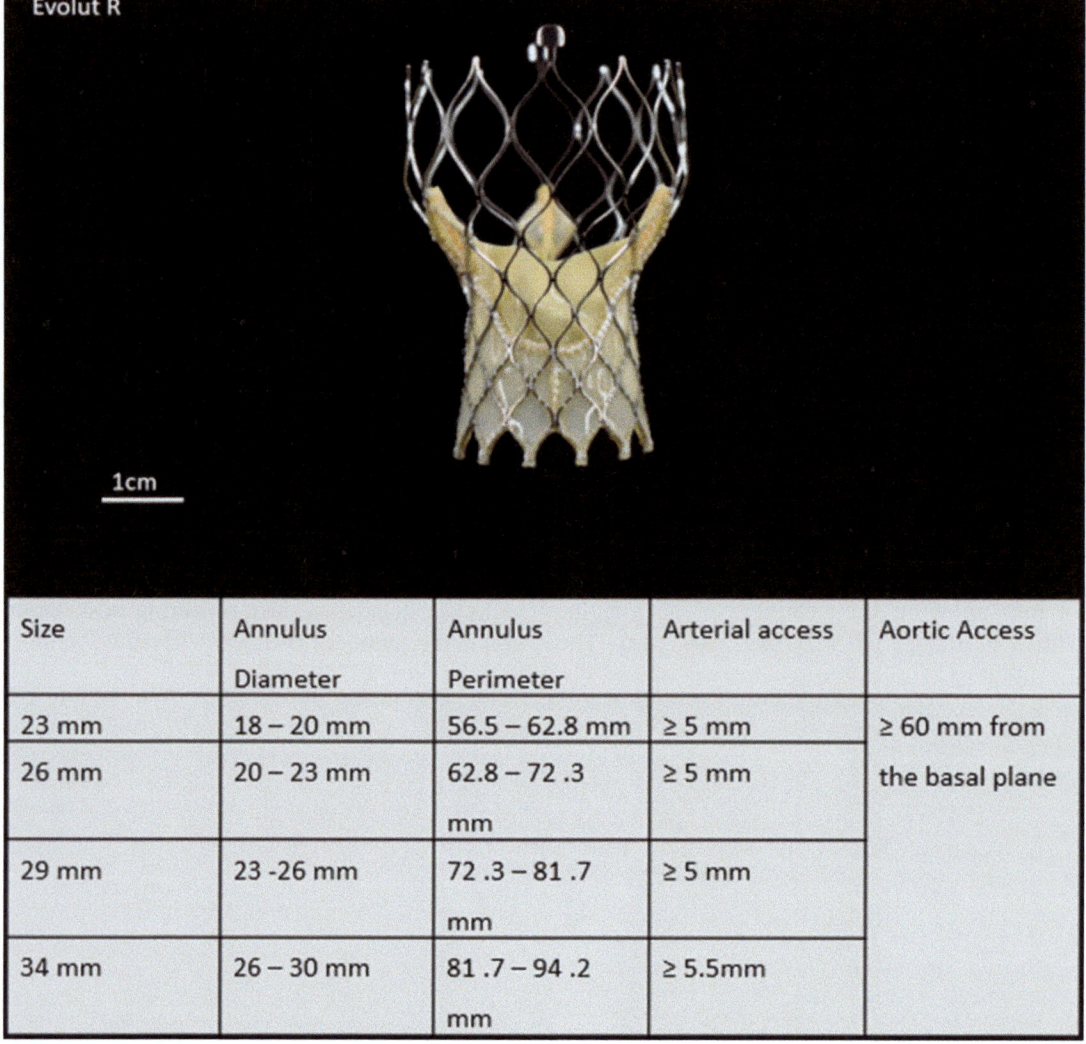

Fig. 12 Adapted from manufacturer instruction document

rupture risk and PVL without the need for post dilatation, self-expanding expanding valves are ideal when there is a heavily calcified landing zone [40].

Preservation of coronary access: In patients with severe aortic stenosis, the prevalence of coronary artery disease (CAD) is high [40]. A TAVI valve in which there is easy coronary access is favored in younger patients and those with existing CAD [40]. Frame mesh density and frame height are principal factors determining the ease of coronary access [40]. Although the S3 and Sapien 3 Ultra extend above the coronary ostia, they have large upper cells and a low density mesh allowing for coronary cannulation [40].

Heart Team Decision

The patient was diagnosed with severe, symptomatic, low flow, low gradient aortic stenosis with preserved ejection fraction requiring aortic valve replacement, however multiple comorbidities rendered him high risk for SAVR as determine by both clinical assessment and calculation of his Society of Thoracic Surgeons (STS) AVR risk score. Pre procedural diagnostic and planning imaging concluded TF TAVR was feasible with no adverse features on aortic root and femoral access assessment. CT parameters demonstrated annular dimension conducive to a 23 mm Sapien S3 or a 26 mm Evolut R. In the absence of significant contraindications for a balloon expandable valve, a Sapien 3 Ultra was utilized.

Intra and Post Procedural Assessment

Fluoroscopy and Vascular or Intravascular Ultrasound

Fluoroscopy in conjunction with vascular ultrasound is preferred for facilitating vascular access. Vascular Access for TF TAVR should be aimed over the iliopubic eminence and confirmed fluoroscopically either by placing a marker at the site of puncture or by performing a femoral angiogram following contralateral femoral access, thus avoiding a high puncture, which places the patient at risk of an intra peritoneal bleed [8]. Ultrasound guided access has a significantly lower total, major and minor vascular complication rate when compared to fluoroscopy [41]. Ultrasound can also be used to identify and avoid severe anterior wall calcification which may hinder percutaneous closure [8]. At the time of vascular access, peripheral intra vascular ultrasound (IVUS) is occasionally performed and provides diagnostic information when CT angiography findings are inconclusive with borderline diameters [42] and in patients with renal failure [8]. Assessment of luminal diameter, plaque burden and plaque composition [8] can be supplemented with information on tortuosity provided by angiography [42]. There is good accuracy and correlation between CTA and IVUS with lower radiation exposure and potentially lower contrast dose in IVUS [42].

Fluoroscopy is the mainstay of intraprocedural imaging, guiding optimal prosthetic positioning to avoid complications of conduction abnormalities, coronary obstruction, paravalvular leak and device embolization [43]. Balloon annular sizing may be required in cases of uncertain annular dimensions by CT or TEE. [44]. Optimal fluoroscopic angulation may be derived from pre procedural CT or the fluoroscopic right cusp rule to provide a projection orthogonal to the annular plane [43, 45]. A cusp overlap view is advantageous in deployment of the self-expanding valves and projections can be determined by pre procedural CT and fluoroscopy [46] (Fig. 13; Videos 6 and 7).

TEE and TTE

With the advent of minimalist TAVR, whereby TAVR implantation is done under moderate sedation guided largely by fluoroscopy and pre-procedure CT ± TTE, TEE during TAVR has become much less frequent and generally relegated to cases in which general anesthesia is being used due to patient comorbidity or airway con-

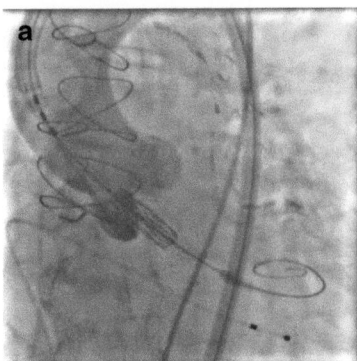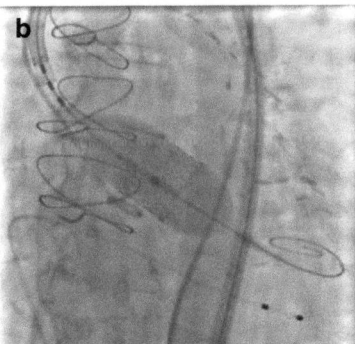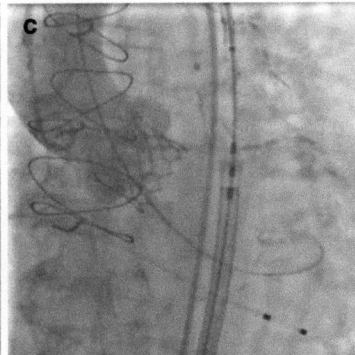

Fig. 13 Intraprocedural fluoroscopy images used to guide placement of THV. (**a**) Pre-deployment positioning of the THV. (**b**) Balloon expansion of the THV during valve deployment. (**c**) Post valve deployment imaging confirming valve positioning

cerns. In minimalist TAVR, valve implantation can be done either solely through fluoroscopy or through fluoroscopy with intermittent TTE imaging [47]. When TAVR implantation is done under general anesthesia, 2D TEE is recommended by the American Society of Echocardiography and 3D TEE is recommended but not required [48]. Routine procedural interpretation along with additional assessment of TAVR position, expansion, shape, leaflet motion and transvalvular gradients are assessed [48]. Due to shortening of the valve (S3) on the ventricular side during deployment, ideal positioning of third generation balloon expandable valves is achieved by aligning the aortic margin of the valve between the STJ and native leaflets [48]. Acute complications including acute valvular and ventricular dysfunction, aortic injury, tamponade, and ventricular injury should be excluded [49]. Alteration in severity of mitral regurgitation should raise the concern of mechanical impedance of the mitral valve apparatus by wires or the prosthetic aortic valve, and a new left or right ventricular wall motion or acute dysfunction may be caused by acute coronary obstruction [49]. Although classically self-expandable valves should ideally be positioned with the ventricular margin 3–5 mm below the annular plane [48], recent efforts have identified the "cusp-overlap" fluoroscopy technique to facilitate higher valve implantation depth and lower post TAVR pacemaker rates [46].

Post Procedural Follow Up

Echocardiography remains the mainstay of TAVR follow up with imaging designed to assess for valve hemodynamics, the presence of both valvular and paravalvular aortic regurgitation, biventricular function, and function of the other three cardiac valves. Assessment of valve hemodynamics and aortic regurgitation are of particular importance due to the association between moderate or greater residual aortic regurgitation and severe patient-prosthesis mismatch with increased risk of 1 year death or heart failure hospitalization [50, 51]. Additionally, elevated aortic valve gradients post TAVR or SAVR with a bioprosthetic valve may be associated with bioprosthetic leaflet thrombosis or hypoattenuated leaflet thickening (HALT), as is discussed further below.

The patient's echocardiogram performed 1 day post TAVI (Fig. 14, Videos 8 and 9) was notable for normal LVEF estimated at 60%.

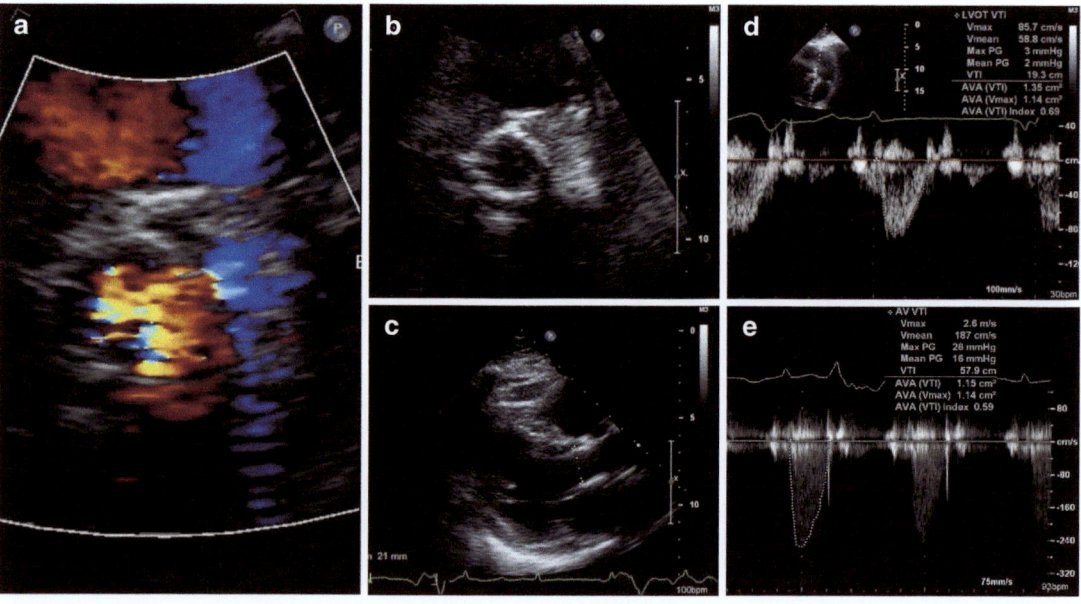

Fig. 14 Day 1 post procedural 2D TTE. Parasternal short axis view (**a**) with and (**b**) without color doppler with a circular valve appearance and no significant AR. (**c–e**) LVOT diameter, AVA and trans valvular gradients and velocities have improved following TAVR

Aortic transcatheter heart valve was well seated with mean gradient: 16 mmHg, an aortic valve area of 1.1 cm^2 and a Vmax of 1.6 m/s. The Doppler velocity index is 0.33. No significant paravalvular or central aortic regurgitation is seen.

The assessment of post procedure paravalvular regurgitation by transthoracic echocardiography is challenging due to metallic shadowing from the valve frame with posterior regurgitation being especially difficult to assess due to the presence of metal shadow in artifact from the valve with anterior echo probe position. Consequently, posterior paravalvular leak is better seen by TEE [4]. Pre procedure risk prediction for paravalvular leak by CT and echocardiography includes the presence of severe and especially protuberant LVOT and aortic valve calcification [15], the presence of a non tubular LVOT [47], increased ellipticity of the annulus [47] and a lower annular cover index [47]. The cover index is defined as 100 × [(THV diameter − TEE annulus diameter)/THV diameter] [52].

Post-TAVR aortic regurgitation can be assessed by TTE, TEE, angiography, or CMR. In the post-procedure setting, TTE is generally the most easily accessible non-invasive test and represents the first line for assessment [4, 47]. The VARC 3 definition for paravalvular regurgitation by TTE, which represents expert consensus, suggests that grading should be based on a combination of color doppler, qualitative spectral doppler, and quantitative doppler, as shown in Table 2. In contrast, angiography can provide semiquantitative and qualitative assessment of PVL and is graded according to the Sellers criteria, assessing the degree of LV opacification [53]. It is easily performed during the TAVR procedure however this subjective assessment leads to increased inter and intra observer variability and there is risk of acute kidney injury due to increase intravenous contrast requirements [53]. Lastly, CMR may provide a more precise assessment of PVL with CMR determination of increasing PVL severity correlating with higher mortality and poorer clinical outcomes [47, 54]. Phase contrast velocity mapping is utilized to obtain flow derived parameters including velocity and gradients [47].

In this case, although the patient's doppler velocity index is somewhat lower and valve gradients somewhat higher than would be expected in the setting of a recent TAVR, given that the patient was clinically stable and recovering well with significant aortic regurgitation, they were discharged for follow-up echocardiography in ~30 days.

A subsequent 30-day echocardiogram showed normal LV size and systolic function with the LVEF estimated at 65% and a mild reduction in

Table 2 VARC recommendations for the evaluation of aortic paravalvular regurgitation after TAVR

	Mild	Moderate	Severe
Semiquantitative parameters			
Diastolic flow reversal in the descending aorta—pulsed wave	Absent or brief early diastolic	Intermediate	Prominent, holodiastolic
Circumferential extent of prosthetic valve paravalvular regurgitation (%)[a]	<10	10–29	≥30
Quantitative parameters[b]			
Regurgitant volume (ml/beat)	<30	30–59	≥60
Regurgitant fraction (%)	<30	30–49	≥50
Effective regurgitant orifice area (cm^2)	0.10	0.10–0.29	≥0.30

Reprinted from The Journal of Thoracic and Cardiovascular Surgery, Vol 145/1, A. Pieter Kappetein, Stuart J. Head, Philippe Généreux, Nicolo Piazza, Nicolas M. van Mieghem, Eugene H. Blackstone, Thomas G. Brott, David J. Cohen, Donald E. Cutlip, Gerrit-Anne van Es, Rebecca T. Hahn, Ajay J. Kirtane, Mitchell W. Krucoff, Susheel Kodali et al. Updated standardized endpoint definitions for transcatheter aortic valve implantation: The Valve Academic Research Consortium-2 consensus document, 6–23, 2013 Copyright 2013, with permission from Elsevier

[a] In conditions of normal or near normal stroke volume (50–70 mL)
[b] These parameters are more affected by flow, including concomitant aortic regurgitation
[c] Adjacent to the effective regurgitant orifice area

the RV function (Fig. 15, Videos 10–12). The aortic transcatheter valve was well positioned, however lack of leaflet motion raised suspicion for stenosis vs. HALT. Of concern the calculated aortic orifice had decreased from 1.1 cm^2 on the prior study to 0.8 cm^2 and DVI was reduced from 0.33 to 0.22. The aortic spectral doppler acceleration time (defined as the time between the onset of flow to maximal velocity) was >100 ms. There was also an increase in the pressure gradient from 16 mmHg on the prior imaging to 26 mmHg on the current study. Taken together, these findings were concerning for prosthetic valve stenosis, as indicated in Fig. 16).

Importantly, bioprosthetic valve stenosis is typically a gradual process characterized by pannus growth, leaflet fibrosis and calcification and would be unlikely to present within 30 days of valve implantation. More likely differential diagnosis given the short timeframe would include valve thrombosis or HALT.

An urgent CT was subsequently performed and demonstrated an expanded valve with a minimal measurement of 21 mm at the mid valve level and hypoattenuating leaflet thickening (HALT) affecting 50–75% of the bioprosthetic valve corresponding to the left and right coronary cusps and 25–50% of the of the bioprosthetic leaflet adjacent to the non-coronary cusp with restricted leaflet motion (Fig. 17).

On the 3 month follow up post contrast CT, HALT had progressed with restricted leaflet motion. Early pannus was also now evident. The bioprosthetic valve was adequately expanded. (Figs. 18 and 19).

The outcomes of HALT are not well defined, with several analyses suggesting that short term outcomes are not impacted [55]. Additionally, treatment for HALT is ill defined, with some suggesting anticoagulation while others suggesting that no change in ongoing antiplatelet therapy is necessary.

Elevated Gradient Post TAVR

Subclinical leaflet thrombosis: Hypoattenuating leaflet thickening (HALT) is defined as meniscal shaped increase in leaflet thickening identified in at least two different multiplanar reformatted projections and in at least two different reconstruction time intervals [56] on CT. It is present in approximately 10–20% of patients following TAVR and SAVR [56]. It originates at the leaflet insertion points with varying extent to the leaflet edges [57] and is graded on a 4 tier scale of less than 25%, 25–50%, 50–75% and greater than 75% [15]. HALT can result in reduced leaflet mobility and should be assessed for on 4D volume rendered CT [58]. CT is the gold standard for assessing leaflet thickness [58] and reduced leaflet motion (RELM) can be graded as not significantly reduced, HAM (Hypoattenuation affecting motion) negative (<50%) or HAM positive with significantly reduced motion (≥50%) [57]. Clinical outcomes show no correlation between HALT and stroke or transient ischemic episode [59] however Garcia et al. described the presence of HALT as associated with increased long term mortality [56].

In the setting of leaflet abnormalities, transvalvular gradients are usually normal on echocardiogram and echo provides limited information

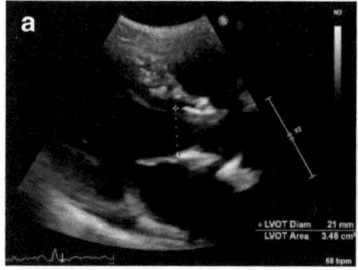
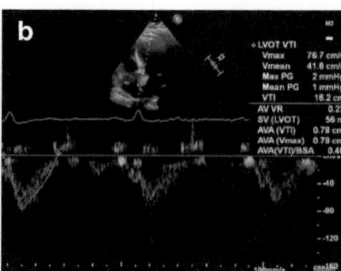
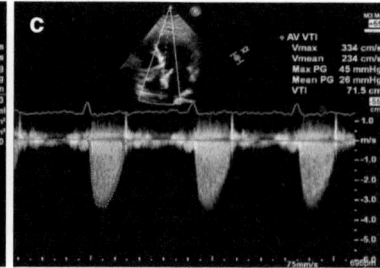

Fig. 15 30 day post procedural 2D TTE. (**a–c**). Aortic bioprosthetic valve is well seated. The cine images demonstrated lack of leaflet motion (Video 10). AVA is 0.8 cm^2 with a peak gradient of 26 mmHg and peak velocity of 3.4 m/s

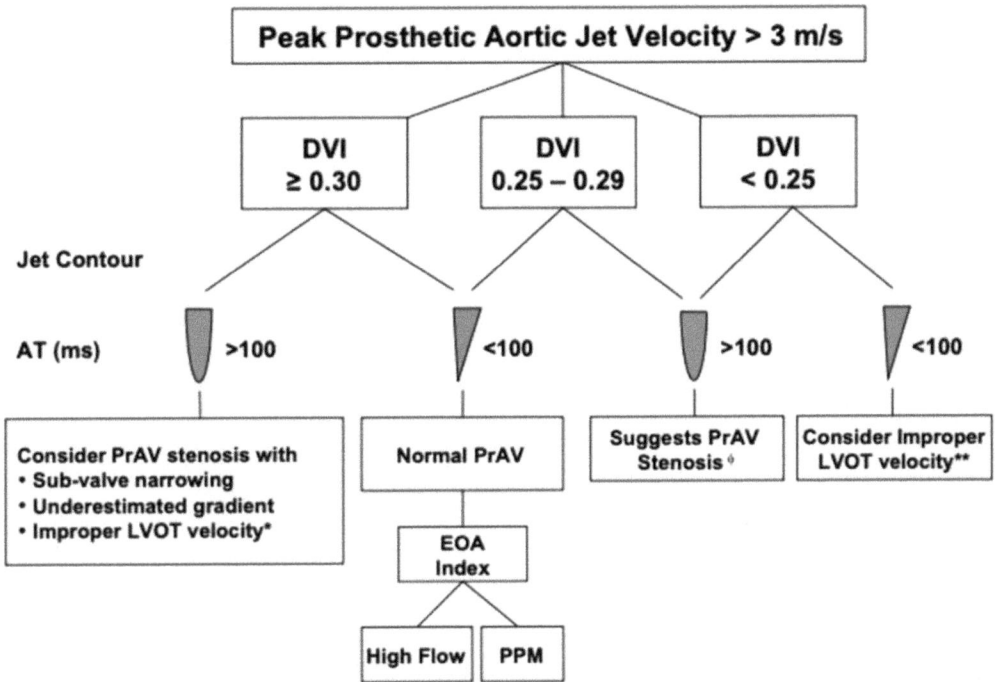

Fig. 16 Approach to the patient with prosthetic aortic valve and elevated aortic jet velocity. (Reprinted from Journal of the American Society of Echocardiography, 22, William A. Zoghbi, John B. Chambers, Jean G. Dumesnil, Elyse Foster, John S. Gottdiener, Paul A. Grayburn, Bijoy K. Khandheria, Robert A. Levine, Gerald Ross Marx, Fletcher A. Miller, Satoshi Nakatani, Miguel A. Quiñones, Harry Rakowski, L. Leonardo Rodriguez et al., Recommendations for Evaluation of Prosthetic Valves With Echocardiography and Doppler Ultrasound A Report From the American Society of Echocardiography's Guidelines and Standards Committee and the Task Force on Prosthetic Valves, Developed in Conjunction With the American College of Cardiology Cardiovascular Imaging Committee, Cardiac Imaging Committee of the American Heart Association, the European Association of Echocardiography, a registered branch of the European Society of Cardiology, the Japanese Society of Echocardiography and the Canadian Society of Echocardiography, Endorsed by the American College of Cardiology Foundation, American Heart Association, European Association of Echocardiography, a registered branch of the European Society of Cardiology, the Japanese Society of Echocardiography, and Canadian Society of Echocardiography, 975–1014, Copyright 2009, with permission from Elsevier)

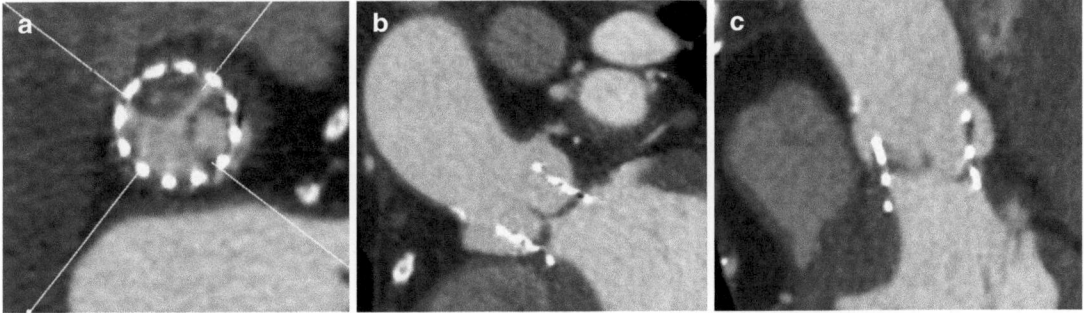

Fig. 17 CT 30-day post TAVR demonstrating HALT of 50–75% on the right and left coronary leaflet with HALT of 25–50% on the non-coronary leaflet

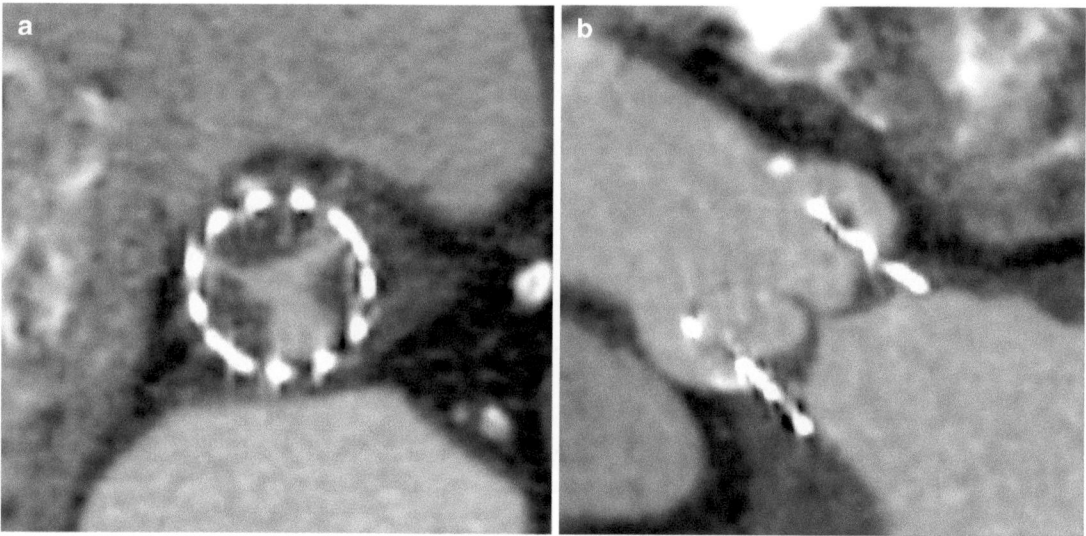

Fig. 18 CT post contrast 3 months post TAVR demonstrating progression in HALT with 50–75% involvement of all three coronary leaflets. Minimal pannus was also appreciated (white open arrow)

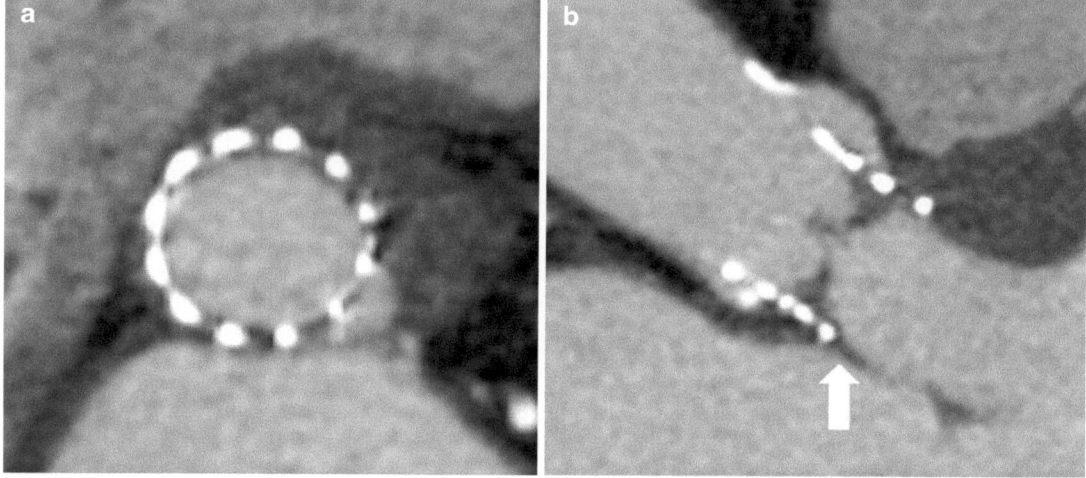

Fig. 19 CT post contrast 3 months post TAVR demonstrating progression in HALT with 50–75% involvement of all three coronary leaflets. Minimal pannus was also appreciated (white open arrow)

on leaflet assessment [60]. CT is uniquely useful in detecting early subclinical thrombosis and echocardiogram detects the valvular stenosis and the late sequelae of thrombosis [60]. TEE may supplement diagnostic information and is capable of detecting RELM [60].

Clinical valve thrombosis: Clinical valve thrombosis is rare and usually occurs in the early postoperative period [58]. Patients present with valve regurgitation or stenosis with progressive dyspnea due to cardiac failure based on the extent of valve obstruction or features of systemic embolic phenomena [58]. In contrast, subclinical leaflet thrombosis presents with hemodynamic derangement of aortic valve function without associated clinical findings. Echocardiography is key in diagnosis with TTE usually being used to TEE the modality of choice [61] usually detecting the thrombus as echo dense structures on the heart valve and increased gradients [58]. Cardiac

CT localises a mobile mass or thrombus on the prosthetic valve [58].

Structural valve degeneration: Structural failure of the prosthetic valve results in permanent or irreversible damage to the THV leaflets with resultant prosthetic valve stenosis or regurgitation [47]. There is restriction of motion of the prosthetic leaflets with calcification of the leaflets on echo [62] and CT [47].

CT has a higher sensitivity than echo in detecting stent frame abnormalities, visualizing HALT and the assessment of leaflet motion [47].

Patient–Prosthesis mismatch (PPM): Patient-prosthetic mismatch is defined as a prosthetic valve of normal size that is too small for the hemodynamic needs of the patient [62]. Patient prosthesis mismatch is defined as an effective orifice area (indexed to body surface area) <0.85 cm^2/m^2 and severe if <0.65 cm^2/m^2 [62]. This definition however is said to overestimate PPM in patients that are obese (BMI >30 kg/m^2) with lower cut-off values of <0.70 cm^2/m^2 and <0.60 cm^2/m^2 used in obese patients [62]. PPM is the most common cause of high TAVR gradients on echocardiography, with other causes including high flow states and acquired valve stenosis [63]. TTE is the primary modality for assessment and may be supplemented by CT or TEE [63]. The valve EOA indexed to body surface area is key in diagnosing and quantifying PPM and the non-indexed measured EOA is usually normal in PPM and reduced in stenoses [63] (Fig. 16). Leaflet mobility and thickness (normal in PPM and reduced in stenosis) also helps in differentiating stenosis from PPM and can be assessed on echocardiogram and CT [63]. Non contrast CT detects leaflet mineralization in bioprosthetic leaflet degeneration [63]. Table 3 shows the role of different imaging modalities in peroprocedural assessment of TAVR.

Table 3 TAVR multimodality imaging

TAVR	Echocardiogram	Fluoroscopy/angiogram	Computed tomography	MRI
Preprocedural	First step and gold standard in diagnosis and quantification of disease severity	Assessment of existing coronary artery disease and feasibility of future coronary access. Assessment of annulus and the presence of adverse root features and trans femoral access	Gold standard in assessment of annular dimension, quantification of annular calcification, risk of coronary artery obstruction and access feasibility	Provides similar information on annular assessment to CT and 2D echo. Can assess valve anatomy, severity of disease and LV function especially in situations where echo assessment is suboptimal. Can be used in scenarios where iodine-based contrast is contraindicated
Intraprocedural	2D or 3D recommended. Assessment of acute aortic root and coronary complications along with THV position and function. Previously done primarily through TEE and now with minimalist TAVR and moderate sedation, typically done with TTE	Preferred intraprocedural imaging. Guides optimal prosthetic position. Visualizes acute complications		
Post procedural	Routine monitoring of THV position and function. Identifies gradient abnormalities along with leaflet morphology and motion		Essential in assessment of HALT, leaflet motion, PPM, THV position and expansion. Also assesses vascular access complications	

Clinical Controversies and Pearls

- Multi-window assessment of aortic gradients, potentially including two separate echocardiographic sonographers can improve correlation with cath-derived aortic valve gradients.
- In the setting of mismatch between aortic valve gradients and calculated aortic valve area (where aortic valve area is <1 cm^2 and mean aortic gradient is <40 mmHg), first assess for measurement error of the left ventricular outflow tract and then consider normal or low flow, low gradient AS.
- Low flow state in patients with AS is frequently associated with cardiac amyloidosis, mitral valve disease, atrial fibrillation, RV dysfunction, or concentric remodeling.
- Elevated gradients after TAVR may be the result of high flow states, prosthetic valve dysfunction, patient-prosthesis mismatch, HALT, or leaflet thrombosis. Consider 4D Cardiac CT after echocardiography to assess further.
- Higher implantation depth of self-expanding TAVR valves using the cusp-overlap fluoroscopy technique may decrease the risk of post-procedure pacemaker implantation.
- Deep implantation of TAVR valve might interference with normal function of MV and leading to mitral regurgitation (Fig. 20a and b, Videos 13 and 14)
- Migrated TAVR valve is another rare complication that should be diagnosed and managed properly. Figure 21 AP (A) and lateral (B) CT scanogram with a bioprosthetic valve in the aortic annulus and a migrated bioprosthetic valve positioned in the distal thoracic aorta at the level of the aortic hiatus of the diaphragm. MPR oblique sagittal (C) and axial (D) post contrast CT scan demonstrating a migrated TAVR valve positioned in the descending thoracic aorta at the level of the aortic hiatus of the diaphragm.

Key Points
- Annulus should be measured at the largest dimension, usually at end systole. In the presence of a hypertrophied septum, the annulus maybe smaller in systole, referred to as inverse dynamism.
- Sinus of Valsalva <30 mm combined with coronary ostial height <12 mm is at risk for coronary occlusion after TAVR.

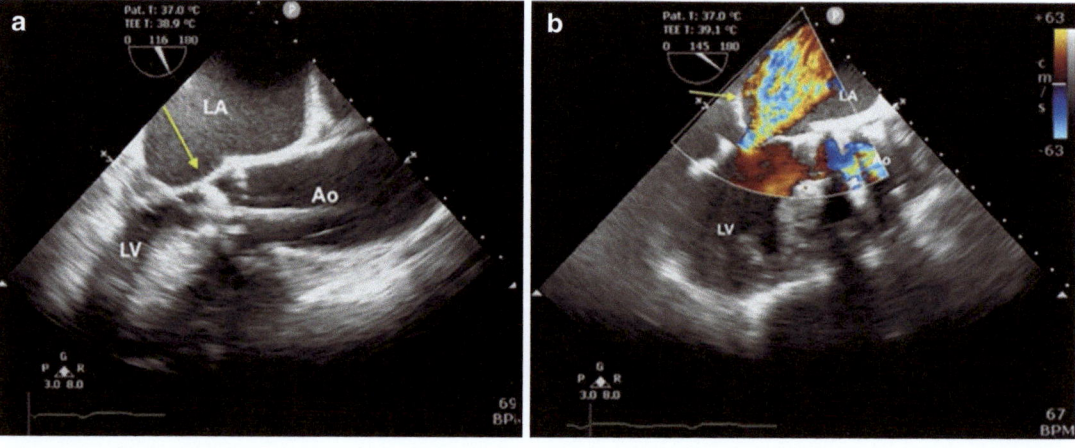

Fig. 20 (a) Deep implantation of TAVR valve (arrow) might interference with normal function of MV and (b) leading to mitral regurgitation (arrow)

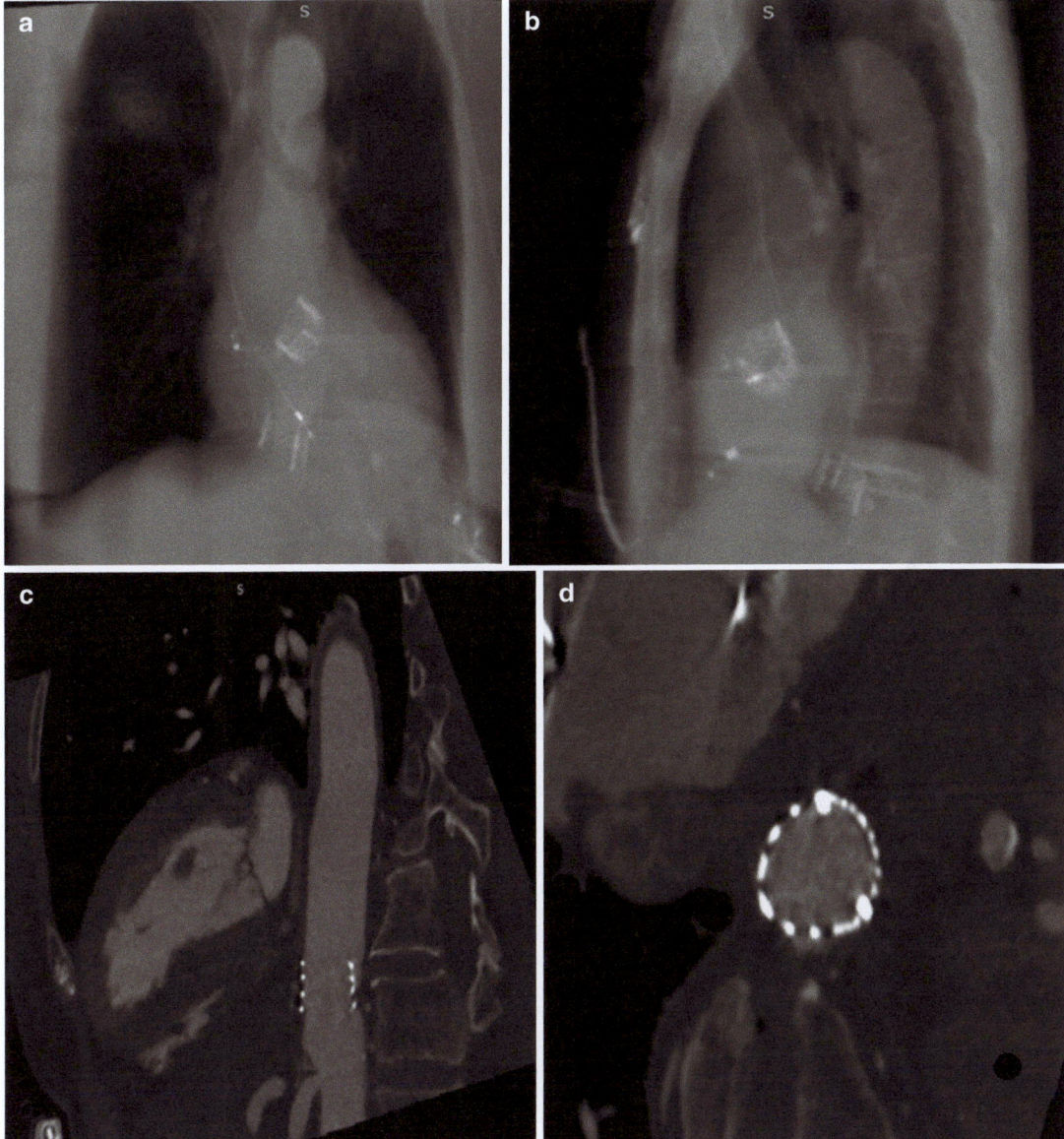

Fig. 21 Migrated TAVR valve in AP (**a**) and lateral (**b**) CT scanogram with a bioprosthetic valve in the aortic annulus and a migrated bioprosthetic valve positioned in the distal thoracic aorta at the level of the aortic hiatus of the diaphragm. MPR oblique sagittal (**c**) and axial (**d**) post contrast CT scan demonstrating a migrated TAVR valve positioned in the descending thoracic aorta at the level of the aortic hiatus of the diaphragm

- LVOT calcification severity must be assessed as increasing calcification increases risk of rupture during TAVR.
- For vascular access, in particular transfemoral access, dimensions and severity of calcification should be assessed in combination with values less than 5.5 mm diameter and increasing calcification burden at higher risk of vascular injury.
- Hypoattenuated leaflet thickening (HALT) is usually asymptomatic and may arise and resolve spontaneously.

Bicuspid Aortic Valve

> **Case Study**
>
> *A 79-year-old female with known hypertension presented with a history of progressive shortness of breath and dizziness (without loss of consciousness). No chest pain or syncope. On clinical examination there was a midsystolic murmur in the second intercostal space radiating to the carotid vessels. The patient had no features of heart failure. ECG was notable for Sinus rhythm, first degree AV block, narrow QRS complex.*

Background and Definitions

Bicuspid aortic valve (BAV) is the commonest congenital cardiac anomaly [64–66] and occurs in 0.5–2% of the general population with a male predominance [67].

The pathophysiology of premature aortic valve disease in patients with bicuspid aortic valve, particularly AS [66], includes increased sheer stress on the leaflets resulting in accelerated calcification and valve degeneration [67]. The annulus is usually ellipsoid with severe calcification [65]. It is approximated that 25% of patients with bicuspid aortic valve will require aortic valve surgery and 5% will require surgery of the ascending aorta over a follow up period of 20 years [67].

Associations of Bicuspid Aortic Valves

Ascending aorta aneurysms occur in up to 50% of patients and correlates directly with increasing age [67]. Dilatation and aneurysms of the ascending aorta are more common in bicommissural when compared to tricommissural BAV morphology [15]. Furthermore, there is an association with a horizontally orientated ascending aorta [65]. The annulus is usually elliptical and larger when compared to tricuspid valves [65].

Leaflets may be heavily calcified [64] and longer with leaflet fusion [65]. This increases the risk of coronary obstruction with greater significance on coronary heights and sinus of Valsalva width [65]. The increased risk of coronary artery obstruction is compounded by one or both coronary ostia approximating the commissures [67]. There is potentially accelerated degeneration of prosthetic leaflets in bicuspid aortic valves [64].

Classifications

Sievers and Schmidtke—Main focus is on the number of raphes (0, 1 or 2 raphes) Table 4 [15].

TAVR—directed simplified BAV classification-focus is on number of commissures (2 or 3) and the presence or absence of a raphe [13]. There are three morphologies [15]:

- Tricommissural: (functional or acquired BAV). This is not included in the Sievers classification.
- Bicommissural raphe-type: (Sievers Type 1).
- Bicommissural non raphe type: (Sievers type 0).

Diagnosis and Pre-procedural Evaluation (Fig. 22)

A TTE was obtained to evaluate the source of the patient's midsystolic murmur and revealed severe aortic stenosis with BAV (Videos 15–18) with an area of 0.4 cm^2, peak velocity of 5.3 m/s and a mean gradient of 70 mmHg. The patient had concentric left ventricular hypertrophy with left ventricular septal (Video 18) and posterior wall dimensions of 13 mm and 12 mm respectively. Function was preserved with an ejection fraction of 65%. The left atrium was severely dilated with mild to moderate mitral regurgitation.

Transoesophageal echocardiography allows for detailed anatomic and physiologic assessment of cardiac valves and is considered the gold standard initial test for cardiac valvular function and anatomy. In addition to ease of access and a lack of ionizing radiation, echocardiography does not require iodinated contrast and therefore can be used in patients with renal insufficiency [67]. Diagnostic findings in bicuspid valves include

Table 4 The heterogeneous spectrum of bicuspid aortic valve morphology

Classification	Characteristics	Double oblique transverse MPR	Volume rendered en face view systole	Volume rendered en face view diastole
Sievers Type 0/ bicommissural non-raphe type	• Two fairly symmetric cusps and two commissures • Each cusp has one most basal insertion point; thus there is a total of two most basal insertion points			
Sievers Type 1/ bicommissural raphe type	• Two of three cusps are conjoined by a raphe • Asymmetric cusp sizes with the cusp opposing the raphe (i.e. cusp not participating in raphe formation) being larger than in a tricuspid aortic valve • Raphe does not extend to the level of the STJ which is the distinguishing characteristics to a non-opening commisure • Size of raphe and degree of calcification can vary *Upper row*: non-calcified raphe *Middle row*: Moderately calcified raphe *Lower row*: Severly calcified raphe			
Acquired/ functional bicuspid valve (underlying tricuspid anatomy)	• Underlying tricuspid anatomy with symmetric Sinus of Valsalva • Non-opening commissure due to degenerative changes (here RL commissure) • Non-opening commissure reaches STJ, which is the distinguishing factor compared to a raphe			

Adapted and reprinted from Journal of Cardiovascular Computed Tomography, Vol 13/1, Philipp Blanke, Jonathan R. Weir-McCall, Stephan Achenbach, Victoria Delgado, Jörg Hausleiter, Hasan Jilaihawi, Mohamed Marwan, Bjarne L. Norgaard, Niccolo Piazza, Paul Schoenhagen, Jonathon A. Leipsic, Computed tomography imaging in the context of transcatheter aortic valve implantation (TAVI)/transcatheter aortic valve replacement (TAVR): An expert consensus document of the Society of Cardiovascular Computed Tomography, 1–20, Copyright 2019, with permission from Elsevier

"fish mouth" appearance and systolic doming of the valve apparatus with color doppler providing further information in differentiating tricuspid from bicuspid valves in the presence of calcification and reduced leaflet mobility [5]. However, anatomic assessment, including bicuspid valve type, annular shape, and calcium distribution is limited by echocardiography [68] (Fig. 23).

Given the diagnosis of severe, symptomatic AS and bicuspid aortic valve, a preprocedural CT scan was ordered and demonstrated an aortic annular area of 394 mm^2 with a bicuspid type 0

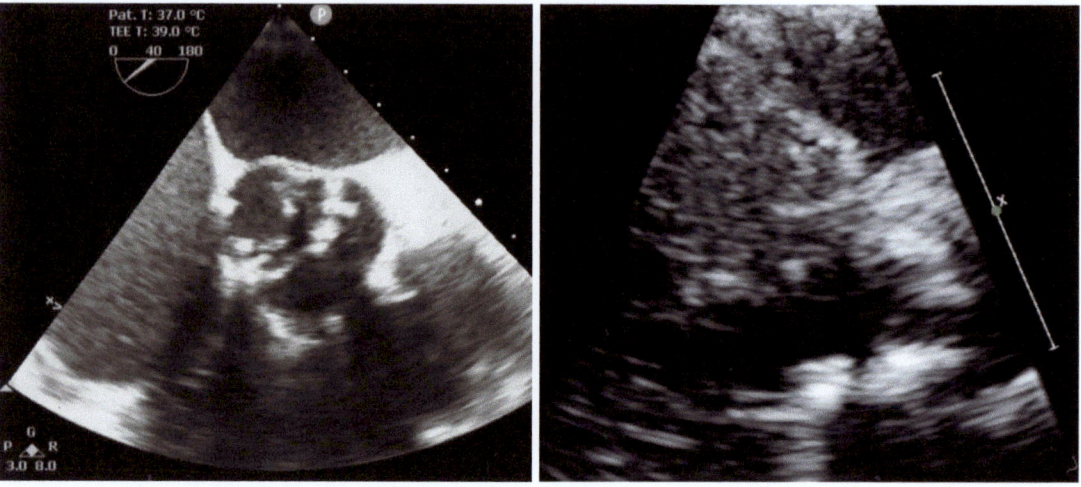

Fig. 22 2D TEE (left panel) 2D TTE parasternal long axis (right panel) demonstrating severely calcified aortic valve

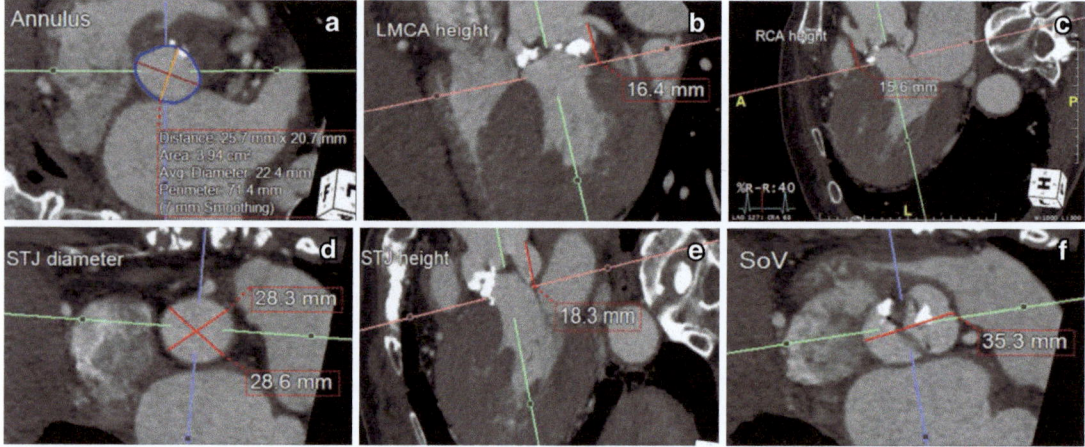

Fig. 23 Post contrast Pre TAVR planning CT images with measurements performed in the systolic phase of the cardiac cycle. (**a**) Annular area of 394 mm² and perimeter of 71.4 mm. (**b**) The Left main coronary artery ostium is located 16.4 mm and the (**c**) right coronary artery ostium is 15.6 mm above the annular plane suggesting low risk for coronary obstruction. (**d**) The sinotubular junction measures 28.3 × 28.6 mm in diameter and is located (**e**) 18.3 mm above the annular plane. (**f**) The Sinus of Valsalva is capacious and measures 35.3 cm in diameter

valve and severe nodular calcification at both leaflets. There was moderate annular calcification with a calcified nodule protruding into the annular lumen and a short intervalvular fibrosa. Risk of coronary artery obstruction was low with both right and left main coronary artery heights of 16 mm, a sinus of Valsalva diameter averaged at 35 mm and an STJ height of 18 mm. The ascending aorta was dilated but less than 45 mm. An orthogonal projection was possible at a left anterior oblique and caudal angulation of 10 and 21° respectively. Femoral access was feasible bilaterally.

CT is integral in the planning for the TAVR procedure particularly in bicuspid aortic valves due to the heterogeneity of the various bicuspid valve morphologies that has a potential to influence the patients outcome [66]. MDCT demonstrates accurate correlation with surgical findings and has improved diagnostic sensitivity when compared to TTE and TEE [68]. CT or MRI are recommended if echocardiographic assessment of the sinus of Valsalva and ascending aorta is suboptimal and inconclusive [4].

CMR provides good assessment of valve morphology with the ability to accurately determine velocities and gradients and annular size [68]. However assessment of calcification is limited [68].

Important features to be assessed by 3D imaging (ideally by CT but possible by CMR, or 3D TEE as well) include valve morphology [15] and the degree of raphe calcification assessed qualitatively as mild, moderate and severe. A raphe particularly if calcified may affect TAVR expansion and apposition at the annulus [66, 69] and increases pacemaker requirement risk, risk of device misplacement and regurgitation [69]. The bicuspid aortic valve annulus is relatively larger, often demonstrating an elliptical shape and more often exhibiting severe eccentric calcification when compared to tricuspid valves [65]. Note should be made that non raphe bicommissural bicuspid aortic valves demonstrates a larger sinus diameter but smaller annuli [15]. Landing zone configuration may be tubular, flared or tapered (classified by relative perimeters of the annulus and at the level of the free edge of the leaflets) [69]. An aortic root with a tapered configuration may require THV under sizing or sizing at dimensions closer to the supra annular measurements [69]. There are two schools of thought regarding annular measurement and include sizing at the annulus and/or supra annular tracing (measuring perimeter and intercommissural distance approximately 4 mm above annulus) [70]. These may be supplemented by balloon sizing [70]. The BAVARD registry states that annular measurements are suitable in almost 90% of cases [70]. Inappropriate oversizing can result in annular rupture and heart block [65]. The annular ellipticity, calcium burden and location should be assessed [67]. Heavy and asymmetric calcifications are a concern and may result in impaired valve expansion or aortic root injury following a countercoup injury from balloon inflation and THV expansion [67]. Calcium located at the commissures can result in perforation whilst bulky calcification located at the tip of a leaflet is a risk for coronary obstruction [69]. Spacious sinuses in patients with BAV is often protective from coronary occlusion [69]. The ascending aorta should be assessed for aortopathy and dilatation [15]. Optimal projection angles can be obtained using MDCT software providing coaxial angles with optimal assessment of calcification [70] (Fig. 24).

In light of the patient's likely suitability for TAVR, a pre-procedural angiogram was obtained to evaluate the coronary arteries and further evaluation of the aortic root. There was no significant coronary artery disease with aortic root calcification (Video 19). The ascending aorta was dilated. Femoral access had favorable imaging features bilaterally.

Differential Diagnosis
Pre echocardiography differentials of lung pathology, mitral valve disease and congestive heart failure were excluded following imaging confirmation of severe aortic stenosis.

Heart Team Approach and Discussion
Based on the diagnoses of severe AS in a patient with bicuspid aortic valve, reasonable root features and maximal aortic dimension of 41 mm on CT and 42 mm on TTE the decision was to proceed with TAVR using a 23 mm SAPIEN 3 Ultra.

Heart Team Decision
Bicuspid valves often have a larger annulus, an asymmetric valve orifice, are heavily calcified, have a dilated and asymmetric aortic root and ascending aorta [40]. Complications such as significant PVL, device migration/embolization, non-uniform non circular valve deployment and annular rupture are more common [40]. Success rates are good with newer generation TAVR valves with improved outcomes in Sievers Type 1 L-R fusion [5]. Similar outcomes were achieved in low surgical risk patients with BAV (without raphe or leaflet calcification), when compared with TAVR patients with similar clinical profile but with tricuspid valves and treated with SAPIEN 3 THV [71]. Patients with BAV and high surgical risk treated with EvolutR/Evolut PRO demonstrated similar outcomes in terms of 1 year post procedural stroke and mortality rates

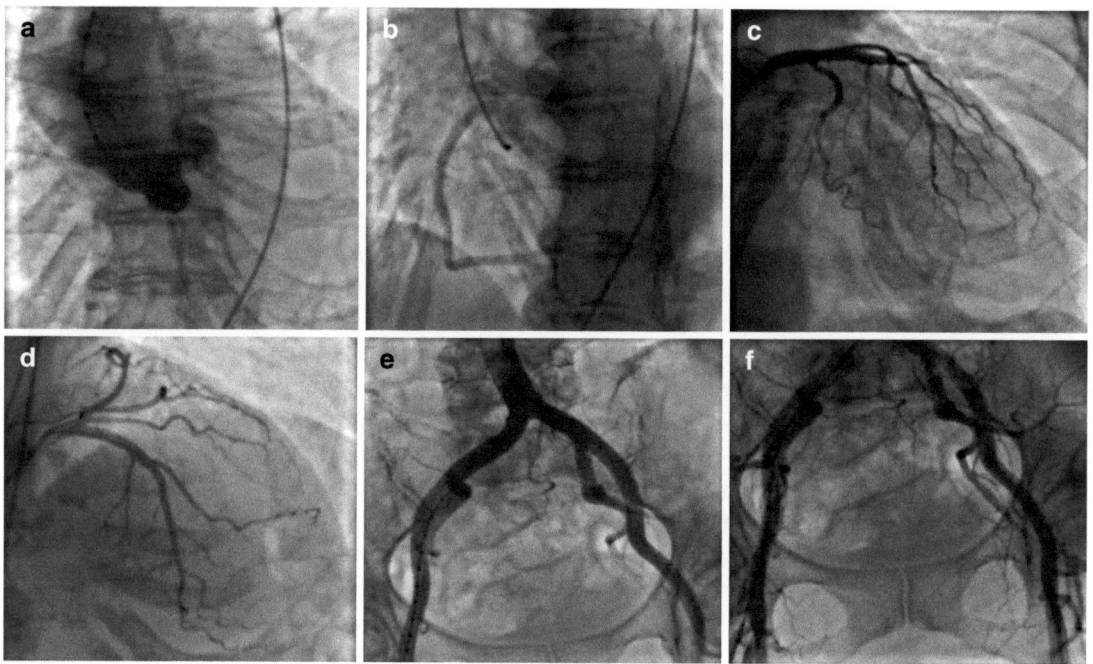

Fig. 24 (**a**) Angiogram of the aortic root with mildly dilated ascending aorta and no significant adverse root features and coronary ostial heights were at low risk for obstruction. (**b–d**) Coronary angiogram of the RCA and LM and its branches showed patent vessels with no requirements for percutaneous intervention or bypass grafts. (**e** and **f**) patent iliofemoral arteries without significant calcification, tortuosity or stenosis

when compared to their tricuspid aortic valve counterparts [72].

Definitive criteria between the choice of SAVR and TAVR is still to be decided with SAVR preferred in young patients, patients with aortopathy and low risk patients [73]. Currently features conducive for TAVR in BAV include a favourable annular dimension, absence of severe leaflet and raphe calcification especially in Sievers type 1 and with Sievers type 0 (in the absence of an extreme ellipsoidal annulus) [73]. Of note, in patients with bicuspid morphology treated with TAVR, there is a higher incidence of conduction abnormalities [5] and the presence of severe calcification of the raphe and leaflets is associated with aortic injury and higher incidence of PVL with a higher 2 year mortality especially if both leaflet and raphe calcification were present [74]. There is however reduced incidence of PVL with newer generation devices [75].

Intra Procedural Assessment

The aortic valve was predilated using a 20 mm balloon (Fig. 25, Video 20). The patient then demonstrated high degree A-V block requiring pacing. A 23 mm Sapien 3 valve (−2 cc) was successfully deployed under rapid pacing (Fig. 25, Video 21) using fluoroscopy.

Balloon Sizing and Pre Dilatation in Bicuspid Valves

Pre-dilatation is recommended for balloon annular sizing in borderline dimensions, in fused right and non-coronary cusps, when considering sizing to the supra annular space and in the presence of heavily calcified bicuspid aortic valve with a calcium score >1000 HU (to assist in crossing the native valve and prosthetic valve deployment) [69]. The region of balloon waisting will identify the position of best sealing whilst approximation of calcified leaflets to the coronary ostia will

Transcatheter Aortic Valve Replacement

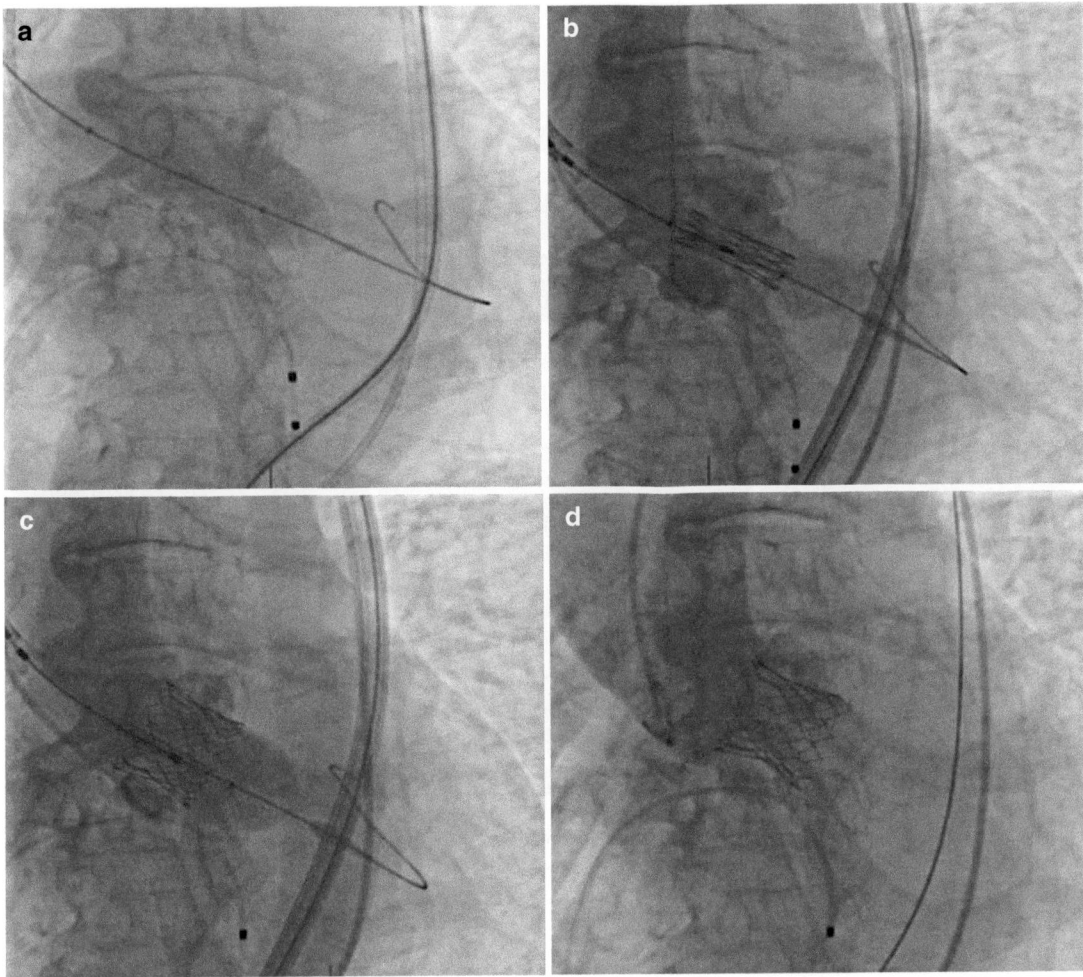

Fig. 25 (a) Pre deployment balloon valvuloplasty with balloon placed across the aortic valve and inflated with displacement of leaflet calcification. (**b–d**) A Sapien 3 bioprosthetic valve was deployed at the annulus with minimal tailoring in its mid portion

assist in determining risk of coronary obstruction [69]. Absence of a leak supports congruent balloon and valve orifice dimensions [69].

Post Procedural Assessment

Formal postprocedural TTE demonstrated a well seated aortic transcatheter heart valve with a mean gradient of 10 mmHg, Peak velocity of 2.3 m/s and an aortic valve area of 1.4 cm^2 (Fig. 26). Mild paravalvular prosthetic regurgitation was present and leaflet motion was poorly visualized.

Postprocedural electrophysiology assessment resulted in permanent pacemaker placement (Fig. 27) 30 days post procedure echocardiogram revealed a well seated aortic valve with poor visualization of leaflet motion. Mild paravalvular regurgitation persisted and was non-progressive. Aortic peak velocity had increased to 3.3 m/s with a mean gradient of 21 mmHg. There was mild mitral regurgitation with no systolic anterior motion of the mitral valve. Concentric hypertrophy of the left ventricle remained stable. No pericardial effusion, septal defects or intracardiac

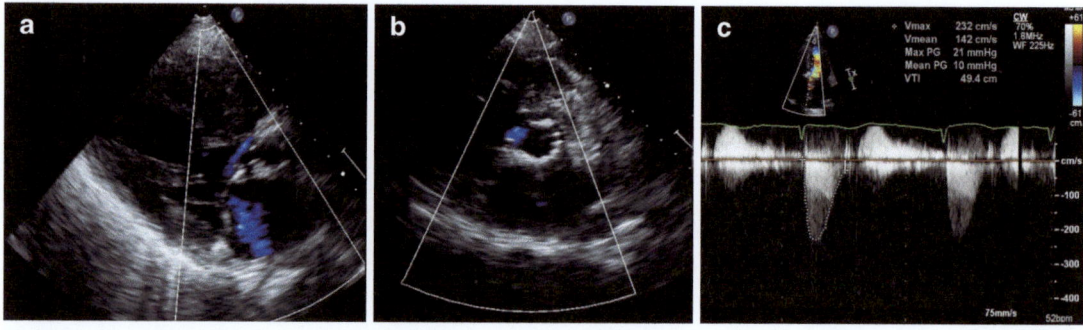

Fig. 26 2D TTE post procedure demonstrating normal valve position (**a**) with mild paravalvular regurgitation (**a** and **b**), mild mitral regurgitation and acceptable hemodynamic parameters (**c**)

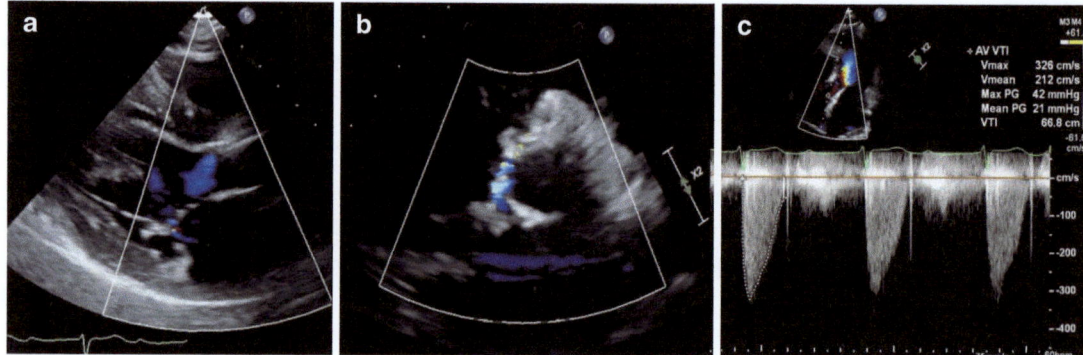

Fig. 27 (**a** and **b**) 2D TTE 30 days post TAVR procedure with (**a** and **b**) demonstrate persistence of mild paravalvular regurgitation. (**c**) Continuous wave doppler echo shows an elevated mean gradient at 21 mmHg

shunts were present. Pacemaker leads identified in the right atrium and right ventricle.

Similar to the post-procedure evaluation of TAVR valves placed for severe, symptomatic AS in tricuspid aortic valves, post-procedure imaging is based initially on echocardiography. Postprocedural echocardiography should be focused on valve hemodynamics, the presence of aortic regurgitation, biventricular function, the function of the other three cardiac valves, and evidence of any intracardiac complications, such as cardiac perforation. Given the often-ovular nature of the bicuspid valve annulus, assessment for aortic valve regurgitation is of particular importance, with posteriorly located regurgitant jets being most difficult to visualize due to metal shadowing from the valve frame. In the present case, an increase in 30-day TAVR gradients as compared to the post-procedure assessment suggested potential valvular dysfunction versus leaflet abnormality and prompted a contrasted cardiac CT.

Valve dimensions demonstrated under-expansion (Fig. 28) of the valve in its midportion (17 mm diameter) with no thrombus or HALT. No VSD or pericardial effusion present and pacemaker leads were appropriately positioned. Aortic dimensions were stable with no aortic root injury.

Complications in Bicuspid Aortic Valves

Patients with BAV have a higher risk of malposition [64], pacemaker rates [70] and paravalvular regurgitation with lower device success rates [15] above and beyond the standard TAVR complication profile.

Paravalvular Regurgitation

Paravalvular leak occurs when the THV incompletely approximates annulus and LVOT [47]. Incidence of moderate to severe paravalvular regurgitation is higher in a bicuspid valve with a calcified raphe and, higher still, if both the raphe

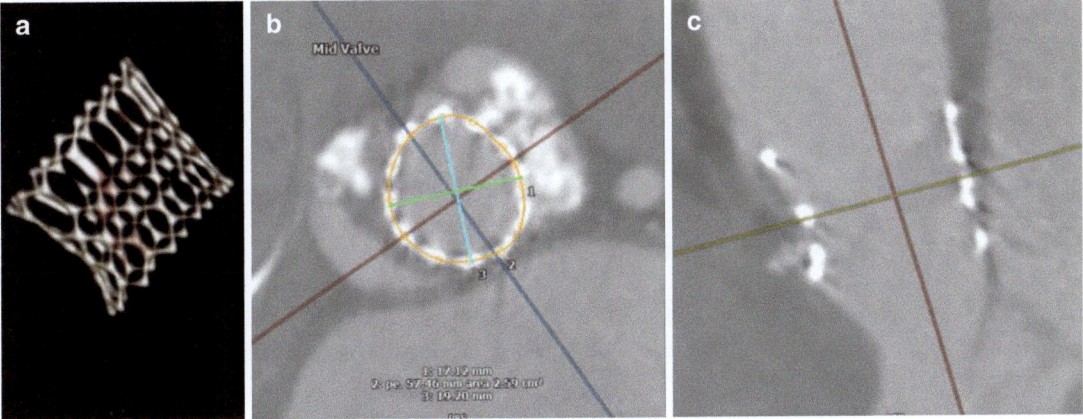

Fig. 28 Post procedure post contrast CT performed to assess for valve expansion and exclude complications. (**a**) Sapien 3 valve 23 mm that was underfilled by 2 cc demonstrates mild tailoring at the mid portion of the valve. (**b**) Short axis image of the valve at the mid portion demonstrates a diameter of 17.12 mm by 19.2 mm. Confirming mild under expansion with no leaflet thickening or thrombosis. (**c**) Long axis view of the valve confirms mild under expansion of the mid portion of the valve

Table 5 Bicuspid aortic valve multimodality imaging

Bicuspid valve ± aortopathy	Echocardiography	Computed tomography	MRI
Pre procedure imaging	First line for valvular assessment with high accuracy especially on TEE. Accurate assessment may be limited in the presence of severe calcification. Limited assessment of co-existant aortopathy	Improved diagnostic sensitivity when compared to echocardiogram. Recommended in assessing sinus of Valsalva and ascending aorta if echo assessment is inconclusive	Good assessment of valve morphology and function as well as aortic morphology and pathology. Limited by calcification
Intraprocedure imaging	Similar to tricuspid aortic valves (see case 1) with the exception that TEE may play a larger role in device positioning in the absence of severe calcification to serve as a landmark on fluoroscopy		
Postprocedure imaging	Similar to tricuspid aortic valves (see case 1)		

and leaflets are calcified [74]. Sievers type 1 BAV was associated with a relatively higher rate of PVL in comparison to other classifications, however there no significant difference in paravalvular regurgitation between the self and balloon expandable valves in all classification types [48]. Table 5 showing role of Multimodality Imaging in TAVR in Bicuspid Aortic Valve.

Post Procedure Pacemaker Requirements

Higher pacemaker rates are documented in patients with bicuspid aortic valves post TAVI more so in balloon expandable instances which has a 23.5% post implantation pacemaker rate [70]. Lack of foreshortening of the stent frame of balloon expandable valves during oversizing and excessive force being applied to the conduction system in self-expanding cases are thought to be aetiological contributory factors [70].

Features predictive of conduction disturbances include calcification of the LVOT, especially below the non-coronary cusp and severe mitral annular calcification (>180°) [47]. The presence of a short membranous septum [47] less than 8 mm in length is a predictor for high degree AV-Block, especially if found in combination with low valve implant and an underlying right bundle branch block [15]. Procedural risks include the use of a self expanding THV [47, 76], low valve placement of greater than 4 mm below the annulus [47] and annular and LVOT oversizing [76]. Low deployment is the most frequent predictor of LBBB with balloon and self-expandable valves [15]. Reduction of the implant depth significantly reduces mortality and pacemaker requirements [15]. The short term effects of edema, inflammation, ischemia or direct trauma may demonstrate recovery thereby negating long term pacemaker dependency post TAVR [76].

Clinical Controversies and Pearls

- Trials of FDA approved TAVR valves excluded patients with bicuspid aortic valves. As a result, randomized comparisons of TAVR vs. SAVR for bicuspid aortic valves is lacking.
- Bicuspid aortic valve disease is associated with aortopathy and other left sided cardiac lesions. As a result, careful evaluation of these structures is necessary when planning for treatment of severe symptomatic bicuspid aortic valve disease.

> **Key Points**
> - The degree of raphe calcification should be assessed qualitatively as mild, moderate, and severe. A raphe especially when calcified may affect expansion and apposition of the TAVR at the annulus, risk of requiring pacemaker, device misplacement, root injury and regurgitation.
> - Non raphe bicommissural bicuspid aortic valve have a larger sinus diameter but smaller annuli.
> - Calcium at the commissures can result in perforation. Bulky calcification at the tip of the leaflet is a risk for coronary obstruction.

Aortic Regurgitation

> **Case Study**
>
> *An 83-year-old male patient presented with NYHA class II symptoms without chest pain or syncope. He has had multiple prior hospitalizations for congestive cardiac failure. Physical examination revealed a grade 2 diastolic murmur loudest in the third intercostal space.*

Background and Definitions

Aortic regurgitation (AR) refers to the retrograde blood flow from the aorta into the left ventricle in diastole secondary to lack of aortic valve leaflet coaptation [77].

Isolated (AR) is less common than symptomatic (AS) and affects approximately 13% of patients with pure left sided native valve disease [78]. The estimated prevalence of at least moderate AR in those older than 70 years is 2.2% [79]. Less than 1% of transcatheter aortic valve implantation is done for AR in the United States [80]. Chronic AR is clinically asymptomatic for prolonged periods. Thereafter patients develop congestive heart failure, secondary to volume overload, left ventricular dysfunction and increased wall stress [81]. Valve replacement should be performed when regurgitation is severe and the patient is symptomatic, or when the left ventricle end systolic dimension is >50 mm (index left ventricular end systolic dimension is >25 mm/m^2) [82] or there is left ventricular systolic impairment [83].

The pathophysiology of AR differs from AS (degeneration and calcific disease [77]) and causes include:

- Congenital [81]
- Bicuspid Valve [80]
- Infectious [81]
- Rheumatic heart disease [80]
- Previous endocarditis [80]
- Vasculitis [81]
- Calcified/myxomatous leaflets [77]
- Connective tissue diseases [80]
- Aortic root dilatation [80] secondary to trauma, dissection, viruses or arteritides [77]
- Radiotherapy [81]

Diagnosis and Pre-procedural Evaluation

A TTE demonstrated a trileaflet, sclerotic aortic valve with mild reduction in cusp motion. There was moderate to severe aortic regurgitation with a regurgitant volume of 45 mL, an EROA of 0.23 cm^2, a P1/2T of 381 ms and a vena contracta of 5 mm. The left ventricle was severely dilated and globally hypokinetic with left ventricular hypertrophy and a reduced systolic function of 25%. The proximal ascending aorta was dilated, indexed at 20 mm/m^2.

Transthoracic Echo

TTE is the gold standard for workup [77] and assesses the mechanism and severity of regurgitation, valve type, and left ventricle remodelling and function [84]. Leaflets are assessed for non-coaptation and prolapse and multiple measures are assessed and integrated to determine the severity of regurgitation [83]. Additionally, left ventricular end systolic dimension, ejection fraction, aortic root and ascending aorta are also assessed [83].

Severe AR:

- Ratio of regurgitant jet width to LVOT width ≥65% [84].
- Vena contracta >0.6 cm [83].
- Effective regurgitant orifice area ≥0.3 cm^2 [84].
- Regurgitant volume >60 mL and regurgitant fraction ≥50% [84].
- Deceleration time (pressure half-time) of the continuous wave aortic regurgitation doppler jet of <200 ms [83].
- Reversal of flow in the descending aorta throughout diastole particularly when in conjunction with end diastolic velocity of >20 cm/s [83].

Caveats:

- Linear measurements are based on the presumption of a circular orifice from a single plane of assessment. The accuracy may therefore be increased with 3D TTE [83].
- Pressure half time varies with blood pressure and LV compliance and is often lower in acute AR [83].

Transoesophageal Echo

TEE is usually performed if a more detailed assessment of the aortic valve or aortic root is required [84]. Both 2D and 3D TEE provide diagnostic value in defining mechanisms of AR [84]. Pre procedural TEE provides information for device sizing whilst intraprocedurally it is used to visualise bioprosthetic valve positioning and assess for immediate complications [83]. TEE can also assess the valve morphology to enable valve preserving repair in some patients, especially those with aneurysms of the aortic root as well as regurgitation in non-calcified bicuspid valves [83]. Of note, doppler angles for assessing aortic regurgitation (for calculations such as aortic pressure ½ time or PISA EROA) are usually suboptimal in TEE as compared to TTE and necessitate deep transgastric imaging.

Cardiac Magnetic Resonance Imaging

CMR is the gold standard for the assessment of left ventricle volumes and ejection fraction [83]. In AR CMR may be used for valve planimetry, to determine the mechanism and quantify the severity of aortic regurgitations and the presence of aortopathy [84]. CMR is indicated when the echo is suboptimal or when there is a discordance between either echo and clinical findings or in determining AR severity between echo and doppler results [84]. CMR is also indicated when echo is limited in assessing aortopathy or in the presence of multiple valvular pathologies [84]. In addition, CMR is useful in follow up assessment with less variability then echo in determining the severity of AR and LV remodeling and is beneficial in long term assessment of aortopathy in coexistent AR and a bicuspid aortic valve [84]. Aortic regurgitant volume and fraction is determined by phase contrast velocity mapping of the aortic valve or in the absence of other valvular lesions by determining the difference between the aortic and pulmonic stroke volumes [84]. An aortic regurgitant orifice of ≥48 cm^2 and a holodiastolic flow reversal in the mid descending aorta where found to be sensitive in detecting and predicting severe AR [84]. Left ventricular dilation with end diastolic volume >246 mL predicts symptom onset and possible requirement of valve surgery whilst a regurgitation fraction >33% on phase contrast predicts surgical need within 3 years [83].

In the present case, the patient had a sufficient quality TTE to obviate the need for TEE or CMR. However, since the etiology of the patient's LV dysfunction wasn't clear, he underwent a coronary artery CT. There was no coronary artery disease, and the patient was categorized as a CAD-RADS 0.

Differential Diagnosis

The possible diagnoses included coronary artery disease which was excluded with a CT coronary angiogram. Echocardiogram demonstrated features of severe aortic regurgitation and excluded leaflet vegetation. Echocardiogram also excluded co existent significant mitral valvular disease or ASD. In light of the patient's worsening aortic regurgitation and the reduced left ventricular function, the work-up for TAVR was commenced (Fig. 29).

A pre TAVR CT was performed and demonstrated a tricuspid non calcified valve with no annular or LVOT calcification. The systolic annular area was measured at 405 mm². The risk for coronary ostial occlusion is low with the left main and the right coronary artery heights measuring 17.6 mm and 17.9 mm respectively. The average SOV dimension is 31 mm. The STJ diameter measured 25.9 mm. The orthogonal view was obtained at LAO 16° and CAU 20°, centered onto the right cusp. There was dilatation of the left ventricle, measured as LVEDD of 66 mm LVESD of 58 mm, and both atria. The ascending aorta was dilated, and this with the arch and descending thoracic and abdominal aorta demonstrated no significant calcifications, stenosis or tortuosity.

Computed Tomography

Computed Tomography is used primarily for pre-procedural planning rather than diagnosis. However, absence of complete coaptation of aortic leaflets during diastole can be used to detect aortic regurgitation [85]. An anatomic regurgitant area may be reliable to quantify severity with a value of 0.27 ± 0.16 cm² suggestive of severe AR [85]. Regardless of symptoms, end—systolic diameter of 55 mm or greater or an ejection fraction below 55% are indications for intervention [85]. Risk assessment for coronary obstruction, valve sizing and aortic dimension are assessed similarly to TAVR for aortic stenosis in the native valve.

Heart Team Approach and Discussion

Only 1 in 5 patients with severe AR and left ventricular ejection fraction between 30 and 50% are referred to surgery [81]. The co-existence of multiple co-morbidities and the advanced patient age

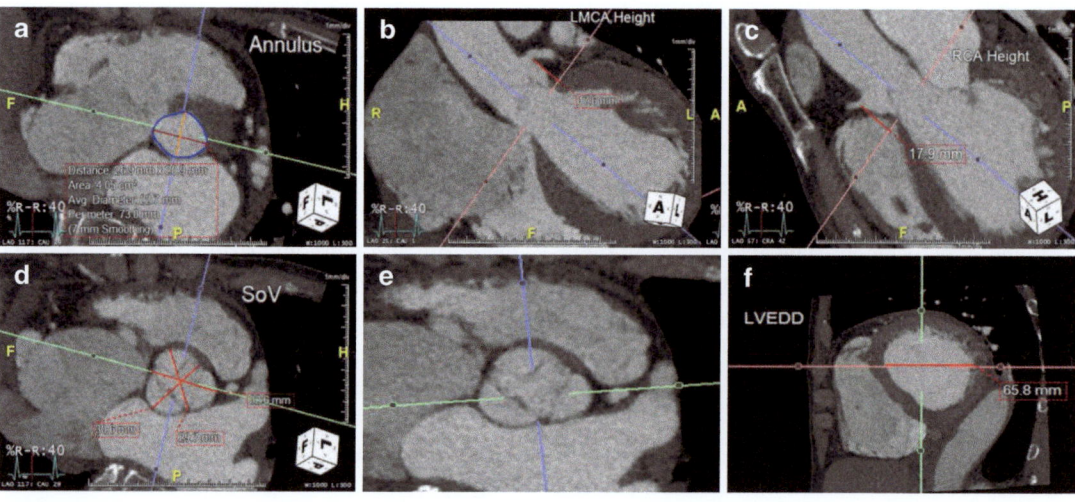

Fig. 29 (a) The annulus measures 405 mm² with a perimeter of 73 mm. (b–d) Low risk of coronary obstruction with coronary artery heights above 12 mm and a capacious sinus of Valsalva. (e) The RCC centered view provided a plane orthogonal to the annulus. (f) The left ventricle is dilated measuring 66 mm on end diastole

result in conservative management rather than surgery with a resultant mortality between 10 to 20% [81]. In patients fit for surgery, valve replacement is the treatment of choice [78]. Patients with aortic regurgitation have a higher lifespan potential then in patients with AS therefore such patients with a co-existing dilated aorta may benefit from surgery for both pathologies [86]. TAVR valves are used off label for the treatment of pure AR [81].

Given the patient's history of shortness of breath and the multiple admissions presenting with features of cardiac failure, worsening AR without significant coronary disease, the patient was recommended for AVR. Pre procedural TAVR CT indicated the feasibility of SAVR or TAVR for AVR in this patient.

However, several challenges exist in the use of TAVR to treat AR:

- There is lack of valvular calcification in most patients with native pure AR [78–81, 86]. This renders the anchorage of the transcatheter valve in the annular plane difficult [77, 78, 80, 81] and increases the risk of valve embolization or paravalvular leak [87].
- The lack of a fluoroscopic landmarks make positioning the valve challenging [77, 78].
- Oversizing the valve [78] reduces the risk of valve migration, embolization [77], malposition, and paravalvular regurgitation, however the risk of annular rupture and valve dislocation is increased [81]. The transcatheter valves that depend on oversizing and radial expansion to anchor the valve may predispose to progressive increase in size of the annulus [86]. Approximately 5–20% of oversizing is advised for the SAPIEN valve in order to balance the risk of annular rupture and paravalvular leak, however during off label use in pure AR 20 to 30% oversizing is sometimes utilised [88]. This however often results in requiring a size greater than the available valves [88]. In addition to aortic root rupture, incomplete expansion of the valve is a further complication of oversizing [87].

- There is often co-existent dilation of the aortic root and/or dilatation of the ascending aorta [78, 79].
- The aortic annulus is larger [80, 86] and dynamic [80] and may be larger than the available sizes of prosthetic valves [81].
- Hyper contractility of the left ventricle due to the high stroke volume as well as the regurgitation jet [80, 81] reduces control of the device whilst positioning and releasing the prosthetic valve [81] with an increased risk of malposition [80].
- The left ventricle is usually dilated [81].

Features improving TAVR success in native AR:

- *Calcified annulus* [80].
- *Calcified aortic leaflets* [80].
- *Mixed AR and AS* [80].

Predictors for TAVR failure in native AR:

- *Residual AR that is moderate to severe* [77].
- *Society of thoracic surgeons (STS) score of >8%* [77].
- *<20 g/m² body mass index* [77].
- *Presence of major vascular complications* [77].

Exclusions for TAVR in native AR:

- *Patients fit for surgery with acceptable risk* [80].
- *Active infective endocarditis* [80].
- *Co-existing ascending aorta aneurysm requiring surgery* [80].
- *Very large aortic annulus that commercial THV's cannot treat* [80].

Heart Team Decision

Based on the patient's age and severe left ventricular dysfunction, he was considered high risk for conventional open cardiac surgery. TAVR with the J-Valve was the preferred choice of treatment.

Valve Options

In general, second generation TAVR devices and beyond are preferred for aortic regurgitation because of self-positioning geometry and the possibility of repositioning with additional fixation devices allowing for better valve function in aortic regurgitation [81] (Fig. 30).

We used a Jena valve in this procedure.

It is a transapical self-expanding valve [81] with nitinol tabs above the leaflets with clips, feelers or claspers to assist with positioning and anchoring of the valve [86]. The three U-shaped graspers allow for the valve to position and clip onto the native leaflets [81]. Currently access is via a transapical route [78] with transfemoral axis systems becoming available [86]. The J valve has a CE mark for on label use in AR [80] but is pending FDA approval for this indication. Imaging is required for correct positioning of the three feelers in the aortic sinuses to adequately anchor the stent [87]. Alignment is necessary as poor alignment and positioning may result in persistent regurgitation or device embolization/migration [87]. The valve does not need annular calcification or oversizing to anchor and has a supra—annular location said to improve haemodynamics [79]. There is no sealing skirt, therefore there may be an increased risk for significant post procedural PVL [79].

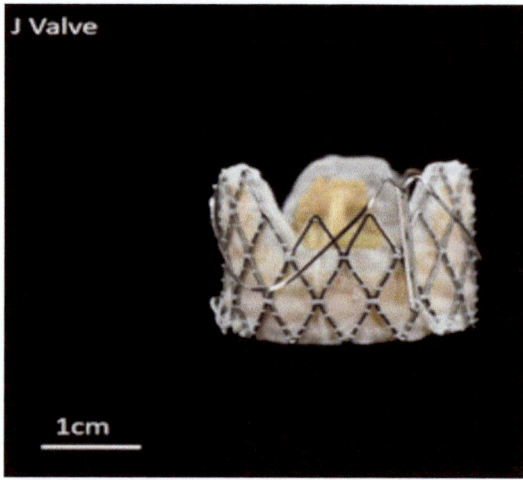

Fig. 30 J valve

Planning for Trans Apical Access

Preoperatively an ECG gated CT [31] is acquired and assessment includes identifying the left ventricular apex and its relationship to the thoracic wall [89], in particular to the fifth and sixth intercostal space [90], whilst immediate preprocedural localization of the apex can be achieved with trans thoracic echo [89]. Chest wall abnormalities including pleural and pericardial calcifications may hinder access [90]. Dimensions of the anterior chest wall to LV apex and apex to the aortic wall are required and the course and location of coronary bypass grafts in relation to the LV apex and chest wall should be noted [90]. A LV thrombus is a contraindication to trans apical access [89] and can be identified both by CT and echocardiography. Furthermore, LV apical myocardial thinning, and calcification may limit access and post procedural repair [90]. An impaired LV function with an EF of less than 20% precludes LV access, this can be quantified via echocardiography or a retrospective ECG gated full cycle cardiac CT [90]. Immediate complications include risk of myocardial tear with a delayed risk of bleeding and pseudo aneurysm formation [90].

Intraprocedural Assessment (Fig. 31)

Intraprocedural TEE demonstrated severe central aortic regurgitation with an aortic annulus measuring 22 mm. The left ventricle was severely dilated with a reduced ejection fraction of 45%. There was reversal of flow in the distal aortic arch during diastole.

The lack of valvular calcification renders the procedure more challenging due to the lack of landmarks of the annulus and root on fluoroscopy [91]. As a result, TEE guidance for TAVR positioning may play a larger role in AR than AS. The fluoroscopic limitation can be minimised by using fixed landmarks in the thorax e.g. vertebrae, sternal or pacemaker wires and using pigtail catheters (Place 1 catheter in the noncoronary sinus and the one in the left sinus) [91]. This assists in correct positioning and reduces contrast or the need of several aortograms [91]. Roy et al. suggest intraprocedural rapid pacing during deployment of the

Transcatheter Aortic Valve Replacement

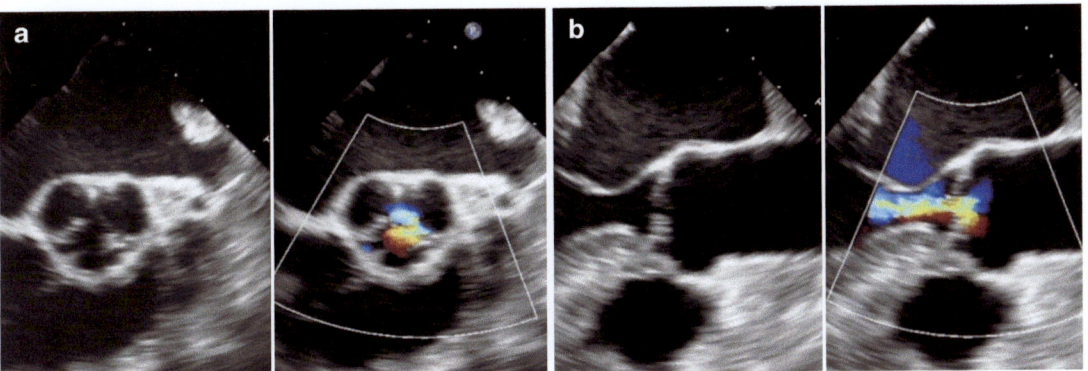

Fig. 31 2D TEE with mid esophageal aortic valve short axis (**a**) and long axis view (**b**) demonstrates a trileaflet aortic valve with mild thickening and moderate to severe central aortic regurgitation

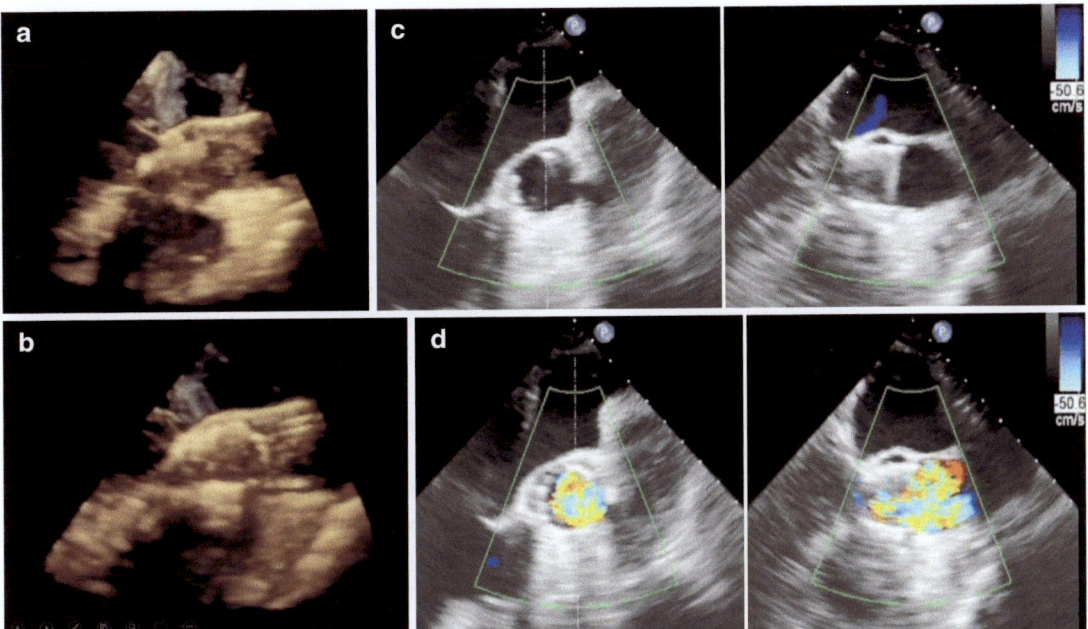

Fig. 32 (**a** and **b**) demonstrate 2D long axis deployment of an appropriately positioned prosthetic valve. (**c** and **d**) short and long axis 2D TEE with (**c**) and without (**d**) color flow doppler with no central aortic regurgitation

CoreValve in severe native aortic regurgitation as this reduces systolic pressure, regurgitant volume and risk of movement of the valve [91]. Intraprocedural rapid ventricular pacing is not essential for best alignment and stability during valve positioning, however this contributes to procedural safety especially in patients with compromised left ventricle function [87].

The patient underwent a trans apical TAVI and a 25 mm Jena-valve was deployed via mini thoracotomy. No pre or post implant dilatation was required (Fig. 32).

A post-deployment TEE demonstrated a well seated and well positioned Jena-Valve with normal leaflet motion, no regurgitation and trivial posterior paravalvular leak. The mean gradient was 10 mmHg. There was no change in the LVEF (Fig. 33).

A post-deployment root angiogram demonstrated a well seated Jena–valve with no aortic

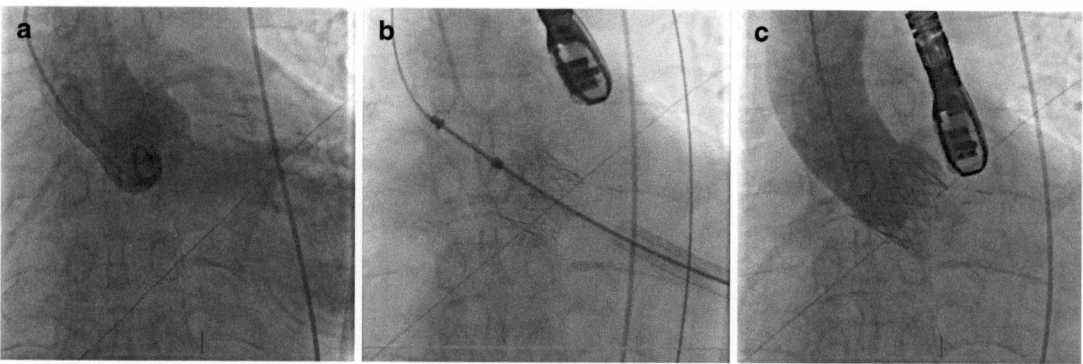

Fig. 33 (a) Aortic root angiogram with central regurgitation. (b) Deployed and expanded bioprosthetic J valve (c) appropriately positioned without significant paravalvular regurgitation

regurgitation. ECG demonstrated sinus rhythm with no features of a new AV block.

Possible complications:

- The anchorage and sealing of the valve may be inadequate [81] with resulting valve regurgitation [77, 81]. There is a high incidence of valve-in valve procedures due to persistent aortic regurgitation [87].
- Paravalvular regurgitation [86].
- Valve malposition or embolization [86] with potential ventricular dislocation occurring several hours post implantation [78].

The rates for valve embolization [79], deployment of a second THV, presence of paravalvular leak or moderate to severe aortic regurgitation as well as the 30 day mortality are higher in TAVI for AR compared to AS [80]. Newer generation valves may have better outcomes [80] and a reduction in mortality [77]. Newer generation devices are able to grasp native leaflets, have a larger variety of sizes, expanded adaptive seals and the capability to be repositioned and recaptured [77].

Postprocedural Assessment

The THV was well seated. The aortic valve area measured 2.1 cm^2 with a Vmax of 1.8 m/s and a mean gradient of 6 mmHg. The LVEF was visually estimated at 45%. When compared to the prior echo, there was interval improvement in systolic function with reduction in the pulmonary artery pressure.

The requirement for permanent pacemaker is lower when compared to TAVR for AS despite the increased use of self-expanding devices. This is due to lack of calcification of the aortic valve and surrounding structures especially at the atrioventricular conduction system [78]. Contradictory to this, Alexis et al. stated that TAVR performed for aortic regurgitation causes a significant number of new left bundle branch blocks and permanent pacemaker requirements similar to the outcome post TAVR for AS even with the new generation valves [77]. Table 6 showing role of Multimodality Imaging in TAVR in Aortic regurgitation.

Transcatheter Aortic Valve Replacement

Table 6 Aortic regurgitation multimodality imaging in aortic regurgitation

Aortic regurgitation	Echocardiography	Fluoroscopy	Computed tomography	MRI
Preprocedure imaging	First line for valvular assessment TTE generally being superior due to doppler angle and TEE reserved for better delineation of mechanism or potentially device sizing		Provides diagnostic and planning information same as in AS	Provides diagnostic and planning information same as in AS
Intraprocedure imaging	TEE optimizes valve positioning especially in the absence annular calcification	Absence of annular and leaflet calcification makes valve deployment more challenging than in AS. Techniques available to optimize device positioning		
Postprocedure imaging	Same as AS (case 1)			

Clinical Controversies and Pearls

- Randomized controlled trials of TAVR valves for AR are lacking.
- The lack of valvular calcification in majority of patients with native pure AR makes anchorage of the transcatheter valve in the annular plane difficult with increased risk of paravalvular leak and valve embolization.

> **Key Points**
> - Only 1 in 5 patients with severe AR and LVEF between 30 and 50% are referred for AVR.
> - There is often co-existent dilatation of the aortic root and or ascending aorta.
> - Moderate to severe post TAVR residual AR is a predictor for TAVR failure in native AR.
> - The presence of a calcified annulus, calcified aortic leaflets and mixed AR and AS improve TAVR success in native AR.

Valve in Valve

> **Case Study**
>
> *90-year-old female presents with new onset worsening exertional dyspnea and fatigue with a history of SAVR with a 21 mm Trifecta bio prosthetic valve 9 years prior.*

Background and Definitions

Increased utilisation of bio prosthetic valves in younger patients predicts higher rates of future re-intervention [92]. The valve academic research consortium (VARC) defines structural valve deterioration as a mean gradient ≥40 mmHg and/or ≥20 mmHg change in baseline values (values obtained within 30 days of procedure or at discharge) [92].

TAVR in valve is the preferred treatment in patients at high risk for redo SAVR or unfavourable anatomy including calcified aorta or hostile chest [92]. Redo SAVR is preferred in patients under 75 years or patients with unfavourable coronary anatomy, patient-prosthesis mismatch, a non fracturable SHV or severe PVL not amenable to percutaneous intervention [92]. There is improved short term and comparable major long term cardiovascular outcomes in VIV TAVR when compared to redo SAVR [93] with reduced hospital stay, morbidity and mortality [94]. Currently, self-expanding (CoreValve/Evolut) and balloon expandable (Sapien XT/Sapien S3) TAVR valves have been approved for VIV in patients at high risk for SAVR [95].

Diagnosis and Pre-procedural Assessment

TTE demonstrates moderate aortic insufficiency with normal left ventricular size (left ventricular inner diameter indexed at 24 mm/m^2), wall thick-

ness and function (EF 60%). The surgical bio prosthetic valve was well seated with a mean gradient of 41 mmHg, V max: 4.1 m/s AVA, AOV VTI 115 cm: Peak gradient AVA: 66 mmHg, EOA: 0.5 cm²; EOA index 0.3 cm²/m²; AR P1/2T: 475 ms. Leaflet excursion was decreased, and the leaflets appeared echodense, suggesting possible calcification. Of note, aortic acceleration time was 150 ms.

Cause of Bio Prosthetic Failure

Echocardiography is the primary modality to determine the aetiology of bioprosthetic failure and resultant LV function and remodelling [96]. Quantitative Doppler echocardiography can be performed to help differentiate between high flow states, improper measurements, prosthetic valve stenosis, and patient-prosthesis mismatch (Fig. 16), although the latter is more likely to present soon after prosthetic valve placement. Planimetry can be performed via short axis views and the EOA should be determined using continuity equation bearing in mind that values may be underestimated in the presence of significant regurgitation [96]. Degenerative stentless valves most commonly present with regurgitation [92] (Fig. 34).

Cardiac catheterization was pursued to rule-out significant coronary disease as an etiology for dyspnea and demonstrated coronary arteries without significant angiographic disease. The right coronary artery was possibly below the upper margin of the Trifecta valve posts. The aortic sinus appeared large at the level of the coronary arteries. The aortic root was normal. Femoral access was adequate for TAVR valve in valve.

Differential Diagnoses

The patient's presentation of exertional dyspnea and fatigue are potentially consistent with coronary disease, heart failure, or valve degeneration, as well as non-cardiac conditions. However, the echocardiogram is most consistent with prosthetic valve degeneration. Bio prosthetic valve failure may result from a combination of factors including pannus, leaflet degeneration and leaflet perforation [97] (Fig. 35).

A preprocedural CT scan was obtained to assess suitability for a potential valve-in-valve (TAVR in SAVR) procedure. CT scan confirmed a 21 mm Trifecta bio prosthetic valve with no significant prosthetic leaflet calcification. Dimensions of a 20 mm S3 valve were simulated with both coronary arteries below the upper margin of the stent posts. The stent posts did not extend to the level of the STJ. Valve to coronary distance (VTC) was 4.8 mm for the right and 5 mm for the left main coronary artery. Trans femoral access was feasible bilaterally with bilateral minimum dimensions of 7 mm and no significant tortuosity. There was mild calcification on the right and no calcification on the left iliofemoral vessels. Importantly, PPM, infective

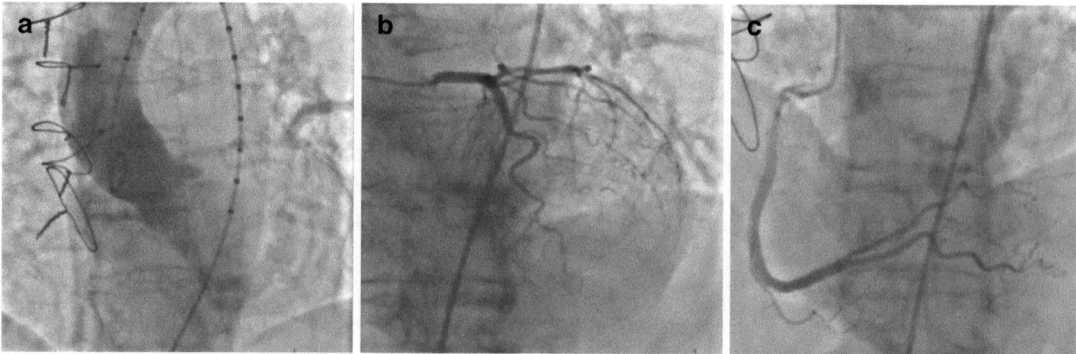

Fig. 34 Aortic root and coronary angiogram demonstrating MAC, mild aortic regurgitation, normal coronary arteries with the RCA ostium at the upper margin of stent post (**a** and **c**) and the LM above the level of the stent posts (**a** and **b**)

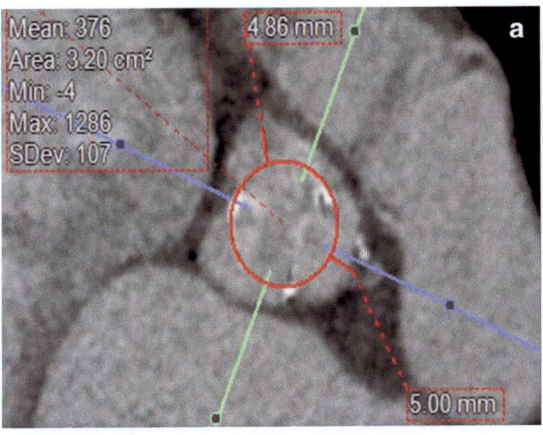 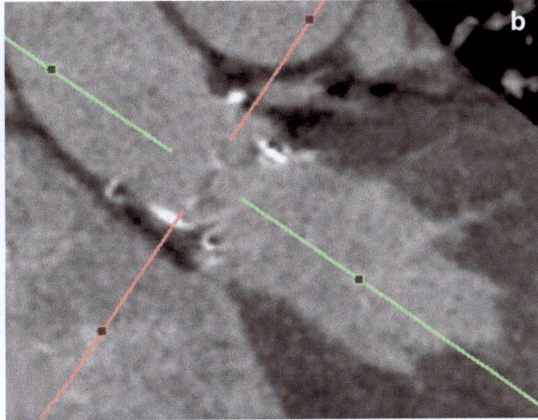

Fig. 35 Post contrast pre procedural planning CT of the aortic root confirmed a Trifecta 21 mm bio prosthetic valve with no significant bioprosthetic leaflet calcification. (**a**) The red annular ring represents a 20 mm S3 valve simulated in the plane of the basal ring and projected to the level of the coronary arteries. A VTC of 4.8 mm for the right and 5 mm for the left main coronary arteries were obtained. (**b**) Long axis images with the cross hairs corresponding to the plane of the short axis in (**a**) confirmed that the coronary arteries arise below the upper margin of the stent posts

endocarditis and valve dehiscence with significant paravalvular regurgitation were ruled out by the TTE, as these are associated with poor outcome after attempted valve-in-valve (TAVR in SAVR) procedures [96].

Heart Team Approach and Discussion

Although TAVR in SAVR and TAVR in TAVR have become the procedures of choice for degenerated bioprosthetic aortic valves in high surgical risk patients, there are a number of valve and anatomic factors that need to be assessed to determine procedural feasibility and likelihood of success.

Bioprosthetic Valve Characteristics

Pertinent knowledge of surgical valve durability, true inner diameter, fracturability and leaflet position are important [98]. Bioprosthetic valves with porcine leaflets tend to retract, reducing the risk of coronary obstruction, whilst Sapien 3 valves tend to flare particularly following valve fracture with increased risk of coronary obstruction [99]. The CoreValve however has a narrowed waist which is narrower than the annulus and accounts for a relatively reduced risk of obstruction [99].

Bio prosthetic valves are divided into stented and stentless SHV (i.e with and without a rigid framework) and transcatheter heart valves [15]. The size of the implanted surgical valve may not be known, but can be easily determined on pre-procedural CT [15, 96] or TEE [96].

On CT this is done by calculating the inner area at the basal sewing ring and comparing with available reference charts [15]. Care should be taken to obtain dimensions as per the technique described in the referenced charts as these may differ and effect accuracy [15]. Intraprocedurally, valves can be identified by their unique fluoroscopic appearance [100, 101].

TEE dimensions are acquired during a single heartbeat and reconstructed in short axis at the plane of the sewing ring [96]. Error in measurement from acoustic noise can be reduced by optimising gain settings and measuring at the most echogenic margin [96].

Aortic valve in valve online and mobile applications are available to confirm radiographic appearance of the SHV and provides information on a suitable VIV THV that may be used [101].

Coronary Artery Obstruction

The incidence of coronary artery obstruction has a mortality rate of up to 50% [102] and is higher for valve in valve procedures when compared to native aortic TAVR occurring in 2.3% of patients with valve in valve [15, 102]. Coronary occlusion more commonly occurs in the LM with an incidence of between 72% [92] and 90% [101], with both coronaries involved in 20% of cases [98].

Obstruction more commonly occurs in stentless valves, valves with externally mounted leaflets [101, 103, 104], lower ostial and STJ to annular heights, narrow sinuses or STJ dimensions and bulky leaflets [96, 104]. Blanke et al. further documented higher rates of coronary occlusion when the bioprosthetic valve is canted with subsequent approximation to either coronary ostium especially in patients with a relatively small aortic root [15].

When implanted into a stented bioprosthetic valve the THV permanently displaces the leaflets of the degenerative bioprosthetic valve to an open position [15, 101] forming a "covered cylinder" with the alignment and position of the THV conforming to the plane/long axis of the bioprosthetic valve [15]. If the degenerative bioprosthetic valve is canted in particular towards either coronary artery, this would result in approximation of the now canted covered cylinder in the direction of either coronary artery increasing the risk of coronary obstruction with limited "protective" effect from a wide sinus of Valsalva [15]. Annibali et al. describes delayed coronary obstruction (DCO) occurring as late as 60 days post procedure [92]. DCO is more common in VIV procedures [101]. Progressive expansion in self-expandable devices, which may continue to expand for days post procedure [92, 101], aortic mural hematoma, and coronary dissection are possible causes in earlier DCO. Late DCO is more commonly secondary to obstruction caused by native or surgical leaflet endothelialisation or thrombus embolization [92].

In stentless valves, coronary ostial heights and SOV dimensions are determined as per native valve bearing in mind the increased risk of coronary obstruction as these valves are usually used in small aortic roots [15]. Lack of radiopaque markers may limit fluoroscopic visualisation, usually necessitating intraprocedural echocardiographic guidance [104].

In stented valves, a VTC distance at the level of the ostium (if below or at the level of the tip of the stent post) and a VTS (virtual valve to sinus distance) at the tip of the stent posts should be obtained [15]. A VTC of less than 4 mm is high risk of obstruction [99, 101]. With low risk if >6 mm and intermediate risk when 4–6 mm, when present bailout procedures should be planned [100]. Blanke et al. described a virtual THV to coronary distance as an independent predictor of risk for coronary obstruction [15]. In situations in which the SHV lies above and in close proximity to the STJ, the displaced leaflets may once again form a covered cylinder and limit flow to the coronary ostium [101]. The leaflets should be accessed for distal bulky calcification (risk of ostial occlusion by calcifications) and its height in plane and relation to the ostium and STJ [99]. A valve to sinotubular junction distance measured at the level of the STJ is significant if circumferentially below normal values [99]. A valve to STJ distance of less than 3 mm correlates with high risk of coronary obstruction [92].

STJ and coronary artery height dimensions are determined as described in native TAVR, bearing in mind that the heights should be measured from the basal plane of the suture ring [101]. Comparatively, coronary artery heights are lower in VIV versus native TAVR as SHV's are frequently sutured in a supra annular location [101]. Normal values have not yet been defined [101]. Coronary artery heights are not as significant in VIV as in native TAVR [105].

Angiographic assessment of potential coronary occlusion can be determined by the relative height and size of the SHV to the coronary artery height and aortic root width [100]. Poor contrast opacification of the aortic root as a result of aortic regurgitation, usually present on degenerative bioprosthetic valves, may require semi selective coronary artery injections [105]. Dominance, collateral flow, and the presence and patency of bypass grafts [105] should be assessed. The basal stent ring provides appropriate radiopaque implantation landmarks and if not appreciated (stentless valve) can be identified with optimal positioning of the pigtail catheter deep into the aortic root followed by contrast injection [100] or balloon valvuloplasty [96].

Heart Team Decision

In view of the patient being symptomatic with imaging demonstrating elevated gradients and bioprosthetic dysfunction it was decided to proceed with TAVR VIV. The decision was to use a smaller THV (20 mm SAPIEN) to minimize the risk of coronary obstruction and this was thought appropriate given the patients' age. Coronary protection with chimney stent would be used if deemed necessary.

Intraprocedural Imaging Modalities and Measurements

A 20 mm S3 Sapien was deployed in a bioprosthetic TAVR valve during rapid pacing via a right transfemoral access. Post valve deployment coronary angiogram demonstrated no coronary artery obstruction in particular the left main was patent.

Coronary Artery Management During Valve in Valve

The TAVR device is deployed in the orthogonal projection to the plane of the basal ring/"neo annulus" [100]. This is easily performed with fluoroscopic guidance however in stentless valves supplemental imaging with echocardiography is useful in identifying the basal ring [96, 100]. Optimal fluoroscopic projections require a plane orthogonal to both the basal ring and ostium of the coronary artery [105]. Due to absence of radio-opaque markers in stentless surgical valves, a perpendicular view is obtained with the three cusps view, demonstrating symmetrical cusps [105]. A plane orthogonal to the coronary ostia can be obtained by a one to two technique in which two stent posts are superimposed and the technique is performed independently for each coronary artery [105].

TEE can assess and determine the height of the coronary ostium above the sewing ring, dimensions of the STJ and SOV, leaflet length and degree of calcification [96]. Balloon valvuloplasty in conjunction with TEE can also determine risk of coronary obstruction in the absence of radiopaque landmarks [96].

Balloon inflation displaces the bio prosthetic valve leaflets similarly to the planned transcatheter valve and should be inflated to the diameter of the planned replacement valve [105]. Contrast opacification of the aortic root should be performed when the compliant balloon is completely inflated in a plane orthogonal to the basal ring [105]. During aortic root opacification the risk of coronary obstruction and information on positioning of the stent especially in non radio-opaque stents may be obtained [105].

New wall motion abnormality should alert the proceduralist to the possibility of significant coronary obstruction whilst other causes of hypotension including haemodynamically significant AR and cardiac tamponade can be assessed with TEE [96].

Precautionary Measures and Strategies in Patients at Risk for Coronary Obstruction

In patients with high risk for coronary obstruction, protective measures may be undertaken prior to valve deployment. Cannulation and placement of a guidewire and non-deployed stent in the coronary artery at risk, with pre-emptive or anticipated deployment in the event of coronary obstruction [101, 104]. Any movement of the segment of wire near the ostium, at the time of TAVR implantation should raise suspicion for possible coronary occlusion (wire sign) [105]. Once The TAVR VIV is deployed assessment should be made for coronary occlusion either by aortography, selective angiography or new wall motion abnormality on echocardiography [101]. If coronary obstruction is present, the stent can be deployed partially within the coronary artery extending into the aorta, the technique known as chimney stenting [101]. If the coronary arteries are not obstructed, the non-deployed stent should be removed with the wire left within the coronary artery with a repeat angiogram as coronary patency may temporarily be preserved by the stent shaft [105]. If obstructed the coronary stent should be placed across the site of obstruction, be it at the ostium or STJ [105].

Coronary obstruction in patients at significant risk may be limited by under expanding a BE valve [105] or using a lower profile TAVR valve which should be balanced with risk of PPM [104, 105]. Further coronary protective strategy includes low implantation depth which may result in less outward displacement of the stent posts and leaflets [105]. The use of a retrievable stent (Evolut R, Lotus or Portico) with flow assessment following partial deployment is another option in high risk patients [101]. If obstruction is detected acutely, the valve may be resheated and repositioned or the procedure abandoned [101]. The risk of DCO should be acknowledged if proceeding with a self-expanding valve [101]. Retrievability depends on valve type, with the Lotus valve retrievable after full implantation and the Portico retrievable prior and not after implantation [105].

A further strategy to reduce coronary obstruction is the BASILICA (bio prosthetic aortic scallop intentional laceration to prevent coronary artery obstruction) procedure. During the procedure the degenerative leaflet either native or bio prosthetic is lacerated using electrocautery, minimising obstruction of the coronary ostium by splaying the leaflets following TAVR deployment [98, 106]. Splaying of the leaflets uncovers the ostium with improved flow whilst maintaining feasibility for future coronary access [98]. BASILICA is considered when the leaflet tip, either prosthetic or native, projects above the coronary ostia extending to the STJ or in the setting of a small SOV [107] with risk of coronary ostial obstruction or sinus sequestration [99]. Khan et al. demonstrated no strokes, myocardial infarctions or deaths related to BASILICA at 1 year and concerns of delayed coronary obstruction from leaflet mobilisation, paravalvular leak or embolised valve were not evident [102].

A classification strategy defining the need for BASILICA was developed from the VIVID registry [92]. With information of the aortic root and coronary ostial height three categories where obtained:

Type I: aortic valve leaflets below the ostium,
Type II: Leaflets above the ostium.
Type IIA: with wide sinuses of Valsalva.
Type IIB: with effaced sinus of Valsalva.
Type III: Leaflets above or very close to the STJ.
Type IIIA: with wide sinuses and STJ.
Type IIIB: with effaced sinuses.
Type IIIC: with narrow STJ.
Types IIB, IIIB and IIIC should be considered for
  BASILICA if VTC is less than 4 mm [92].

Pre procedural TEE guidance for BASILICA includes routine TEE assessment supplemented by exclusion of valve pathology including thrombus, vegetations, target leaflet tears and identification of patient specific valve anatomy (relative location of coronary ostia and views necessary for procedural guidance) [107]. 3D TEE complements anatomical findings and spatial relationships [107]. Bulky calcification at the leaflet tips are at risk for embolization and may preclude BASILICA [99].

The success of the procedure depends on the relative position of the coronary ostia to the gap between the edges of the lacerated leaflet with malalignment resulting in a risk of the coronary ostium covered by the deflected leaflet and potentially difficult future coronary access [108]. Greenbaum et al. described suboptimal splaying of the lacerated leaflet posing a higher risk for coronary obstruction in scenarios with a heavily calcified leaflet, TAV in TAV and very small VTC and proposes balloon dilatation at the points of leaflet crossing prior to leaflet laceration as a method for risk reduction [109].

Following leaflet laceration and TAVR placement post procedural imaging includes routine assessment complemented by assessment of coronary perfusion and exclusion of aortic root injury/dissection, intracardiac shunts/pericardial effusion (raising the suspicion of possible chamber/aortic penetration with stiff or electrocautery wires) and exclusion of wall motion abnormalities [107]. Ostial occlusion, complete or partial may still occur in a canted prosthetic valve or partial valve prolapse into the coronary ostium [107].

Positioning of Valve in Valve Bioprosthesis

Along with fluoroscopic and angiographic determination of the sewing ring position, echocardiography is useful especially in non-radiopaque SHV. When positioning and deploying the THV, appropriate fluoroscopic angles should be perpendicular to the basal ring of the SHV with angles determined by pre procedural CT/angiography or intraprocedurally [95]. High implantation is associated with risk for embolization and coronary obstruction in both self and balloon expandable valves but has an advantage of reduced gradients [96]. Low implantation of balloon-expanding valves are at risk for paravalvular regurgitation and bioprosthetic SHV leaflet overhang (unlikely in the longer S3) with risk of anterior mitral leaflet impingement and suboptimal lower annular position in self expanding valves [96]. Note should be made that coplanar fluoroscopic views do not correlate with long axis views on echo [96]. Optimal positioning on TEE is achieved with the THV implanted within 5 mm from the inferior margin of the suture ring for SE valves and 10% below the suture ring for BE valves [96]. Fluoroscopic and echocardiographic landmarks are different [96]. Manufacturer recommendations are for the central marker on the balloon to be aligned with the base of the right coronary cusp during Sapien implantation [110]. Ramanathan et al. describes a 100% success rate with no new pacemaker requirement, procedure related death or valve embolization when the lucent line at the inflow of the Sapien valve was aligned with the radiopaque basal ring [110]. The larger height of third generation BE THV's (compared to any SHV) require echocardiographic confirmation of the upper margin positioned below the STJ and above the SHV leaflets with automatic appropriate positioning of its lower margin below the suture ring [96].

Following valve implantation echocardiographic assessment for valve position, leaflet motion, gradients, valve area, intra and inter valvular regurgitation, ventricular function and size and new or increasing size of any pericardial effusion should be performed [96]. Table 7 showing role of Multimodality Imaging in aortiv valve in valve implantation.

Post Procedural Assessment

Immediate post procedural transthoracic echocardiogram demonstrated a well seated trans catheter heart valve, however leaflet motion was not well seen. The AVA measured 0.7 cm², indexed AVA = 0.42 cm²/m² Vmax measured 3.5 m/s with a peak gradient of 49 mmHg and mean gradient was 26 mmHg. Left ventricle demonstrated mild concentric hypertrophy with an ejection fraction of 60%. Trivial PVL was present. Elevated gradients and velocities post procedure, while improved as compared to pre-procedure, likely represent PPM due to the use of a 20 mm SAPIEN valve (Fig. 36).

To rule out leaflet abnormality, a post procedure CT was obtained and demonstrated an under expanded Sapien 3 valve with an area of 2.44 cm² at the stent inflow, 2.02 mm² at the mid

Table 7 Valve-in-valve multimodality imaging

Valve in valve	Echocardiography	Fluoroscopy	Computed tomography	MRI
Preprocedure imaging	First line for diagnostic assessment of a prosthetic valve and quantification of severity		Essential in determining risk of coronary artery obstruction and determining size and type of SHV (if information not already provided)	Limited due to metal artifact from degenerated bioprosthetic valve
Intraprocedural imaging	TEE is of greater intraprocedural utility in stentless valves. Can assist in determining risk of coronary obstruction	Visualization of indwelling valve optimizes deployment		
Postprocedural imaging	Same as AS (case 1)			

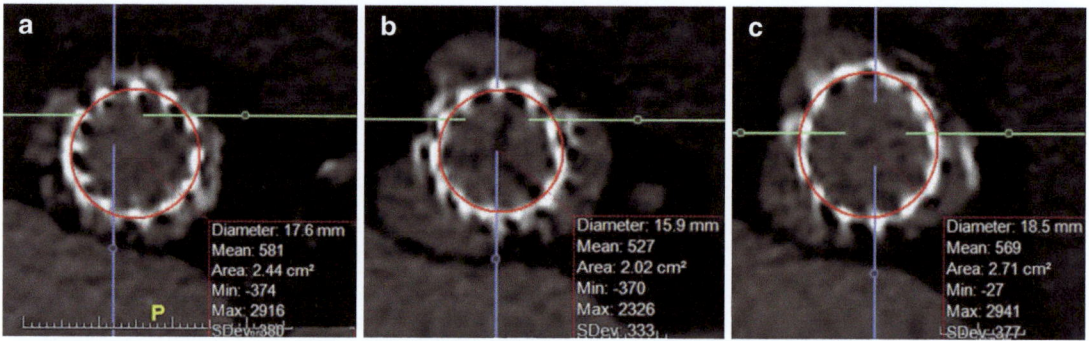

Fig. 36 Post contrast CT at 30 days following TAVR VIV with coplanar images at the inflow (**a**), mid (**b**) and outflow (**c**) demonstrating an under expanded S3 with the areas obtained less than expected for a 20 mm S3

portion of the stent and 271 mm² at the stent outflow. No evidence of HALT or leaflet thrombosis.

30-day TEE revealed a well seated transcatheter heart valve and poorly visualized leaflet motion, AVA of 0.7 cm², Vmax of 3.5 m/s and a mean gradient of 28 mmHg. There was concentric left ventricle hypertrophy with an ejection fraction of 65%. This was essentially unchanged as compared to the immediate post-procedure TTE.

Complications Following VIV TAVR

Leaflet Thrombosis and Thickening
Computational modelling demonstrates relative increase in blood stasis within the neo sinus as a potential mechanism to leaflet thrombosis following VIV TAVR [98]. Other causes of leaflet thickening and altered motion include incomplete valve frame expansion, endocarditis, HALT and leaflet degeneration [58, 111].

Elevated Gradients and PPM
PPM results from a normally functioning bioprosthetic valve with an EOA relatively smaller than required for the patient's body size with subsequent elevated post procedural gradients [92]. An indexed EOA of <0.65 cm²/m² defines severe PPM. Post TAVR valve in valve mean gradients are higher than mean gradient post native TAVR, averaging 12.4–16 mmHg [104]. A gradient of greater than 20 mmHg following TAVR VIV is associated with poor clinical outcomes and 1 year mortality rates [95]. Supra annular morphology of the core valve, inner versus externally mounted leaflets, higher implantation depth (allowing for better coaptation and leaflet motion, unrestricted by the basal ring of the SHV [98]) and larger THV sizes confer lower valve gradients [104]. The effective orifice area is not necessarily larger with a larger THV choice with in vitro results demonstrating different EOA in similar sized THV by different SHV manufacturers [98]. Pre dilation of the bioprosthetic valve to increase the inner diameter in the setting of calcification, thickened leaflets and fibrotic pannus is an available option but seldom used due to the risk of embolization or haemodynamic compromise following acute aortic regurgitation [104]. Appropriate THV choice (supra annular valve in SE THV) should be considered with smaller SHV [96]. VIV THV in small SHV (e.g. 19 mm SHV) should be avoided [96] with poor outcomes in SHV's less than 21 mm due to persistent high gradients [95]. Valve fracture, in the appropriate setting, and post implantation dilatation are further available options to minimise risk of patient prosthesis mismatch [104].

Permanent Pacemaker Requirements
The stable and firm nature of the surgical valve limits injury and compression to the conduction system with reduced post procedural pacemaker requirements [104], especially with new generation devices with no significant difference

between the balloon or self-expandable valves [112]. Pre-existing RBBB, increased age and larger THVs have increased pacemaker requirement risks [112].

Paravalvular Leak

The firm and regular surface provided by the surgical valve reduces the risk of PVL and annular rupture, unless balloon expansion is aggressive [104].

Clinical Controversies and Pearls

- In stented valves measure VTC, if the ostium is below or at the level of the tip of the stent post, and a VTS at the tip of the stent posts should be measured. A VTC <4 mm is high risk for obstruction, intermediate risk when 4–6 mm and low risk when >6 mm.
- If the SHV valve lies above and in close proximity to the STJ, a valve to STJ distance should be measured and is significant if circumferentially below normal. A valve to STJ less than 3 mm is high risk for coronary obstruction.

> **Key Points**
> - A key assessment in evaluation of degenerative bioprosthetic aortic valve disease is the risk of early or delayed coronary obstruction, which is largely based on CT measurements.
> - Outcomes of valve-in-valve after implantation of a TAVR valve of 21 mm or less are suboptimal, likely due to elevated gradients and patient-prosthesis mismatch.
> - With the exception of the risk for coronary obstruction, early outcomes after valve-in-valve (TAVR in SAVR) are generally superior to native valve TAVR because of the presence of a regular, rigid structure (degenerated bioprosthetic valve) upon which to expand the TAVR valve.

Valvuloplasty

> **Case Study 1**
>
> *An elderly patient presented with significant shortness of breath on mild exertion worsening in the last 6–8 months (NYHA 3) without syncope or pre syncope. The clinical examination revealed a systolic ejection murmur, loudest in the right parasternal region.*

Background and Definitions

Initial optimism for standalone balloon valvuloplasty for AS in the pre-TAVR era was tempered by recurrence of symptoms and restenosis with mortality rates equivalent to those in patients managed conservatively [113]. With the advent of TAVR there has been a resurgence of balloon valvuloplasty procedures with up to 40% of patients progressing from balloon valvuloplasty to TAVR [114].

Balloon valvuloplasty serves as a bridge to more definitive TAVR and SAVR in haemodynamically unstable patients and may be utilised in patients requiring urgent noncardiac surgery but have comorbid severe aortic stenosis [82, 113, 115]. Both the self-expandable valve (Evolut R generation) and balloon expandable valve (Sapien 3, Edwards Life Sciences) demonstrate similar outcomes with non-inferiority of the direct to TAVR procedures when compared to pre TAVR valvuloplasty [116]. It should be noted however that during direct to TAVR procedures, 5.8% of procedures had to be preceded by balloon valvuloplasty due to difficulty in traversing the aortic valve in the presence of severe valve calcification, small valve area and variant valve morphology e.g. bicuspid valves [116].

Balloon valvuloplasty may be used to determine the contribution of severe AS to the presence and severity of symptoms in a patient with multiple co morbidities with any co morbidity as a possible cause to symptoms [113, 114]. Patients with advanced co morbidities, low left ventricular systolic function, chronic obstructive pulmonary disease and significant frailty whom develop improved transvalvular gradient post balloon valvuloplasty are likely to demonstrate improvement in left ventricular function following TAVR [113].

Currently, balloon valvuloplasty is the preferred treatment option of young adults and children with congenital aortic stenosis in the absence of severe calcification [115]. Balloon valvuloplasty may also be utilised post THV deployment. Balloon dilation improves apposition of the prosthetic valve with the annular wall and generally increases the smallest diameter by 1.9 mm [113] subsequently enlarging the effective orifice area, minimising PVL and reducing the risk of PPM [113, 116]. Risk of annular rupture and post dilation requirements should be balanced when using a non-compliant balloon which should subsequently be at least 1 mm smaller than the average annular diameter obtained from pre procedural CT and the procedure continued depending on patients response [113, 116]. Complications associated with balloon post dilatation include annular rupture, stroke, left bundle branch block [116] and valve embolization [117]. Both TEE and fluoroscopy can identify valve infolding requiring post deployment valvuloplasty, which has been described with the Core valve and Evolut R [118, 119]. In valve in valve procedures, balloon valvuloplasty may improve the effective orifice area and transvalvular gradients by cracking the implanted surgical prosthetic valve [116].

Diagnoses and Preprocedural Assessment

Initial TTE revealed a moderately thickened trileaflet aortic valve with severely restricted cusp motion. The aortic valve area measured 0.8 cm² with a peak velocity of 4.2 m/s and a mean gradient of 43 mmHg with trivial valvular regurgitation. The left ventricular ejection fraction was 60%.

A pre prosthetic valve work up CT was performed. The patient has a tricuspid calcified aortic valve with an annular area of 413 mm², with moderate annular calcification and a mildly protruding nodule below the left coronary sinus. Risk for coronary obstruction was low and transfemoral was route chosen as the preferred access site (Fig. 37).

Cardiac catheterization demonstrated mild coronary artery disease with no revascularization requirements. The aortic valve and aortic root were moderately calcified. No significant coronary artery disease was present, but the patient had moderate pulmonary hypertension and borderline femoral dimensions for large sheaths at 6 mm in narrowest diameter (Fig. 38).

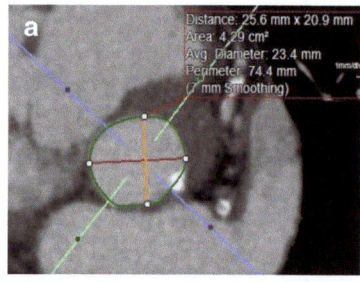 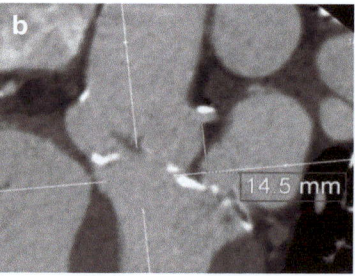 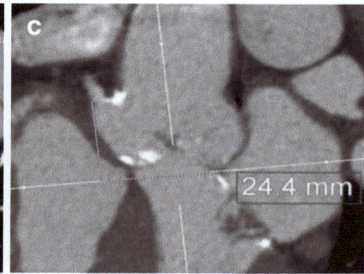

Fig. 37 (**a**) Annulus is drawn ensuring to be oblivious to calcium during measurement. Leaflets are moderately calcified with a protruding nodule below the left coronary cusp. Annulus area of 429 mm² and perimeter of 74.4 mm suggests use of a 23 mm S3 valve. (**b**) LM height of 14.5 mm. (**c**) RCA Height of 24.4 mm. Suggests low risk for coronary artery obstruction

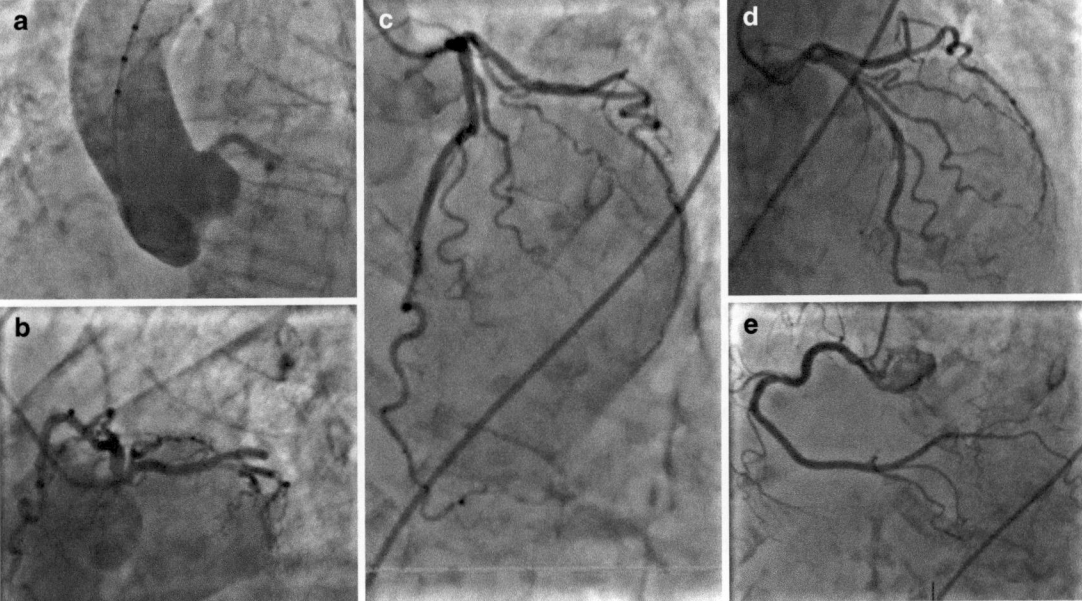

Fig. 38 Conventional cardiac catheterization via transfemoral access. (**a**) The aortic root is normal with mild calcification. (**b–d**) Left main coronary artery and (**e**) Right coronary artery demonstrated mild coronary artery disease

Differential Diagnosis

The patients' symptomatology followed by echocardiogram confirmed severe AS and concurrent pulmonary arterial hypertension. No exacerbating lung pathology or superimposed pneumonia was present. No clinical, biochemical or ECG features of heart failure or myocardial ischemia.

Heart Team Approach and Discussion

In view of her age and co morbidities in the setting of severe symptomatic AS trans catheter aortic valve replacement with a 23 mm Sapien valve was the treatment of choice.

Heart Team Decision

Indications for balloon valvuloplasty in relation to TAVR.

Balloon Valvuloplasty Prior to TAVR

Balloon valvuloplasty may be performed immediately prior to transcatheter valve placement to assist with the valve delivery system negotiating the annulus and valve orifice [113, 116]. Balloon valvuloplasty increases the aortic valve area ensuring a uniform and consistent shape of the orifice allowing for equable prosthetic expansion and reducing the risk of valve malposition and PVL [116]. Improved radial force and delivery system profiles of the later generation valves, institution expertise with direct TAVR and pre-procedural annular sizing with CT and/or TEE has limited the need for balloon valvuloplasty [120].

Annular Sizing

Intra procedural balloon sizing of the annulus provides complementary information when annular sizing by MDCT is not conclusive but rather borderline between two consecutive valve sizes [113, 121]. Condado et al. described similar rates of mild PVL, annular rupture, and acute kidney injury when annular sizing is done by CT or balloon valvuloplasty, however balloon valvuloplasty demonstrates a slightly higher (7% versus 5.7%) rate of moderate PVL [121]. Babilaros et al. described balloon valvuloplasty as an important, safe and efficient supplement to TEE sizing of the annulus with no coronary obstruction, THV embolization or annular damage and in 26% of patients an alternate THV was used based on balloon valvuloplasty findings [44]. Annular sizing is usually performed with rapid pacing, following injection of iodine contrast with opacification at the aortic root and simultaneous maximal insufflation of an appropriately sized balloon, consistent with pre procedural imaging derived annular dimensions [28]. Under sizing is described as the balloon not reaching the annular hinge points or if there is significant contrast leak around the balloon into the left ventricle [28]. There should be precautionary preparation for expedited TAVR placement post valvuloplasty in the event of acute aortic regurgitation with haemodynamic compromise [28].

Coronary Occlusion

Concurrent balloon valvuloplasty, inflated to a size similar to the predicted TAVR valve, and root aortography can help determine risk of coronary artery occlusion [113] by simulating leaflet displacement and position relative to the coronary ostia, as if the TAVR valve was utilised [28].

Crossing the Valve

Pre TAVR balloon valvuloplasty may assist in certain situations which predispose to difficulty in crossing the valve with the delivery device. Situations include highly calcified leaflets with high calcium scores and low AVA [116]. Echocardiographic findings for an unfavourable direct TAVR procedure include severe leaflet calcification, presence of calcification nodules, AVA less than 0.4 cm^2 and an irregular valve orifice [116].

Bicuspid Aortic Valve

Pre TAVR dilation occurs with balloon valvuloplasty in almost all patients with bicuspid aortic valves to minimise asymmetrical valve expansion and valve migration [116].

Contraindications to Balloon Valvuloplasty

Balloon valvuloplasty is contraindicated in the absence of severe AS [113] and in the presence of infective endocarditis [113, 115], moderate [115] to severe aortic valve regurgitation [113, 115], presence of LV thrombus [113], significant left main coronary artery stenosis [113], tumour [115], or life limiting non cardiac co morbidities [113, 115]. Furthermore, exclusive valvuloplasty in the presence of a mechanical or bioprosthetic valve can be complicated by prosthesis fragmentation [113]. Valvuloplasty in patients with reduced intravascular volumes and concentric LV hypertrophy may exhibit persistent hemodynamic instability [28]. Annular dimensions not compatible with balloon specifications, i.e. significantly smaller or significantly larger, and active bleeding preclude the use of intraprocedural heparin and are also a contraindication [113].

Intra and Post Procedural Assessment

Right femoral access was achieved as per protocol and pre deployment valvuloplasty was performed. (Fig. 39, Video 22). This was uneventful with no evidence of haemodynamic instability. The bio prosthesis was then advanced and deployed under rapid pacing at nominal volume with a good result. (Fig. 40).

Whilst still on the table, patient complained of nausea and ECG showed ST elevation. An urgent coronary angiogram was performed showing a filling defect in the left main, presumably thrombus, with slow flow in the LAD and circumflex arteries. A balloon was then inflated in the LAD and circumflex with no visualized thrombus flow was reestablished at the end of the procedure. The patient was transferred to the intensive care unit on dual antiplatelet therapy (Fig. 41).

A same day post procedural echo showed a well seated 23 mm Sapien 3 trans catheter heart valve with trivial valvular and mild paravalvular regurgitation. The peak velocity was measured at 1.8 m/s, the peak gradient was 13 mmHg, with a mean gradient of 7 mmHg and a VTI of 36 cm. A 3 × 10 mm mobile echogenic structure of unknown origin was visualized in the aortic root (Fig. 42, Video 23).

To further investigate the mobile echogenic structure in the aortic root, a CT scan was performed. CT showed a linear filling defect extend-

Transcatheter Aortic Valve Replacement

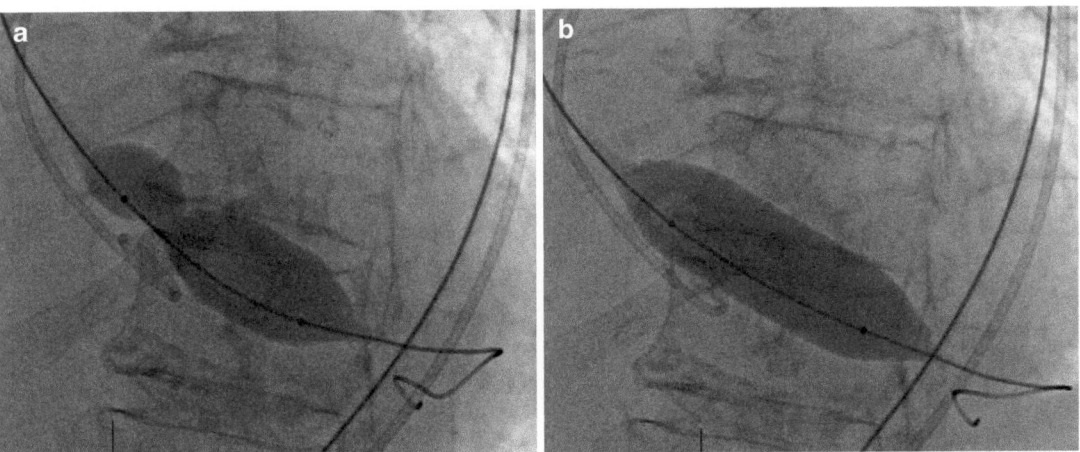

Fig. 39 Intra procedural, pre deployment valvuloplasty shows (**a**) Balloon waist at the site of the valve with (**b**) expansion of the balloon waist post successful valvuloplasty

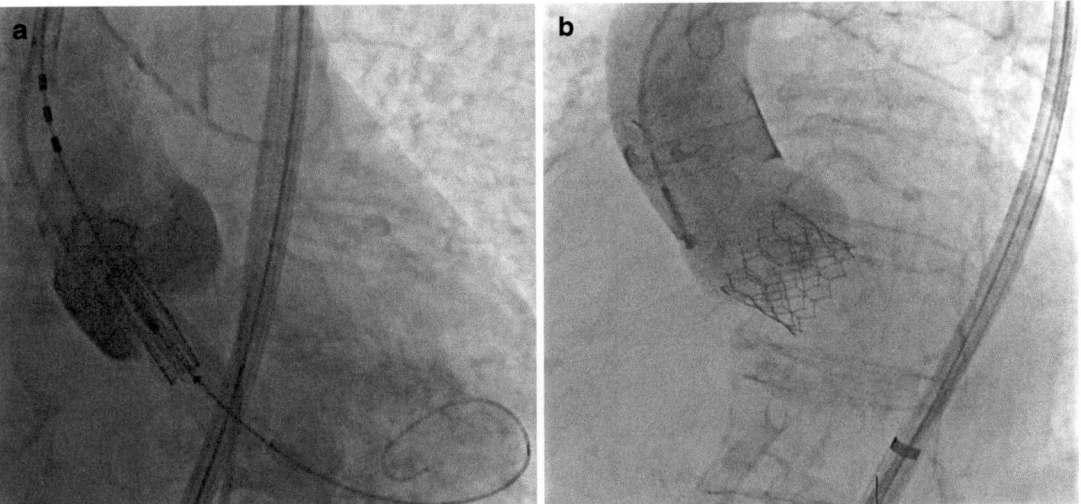

Fig. 40 Transfemoral catheterization of the aortic root. (**a**) Intraprocedural contrast injection with the THV advanced and (**b**) deployed under rapid pacing. Adequately positioned and expanded valve

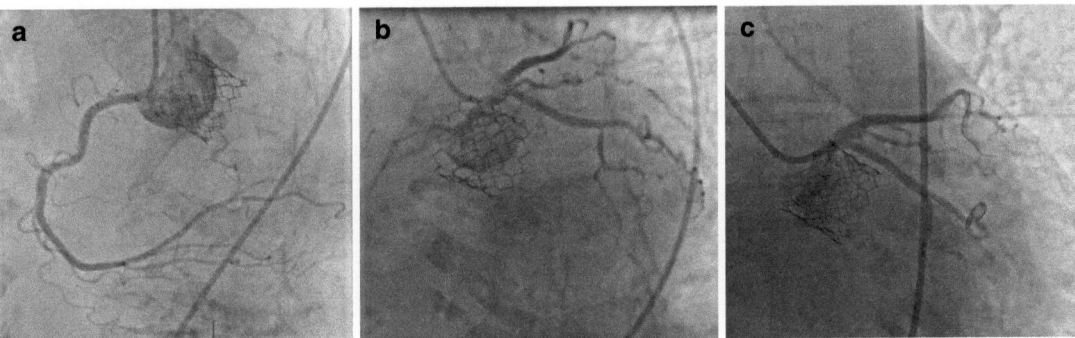

Fig. 41 Urgent on intra procedural conventional coronary angiogram. (**a**) Patent RCA. (**b**) Thrombus in the left main with slow flow in the LAD and circumflex arteries. A balloon was then inflated in the LAD and circumflex with no visualized thrombus. (**c**) Reestablished flow at the end of the procedure

ing from the non-coronary/left coronary commissure traversing through the sinus of Valsalva and into the left main coronary artery and LCX ostium (Fig. 43). There was at least a moderate degree of luminal narrowing of the left main with subtotal occlusion of the LCX ostium. The valve was well expanded with no hypo attenuating leaflet thickening (HALT) or leaflet thrombus (Fig. 44).

During an urgent coronary angiogram, a filling defect in the LM and LCX was appreciated.

PCI with DES's from the LM to CX and from the LM to LAD (simultaneous kissing stents) were deployed (Fig. 45).

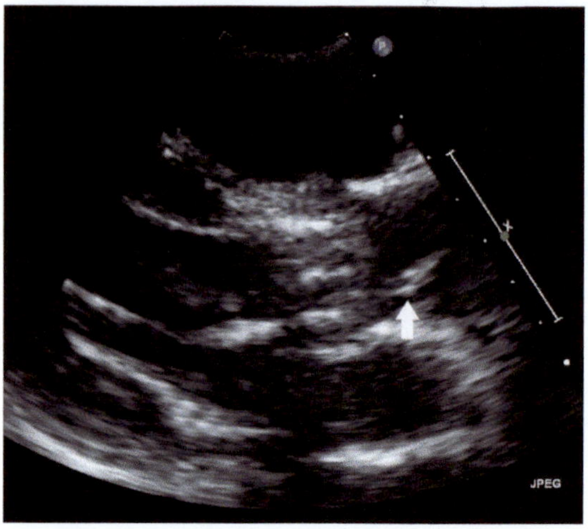

Complications Post Isolated BAV and Pre TAVR BAV

In this patient, a post balloon valvuloplasty (and TAVR) echocardiogram showed an echogenic mobile structure corresponding, on CT, to a filling defect in the aortic root extending into the left main coronary artery, with subtotal occlusion of the left circumflex artery. Possible considerations include focal dissection or a torn leaflet extending into the coronary ostium. Prior descriptions of coronary ostial occlusion by a perforated leaflet following balloon valvuloplasty have been described. The incidence is extremely low and with an unfavourable 30 day mortality rate of 41% [122]. Clinical features include hypotension with ECG and biochemical features of ischemia [122, 123], ventricular arrhythmias or cardiac

Fig. 42 Zoomed Long axis TTE with an echogenic flap distal to the THV outflow

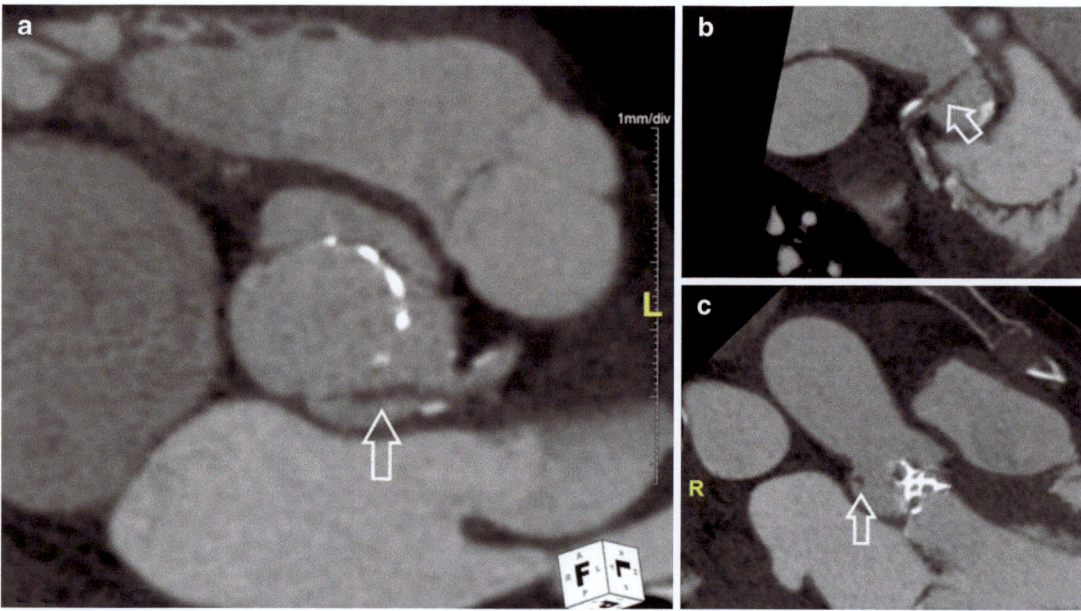

Fig. 43 (a–c) Linear filling defect (open arrow) (viewed in orthogonal planes centred on the filling defect) seen extending from the Sinuses of Valsalva into the left main coronary artery

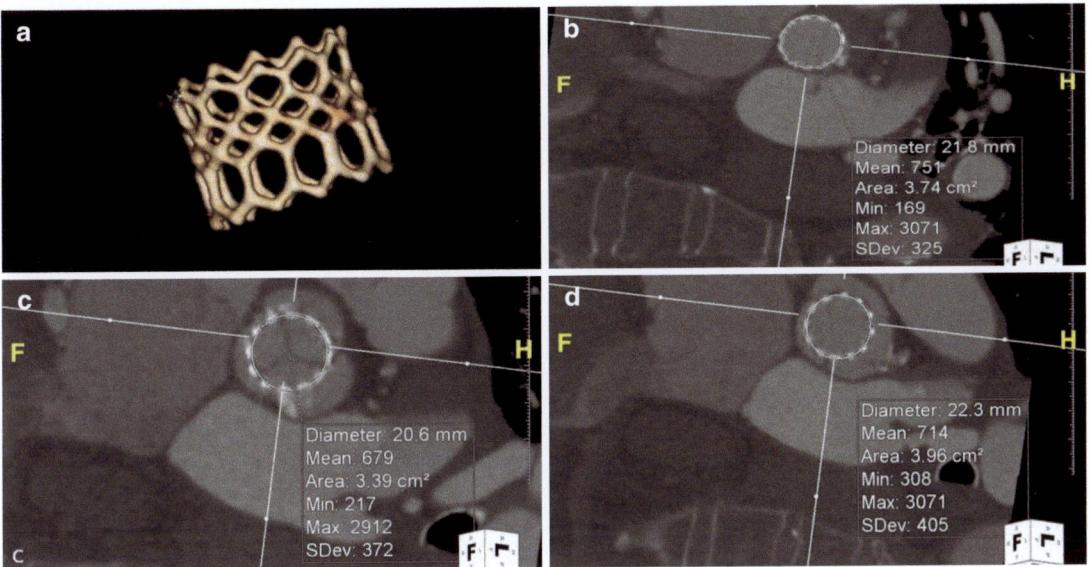

Fig. 44 (a) Sapien 3 ultra 23 mm valve with expansion measured at (b) inflow, (c) mid and (d) outflow demonstrating good valve expansion

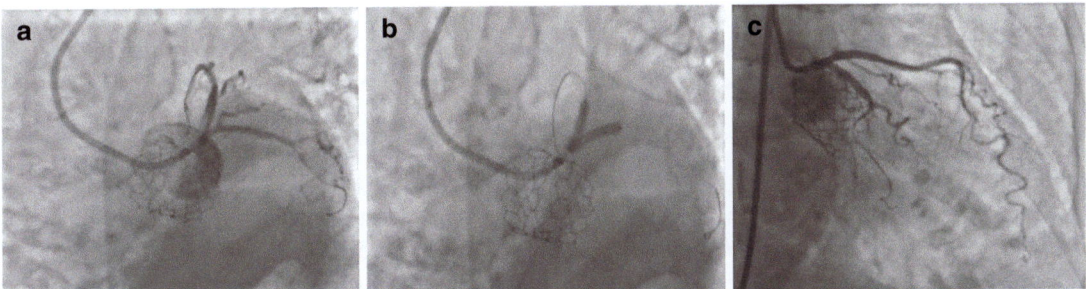

Fig. 45 Emergency post procedural coronary angiogram performed. (a) Shows a filling defect in the LM and LCX. (b) PCI with DES's from the LM to CX and from the LM to LAD (simultaneous kissing stents) were performed. (c) Flow was reestablished in the LM and LCX

arrest [123], and should be treated with emergency percutaneous intervention or bypass graft [122, 123]. Although uncommon, coronary ostial occlusion by an avulsed leaflet, aortic root dissection, mural haematoma or embolised leaflet material do occur [123, 124]. Common predictors of coronary artery occlusion risk during the TAVR procedure are a narrowed sinus of Valsalva in combination with a low lying coronary height and bulky leaflet calcification which are easily detectable on CT and MRI [123].

Other complications associated with balloon valvuloplasty include stroke, ventricular perforation, annular rupture [113–115], aortic regurgitation [114, 115], death [113, 114], dysrhythmias [113, 115], myocardial infarction, acute mitral regurgitation [113] and contrast allergies [115]. Haemodynamic instability may occur as a result of rapid pacing or severe aortic insufficiency following leaflet and commissural separation [116]. Severe aortic insufficiency occurred in 1–2% of patients when balloon valvuloplasty was used in isolation to treat AS, prior to the TAVR era [116]. Echocardiographic assessment of hemodynamic instability is directed at identifying AR, annular rupture and cardiac tamponade with aortofemoral angiograms accessing for the presence of contrast extravasation in aortofemoral injury [113]. Other potential complications include vascular and access site complications (pseudo aneurysm, dissection, vascular ischemia [113–115]) and access site haematomas and infection [115]. There are increased rates of new conduction disorders, often persistent following valvuloplasty [116]. Periprocedural stroke is thought to result from excessive native valve manipulation with rates of stroke at 30 days post procedure ranging from 2 to 4% [116]. There is no significant increase in stroke rates with pre procedural valvuloplasty however higher rates are described with balloon post dilation [116]. Contrasting evidence currently describes reduced PVL in patients with and without preprocedural balloon valvuloplasty, with one school of thought stating that patients who do not have pre TAVR balloon valvuloplasty have reduced PVL due to better prosthetic valve anchorage, and the other that patients with pre TAVR valvuloplasty have reduced PVL due to circular valve expansion and lower incidence of under expansion [116].

> **Case Study 2: VIV Valvuloplasty**
>
> *An elderly patient presented with productive cough, shortness of breath, orthopnea and effort intolerance (NYHA III) for 2 weeks. Prior history was significant for CABG and SAVR. On physical examination the patient had pitting sacral oedema and a non-radiating early systolic murmur at the left upper sternal border. Troponin: 0.04 ng/mL, ECG: atrial fibrillation without ischemic changes.*

Background and Definitions

Bioprosthetic valve fracture (BVF) and remodelling.

Bioprosthetic valve fracture is performed to reduce transvalvular gradients and increase the effective aortic valve area [103] reducing the risk of PPM and possible leaflet pin wheeling (which may result in premature leaflet degeneration of an under expanded THV) [125, 126]. Patient prosthetic mismatch, when defined as a post procedural gradient >20 mmHg, occurs more commonly after VIV TAVR and is due to under expansion of the TAVR valve which is limited by the true inner diameter of the failing surgical valve [125, 126]. Following VIV TAVR, 1 year mortality rates in patients with small (≤21 mm) valves was significantly higher at 25% when compared to intermediate (18%) and large (7%) surgical prosthetic valves with PPM hypothesised as a possible contributory factor [125, 126]. Bioprosthetic valve fracture entails fracturing the valve by insufflation of a non-compliant high pressure balloon, placed across the valve during rapid pacing [98]. Visual sudden expansion at the balloon waist with a reduction in inflation pressure and/or an audible click occurs with successful fracture [95]. On the other hand sudden reduction in pressure with deflation of the balloon is regarded as an unsuccessful fracture with balloon rupture [95].

The risk of annular injury as a consequence of the valve fracture procedure is low and explained by most SHV's positioned in a slight supra valvular location [125, 126]. In the setting of an intra annular implantation, SHV fracture should be avoided [125, 126].

BVF prior to TAVR deployment facilitates the use of a larger TAVR valve and limits potential injury to the new TAVR valve leaflets [98]. BVF post deployment has the advantage of a reduced risk of particulate embolization, greater valve expansion and limits the risk of haemodynamic compromise [98].

In patients with increasing gradients with initially normal valve haemodynamics, and no evidence of leaflet thrombosis, balloon valve fracture may also be performed within 1 year post VIV procedure [125, 126]. Most but not all SHV's are amenable to remodelling or fracture [125, 126].

Aortic surgical valves that can be fractured include the Magna (Edwards Lifesciences), Magna Ease (Edwards Lifesciences), Perimount 2800 (Edwards Lifesciences), Mitroflow (Sorin Group), Mosaic (Medtronic), and Biocor Epic (Abbott) [125, 126]. Surgical valves that can be remodelled or stretched, but not fractured, include Trifecta (Abbott), Carpentier-Edwards standard and supra-annular (Edwards Lifesciences), Inspiris (Edwards Lifesciences) and, Perimount 2700 (Edwards Lifesciences) [15, 27]. Surgical valves that cannot be fractured or remodelled include the Hancock II (Medtronic) and Avalus (Medtronic) surgical valves. Stentless and suture less valves can be remodelled but not fractured [92].

An achievable increase in internal valve diameters of up to 3–4 mm in 19–21 mm surgical valve has been demonstrated on in vitro testing with up to 6 mm increase in inner diameter with ≥ 27 mm valve [125, 126]. The size of balloon to be used should be determined by the true inner diameter of the SHV, anticipated increase in size of the valve, location of the coronary arteries (VTC) and anatomy of the aortic root [125, 126]. The aortic root and LVOT should be carefully accessed for calcification and although usually debrided [125, 126] if present the procedure should be avoided [98].

Procedural associated complications include THV damage and embolization, coronary artery obstruction, annular rupture, mitral valve injury [92, 125, 126], VSD [125, 126], hemodynamic instability, accelerated leaflet degeneration and leaflet tearing [92]. A new surgical valve (Inspiris Resilia, by Edwards Lifesciences) has inherent ability to expand during VIV TAVR thereby accommodating a larger TAVR valve [92].

Diagnoses and Preprocedural Assessment

Trans Thoracic Echocardiography
Surgical bio prosthesis in situ with moderate valvular regurgitation. Reversal of flow in the distal aortic arch during diastole with a mean transvalvular gradient of 15 mmHg, peak velocity of 2.7 m/s AVA, VTI 2.3 cm^2 and VTI indexed at 1.1 cm^2/m^2. The left ventricle is normal in size with normal systolic function. Concentric remodeling with septal flattening present. The aorta shows normal sinus of Valsalva (index at 16 mm/m^2; 33 mm). Ascending aorta measures 43 millimeters.

CT Planning for TAVR
The patient had a 27 mm Magna Ease with prosthetic leaflet thickening and the bio prosthesis appears canted (Figs. 46 and 47). Simulating a 26 mm THV the VTC was 10 mm at the LM and 4 mm at the RCA (Fig. 48) A STJ dimension of 35 × 35 mm and the surgical posts did not reach the STJ. The dimension at the sewing ring was 26 mm. There was mild calcification of the proximal dilated ascending aorta which measured 42 mm × 41 mm. There was horseshoe calcification in the right ilio femoral system however in the presence of a minimum diameter of 8 mm and lack of significant tortuosity access was deemed feasible. Left sided femoral access not feasible due to bulky severe calcification.

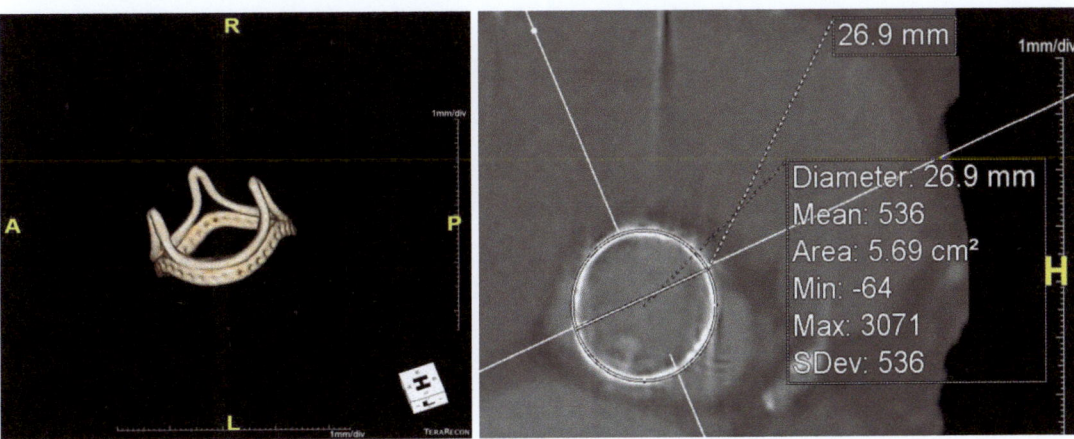

Fig. 46 27 mm Magna Ease visualised on preprocedural CT with the sewing ring diameter measuring 26.9 mm

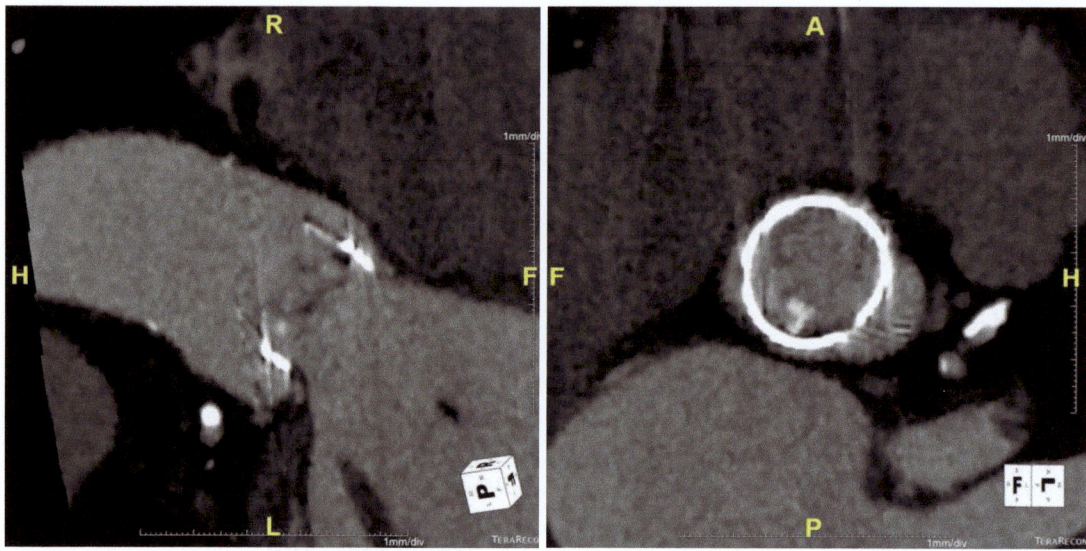

Fig. 47 Degenerative valve changes with leaflet calcification

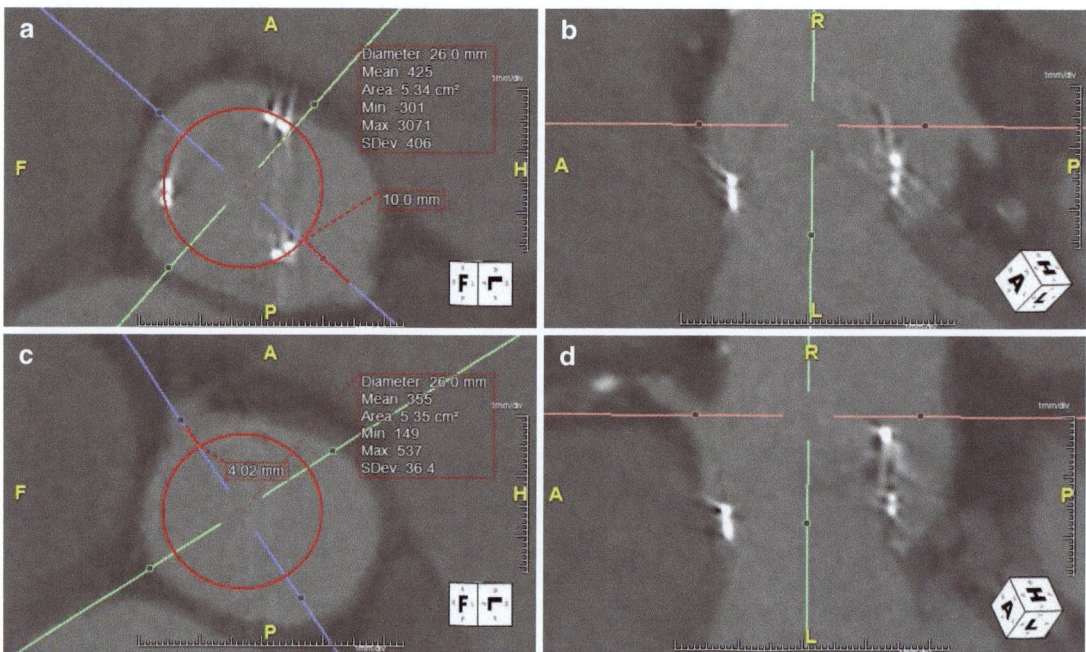

Fig. 48 Simulating a 26 mm THV (**a**) VTC was 10 mm at the left main coronary with the (**b**) stent post extending above the left main coronary ostium. (**c**) The VTC measures 4 mm at the RCA with the (**d**) stent post at the level of the right coronary artery

Differential Diagnosis

The patient's symptoms were attributed to heart failure with moderate aortic regurgitation. Myocardial ischemia was excluded with normal troponins and a non-ischemic ECG pattern. Pneumonia was excluded in the absence of pyrexia and normal inflammatory markers. There were no features or biochemical markers to suggest a pulmonary embolism. A possible prosthetic leaflet vegetation as the cause of AR was suspected on TEE however this was excluded on CT. The final diagnoses was a failed SAVR with clinical deterioration.

Heart Team Approach and Discussion

In view of the patient's acute clinical decline secondary to acute aortic insufficiency in a failed 27 mm Magna Ease a decision was made to replace the aortic valve. Considering his co morbidities and high surgical risk, percutaneous transcatheter heart valve in valve procedure with the possibility of balloon valvuloplasty was planned.

Intra and Post Procedural Assessment

Following routine right sided trans femoral access, the implanted surgical aortic valve was crossed with a J-wire then exchanged for an extra stiff wire. The prosthetic valve was then cracked with a 26 mm non-compliant balloon (Fig. 49) Immediately thereafter the patient became hypotensive due to leaflet tear and torrential AR. The Sapien 3 was rapidly advanced and deployed under rapid pacing with good results. Haemodynamic stability was restored, and the procedure continued and completed uneventfully.

Immediate post procedural trans thoracic echocardiogram demonstrated a well seated trans catheter aortic heart valve in surgical valve with a peak velocity of 2.5 m/s and a mean gradient 12 mmHg. There was no valvular or paravalvular regurgitation. No pericardial effusion was present and left ventricular function was normal without a shunt.

Thirty-day transthoracic echocardiogram demonstrated a well seated TAVR valve with a valve area of 1.5 cm^2, peak velocity of 2.6 m/s, VTI 1.5 cm^2 and a mean gradient of 12 mmHg. No valvular prosthesis regurgitation and trivial paravalvular regurgitation was present. LVEF was low normal at 52%.

Post procedure CT demonstrated an S3 in Magna Ease in good position and adequately expanded (Fig. 50) without coronary artery obstruction (Fig. 51).

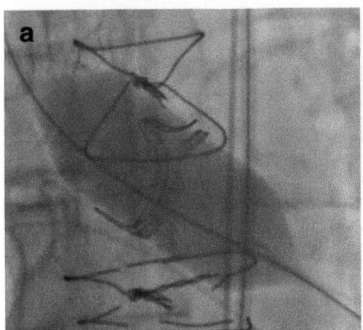 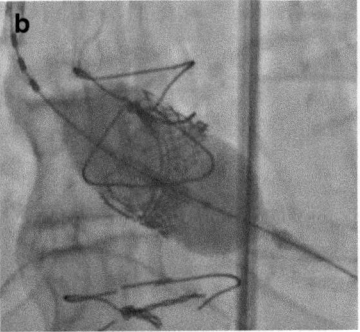 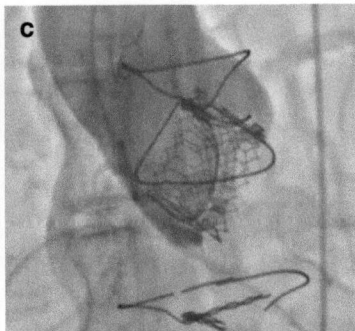

Fig. 49 Intra procedural fluoroscopy demonstrates (**a**) balloon dilatation to fracture surgical valve. (**b**) Deployment of TAVR (S3) into fractured SAVR. (**c**) Post TAVR deployment contrast injection suggests good position

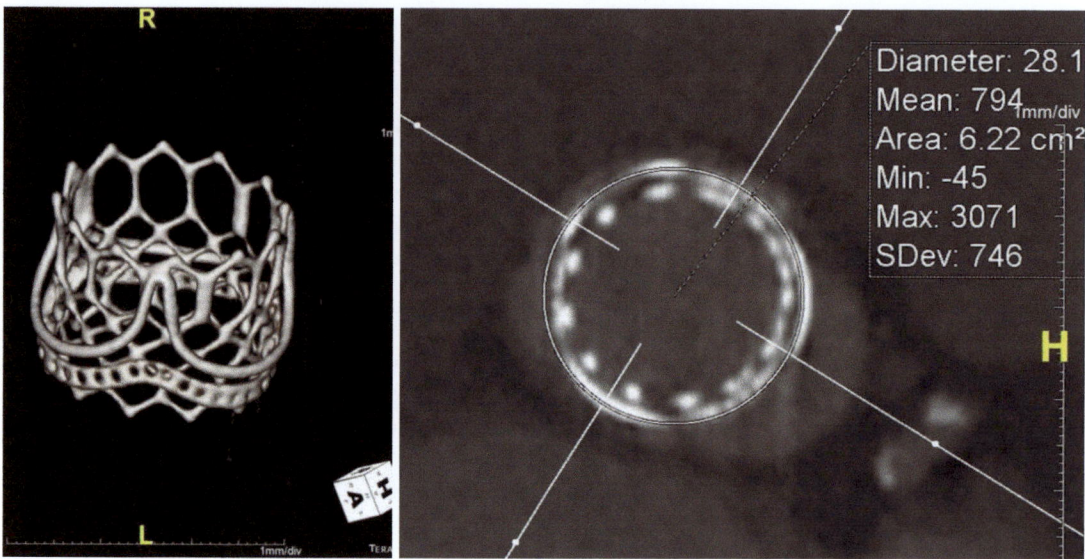

Fig. 50 Post procedure CT demonstrates an S3 in Magna in good position and adequately expanded

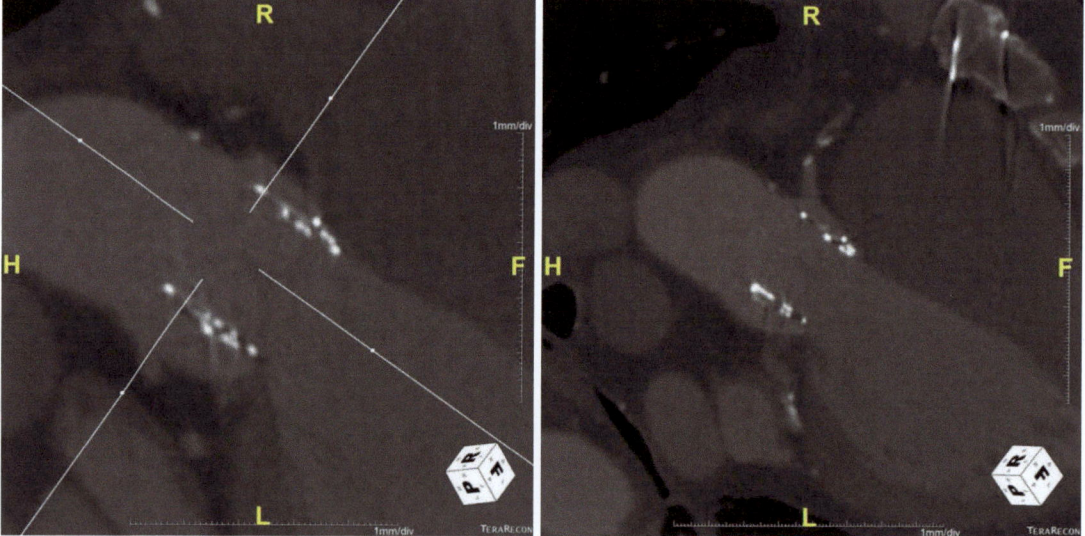

Fig. 51 Orthogonal views demonstrating good expansion and no coronary artery obstruction

Clinical Controversies and Pearls

- Pre-TAVR valvuloplasty may either increase the rate of PVL (due to reduced prosthetic valve anchorage) or reduce the rate of PVL due to more circular TAVR valve expansion and reduction of under-expansion.

Key Points
- Balloon valvuloplasty has been used more commonly following the advent of TAVR.
- Intraprocedural balloon sizing of the annulus provides complementary information when CT sizing of the annulus is borderline between two valve sizes.

- Balloon valvuloplasty inflated to a size similar to the predicted TAVR valve and aortography of the root can help determine risk of coronary artery occlusion.
- Although leaflet laceration during valvuloplasty is rare, mortality is high at 41%.

Chapter Review Questions

Aortic Stenosis

1. What are the factors to be considered and reported on during the pre-procedure TAVR to reduce the risk of coronary artery obstruction?
   A. Coronary ostial height
   B. Sinus of Valsalva diameter
   C. Leaflet heights
   D. Aortic root dimensions
   E. Choice of prosthetic valve
   F. All of the above **Answer: F**

   Explanation: A combination of coronary ostial height (concerning if less than 12 mm) and Sinus of Valsalva diameter (<30 mm predicts risk of coronary artery occlusion). Additional considerations include leaflet heights, aortic root dimensions and choice of prosthetic valve.

   Any accessory coronary artery and separate ostium of the any coronaries must be identified and assessed for risk of occlusion.

Bicuspid Aortic Valve

2. Which of the following complications are NOT more likely in TAVR of Bicuspid aortic valves?
   A. Malposition
   B. Paravalvular regurgitation
   C. Device migration/embolization
   D. Pacemaker requirements
   E. Peripheral vascular injury
   F. Annular rupture

Answer: E

Explanation: Ascending aortic dilatation and aortopathy is more common in patients with bicuspid aortic valves, however there is no higher risk for peripheral vascular injury in patients with bicuspid aortic valves.

Aortic Regurgitation

3. Which of the following is NOT a feature of severe AR on TTE?
   A. Ratio of regurgitant jet width to LVOT width $\geq 65\%$.
   B. Regurgitant volume >50 mL and regurgitant fraction $\geq 60\%$.
   C. Effective regurgitant orifice area ≥ 0.3 cm^2.
   D. A vena contracta >0.6 cm.
   E. All the above.
   F. None of the above **Answer: B**

   Explanation: Regurgitant volume >60 mL and regurgitant fraction $\geq 50\%$ are indicative of severe aortic regurgitation.

Valve in Valve

4. Which of the following statements about valve in valve procedures is INCORRECT?
   A. The incidence of coronary artery obstruction is higher for valve in valve compared to native aortic TAVR.
   B. When implanted into a stented bioprosthetic valve the THV displaces the leaflets of the degenerated bioprosthetic valve into an open position forming a covered cylinder.
   C. In stentless valves, the coronary ostial heights and Sinus of Valsalva dimensions are determined as per the native valve
   D. Obstruction occurs more commonly in stented valves compared to stentless valves. **Answer: D**

   Explanation: Obstruction occurs more commonly in stentless valves which are usually utilized in small aortic roots.

Valvuloplasty

5. Which of the following is not a contraindication to the aortic balloon valvuloplasty
   A. Presence of severe AS.
   B. Presence of infective endocarditis
   C. Presence of LV thrombus
   D. Presence of significant left main coronary artery stenosis
   E. None of the above

Answer: A

Explanation: Aortic balloon valvuloplasty is contraindicated in the absence of severe AS.

References

1. Carabello BA. Introduction to aortic stenosis. Circ Res. 2013;113(2):179–85.
2. Thaden JJ, Nkomo VT, Enriquez-Sarano M. The global burden of aortic stenosis. Prog Cardiovasc Dis. 2014;56(6):565–71.
3. Grimard BH, Safford RE, Burns EL, School MM. Aortic stenosis: diagnosis and treatment. Aortic Stenosis. 2016;93(5):8.
4. Otto CM, Nishimura RA, Bonow RO, Carabello BA, Erwin JP, Gentile F, et al. 2020 ACC/AHA guideline for the management of patients with valvular heart disease: a report of the American College of Cardiology/American Heart Association Joint Committee on Clinical Practice Guidelines. Circulation. 2021;143(5):e72–e227. https://doi.org/10.1161/CIR.0000000000000923.
5. Hahn RT, Nicoara A, Kapadia S, Svensson L, Martin R. Echocardiographic imaging for transcatheter aortic valve replacement. J Am Soc Echocardiogr. 2018;31(4):405–33.
6. Samad Z, Minter S, Armour A, Tinnemore A, Sivak JA, Sedberry B, et al. Implementing a continuous quality improvement program in a high-volume clinical echocardiography laboratory: improving care for patients with aortic stenosis. Circ Cardiovasc Imaging. 2016;9(3):e003708.
7. Silva I, Salaun E, Côté N, Pibarot P. Confirmation of aortic stenosis severity in Case of discordance between aortic valve area and gradient. JACC Case Rep. 2022;4(3):170–7.
8. Foley TR, Stinis CT. Imaging evaluation and interpretation for vascular access for transcatheter aortic valve replacement. Interv Cardiol Clin. 2018;7(3):285–91.
9. Abramowitz Y, Jilaihawi H, Pibarot P, Chakravarty T, Kashif M, Kazuno Y, et al. Severe aortic stenosis with low aortic valve calcification: characteristics and outcome following transcatheter aortic valve implantation. Eur Heart J Cardiovasc Imaging. 2017;18(6):639–47.
10. Pawade T, Sheth T, Guzzetti E, Dweck MR, Clavel MA. Why and how to measure aortic valve calcification in patients with aortic stenosis. JACC Cardiovasc Imaging. 2019;12(9):1835–48.
11. Perry TE, George SA, Lee B, Wahr J, Randle D, Sigurðsson G. A guide for pre-procedural imaging for transcatheter aortic valve replacement patients. Perioper Med. 2020;9(1):36.
12. Salgado RA, Leipsic JA, Shivalkar B, Ardies L, Van Herck PL, Op de Beeck BJ, et al. Preprocedural CT evaluation of transcatheter aortic valve replacement: what the radiologist needs to know. Radiographics. 2014;34(6):1491–514.
13. Toggweiler S, Leipsic J, Binder RK, Freeman M, Barbanti M, Heijmen RH, et al. Management of vascular access in transcatheter aortic valve replacement. JACC Cardiovasc Interv. 2013;6(7):643–53.
14. Tzolos E, Andrews JP, Dweck MR. Aortic valve stenosis—multimodality assessment with PET/CT and PET/MRI. Br J Radiol. 2020;93(1113):20190688.
15. Blanke P, Weir-McCall JR, Achenbach S, Delgado V, Hausleiter J, Jilaihawi H, et al. Computed tomography imaging in the context of transcatheter aortic valve implantation (TAVI)/transcatheter aortic valve replacement (TAVR). JACC Cardiovasc Imaging. 2019;12(1):1–24.
16. Suchá D, Tuncay V, Prakken NHJ, Leiner T, van Ooijen PMA, Oudkerk M, et al. Does the aortic annulus undergo conformational change throughout the cardiac cycle? A systematic review. Eur Heart J Cardiovasc Imaging. 2015:jev210.
17. Blanke P, Weir-McCall JR, Achenbach S, Delgado V, Hausleiter J, Jilaihawi H, et al. Computed tomography imaging in the context of transcatheter aortic valve implantation (TAVI)/transcatheter aortic valve replacement (TAVR): an expert consensus document of the Society of Cardiovascular Computed Tomography. J Cardiovasc Comput Tomogr. 2019;13(1):1–20.
18. Kulkarni JP, Jyoti, Paranjpe V. Topography, morphology and morphometry of coronary ostia—a cadaveric study. Eur J Anat. 2015;19:165–70.
19. Ishizu K, Murakami N, Morinaga T, Hayashi M, Isotani A, Arai Y, et al. Impact of tapered-shape left ventricular outflow tract on pacemaker rate after transcatheter aortic valve replacement. Heart Vessel. 2022;37(6):1055–65. https://doi.org/10.1007/s00380-021-01999-5.
20. Medranda GA, Musallam A, Zhang C, Rappaport H, Gallino PE, Case BC, et al. The impact of aortic angulation on contemporary transcatheter aortic valve replacement outcomes. JACC Cardiovasc Interv. 2021;14(11):1209–15.
21. Abramowitz Y, Maeno Y, Chakravarty T, Kazuno Y, Takahashi N, Kawamori H, et al. Aortic angulation attenuates procedural success following self-

22. Bob-Manuel T, Pour-Ghaz I, Sharma A, Chinta VR, Abader P, Paulus B, et al. Correlation between aortic angulation and outcomes of transcatheter aortic valve replacement with new-generation valves. Curr Probl Cardiol. 2021;46(2):100415.
23. Kerneis C, Pasi N, Arangalage D, Nguyen V, Mathieu T, Verdonk C, et al. Ascending aorta dilatation rates in patients with tricuspid and bicuspid aortic stenosis: the COFRASA/GENERAC study. Eur Heart J Cardiovasc Imaging. 2018;19(7):792–9.
24. Wilton E, Jahangiri M. Post-stenotic aortic dilatation. J Cardiothorac Surg. 2006;1:7. https://doi.org/10.1186/1749-8090-1-7.
25. Ochiai T, Yoon SH, Sharma R, Miyasaka M, Maeno Y, Raschpichler M, et al. Prevalence and prognostic impact of ascending aortic dilatation in patients undergoing TAVR. JACC Cardiovasc Imaging. 2020;13(1):175–7.
26. Díaz-Peláez E, Barreiro-Pérez M, Martín-García A, Sanchez PL. Measuring the aorta in the era of multimodality imaging: still to be agreed. J Thorac Dis. 2017;9(S6):S445–7.
27. Michail M, Ihdayhid AR, Comella A, Thakur U, Cameron JD, McCormick LM, et al. Feasibility and validity of computed tomography-derived fractional flow reserve in patients with severe aortic stenosis: the CAST-FFR study. Circ Cardiovasc Interv. 2021;14(1):e009586.
28. Otto CM, Kumbhani DJ, Alexander KP, Calhoon JH, Desai MY, Kaul S, et al. 2017 ACC expert consensus decision pathway for transcatheter aortic valve replacement in the management of adults with aortic stenosis. J Am Coll Cardiol. 2017;69(10):1313–46.
29. Harloff MT, Percy ED, Hirji SA, Yazdchi F, Shim H, Chowdhury M, et al. A step-by-step guide to trans-axillary transcatheter aortic valve replacement. Ann Cardiothorac Surg. 2020;9(6):510–21.
30. Fröhlich GM, Baxter PD, Malkin CJ, Scott DJA, Moat NE, Hildick-Smith D, et al. Comparative survival after transapical, direct aortic, and subclavian Transcatheter aortic valve implantation (data from the UK TAVI registry). Am J Cardiol. 2015;116(10):1555–9.
31. Litmanovich DE, Ghersin E, Burke DA, Popma J, Shahrzad M, Bankier AA. Imaging in Transcatheter aortic valve replacement (TAVR): role of the radiologist. Insights Imaging. 2014;5(1):123–45.
32. Mayr A, Klug G, Reinstadler SJ, Feistritzer HJ, Reindl M, Kremser C, et al. Is MRI equivalent to CT in the guidance of TAVR? A pilot study. Eur Radiol. 2018;28(11):4625–34.
33. Kallianos K, Henry TS, Yeghiazarians Y, Zimmet J, Shunk KA, Tseng EE, et al. Ferumoxytol MRA for transcatheter aortic valve replacement planning with renal insufficiency. Int J Cardiol. 2017;231:255–7.
34. Pamminger M, Klug G, Kranewitter C, Reindl M, Reinstadler SJ, Henninger B, et al. Non-contrast MRI protocol for TAVI guidance: quiescent-interval single-shot angiography in comparison with contrast-enhanced CT. Eur Radiol. 2020;30(9):4847–56.
35. Zamorano JL, Goncalves A, Lang R. Imaging to select and guide transcatheter aortic valve implantation. Eur Heart J. 2014;35(24):1578–87.
36. Abdel-Wahab M, Mehilli J, Frerker C, Neumann FJ, Kurz T, Tölg R, et al. Comparison of balloon-expandable vs self-expandable valves in patients undergoing transcatheter aortic valve replacement: the CHOICE randomized clinical trial. JAMA. 2014;311(15):1503–14.
37. Binder RK, Rodés-Cabau J, Wood DA, Mok M, Leipsic J, De Larochellière R, et al. Transcatheter aortic valve replacement with the SAPIEN 3. JACC Cardiovasc Interv. 2013;6(3):293–300.
38. Nijhoff F, Abawi M, Agostoni P, Ramjankhan FZ, Doevendans PA, Stella PR. Transcatheter aortic valve implantation with the new balloon-expandable Sapien 3 versus Sapien XT valve system: a propensity score–matched single-center comparison. Circ Cardiovasc Interv. 2015;8(6):e002408. https://doi.org/10.1161/CIRCINTERVENTIONS.115.002408.
39. Todaro D, Picci A, Barbanti M. Technical characteristics and evidence to date for FDA- and CE mark-approved valves. Cardiac Interv Today. 2017;11(2):53–8.
40. Ali N, Blackman DJ. TAVI: which valve for which patient? Cardiac Interv Today. 2019;13(2):72–8.
41. Kotronias RA, Bray JJH, Rajasundaram S, Vincent F, Delhaye C, Scarsini R, et al. Ultrasound- versus fluoroscopy-guided strategy for transfemoral transcatheter aortic valve replacement access: a systematic review and meta-analysis. Circ Cardiovasc Interv. 2021;14(10):e010742. https://doi.org/10.1161/CIRCINTERVENTIONS.121.010742.
42. Essa E, Makki N, Bittenbender P, Capers Q 4th, George B, Rushing G, Crestanello J, Boudoulas KD, Lilly SM. Vascular assessment for transcatheter aortic valve replacement: intravascular ultrasound compared with computed tomography. J Invasive Cardiol. 2016;28(12):E172–8.
43. Hussain MA, Nabi F. Complex structural interventions: the role of computed tomography, fluoroscopy, and fusion imaging. Methodist Debakey Cardiovasc J. 2017;13(3):98–105.
44. Babaliaros VC, Junagadhwalla Z, Lerakis S, Thourani V, Liff D, Chen E, et al. Use of balloon aortic valvuloplasty to size the aortic annulus before implantation of a balloon-expandable transcatheter heart valve. JACC Cardiovasc Interv. 2010;3(1):114–8.
45. Kasel AM, Cassese S, Leber AW, von Scheidt W, Kastrati A. Fluoroscopy-guided aortic root imaging for TAVR. JACC Cardiovasc Imaging. 2013;6(2):274–5.
46. Tang GHL, Zaid S, Michev I, Ahmad H, Kaple R, Undemir C, et al. "Cusp-overlap" view simplifies fluoroscopy-guided implantation of self-expanding valve in transcatheter aortic valve replacement. JACC Cardiovasc Interv. 2018;11(16):1663–5.

47. Corrigan FE, Gleason PT, Condado JF, Lisko JC, Chen JH, Kamioka N, et al. Imaging for predicting, detecting, and managing complications after Transcatheter aortic valve replacement. JACC Cardiovasc Imaging. 2019;12(5):904–20.
48. Hahn RT, Little SH, Monaghan MJ, Kodali SK, Williams M, Leon MB, et al. Recommendations for comprehensive intraprocedural echocardiographic imaging during TAVR. JACC Cardiovasc Imaging. 2015;8(3):261–87.
49. Hahn RT, Kodali S, Tuzcu EM, Leon MB, Kapadia S, Gopal D, et al. Echocardiographic imaging of procedural complications during balloon-expandable transcatheter aortic valve replacement. JACC Cardiovasc Imaging. 2015;8(3):288–318.
50. Pibarot P, Hahn RT, Weissman NJ, Arsenault M, Beaudoin J, Bernier M, et al. Association of Paravalvular Regurgitation with 1-year outcomes after Transcatheter aortic valve replacement with the SAPIEN 3 valve. JAMA Cardiol. 2017;2(11):1208–16.
51. Herrmann HC, Daneshvar SA, Fonarow GC, Stebbins A, Vemulapalli S, Desai ND, et al. Prosthesis–patient mismatch in patients undergoing transcatheter aortic valve replacement. J Am Coll Cardiol. 2018;72(22):2701–11.
52. Daneault B, Koss E, Hahn RT, Kodali S, Williams MR, Généreux P, et al. Efficacy and safety of postdilatation to reduce paravalvular regurgitation during balloon-expandable transcatheter aortic valve replacement. Circ Cardiovasc Interv. 2013;6(1):85–91.
53. Bhushan S, Huang X, Li Y, He S, Mao L, Hong W, et al. Paravalvular leak after transcatheter aortic valve implantation its incidence, diagnosis, clinical implications, prevention, management, and future perspectives: a review article. Curr Probl Cardiol. 2021;2021:100957.
54. Ribeiro HB, Orwat S, Hayek SS, Larose É, Babaliaros V, Dahou A, et al. Cardiovascular magnetic resonance to evaluate aortic regurgitation after transcatheter aortic valve replacement. J Am Coll Cardiol. 2016;68(6):577–85.
55. DeAnda A, Jneid H. Putting a HALT to HALT: does anticoagulation matter? J Am Heart Assoc. 2022;11(23):e028275.
56. Garcia S, Fukui M, Dworak MW, Okeson BK, Garberich R, Hashimoto G, et al. Clinical impact of hypoattenuating leaflet thickening after transcatheter aortic valve replacement. Circ Cardiovasc Interv. 2022;15(3):e011480. https://doi.org/10.1161/CIRCINTERVENTIONS.121.011480.
57. Jilaihawi H, Asch FM, Manasse E, Ruiz CE, Jelnin V, Kashif M, et al. Systematic CT methodology for the evaluation of subclinical leaflet thrombosis. JACC Cardiovasc Imaging. 2017;10(4):461–70.
58. Martín M, Cuevas J, Cigarrán H, Calvo J, Morís C. Transcatheter aortic valve implantation and subclinical and clinical leaflet thrombosis: multimodality imaging for diagnosis and risk stratification. Eur Cardiol Rev. 2021;16:e35.
59. Vollema EM, Kong WKF, Katsanos S, Kamperidis V, van Rosendael PJ, van der Kley F, et al. Transcatheter aortic valve thrombosis: the relation between hypo-attenuated leaflet thickening, abnormal valve haemodynamics, and stroke. Eur Heart J. 2017;38(16):1207–17.
60. Testa L, Latib A. Assessing the risk of leaflet motion abnormality following transcatheter aortic valve implantation. Interv Cardiol Rev. 2017;13(1):1.
61. Leetmaa T, Hansson NC, Leipsic J, Jensen K, Poulsen SH, Andersen HR, et al. Early aortic transcatheter heart valve thrombosis: diagnostic value of contrast-enhanced multidetector computed tomography. Circ Cardiovasc Interv. 2015;8(4):e001596. https://doi.org/10.1161/CIRCINTERVENTIONS.114.001596.
62. Pislaru SV, Nkomo VT, Sandhu GS. Assessment of prosthetic valve function after TAVR. JACC Cardiovasc Imaging. 2016;9(2):193–206.
63. Pibarot P, Magne J, Leipsic J, Côté N, Blanke P, Thourani VH, et al. Imaging for predicting and assessing prosthesis-patient mismatch after aortic valve replacement. JACC Cardiovasc Imaging. 2019;12(1):149–62.
64. Tchetche D, de Biase C, van Gils L, Parma R, Ochala A, Lefevre T, et al. Bicuspid aortic valve anatomy and relationship with devices: the BAVARD multicenter registry: a European picture of contemporary multidetector computed tomography sizing for bicuspid valves. Circ Cardiovasc Interv. 2019;12(1):e007107.
65. Frangieh AH, Kasel AM. TAVI in bicuspid aortic valves 'made easy'. Eur Heart J. 2017;38(16):1177–81.
66. Jilaihawi H, Chen M, Webb J, Himbert D, Ruiz CE, Rodés-Cabau J, et al. A bicuspid aortic valve imaging classification for the TAVR era. JACC Cardiovasc Imaging. 2016;9(10):1145–58.
67. Rahim H, Wolbinski M, Bapat V, Nazif TM. TAVR for bicuspid aortic valve disease. Cardiac Interv Today. 2020;14(2):41–5.
68. Hayashida K, Bouvier E, Lefèvre T, Hovasse T, Morice MC, Chevalier B, et al. Potential mechanism of annulus rupture during transcatheter aortic valve implantation: annulus rupture in TAVI. Catheter Cardiovasc Interv. 2013;82(5):E742–6.
69. Blackman D, Gabbieri D, Del Blanco BG, Kempfert J, Laine M, Mascherbauer J, et al. Expert consensus on sizing and positioning of SAPIEN 3/ultra in bicuspid aortic valves. Cardiol Ther. 2021;10(2):277–88.
70. Tchétché D. TAVI in bicuspid aortic valves. Cardiac Interv Today. 2019;13(2):70–1.
71. Williams MR, Jilaihawi H, Makkar R, O'Neill WW, Guyton R, Malaisrie SC, et al. The PARTNER 3 bicuspid registry for transcatheter aortic valve replacement in low-surgical-risk patients. JACC Cardiovasc Interv. 2022;15(5):523–32.
72. Forrest JK, Kaple RK, Ramlawi B, Gleason TG, Meduri CU, Yakubov SJ, et al. Transcatheter aortic valve replacement in bicuspid versus tricuspid aortic valves from the STS/ACC TVT registry. JACC Cardiovasc Interv. 2020;13(15):1749–59.

73. Vincent F, Ternacle J, Denimal T, Shen M, Redfors B, Delhaye C, et al. Transcatheter aortic valve replacement in bicuspid aortic valve stenosis. Circulation. 2021;143(10):1043–61.
74. Yoon SH, Kim WK, Dhoble A, Milhorini Pio S, Babaliaros V, Jilaihawi H, et al. Bicuspid aortic valve morphology and outcomes after transcatheter aortic valve replacement. J Am Coll Cardiol. 2020;76(9):1018–30.
75. Perlman GY, Blanke P, Webb JG. Transcatheter aortic valve implantation in bicuspid aortic valve stenosis. EuroIntervention. 2016;12:Y42–5.
76. Mas-Peiro S, Fichtlscherer S, Walther C, Vasa-Nicotera M. Current issues in transcatheter aortic valve replacement. J Thorac Dis. 2020;12(4):1665–80.
77. Alexis SL, Sengupta A, Tang GHL. TAVR in aortic insufficiency. Cardiac Interv Today. 2020;14(2):35–9.
78. Praz F, Windecker S, Huber C, Carrel T, Wenaweser P. Expanding indications of transcatheter heart valve interventions. JACC Cardiovasc Interv. 2015;8(14):1777–96.
79. Inglessis-Azuaje I. Transcatheter aortic valve replacement for pure aortic insufficiency. JACC Case Rep. 2021;3(4):650–2.
80. Huded CP, Allen KB, Chhatriwalla AK. Counterpoint: challenges and limitations of transcatheter aortic valve implantation for aortic regurgitation. Heart. 2021;107(24):1942–5.
81. Franzone A, Piccolo R, Siontis GCM, Lanz J, Stortecky S, Praz F, et al. Transcatheter aortic valve replacement for the treatment of pure native aortic valve regurgitation. JACC Cardiovasc Interv. 2016;9(22):2308–17.
82. Vahanian A, Beyersdorf F, Praz F, Milojevic M, Baldus S, Bauersachs J, et al. 2021 ESC/EACTS guidelines for the management of valvular heart disease. Eur Heart J. 2022;43(7):561–632.
83. Everett RJ, Newby DE, Jabbour A, Fayad ZA, Dweck MR. The role of imaging in aortic valve disease. Curr Cardiovasc Imaging Rep. 2016;9(7):21.
84. Zoghbi WA, Adams D, Bonow RO, Enriquez-Sarano M, Foster E, Grayburn PA, et al. Recommendations for noninvasive evaluation of native valvular regurgitation. J Am Soc Echocardiogr. 2017;30(4):303–71.
85. Jassal DS, Shapiro MD, Neilan TG, Chaithiraphan V, Ferencik M, Teague SD, et al. 64-slice multidetector computed tomography (MDCT) for detection of aortic regurgitation and quantification of severity. Investig Radiol. 2007;42(7):507–12.
86. Webb JG, Sathananthan J. Transcatheter aortic valve replacement for pure noncalcific aortic regurgitation is coming, but not yet primetime. JACC Cardiovasc Interv. 2016;9(22):2318–9.
87. Seiffert M, Bader R, Kappert U, Rastan A, Krapf S, Bleiziffer S, et al. Initial German experience with transapical implantation of a second-generation transcatheter heart valve for the treatment of aortic regurgitation. JACC Cardiovasc Interv. 2014;7(10):1168–74.
88. Orzalkiewicz M, Bruno AG, Taglieri N, Ghetti G, Marrozzini C, Galiè N, et al. Transcatheter aortic valve replacement for pure aortic regurgitation in a large and noncalcified annulus. JACC Cardiovasc Interv. 2021;14(19):e271–3.
89. Biasco L, Ferrari E, Pedrazzini G, Faletra F, Moccetti T, Petracca F, et al. Access sites for TAVI: patient selection criteria, technical aspects, and outcomes. Front Cardiovasc Med. 2018;5:88.
90. Raptis DA, Beal MA, Kraft DC, Maniar HS, Bierhals AJ. Transcatheter aortic valve replacement: alternative access beyond the femoral arterial approach. Radiographics. 2019;39(1):30–43.
91. Roy DA, Schaefer U, Guetta V, Hildick-Smith D, Möllmann H, Dumonteil N, et al. Transcatheter aortic valve implantation for pure severe native aortic valve regurgitation. J Am Coll Cardiol. 2013;61(15):1577–84.
92. Annibali G, Scrocca I, Musumeci G. Valve-in-valve transcatheter aortic valve replacement: the challenge of the next future. Mini-Invasive Surg. 2022;6:12. https://misjournal.net/article/view/4635.
93. Deharo P, Bisson A, Herbert J, Lacour T, Etienne CS, Porto A, et al. Transcatheter valve-in-valve aortic valve replacement as an alternative to surgical re-replacement. J Am Coll Cardiol. 2020;76(5):489–99.
94. Tam DY, Dharma C, Rocha RV, Ouzounian M, Wijeysundera HC, Austin PC, et al. Transcatheter ViV versus redo surgical AVR for the management of failed biological prosthesis. JACC Cardiovasc Interv. 2020;13(6):765–74.
95. Salem SA, Foerst JR. Valve-in-valve transcatheter aortic valve replacement, with present-day innovations and up-to-date techniques. Interv Cardiol Clin. 2021;10(4):491–504.
96. Hamid NB, Khalique OK, Monaghan MJ, Kodali SK, Dvir D, Bapat VN, et al. Transcatheter valve implantation in failed surgically inserted bioprosthesis. JACC Cardiovasc Imaging. 2015;8(8):960–79.
97. Kostyunin AE, Yuzhalin AE, Rezvova MA, Ovcharenko EA, Glushkova TV, Kutikhin AG. Degeneration of bioprosthetic heart valves: update 2020. J Am Heart Assoc. 2020;9(19):e018506.
98. Edelman JJ, Khan JM, Rogers T, Shults C, Satler LF, Ben-Dor II, et al. Valve-in-valve TAVR: state-of-the-art review. Innov Technol Tech Cardiothorac Vasc Surg. 2019;14(4):299–310.
99. Lederman RJ, Babaliaros VC, Rogers T, Khan JM, Kamioka N, Dvir D, et al. Preventing coronary obstruction during transcatheter aortic valve replacement. JACC Cardiovasc Interv. 2019;12(13):1197–216.
100. Bapat V. Technical pitfalls and tips for the valve-in-valve procedure. Ann Cardiothorac Surg. 2017;6(5):541–52.
101. Bernardi FLM, Dvir D, Rodes-Cabau J, Ribeiro HB. Valve-in-valve challenges: how to avoid coronary obstruction. Front Cardiovasc Med. 2019;6:120.
102. Khan JM, Greenbaum AB, Babaliaros VC, Dvir D, Reisman M, McCabe JM, et al. BASILICA trial: one-year outcomes of transcatheter electrosurgical

leaflet laceration to prevent TAVR coronary obstruction. Circ Cardiovasc Interv. 2021;14(5):e010238.
103. Hamandi M, Nwafor I, Hebeler KR, Crawford A, Lanfear AT, Schaffer J, et al. Bioprosthetic valve fracture during valve-in-valve transcatheter aortic valve replacement. Bayl Univ Med Cent Proc. 2020;33(3):317–21.
104. Reul RM, Ramchandani MK, Reardon MJ. Transcatheter aortic valve-in-valve procedure in patients with bioprosthetic structural valve deterioration. Methodist Debakey Cardiovasc J. 2017;13(3):132–41.
105. Dvir D, Leipsic J, Blanke P, Ribeiro HB, Kornowski R, Pichard A, et al. Coronary obstruction in transcatheter aortic valve-in-valve implantation: preprocedural evaluation, device selection, protection, and treatment. Circ Cardiovasc Interv. 2015;8(1):e002079.
106. Edelman JJ, Khan JM. BASILICA to prevent coronary obstruction in transcatheter aortic valve replacement. Ann Cardiothorac Surg. 2020;9(6):508–9.
107. Protsyk V, Meineri M, Kitamura M, Flo Forner A, Holzhey D, Thiele H, et al. Echocardiographic guidance of intentional leaflet laceration prior to transcatheter aortic valve replacement: a structured approach to the bioprosthetic or native aortic scallop intentional laceration to prevent iatrogenic coronary artery obstruction procedure. J Am Soc Echocardiogr. 2021;34(6):676–89.
108. Komatsu I, Leipsic J, Webb JG, Blanke P, Mackensen GB, Don CW, et al. Coronary ostial eccentricity in severe aortic stenosis: guidance for BASILICA transcatheter leaflet laceration. J Cardiovasc Comput Tomogr. 2020;14(6):516–9.
109. Greenbaum AB, Kamioka N, Vavalle JP, Lisko JC, Gleason PT, Paone G, et al. Balloon-assisted BASILICA to facilitate redo TAVR. JACC Cardiovasc Interv. 2021;14(5):578–80.
110. Ramanathan PK, Nazir S, Elzanaty AM, Nesheiwat Z, Mahmood M, Rachwal W, et al. Novel method for implantation of balloon expandable transcatheter aortic valve replacement to reduce pacemaker rate—line of Lucency method. Struct Heart. 2020;4(5):427–32.
111. Khodaee F, Barakat M, Abbasi M, Dvir D, Azadani AN. Incomplete expansion of transcatheter aortic valves is associated with propensity for valve thrombosis. Interact Cardiovasc Thorac Surg. 2020;30(1):39–46.
112. Alperi A, Rodés-Cabau J, Simonato M, Tchetche D, Charbonnier G, Ribeiro HB, et al. Permanent pacemaker implantation following valve-in-valve Transcatheter aortic valve replacement. J Am Coll Cardiol. 2021;77(18):2263–73.
113. Keeble TR, Khokhar A, Akhtar MM, Mathur A, Weerackody R, Kennon S. Percutaneous balloon aortic valvuloplasty in the era of transcatheter aortic valve implantation: a narrative review. Open Heart. 2016;3(2):e000421.
114. Kawsara A, Alqahtani F, Eleid MF, El-Sabbagh A, Alkhouli M. Balloon aortic valvuloplasty as a bridge to aortic valve replacement. JACC Cardiovasc Interv. 2020;13(5):583–91.
115. Bykowski A, Perez OA, Kanmanthareddy A. Balloon valvuloplasty. In: StatPearls. StatPearls Publishing; 2021. https://www.ncbi.nlm.nih.gov/books/NBK519532/.
116. McInerney A, Vera-Urquiza R, Tirado-Conte G, Marroquin L, Jimenez-Quevedo P, Nuñez-Gil I, et al. Pre-dilation and post-dilation in Transcatheter aortic valve replacement: indications, benefits and risks. Interv Cardiol Rev Res Resour. 2021;16:e28.
117. Kim WK, Schäfer U, Tchetche D, Nef H, Arnold M, Avanzas P, et al. Incidence and outcome of periprocedural transcatheter heart valve embolization and migration: the TRAVEL registry (TranscatheteR HeArt valve EmboLization and Migration). Eur Heart J. 2019;40(38):3156–65.
118. Kataoka A, Watanabe Y, Nagura F, Okabe R, Kawashima H, Nakashima M, et al. Balloon valvuloplasty for Evolut R Infolding. JACC Cardiovasc Interv. 2018;11(17):e135–6.
119. Kaple RK, Salemi A, Wong SC. Balloon valvuloplasty treatment of an infolded CoreValve: balloon valvuloplasty of an Infolded CoreValve. Catheter Cardiovasc Interv. 2017;89(3):499–501.
120. Boe BA, Zampi JD, Kennedy KF, Jayaram N, Porras D, Foerster SR, et al. Acute success of balloon aortic valvuloplasty in the current era. JACC Cardiovasc Interv. 2017;10(17):1717–26.
121. Condado JF, Stewart J, Jensen HA, Lerakis S, Ko SM, Stillman A, et al. TCT-654 balloon vs computed tomography sizing of the aortic annulus for transcatheter aortic valve replacement. J Am Coll Cardiol. 2015;66(15):B267–8.
122. Parekh A, Sengupta V, Hunyadi V, Ianitelli M, Zainea M. Aortic valve leaflet rupture causing delayed left main coronary ostial obstruction during valvuloplasty preceding TAVR. JACC Case Rep. 2021;3(17):1822–7.
123. Spina R, Khalique O, George I, Nazif T. Acute left main stem coronary occlusion following transcatheter aortic valve replacement in a patient without recognized coronary obstruction risk factors: a case report. Eur Heart J Case Rep. 2018;2(4):yty112. https://doi.org/10.1093/ehjcr/yty112/5144004.
124. Gitto M, Leone PP, Regazzoli D, Gasparini G, Pagnotta P, Stefanini GG, et al. Left anterior descending coronary artery occlusion after balloon aortic valvuloplasty. Cardiovasc Revasc Med. 2022;40S:126–9.
125. Allen KB, Chhatriwalla AK, Saxon JT, Huded CP, Sathananthan J, Nguyen TC, et al. Bioprosthetic valve fracture: a practical guide. Ann Cardiothorac Surg. 2021;10(5):564–70.
126. Zoghbi WA, Chambers JB, Dumesnil JG, Foster E, Gottdiener JS, Grayburn PA, et al. Recommendations for evaluation of prosthetic valves with echocardiography and Doppler ultrasound. J Am Soc Echocardiogr. 2009;22(9):975–1014.

Multimodality Imaging of Mitral Valve Diseases: TEER, Valve in Valve, and Beyond

Taimur Safder, Gloria Ayuba, and Vera H. Rigolin

Abstract

The mitral valve apparatus is a complex structure that requires harmonious interplay of several key components to function properly. As such, diseases of the mitral valve can present a significant challenge for clinicians to diagnose and manage. Innovation in cardiac imaging techniques, transcatheter based interventions and study of clinical outcomes has transformed the care available for patients with mitral valve disorders. In this chapter, a case-based review of the optimal imaging approach to patients being evaluated for transcatheter mitral valve intervention will be presented. More specifically, imaging considerations for the following interventions will be reviewed:

1. Transcatheter edge to edge repair for mitral regurgitation
2. Percutaneous balloon mitral valvuloplasty in mitral stenosis
3. Transcatheter mitral valve in valve

Supplementary Information The online version contains supplementary material available at https://doi.org/10.1007/978-3-031-50740-3_2.

T. Safder · G. Ayuba · V. H. Rigolin (✉)
Bluhm Cardiovascular Institute, Northwestern University Feinberg School of Medicine, Chicago, IL, USA
e-mail: Vrigolin@nm.org

Keywords

Mitral stenosis · Mitral regurgitation · Transcatheter intervention · Mitral valve in valve · Valvular disease · Valvular intervention · Mitral valve disease · Transcatheter mitral valve treatment · Mitral valve replacement · Transcatheter edge-to-edge repair · Mitral balloon valvuloplasty · Valve-in-valve · Transcatheter mitral valve replacement · Prosthetic stenosis · Cardiac imaging

Abbreviations

ACC	American College of Cardiology
AHA	American Heart Association
BMI	Body mass index
CT	Computed tomography
DVI	Dimensionless velocity integral
EOA	Effective Orifice Area
EROA	Effective regurgitant orifice area
GDMT	Goal directed medical therapy
HF	Heart failure
LA	Left atrium
LAA	Left atrial appendage
LV	Left ventricle
LVEF	Left ventricle ejection fraction

© The Author(s), under exclusive license to Springer Nature Switzerland AG 2024
A. M. Kelsey et al. (eds.), *Cardiac Imaging in Structural Heart Disease Interventions*,
https://doi.org/10.1007/978-3-031-50740-3_2

LVESD	Left ventricle end systolic diameter
LVOT	Left ventricular outflow tract
ME	Mid-esophageal
MG	Mean gradient
MR	Mitral regurgitation
MS	Mitral stenosis
MV	Mitral valve
MVA	Mitral valve area
MViV	Mitral valve-in-valve
NYHA	New York Heart Association
PASP	Pulmonary artery systolic pressure
PBMV	Percutaneous balloon mitral valvuloplasty
PHT	Pressure half time
PISA	Proximal isovelocity surface area
PLAX	Parasternal long axis
PV	Pulmonary vein
RF	Regurgitant fraction
RV	Right ventricle
Rvol	Regurgitant volume
RVSP	Right ventricular systolic pressure
SLD	Single leaflet detachment
STS	Society of Thoracic Surgeons
TEE	Transesophageal echocardiography
TEER	Transcatheter edge to edge repair
TMVR	Transcatheter mitral valve replacement
TTE	Transthoracic echocardiography

> Test your learning and check your understanding of this book's contents: use the "Springer Nature Flashcards" app to access questions using ▶ https://sn.pub/ambACS.
>
> To use the app, please follow the instructions in the chapter "Transcatheter Aortic Valve Replacement."

Learning Objectives
1. Review initial approach and indications for transcatheter intervention for patients with significant mitral regurgitation presenting to valve clinic for evaluation.
2. Review pre-procedural, procedural and post procedural imaging considerations for patients with significant MR being evaluated for transcatheter edge-to-edge repair.
3. Review initial approach, indications and anatomic suitability for PBMV in patients with mitral stenosis.
4. Review pre-procedural, procedural and post procedural imaging considerations for patients undergoing PBMV for mitral stenosis.
5. Be able to diagnose mitral prosthetic valve dysfunction.
6. Understand the preprocedural considerations of transcatheter mitral valve-in-valve intervention including inclusion and exclusion factors.
7. Understand the role of multimodality imaging in diagnosis, planning and procedural guidance.

Mitral Regurgitation and Transcatheter Edge-to-Edge Repair (TEER)

Mitral regurgitation (MR) is a complex disease process that can present a significant challenge for clinicians to manage. From initial non-invasive evaluation to indications for surgical vs. transcatheter interventions, the decision tree for management of MR continues to branch out. As mitral valve transcatheter interventions become more widely available, a multidisciplinary team approach with integration of multimodality imaging will be key in optimizing and standardizing outcomes across a diverse set of practice settings. Furthermore, it is becoming increasingly clear that expertise in non-invasive imaging for evaluation of MR will be the central tenet of any multidisciplinary team hoping to optimize patient outcomes. In this section, a patient with severe MR presenting to the valve clinic for evaluation of candidacy for a transcatheter intervention will be discussed.

Case Study

A 62 year old male with history of severe MR presents to valve clinic for evaluation. Patient's past medical history is significant for hypertension, hyperlipidemia, obesity (BMI 40), chronic kidney disease and chronic obstructive pulmonary disease and significant anxiety/depression. Exam is significant for elevated jugular venous pulse, 3/6 holosystolic murmur best heard at apex which radiates to axilla, 3+ bilateral lower extremity edema. The patient was initially evaluated at an outside hospital for surgical mitral valve replacement but due to his overwhelming anxiety to undergoing surgery, he was referred for transcatheter edge to edge repair (TEER) evaluation.

The patient was initially diagnosed with significant MR 3 years ago at which time transesophageal echocardiography (TEE) showed normal left ventricular (LV) size and function [LV ejection fraction (EF) 61%] and flail posterior leaflet of the mitral valve. LV end diastolic volume was 102 mL (indexed 45.1 mL/m^2) while LV end systolic volume was 30 mL (indexed 13.3 (mL/m^2). At that time, he was recommended to undergo mitral valve surgery but due to severe anxiety, he declined and was lost to follow up. The patient now presents again for evaluation due to worsening symptoms. He now notes severe dyspnea on exertion and needs to stop and rest several times when climbing three flights of stairs in his apartment building. He also notes lower extremity edema and orthopnea. Symptoms mildly improved with furosemide. Due to the patient's previous aversion to surgical intervention leading to lost to follow up, patient was referred directly for TEER evaluation.

Background and Definitions

The initial evaluation of any patient being considered for an intervention starts with the appropriateness of the indication of the procedure. Once the diagnosis of severe MR has been agreed upon by the valve team, the most impactful factors that determine the patient's eligibility for MR intervention are the etiology of the MR (primary vs. secondary), the status of left ventricular (LV) size and function and the presence or absence of symptoms. The 2020 ACC/AHA practice guideline for patients with valvular heart disease incorporates these factors into the recommendations for valve intervention [1]. A simplified version of these recommendations is shown in Tables 1 and 2.

TEER is a technique which relies on approximating the edges of MV leaflets to reduce the degree of MR. It is modeled after the surgical MV repair technique of the Alfieri Stich credited to Dr. Ottavio Alfieri [2]. The Everest II trial lent initial support for TEER as a viable treatment option for degenerative MR [3]. Currently, no class I indications exist for TEER for treatment of severe MR regardless of etiology or symptoms. For primary MR, the 2020 ACC/AHA practice guideline for valvular heart disease gives TEER a class 2a recommendation for patients with favorable anatomy at high or prohibitive surgical risk (Table 1) [1]. The more recent COAPT and MITRA-FR trials evaluated TEER for treatment of secondary MR [4, 5]. While the former trial showed improved outcomes with TEER in patients with secondary MR, the latter did not. Divergent outcomes are largely driven by differences in the baseline characteristics of the subjects enrolled in the two trials [6]. The 2020 ACC/AHA practice guideline for valvular heart disease gives a 2a indication for TEER for patients with severe secondary MR who have persistent symptoms (NYHA II or greater), are on optimal heart failure (HF) guideline directed

Table 1 Adapted from ACC/AHA 2020 practice guideline for management of patients with valvular heart disease [1]

ACC/AHA chronic primary MR intervention recommendations			
Class of recommendation	I	IIa	IIb
	Symptomatic severe MR, irrespective of LV function	Symptomatic (NYHA class III or IV) severe MR with high/prohibitive surgical risk, TEER is reasonable if anatomy is favorable and life expectancy ≥1 year	
	Asymptomatic severe MR with LV dysfunction (LVEF ≤60%, LVESD ≥40 mm)	In asymptomatic, severe MR with normal LV function (LVEF ≥60%, LVESD ≤40 mm), MV repair is reasonable when likelihood of successful and durable repair without residual MR is >95% and mortality rate <1%) and when done at a comprehensive valve center	Asymptomatic, severe MR with normal LV function but with progressive increase in LV size or decrease in function (on ≥3 serially done imaging studies)

Table 2 Adapted from ACC/AHA 2020 practice guideline for management of patients with valvular heart disease [1]

ACC/AHA chronic secondary MR intervention recommendations			
Class of recommendation	I	IIa	IIb
	N/A	TEER for severe MR, persistent symptoms ≥ NYHA II, on optimal HF GDMT, LVEF between 20–50%, LVESD ≤70 mm, PASP ≤70 mmHg	MV surgery for severe MR due to atrial annular dilation, LVEF ≥50%, NYHA III or IV symptoms despite GDMT for HF
	N/A	MV surgery for severe MR at time of CABG	MV surgery for severe MR related to LVEF ≤50%, NYHA III or IV symptoms despite GDMT for HF

medical therapy (GDMT), have an LV EF between 20 and 50%, have an LV end systolic dimension (LVESD) <70 mm, and pulmonary artery systolic pressure (PASP) <70 mmHg [1]. These criteria are based on the positive results from the COAPT trial population and the lessons learned from the negative results of the MITRA-FR trial.

Diagnosis and Pre-procedural Assessment

Initial Patient Assessment

The clinical presentation of a patient with severe MR can be variable. Symptoms can range from significant to subtle to lacking entirely [7]. Furthermore, the patient may underestimate their functional capacity or subtly decrease their activity level as they adjust to their symptoms slowly over time. Physical exam findings, such as presence and severity of murmur, have been shown to be predictive of severe MR [8]. For these reasons, a comprehensive history and physical exam is crucial in gaining clinical context for the non-invasive findings when assessing patients with MR for the first time.

Our patient has given us a history of symptoms that are typically seen with progression of severity of MR. He reports worsening exertional dyspnea, orthopnea and new lower extremity edema, which are suggestive of fluid overload and heart failure. While the patient's symptoms are somewhat difficult to attribute solely to his MR in the context of BMI of 40, the overall worsening of symptoms (while the weight has stayed stable) gives us more confidence that the MR is a significant factor in his symptomatology. Exam findings of elevated JVP and bilateral lower extremity edema support our concerns about fluid overload and HF and further support a diagnosis of severe MR. The holosystolic murmur radiating to the axilla may suggest a posterolateral direction of the MR jet. This information helps to form a clinical picture of our patient and will later be helpful when reviewing our patient's imaging studies.

Non-invasive Imaging

Transthoracic Echocardiography

Transthoracic echocardiography (TTE) is the gateway imaging modality for the diagnosis and evaluation of MR. TTE can help inform on several important characteristics of the mitral valve pathology that can aid in determining the appropriate management plan.

The first step in the echocardiographic evaluation of MR is to determine the mechanism of the regurgitation. When assessing mechanism, it is important to evaluate the entire mitral valve anatomy including the leaflets, annulus, subvalvular apparatus and the surrounding myocardium. A careful assessment of the anatomy provides not only structural information but also assists in procedural planning. Specific findings, such as leaflet calcification or perforation, may limit a TEER as a treatment option (Table 3). The Carpentier classification is a frequently used classification scheme that groups the etiology of MR into 4 subtypes. Type 1 is MR due to a dilated annulus or perforated leaflet. Type 2 is MR due to excessive leaflet motion. Type 3a is MR due to leaflet restriction in systole and diastole. Type 3b is MR due to leaflet restriction in systole only [8].

The initial TTE for this patient was challenging due to patient's body habitus. Despite this, primary mitral valve disease due to a flail posterior MV leaflet flail was identified (Videos 1, 3 and Fig. 1). Because of the technically challenging nature of the TTE, other important MV structural information could not be assessed (Table 4). MV vegetations, calcification and perforation are just a few characteristics that, if present, would have a significant impact on the patient's candidacy for TEER.

Once the mechanism of mitral regurgitation is identified, quantification of MR severity is the next step. Quantification should not rely solely on color Doppler imaging. There are multiple parameters that are useful to determine the severity of MR and each has pros and cons. MR severity must therefore be assessed using a comprehensive approach. Quantitative parameters such as effective regurgitant orifice area (EROA), regurgitant volume (Rvol) and regurgitant fraction (RF) are particularly useful in patients being considered for TEER. Secondary markers of MR severity, such as left atrial (LA) size and LV chamber size and function, can also be helpful determining MR severity (Table 5).

MR severity in this patient's TTE was difficult to assess because of his large body habitus. A significant color flow Doppler MR jet was not appreciated and only a partial flow convergence zone was visualized (Videos 2, 4, Fig. 2). MR continuous wave (CW) Doppler was also attempted with and without an echo enhancing agent and showed a faint and incomplete MR signal with a possible early MR peak velocity (Figs. 3a and b). Clues to the presence of significant MR included an elevated MV E wave velocity and a dilated LA (Figs. 4a and b). An adequate Doppler signal in the pulmonary veins could not be obtained. LV chamber size was dilated but normalized when corrected for his large body size.

After initial clinical and TTE evaluation, it is reasonable to refer for a TEER procedure if the

Table 3 Unfavorable echocardiographic characteristics for TEER

	Unfavorable echo features
Location of pathology	Within body of leaflet (i.e., perforation, cleft)
Calcification	If severe and at site of grasping zone
MV gradient, MVA	Mitral stenosis (≥5 mmHg), MVA <4 cm^2
Grasping leaflet length	<7 mm
Primary MR	Flail width >15 mm Flail gap >10 mm LVESD >55 mm Highly mobile flail leaflet Severely thickened and redundant leaflet (i.e., Barlow's type valve)
Secondary MR	LVESD >70 mm Coaptation depth >11 mm

Adapted from Badhwar V, JACC 2020: 2236–70 [8]

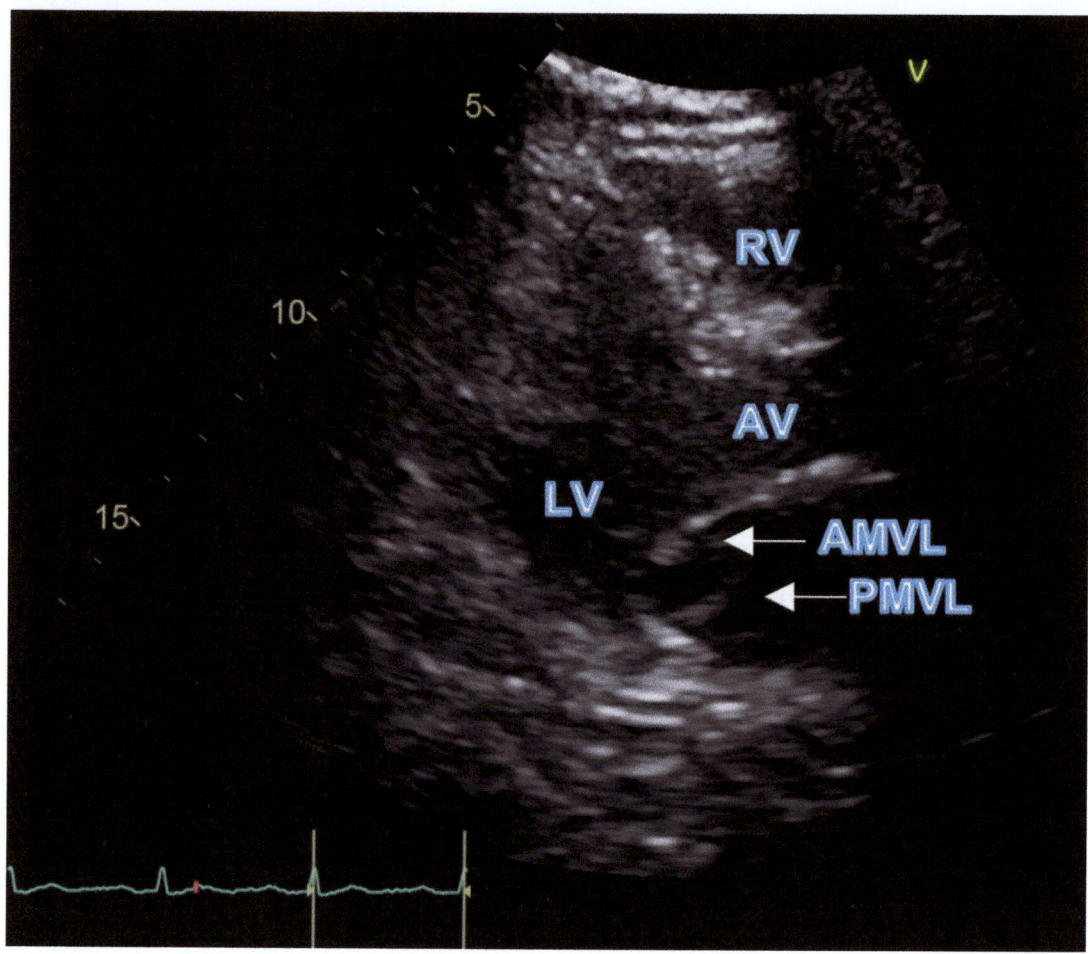

Fig. 1 TTE PLAX view. A flail posterior segment can be appreciated and is labeled

Table 4 Etiology of primary and secondary MR

Primary MR	Secondary MR
Myxomatous changes (prolapse, flail, ruptured chordae)	Ischemic MR
Degenerative changes (calcification, thickening)	Non-ischemic cardiomyopathy
Infectious (perforations, vegetations due to endocarditis)	Annular dilation (atrial fibrillation, restrictive disease)
Inflammatory (rheumatic, radiation, collagen, vascular)	
Congenital (cleft, parachute MV)	

Adapted from Zoghbi WA, et al. J Am Soc Echocardiogr 2017; 30(4): 303–371 [9]

Table 5 Severe MR criteria

Quantitative criteria	Secondary markers
EROA ≥ 0.4 cm^2	Pulmonary vein systolic flow reversal
Regurgitant fraction $\geq 50\%$	LA/LV dilation
Regurgitant volume ≥ 60 mL	Increased MV E velocity and E/A ratio

following questions have been answered with confidence:

1. Indication for procedure (Tables 1 and 2)
2. Severity and mechanism for MR (Tables 4 and 5)
3. Anatomy unfavorable for TEER (Table 3)

Fig. 2 A baseline shifted color Doppler image is seen with a partial flow convergence (FC) signal

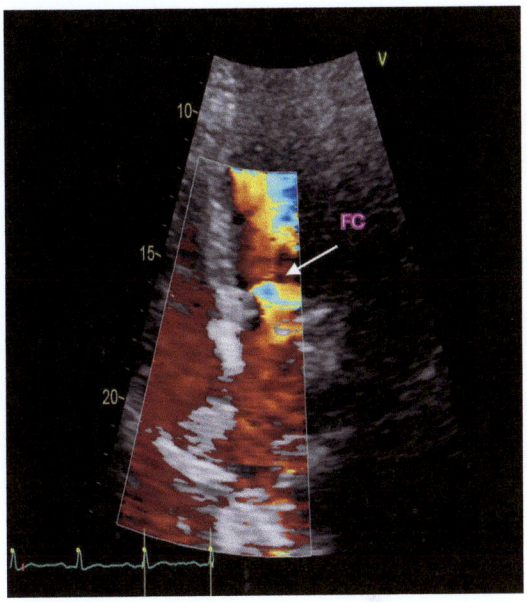

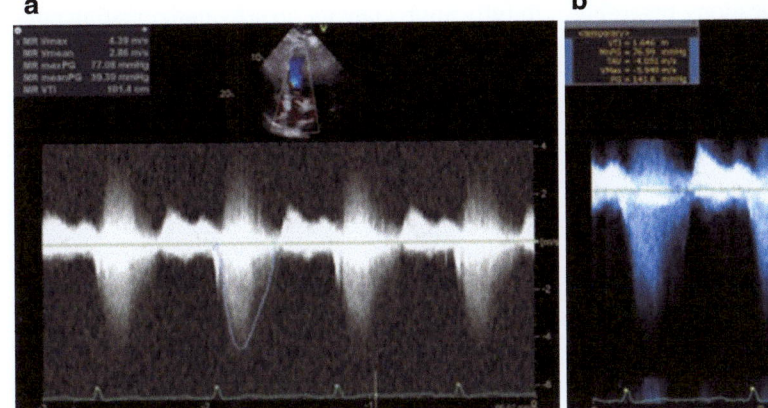

Fig. 3 TTE CW MR Doppler. An incomplete MR CW Doppler signal is seen due to an eccentric jet before (**a**) and after (**b**) administration of an echo enhancing agent. The signal appears to be consistent with an early MR peak velocity

If any of those questions remain unanswered then further testing is warranted.

Symptomatic severe MR is a Class I indication for MV surgery. For our patient to be eligible for a commercial TEER (Class IIa), a surgical evaluation with a designation of high surgical risk is needed. The TTE shows evidence for a flail posterior leaflet, a specific marker for severe MR, but color flow Doppler and quantification measures are unable to confirm severity of

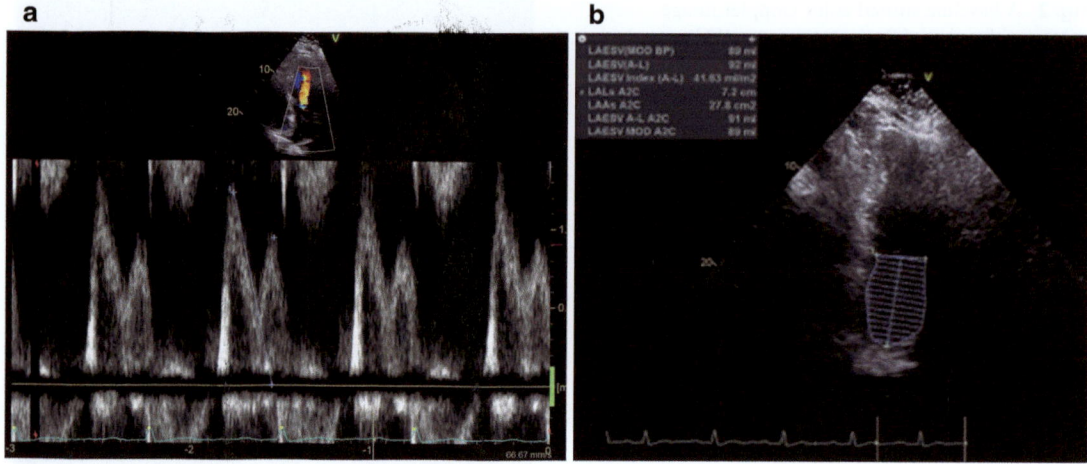

Fig. 4 MR secondary measures. (**a**) With MV PW Doppler showing increased E velocity of 1.23 m/s and (**b**) with biplane method measurement of left atrium showing enlarged LA with an index volume of 41.6 mL/m²

MR. Some secondary markers also suggest presence of significant MR. The MV leaflet morphology is also poorly seen so questions regarding favorable anatomy for TEER remain unanswered in our patient.

Additional Testing

When important questions regarding severity, mechanism of MR and morphology of the MV are not fully answered, further imaging should be undertaken. There are several different imaging modalities that may serve as an appropriate next step depending on the specific situation.

Stress Testing

Stress testing can serve as a valuable tool in the assessment of MR. In asymptomatic patients, stress testing can help to identify a truly asymptomatic patient from a patient whose symptoms are masked by their gradual reduction in physical exertion. Furthermore, in the truly asymptomatic patients with severe MR who may not yet meet indication for intervention, stress testing can help provide an objective baseline measure of functional capacity that can then be followed over time. Besides exercise capacity, stress testing can yield echocardiographic information about a patient's MR that may not be appreciated in baseline echocardiography imaging. The dynamic nature of MR due to alterations in loading conditions can make it difficult to fully appreciate its severity under resting conditions [10]. Hemodynamic stress testing may show worsening of MR with exercise along with other findings such as increased pulmonary artery systolic pressure, failure of left or right ventricle function to augment properly, and failure of appropriate augmentation of LV systolic function.

Transesophageal Echocardiography

The role of transesophageal echocardiography (TEE) in MR evaluation is in the setting of discordant or incomplete TTE findings. TEE can help in obtaining more precise information about valve anatomy and function when not well defined by TTE. It is important to note that TEE may underestimate MR severity due to procedural anesthesia and its effects on loading conditions. Enface views of the MV (surgeon's view) obtained with three-dimensional (3D) TEE can further help localize and identify MR pathology. TEE is essential for procedural planning in patients being considered for TEER.

In our patient, due to incomplete information regarding MR severity and MV morphology obtained via TTE images, a decision was made to order a TEE to make sure the valve team had all the information needed to make an appropriate recommendation.

Cardiac CT and MRI

Cardiac CT may be used in pre-procedural planning depending on type of MV intervention planned. For transcatheter approach, CT imaging can define level of aortic calcifications (typically in patients >65 years old) or define anatomy in the case of any other thoracic aortic disease. If MV surgery is being considered, CT imaging is particularly important in high risk patients as it can define mediastinal anatomy, cannulation strategy, and can exclude aberrant cardiovascular anatomy. CT coronary angiogram can also be used in lieu of left heart catheterization in low risk patients to define coronary artery disease [2].

In cases where there is conflicting or incomplete information on TTE or TEE, CMR can help define LV size/function, MV morphology and MR severity. It can also be used in patients with cardiomyopathies to help with risk assessment.

Other Testing

Invasive hemodynamic testing can be considered in patients with severe pulmonary hypertension and to guide medical optimization prior to MV intervention.

Heart Team Approach and Discussion

Prior to case evaluation by the valve team, all pre-requisite imaging should be completed. The heart valve team should ideally consist of a cardiac interventionalist, cardiac surgeon, cardiac imaging specialist as well as supporting staff including nurse practitioners or physician assistants. Ancillary staff, such as an administrative team, also play a key role in the function of a successful valve team.

With the addition of TEE images, this patients MV morphology and MR severity is now clear. The significant posterior leaflet flail seen on TTE is confirmed (Fig. 5a). Biplane sweep of the 2D MV commissural view allows for the identification of flail P2 scallop. Furthermore, several important leaflet characteristics are noted. Significant leaflet calcification is absent, a significant flail gap is present and the posterior leaflet length is measured (Fig. 5b, c, d, e and f). Color flow Doppler evaluation demonstrates a significant anteriorly directed MR jet but without any evidence of leaflet perforation (Video 5). MR severity is quantified using the proximal isovelocity surface area (PISA) method (Fig. 6a). It is important to note that PISA can overestimate MR severity in this patient due to constraint of the eccentric jet against the posterior wall. Angle of correction due to constrained PISA should be utilized to get a more accurate estimation of MR severity (Fig. 6b). The resulting MR regurgitation volume (Rvol) of 105 mL and MR effective regurgitant orifice area (EROA) of 1.1 cm^2 confirm that the MR in our patient is in the severe range (Table 6). PV flow reversal is also seen further supporting severe MR (Fig. 6c).

3D TEE imaging of the MV (best reconstructed from the MV commissural view) can also aid in confirming MV pathology and morphology. The location of P2 flail in this patient can be appreciated with and without color (Videos 6 and 7) as well as the extent of flail with flail width measurement of 23 mm (Fig. 7). Increasing of the wall filter setting on 3D imaging can allow for simultaneous assessment of the underlying MV anatomy along with the color Doppler MR jet, (Fig. 8). Utilizing 2D and 3D echocardiographic imaging to their full extent can help give a complete picture of MV pathology and aid in procedural planning.

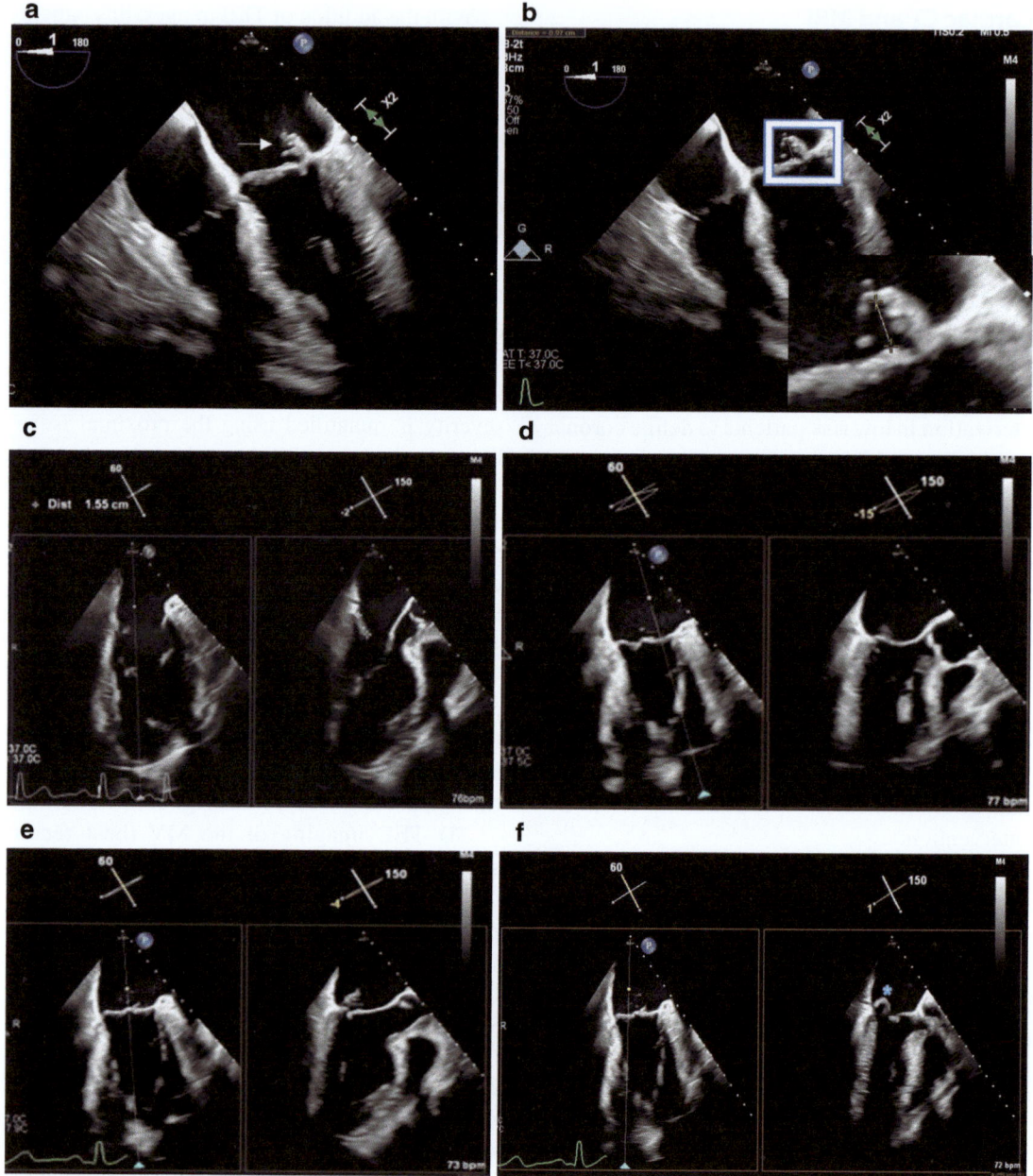

Fig. 5 TEE ME view. The four-chamber view visualizes the flail P2 scallop (arrow, **a**). The flail gap measures 9.7 mm (**b**) and posterior leaflet length measures 15.5 mm (**c**). ME MV commissural view allows for the identification of the flail segment as one sweeps the biplane view from lateral (A1–P1, **d**) to middle (A2–P2. **e**) to medial (A3–P3, **f**). P3 prolapse is also seen (asterisk, figure **f**) in addition to the P2 flail

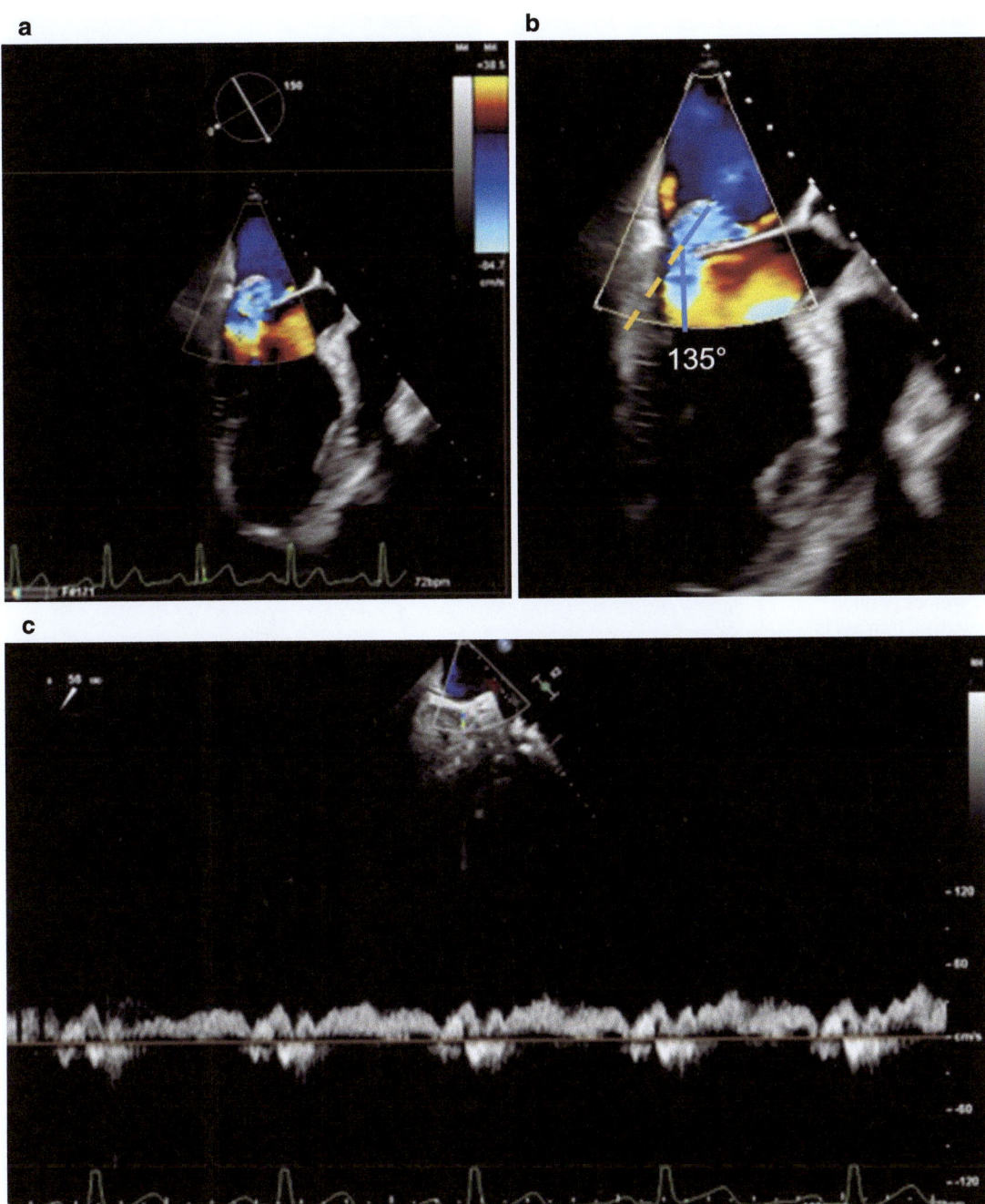

Fig. 6 PISA measurement with color Doppler baseline shift seen on (**a**) (1.6 cm) with angle of correction consideration due to constrained jet (**b**). Reversal of PV flow with PW Doppler seen on (**c**) (arrow)

Table 6 Our patient's echo measures and MR severity calculations

Echo measures	With angle correction	Without angle correction
PISA 1.6 cm MR Vmax 4.2 m/s MR VTI 96 cm Va 0.39 m/s Angle of correction = 135°	$Q = 2\prod (1.6)^2 \times 39 \times (135/180)$ EROA = 1.1 cm² Rvol = 105 mL	$Q = 2\prod (1.6)^2 \times 39$ EROA = 1.5 cm² Rvol = 144 mL

Va aliasing velocity, *Q* regurgitant flow, *MR VTI* MR jet velocity time integral, *Vmax* maximal MR jet velocity

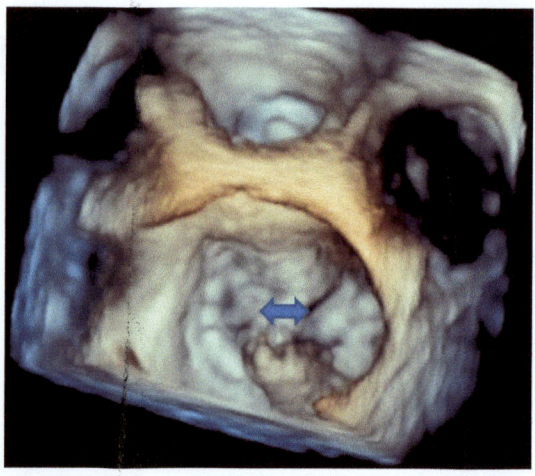

Fig. 7 Flail width measurement of 23 mm on MV enface 3D view

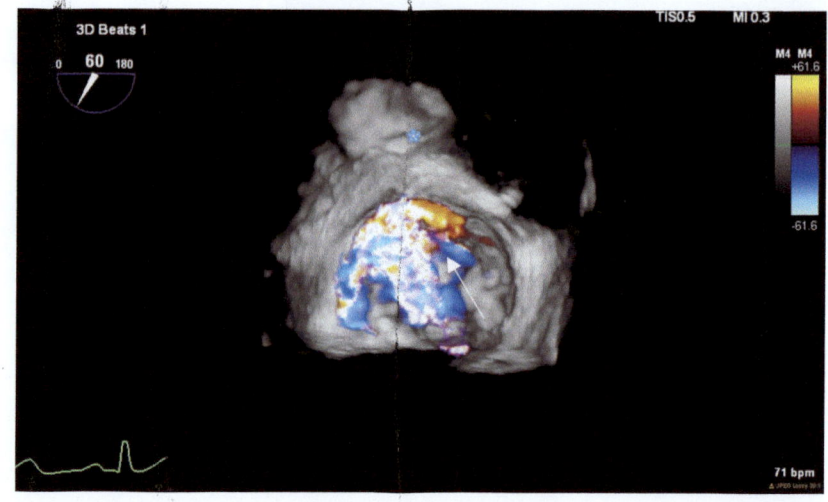

Fig. 8 TEE 3D. MV enface view with AV at 12 o'clock position (asterisk). Increase in the wall filter setting allowing for simultaneous visualization of MV anatomy and the jet of MR (arrow)

Heart Team Decision

The ACC/AHA 2020 practice guideline on valvular heart disease provides a framework for decision making for MV surgical vs. transcatheter approach primarily based on mechanism of MR (Tables 1 and 2) [1]. Surgical MV repair is considered the gold standard for primary MR due to the ability to provide a more complete repair when compared to TEER. Thus, TEER for primary MR is suitable only when the patient is demonstrated to be high surgical risk or a poor candidate for surgical repair due to other factors (i.e. anatomical). Despite our patient's anxiety over surgical repair, a formal cardiothoracic surgery evaluation is required and was ordered to assess for eligibility for TEER. Due to patient's comorbidities, he was determined to be of high surgical risk for surgical MV repair with a calculated STS score of 9.5%. With a designation of high surgical risk, our patient can now be considered for TEER if his anatomy proves favorable.

Several anatomical factors need to be reviewed when deciding this patient's suitability for TEER (Table 3). The central location of leaflet pathology is favorable for TEER due to ease of access of the A2–P2 location for the TEER system. Lack of any degree of mitral stenosis and minimal leaflet calcification also favor a TEER approach in this patient. Furthermore, adequate posterior leaflet length measurements also assure us of good grasping zones. But a significant flail width (Fig. 7) and flail gap (Fig. 5b) are less favorable features. A large and/or highly mobile flail segment can lead to an unstable clip attachment and a poor TEER result.

Further discussion within the heart team led to the decision to move forward with TEER. The favorable features that allowed for a successful TEER were thought to outweigh the less favorable ones (Table 7). Additionally, as experience is gained, it is recognized that placement of multiple MV clips during TEER can allow for stabilization of larger more mobile flail leaflets. But this is undertaken at the risk of procedural complications, such as MV clip single leaflet detachment (SLD).

Table 7 Our patients MV characteristics as it pertains to TEER

Favorable	Less favorable
Middle location of pathology	Flail width >15 mm
Minimal leaflet calcification	Flail gap of 9.7 mm
No significant mitral stenosis	
Large grasping zone	

Intraprocedural Imaging Modalities and Measurements

Crucial procedural steps	Imaging highlights	Optimal TEE views
Transseptal puncture	– The transseptal puncture must be at least >3.5 cm (ideally >4 cm) above the MV annular plane (as shown measured in Fig. 9b) – Optimal position of transseptal puncture in midposterior fossa with inferior and posterior positioning – Adequate atrial septal tenting is needed to assess catheter positioning (Video 9 and Fig. 9b) – Confirm crossing of tip of catheter into LA	– 2D ME bicaval view for superior-inferior positioning with biplane which allows for anterior-posterior positioning (Video 8 and Fig. 9a) – Rotating of transducer will likely be needed to locate and follow the catheter
Delivery system guidance	– Guide delivery system and clip into the left atrium as it advances to clear surrounding anatomy	– 2D ME 4Ch and 2Ch views with biplane (Video 10)
Clip arm positioning above the valve	– Aid in positioning of the clip perpendicularly above the known regurgitant orifice based on pre-procedural imaging – Partial opening of clip arms with movement of grasping mechanism to identify clip arm orientation – Confirm clip position above regurgitant orifice by use of color Doppler	– 3D ME enface view (Video 11)
Clip arm positioning below the valve	– Confirm orientation of clip arms has not changed after passing through the MV (reducing 2D/3D gain until MV leaflets are not visible is needed to visualize clip below the MV)	– Combination of 2D and 3D enface ME view (Video 12)
Grasping of leaflets	– The 2 clip arms must be visualized as clearly as possible as the clip is retracted towards the MV in an attempt to capture both leaflets in their appropriate anterior and posterior grippers – Verify each leaflet capture (release and re-capture if necessary due to poor capture, Video 13)	– 2D ME long-axis and higher omniplane (~120°–150°) views (Videos 14 and 15)
Clip closure	– Close clip with concomitant color Doppler evaluation as to note the reduction in MR in real time	– 2D and 3D enface ME views with color Doppler (Videos 16, 17 and Fig. 10)
Evaluation post deployment	– Residual MR location and severity evaluation by color Doppler – PV flow reversal and transmitral peak and mean gradient evaluation – Assess need for additional clip	– 2D ME commissural views for PV PW and MV CW evaluation (Fig. 11a) – 3D ME enface views (Videos 18, 19 and Fig. 11b) – TEE imaging views and approach for second clip similar to first clip (Videos 20, 21, 22, 23, 24, 25 and 26 and Fig. 12)
Delivery system withdrawal	– Continuously image the distal end of delivery catheter to assure clearance of any adjacent anatomy as it is withdrawn – Evaluate shunt flow from resulting iatrogenic interatrial defect	– 2D ME views with biplane (Video 27 and Fig. 13) – 2D ME bicaval view with color Doppler and CW (Fig. 14)

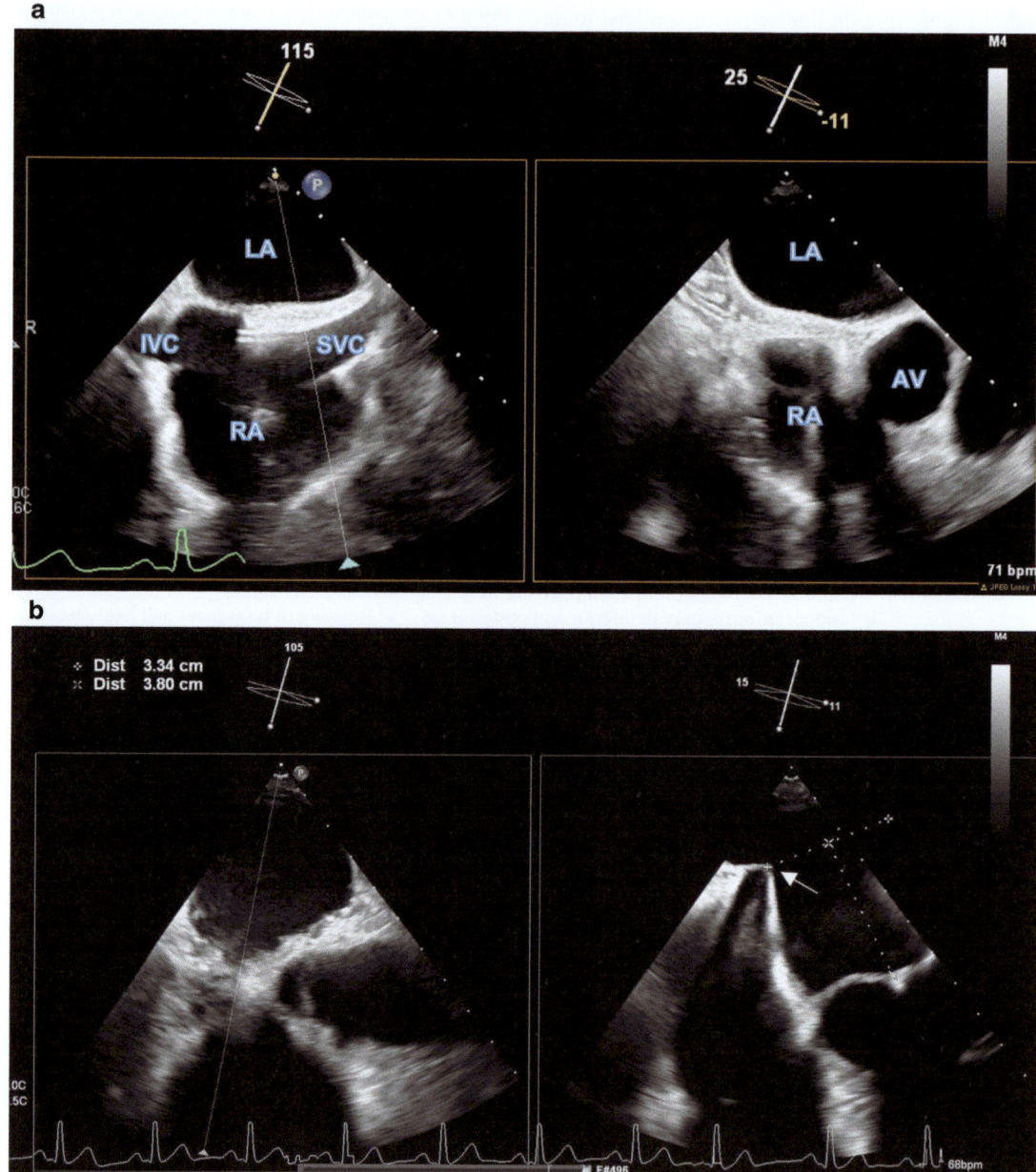

Fig. 9 TEE procedure guidance with ME biplane using the bi-caval view. Optimal superior-inferior and anterior-posterior positioning of the catheter for transeptal puncture can be determined in this view (**a**). Left atrial height should be measured from the coaptation point of the MV in a straight line to the transeptal puncture site (**b**). Atrial septal tenting is crucial in locating catheter position (arrow). Inferior vena cava (IVC), superior vena cava (SVC), left atrium (LA), right atrium (RA), aortic valve (AV)

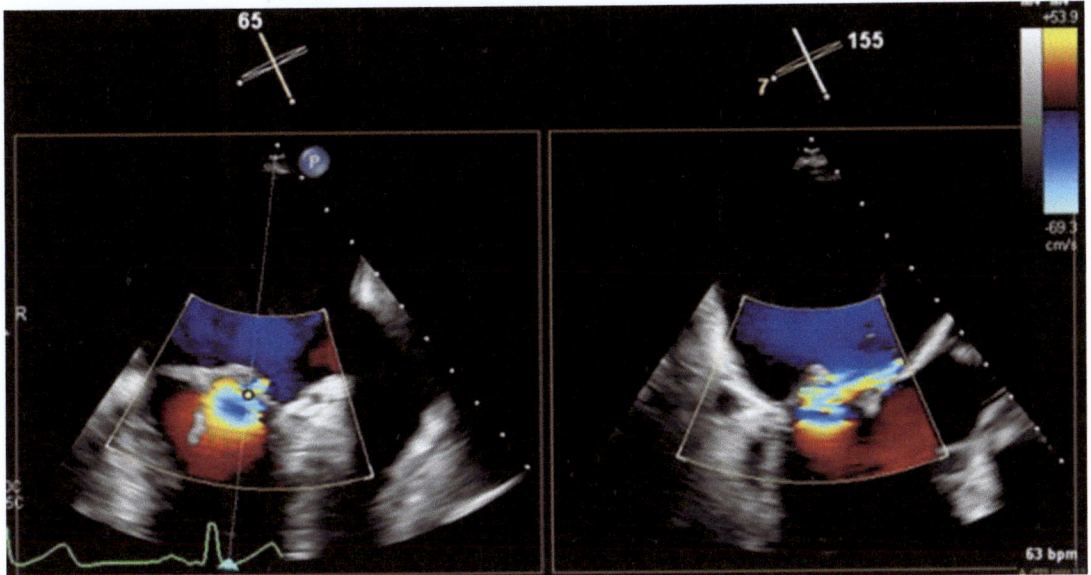

Fig. 10 Color flow Doppler evaluation shows presence of a significant MR jet lateral to the clip with the PISA radius measuring 0.8 cm

Fig. 11 MV gradient with CW Doppler is noted to be 2 mmHg (**a**). Color flow Doppler demonstrates the significant MR jet lateral to the clip (**b**)

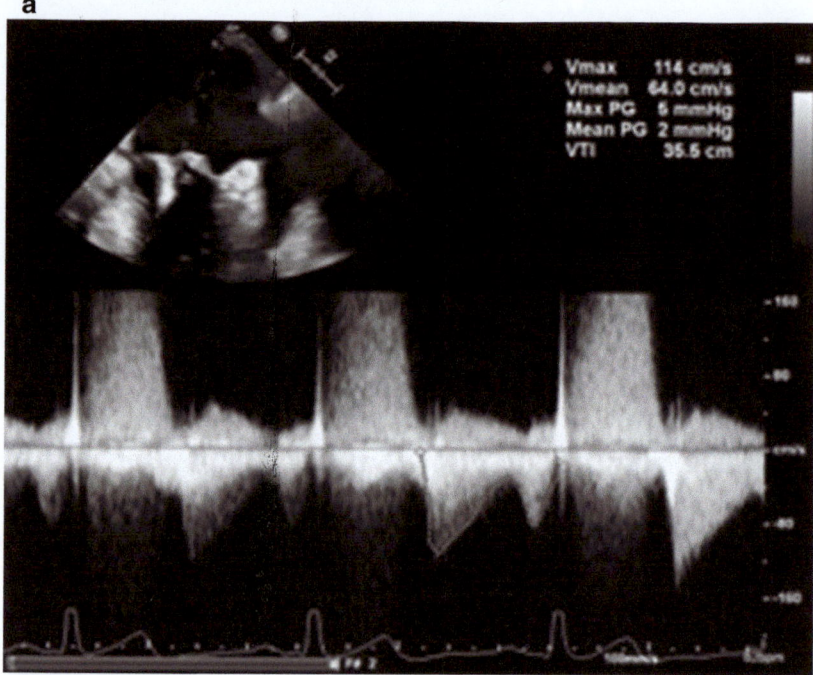

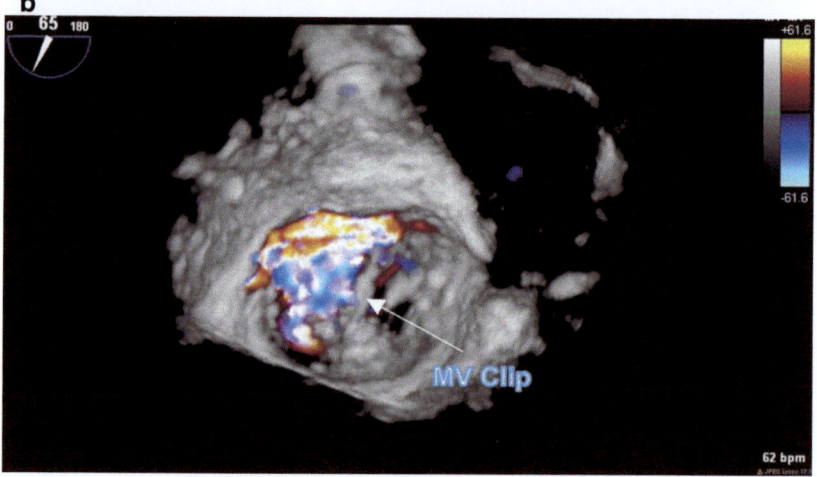

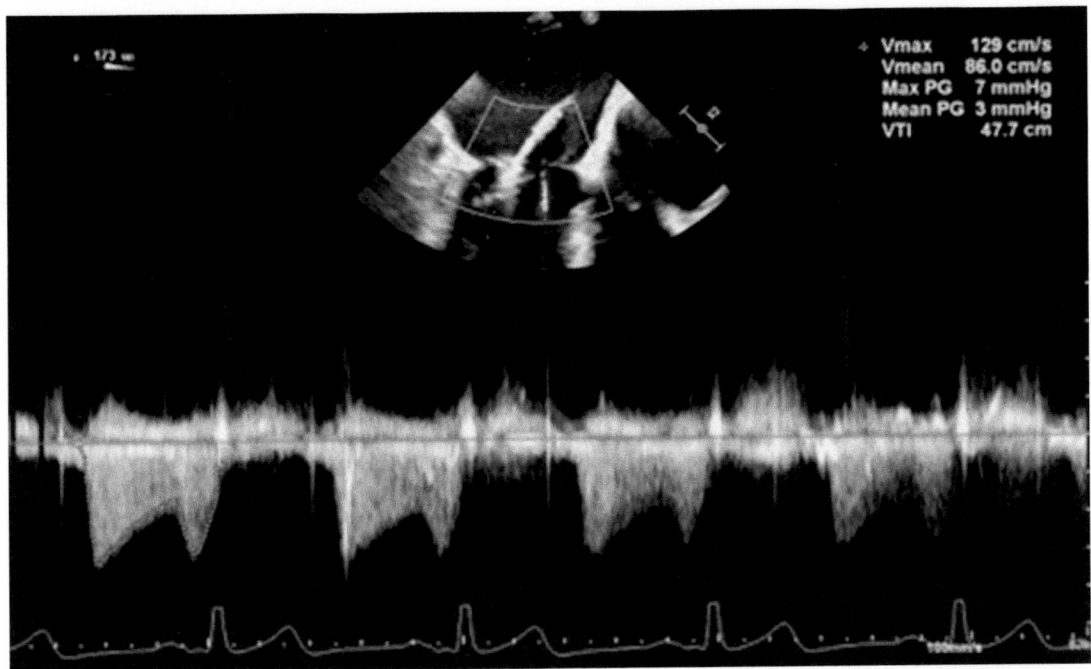

Fig. 12 TEE procedure guidance. MV gradient with CW Doppler after second MV clip is noted to be 3 mmHg

Fig. 13 The Mitraclip by Abbott delivery system has a sharp tip (arrow) that is uncovered post deployment. This sharp tip must be retracted into the delivery system catheter carefully under direct visualization of 2D echocardiographic imaging

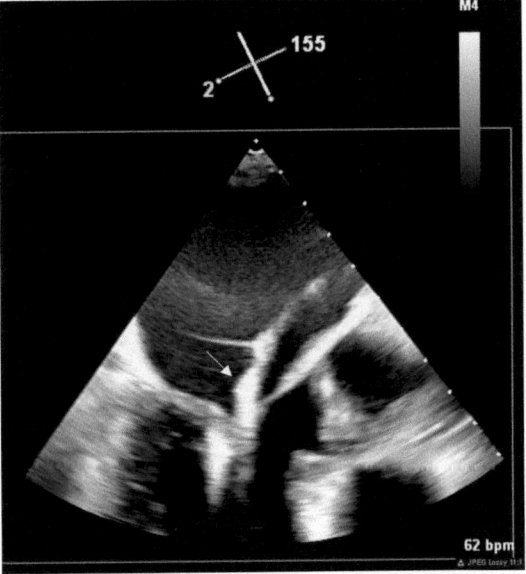

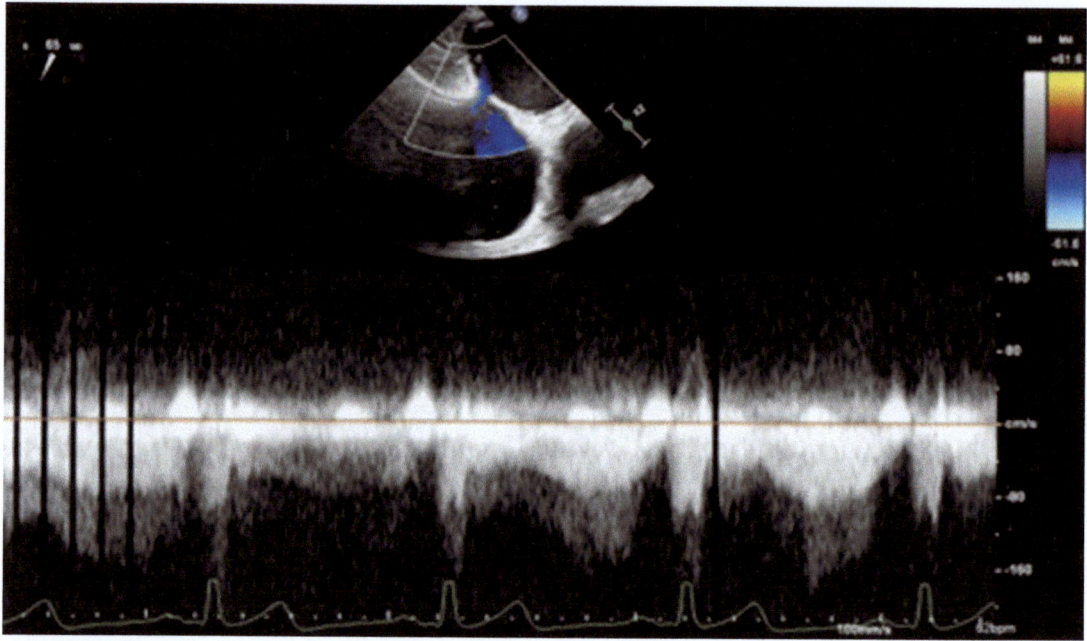

Fig. 14 TEE procedure guidance. Color Doppler and CW of iatrogenic interatrial defect showing predominantly left to right shunt flow

Follow Up Assessment

A comprehensive follow up TTE for patients undergoing TEER is recommended at 1 day, 30 days and again at 6–12 months after their procedure. TTEs at 1 and 30 days aid in identifying any possible complications post procedure while TTE at 6–12 months can help in evaluation of effectiveness of procedure and identify favorable outcomes such reverse remodeling of LV and LA. Our patient's 1 day post procedure TTE showed stable device position and no significant increase in MR. At 30 days and 6 month follow up, our patient reported significant symptom improvement. A TTE was scheduled for 1 year post procedure for our patient.

Multimodality imaging comparison

Modality	Clinical application	Limitations
Transthoracic echocardiography (TTE)	– First line test for assessment of etiology, mechanism and severity of mitral regurgitation – Can refer for TEER procedure after initial TTE if the TTE is of high quality and is able to definitively answer key questions regarding patient's candidacy for TEER	– Lower spatial resolution compared to TEE – Body habitus and artifact may limit adequate assessment of mitral valve
Transesophageal Echocardiography (tee)	– Preprocedural evaluation of MR, especially in the setting of incomplete evaluation or discordant findings on TTE – Can obtain more precise information about valve anatomy and pathology – Intraprocedural imaging guidance – Immediate post procedure evaluation and evaluation for complications	– Some absolute contraindications include upper GI anatomical considerations, active upper GI bleeding – Requires sedation – May underestimate MR severity due to anesthesia and its effect on loading conditions

Modality	Clinical application	Limitations
Exercise stress echocardiography	– Can aid in pre-procedural planning when discordant findings between clinical symptoms and echocardiographic findings	– Mobility limitations of patient
Cardiac computed tomography (CT)	– Can aid in pre-procedural planning if any concern for atypical anatomy – Can aid in MV surgery planning if patient is not a candidate for TEER with evaluation of mediastinal anatomy, cannulation strategy and coronary artery disease	– Unable to fully assess etiology and mechanism of MR – No hemodynamic assessment – Radiation exposure
Fluoroscopy	– Intraprocedural guidance – Pre-procedural hemodynamic testing can be considered in patients with pulmonary hypertension to guide medical optimization prior to MV intervention	– Limited anatomic assessment – Invasive testing – Radiation exposure
Cardiac magnetic resonance imaging (CMR)	– Can aid in pre-procedural planning when discordant findings on TTE/TEE – Can assess LV size and function, MV morphology and MR severity – Can further aid in assessing underlying cardiomyopathy, if present	– Cost – Patient discomfort

Clinical Controversies and Clinical Pearls

- Patient selection, based on both clinical and anatomical features, is key in increasing the odds of a good outcome.
- TEER for primary MR is suitable only when patient is demonstrated to be a high surgical risk, otherwise MV surgical repair is the gold standard.
- Exercise stress testing can serve as a valuable tool to assess asymptomatic patients with MR and can shed light on the dynamic nature of MR in patients with discordant clinical findings.
- Multi-modality imaging (i.e. cardiac MRI) can be useful if used in the proper context such as discordant findings on echocardiogram.

Key Points

- Mitral regurgitation is a complex disease process and transthoracic echocardiography can serve as the cornerstone imaging modality to provide the clinician with a comprehensive evaluation of the mitral valve.
- Transesophageal echocardiography may be needed if TTE findings are incomplete, discordant with clinical findings or more precise information is needed about MV anatomy to ascertain eligibility for transcatheter intervention.
- A careful consideration of clinical and anatomical features that pertain to a favorable outcome for patients being considered for TEER should be undertaken in pre-procedural planning.
- Familiarity with the key TEER procedural steps and experience with TEE image optimization techniques is crucial to a successful TEER.
- Follow up imaging at 1 day, 30 days and at 6–12 months is recommended to evaluate for post procedure complications and effectiveness of procedure.

Percutaneous Balloon Mitral Valvuloplasty for Mitral Stenosis

> **Case Study**
>
> Ms. K is a 56 year old female who moved from Mexico to the U.S. 20 years ago. She has known mitral stenosis (MS) and has followed with cardiology for the last 10 years with intermittent transthoracic echocardiography (TTE) imaging. At the most recent clinic visit, the patient reports worsening exertional dyspnea when climbing the stairs in her home during the last 6 months. She also reports worsening dyspnea and fatigue when working around the house doing her household chores. Her past medical history is significant for hypertension and paroxysmal atrial fibrillation.

Background and Definitions

While MS remains a significant cause of valvular heart disease around the world, its incidence remains low in high-income countries and is declining in low and middle-income countries. MS presentation and management can vary depending on rheumatic versus non-rheumatic etiology (Table 8) [11]. For this reason, it is important to delineate MS etiology and anatomy at time of diagnosis.

Complete and accurate evaluation of patients with MS is key in ensuring appropriate patient selection for possible intervention. The 2020 ACC/AHA practice guideline for patients with valvular heart disease provides the most up to date classification for MS (Table 9) [1]. As is true with all valvular lesions, no one specific parameter or measurement can assess MS completely. Multiple hemodynamic parameters along with valve anatomy, symptoms and secondary cardiac characteristics must be evaluated to accurately assess the presence and severity of MS. Understanding the limitations of the commonly used hemodynamic MS parameters can also help in reconciling conflicting findings (Table 10) [12].

Once a diagnosis of severe MS has been made, the patient should be referred to an experienced center to be evaluated by a multidisciplinary valve team for eligibility for possible intervention. Treatment options may differ

Table 8 Key characteristics of rheumatic vs. non-rheumatic MS

Rheumatic	Non-rheumatic
Significantly more common in women (~80% of cases)	More common in women but ratio not as high as rheumatic
Can present at any age	Typically presents in elderly
Can have minimal or significant valvular calcification	Typically with significant annular and valvular calcification
Commissural fusion often present	No commissural fusion

Table 9 MS classification, adapted from 2020 ACC/AHA practice guideline for valvular disease [1]

	Valve area	Valve hemodynamics	Secondary findings
At risk of MS	≥ 1.5 cm^2	Normal	None
Progressive MS	≥ 1.5 cm^2	Increased transmitral flow velocities but MG <5 mmHg[a] PHT <150 ms	Mild to moderate LA dilation Normal pulmonary pressures at rest
Asymptomatic severe MS	≤ 1.5 cm^2	Typically MG >5 mmHg[a] PHT ≥ 150 ms	Severe LA dilation PASP >50 mmHg
Symptomatic severe MS	≤ 1.5 cm^2	Typically MG >5 mmHg[a] PHT ≥ 150 ms	Severe LA dilation PASP >50 mmHg

MS mitral stenosis, *LA* left atrium, *PASP* pulmonary artery systolic pressure, *MG* mean gradient
[a]At HR 60–70 bpm

considerably depending on valve anatomy and mechanism of disease (i.e. rheumatic versus non-rheumatic).

Patients with rheumatic disease may qualify for one of several possible treatment options. One such option is percutaneous mitral balloon valvuloplasty (PBMV). When compared to surgical techniques, PBMV has shown to be safe and effective with comparable long term outcomes and as such has become the preferable treatment option [13]. The decision regarding PBMV versus surgery is predominantly decided by anatomical suitability.

The most widely used parameter to assess anatomic suitability is the Wilkins score first proposed by Dr. Wilkins in 1988 (Table 11) [14]. It allows for grading of MV leaflet calcification, thickening, mobility as well as subvalvular thickening. Generally, a score of ≤8 with no more than moderate MR is thought to be the ideal candidate for PBMV [15]. Patients with higher scores should be considered for surgical interventions if surgical risk is not prohibitive. One notable limitation of the Wilkins score is the lack of inclusion of information regarding commissural fusion or calcification. If the restrictive pathology lies more in the MV leaflets without significant commissural fusion or if there is presence of significant commissural calcifications, the effectiveness of PBMV is likely to be limited and may potentially be harmful.

Patients with non-rheumatic disease generally have significant annular and valvular calcification and thus make poor candidates for PBMV or surgery. Intervention is only recommended as a last resort and after extensive discussions with patient and family regarding high procedural risk.

Table 10 Common MS hemodynamic parameters used to assess severity

	Advantages	Disadvantages
Planimetry (by 2D or 3D)	– Direct measurement – Independent from other cardiac factors	– Not always feasible due to imaging quality or calcifications – User experience dependent
Pressure half-time (PHT)	– Easy to obtain – Can help derive MVA	– Can be affected by other cardiac factors (i.e. AI, LA/LV compliance)
Mean gradient (MG)	– Easy to obtain	– Can be affected by other cardiac factors (i.e. HR, forward flow)
Systolic pulmonary artery pressure	– Readily available in most studies	– Indirect estimate of RA pressure – No estimation of pulmonary vascular resistance
PISA	– Independent of flow conditions	– Technically difficult – User experience dependent

Adapted from Baumgartner et al. [12]
LA left atrium, *LV* left ventricle, *AI* aortic insufficiency, *RA* right atrium, *MVA* mitral valve area, *PHT* pressure half-time, *PISA* proximal isovelocity surface area

Table 11 Wilkins score adapted from Wilkins et al. [14]

Grade	Leaflet mobility	Leaflet calcification	Leaflet thickness	Subvalvular thickening
0	Normal	None	Normal	None
1	Highly mobile leaflets with only leaflet tips restricted	Single area of increased echo brightness	Leaflets near-normal thickness (4–5 mm)	Minimal thickening just below leaflets (i.e. mild chordal thickening)
2	Leaflet mid- and basal portions have normal mobility	Scattered areas of brightness limited to leaflet margins	Midleaflets normal, considerable leaflet tip thickening (5–8 mm)	Thickening of chordal structures extending to one-third of chordal length
3	Valve continues to move in diastole, mainly from the base	Brightness extending into mid leaflets	Extension of thickening through entire leaflet (5–8 mm)	Thickening of chordal structures extending to the distal third of chordae
4	No or minimal forward leaflet motion in diastole	Extensive brightness throughout the leaflet tissue	Significant thickening of entire leaflet (>8–10 mm)	Extensive chordal thickening and shortening extending down to the papillary muscles

Diagnosis and Pre-procedural Assessment

When assessing any patient for possible intervention for their MS, their indication as well as anatomical suitability for intervention must be thoroughly investigated. The ACC/AHA practice guideline for patients with valvular heart disease recommendations for intervention for severe MS can be seen in Fig. 15.

The evaluation process starts with confirming the diagnosis and severity of MS. On review of the most recent TTE of our patient, we can appreciate thickened MV leaflets with restricted opening on both the PLAX and apical four chamber view but without significant annular or valvular calcifications (Videos 28 and 29). The classic "hockey stick" appearance seen in rheumatic MS is noted on the PLAX view (Fig. 16). Color Doppler evaluation shows flow acceleration through the MV as well as flow convergence zone where a PISA can be measured even without baseline shifting the color Doppler scale (Fig. 17). These findings strongly suggest significant MS along with a likely rheumatic etiology.

For further evaluation of severity of MS, quantitative evaluation is needed (Fig. 18). Some measures of MS severity for our patient are noted in Table 12 and demonstrate a significantly abnormal MG, PHT and MVA. These findings classify our patient as stage D (Table 9). The morphology of the valve seen on TTE fits with the severity

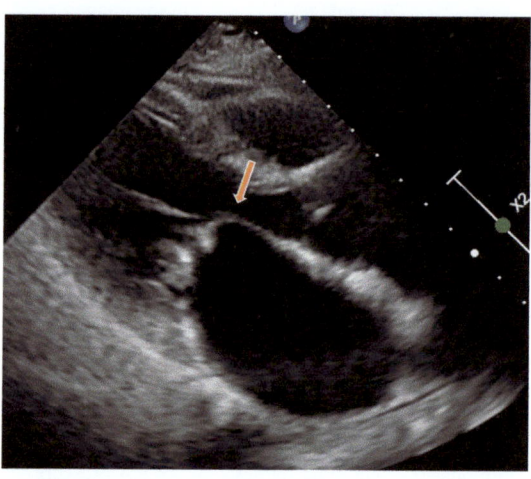

Fig. 16 Classic "hockey stick" appearance of the anterior leaflet (arrow) of the rheumatic MV during valve opening

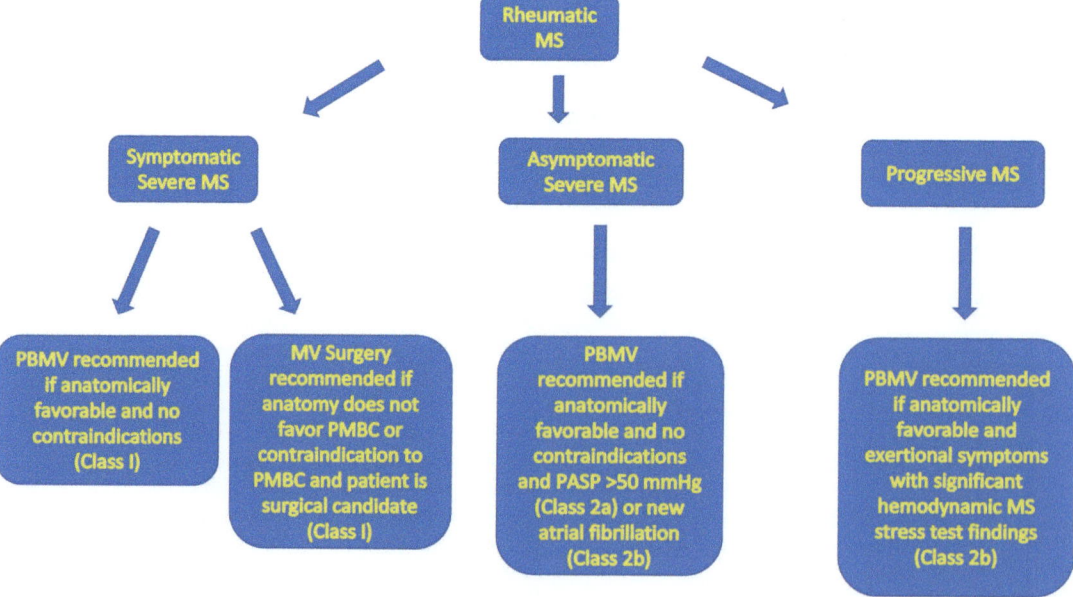

Fig. 15 Indication for intervention for rheumatic MS adapted from the 2020 ACC/AHA practice guideline for valvular guidelines [1]

markers measured on TTE and furthermore, these findings provide a reasonable explanation of our patients worsening symptoms. The next step after confirmation of severe, symptomatic MS due to a rheumatic etiology is to refer our patient to a multi-disciplinary valve team for further evaluation for suitability of intervention.

If a patient with MS presents with discrepancies between clinical symptoms and echocardiographic findings, an exercise stress echo with hemodynamic assessment should be considered (class I, level of evidence C-LD) [1]. Exercise testing may unmask significant MS with increased cardiac workload.

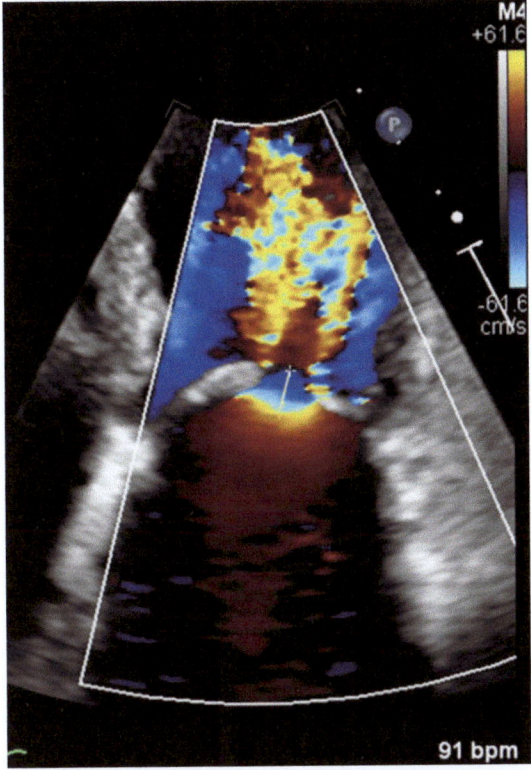

Fig. 17 Zoom view of the apical 4C demonstrating a flow convergence zone at the MV even without baseline shift in Doppler scale

Table 12 Relevant pre-procedural MV Echocardiographic findings for our patient

Transthoracic echocardiogram parameter	Patient's findings
Mean gradient	15 mmHg (at HR 85)
PHT	173 ms
MVA by planimetry (TEE)	0.86 cm^2
Wilkins score	6/16
Mitral regurgitation	Mild

PHT pressure half-time, *MVA* mitral valve area

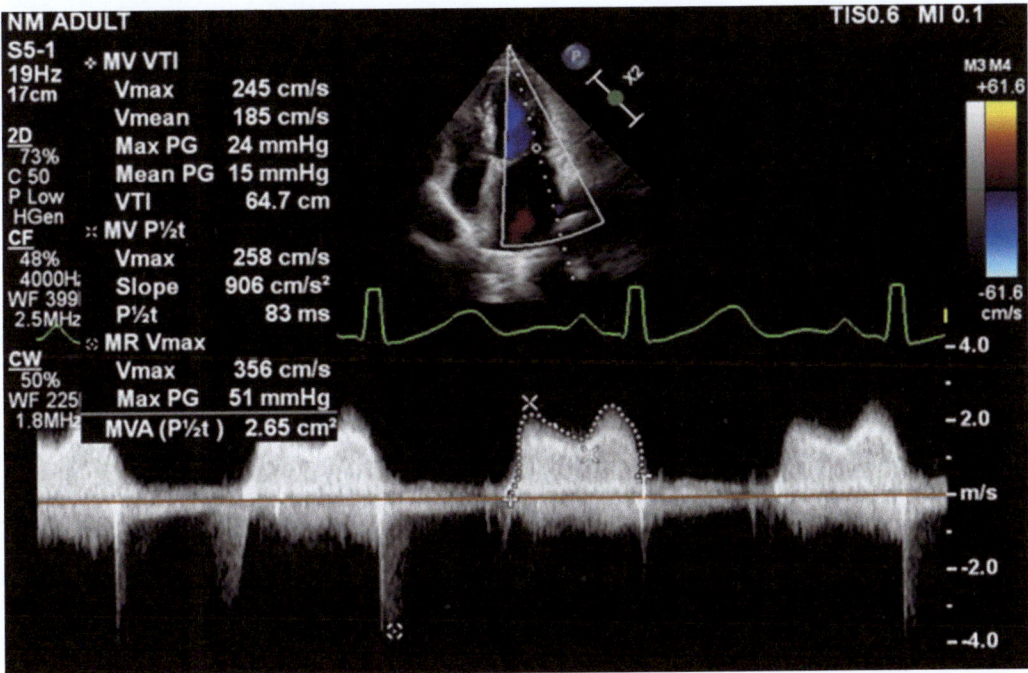

Fig. 18 CW Doppler evaluation through the MV showing MG 15 mmHg at HR 85. PHT is noted to be 173 ms which would lead to a calculated MVA of 1.3 cm^2. All these criteria classify this patient in the severe MS range

Heart Team Approach and Discussion

With a diagnosis of severe symptomatic MS, our patient has a class I recommendation for undergoing PBMV if her MV is anatomically favorable and she is without any contraindications to the procedure [1]. Our patient's Wilkins score was 6/16 with commissural fusion and without significant commissural calcifications. She was noted to have mild MR and was without any other significant valvular lesions.

A TEE is needed prior to a patient proceeding to a PBMV to assure there is no thrombus in the LA and LAA. A TEE can also help further define MV morphology and anatomic suitability as well as evaluating MS severity (Videos 30 and 31 and Figs. 19a, b and 20). A TEE in our patient confirmed the TTE findings of severe MS and ruled out presence of LA or LAA thrombus (Fig. 19c).

Selection of an appropriate balloon size is a critical factor during procedure planning. Balloon size has been shown to be predictive of both post procedure MR severity as well as MS gradient reduction [16]. Some literature has advocated sizing based on height or body surface area. Another approach is to measure the MV annular diameter and use it as a reference for the maximal balloon size for the procedure [15]. For our patient, the MV annular size was measured ~27 mm and so the decision was made to use a 26 mm balloon (Fig. 21a and b).

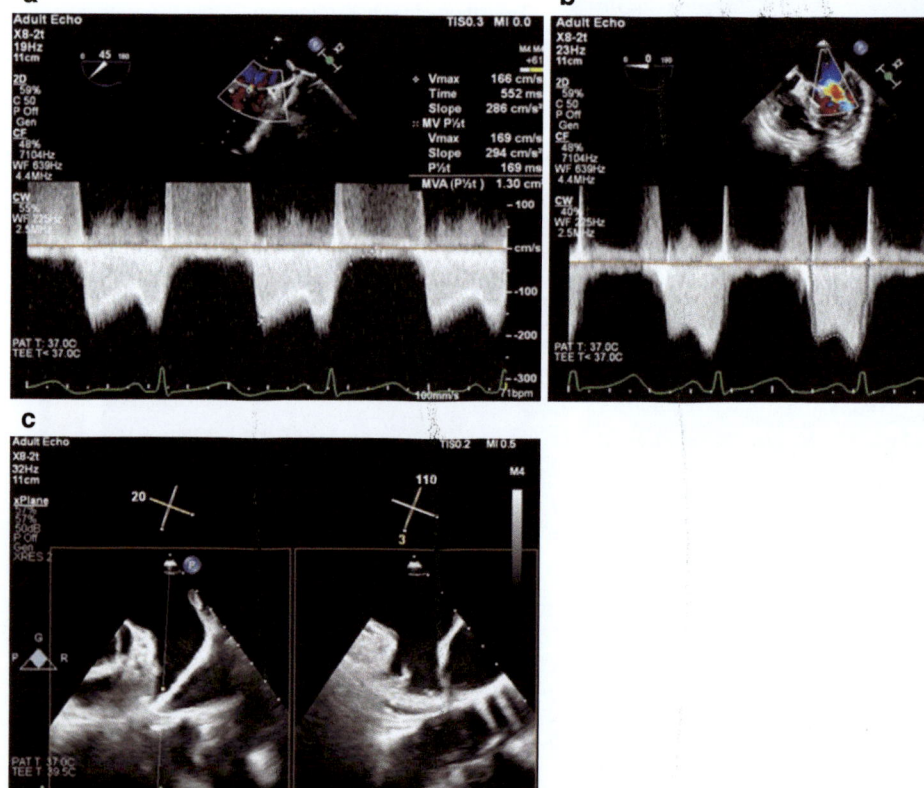

Fig. 19 Figure demonstrates key images from our patient's TEE. Severe MS is confirmed by pressure half time (**a**) and mean mitral valve gradient (**b**). It is important to note the hemodynamic measures can be underestimated during TEE in the presence of anesthesia. (**c**) Shows no thrombus in the LAA

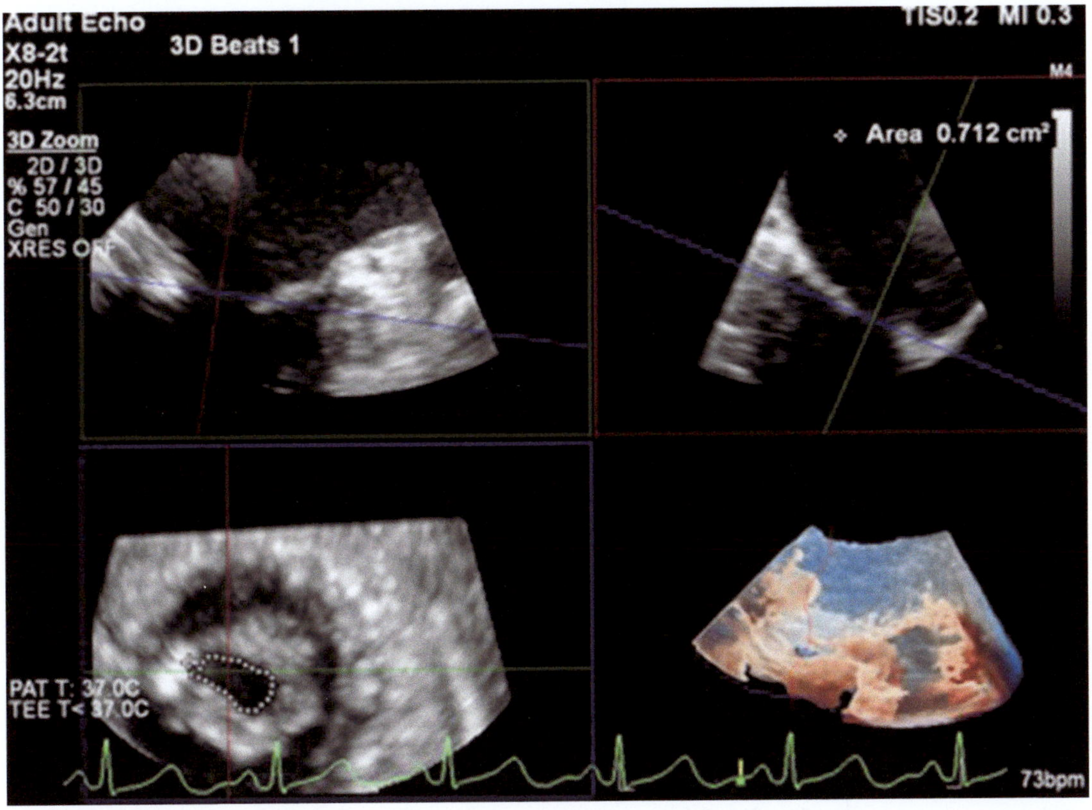

Fig. 20 3D multi-planar reconstruction of MV with TEE demonstrates MVA of 0.712 cm² by planimetry

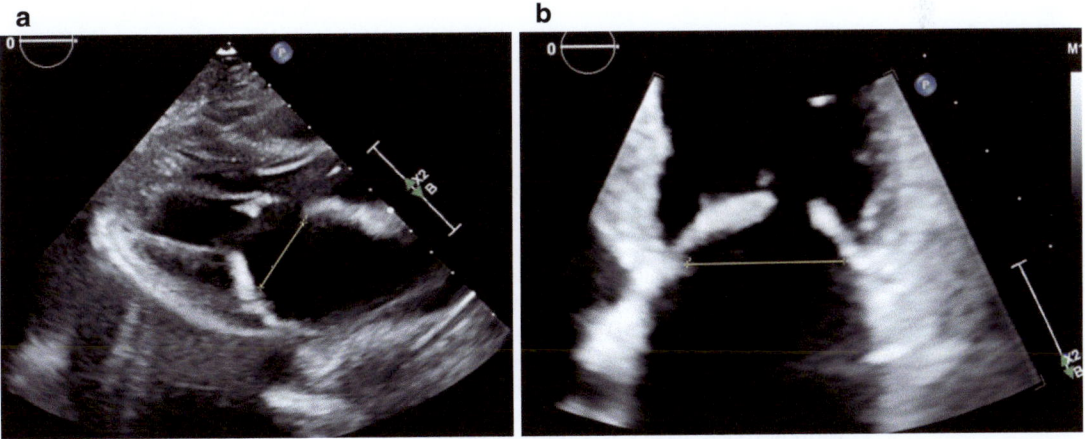

Fig. 21 MV annular size measured at 27 mm on both the PLAX view (**a**) and a zoomed in apical 4C (**b**)

Heart Team Decision

Having a Wilkins score ≤8, commissural fusion without significant calcification along with mild MR makes our patient an ideal candidate for PBMV. She has no contraindications for PBMV (Table 13). MV replacement surgery is a Class I recommendation for patients with severe symptomatic MS with unfavorable anatomic features for PBMV and who are not at prohibitive surgical risk (Class I recommendation). The same recommendation applies for patients who have failed prior PBMV or have an another indication for cardiac surgery [1].

Table 13 Contraindications to PBMV

Contraindications to PBMV
Significant valvular or commissural calcification
MS without commissural fusion
Another indication for cardiothoracic surgery (i.e. severe CAD)
Greater than moderate MR
LA or LAA thrombus
Concomitant significant AV or TV disease

Intraprocedural Imaging Modalities and Measurements

Intraprocedural imaging guidance can be provided using TEE or intracardiac echocardiography (ICE). In our patient, TEE was used for intraprocedural guidance. Below are the key steps and imaging highlights of a typical PBMV procedure.

Key procedural steps	Key imaging highlights	Correlated video/figure
Transeptal puncture	– Optimal position of transeptal puncture is the center of fossa ovalis – Adequate atrial septal tenting is needed to assess catheter positioning – Confirm crossing of tip of catheter into LA	– 2D ME bicaval view for superior-inferior positioning with biplane which allows for anterior-posterior positioning – Figure 22a and b
Delivery system guidance	– Aid in guidewire positioning in to the LA followed by advancing of delivery system over the wire and into the LA	– 2D ME 4Ch and 2Ch views with biplane
Device positioning	– Aid in placing the balloon across the MV where the distal half of the balloon rests in the LV	– 3D ME enface view and ME 2C with biplane can also be utilized – Videos 32, 33 and 34
Balloon inflation	– Once proper positioning is confirmed, the balloon is inflated across the MV for a few seconds only and then deflated – Multiple balloon inflations can be attempted until a successful outcome is achieved as long as there is no worsening of MR. For each subsequent attempt, the balloon is repositioned across the MV with imaging guidance, and generally inflated to a larger size (typically in increments of 1 mm) – Careful MV TEE evaluation is needed after every balloon inflation. A successful outcome is when >50% reduction in the MV gradient or MVA >1.5 cm² is achieved without significant worsening of MR – For our patient, the balloon was inflated to 24 mm (maximum 26 mm). No further inflations were performed since there was >50% reduction in the mean gradient and MR appeared to worsen (Videos 36, 37 and 38, Fig. 24a and b)	– 3D ME enface view and ME 2C with biplane can also be utilized. Fluoroscopy imaging can also be helpful in visualizing balloon expansion – Videos 32, 33, 34, 35, 36, 37 and 38 – Figures 23a–c and 24a–c
Delivery system withdrawal	– Under echocardiographic guidance, confirm slow withdrawal of the device across the septum into the RA – Once in the RA, the device can be fully removed	– 2D ME 4Ch and 2Ch views with biplane
Immediate post procedure evaluation	– The residual atrial septal shunt with left to right flow should be evaluated and documented – Pericardial space should be evaluated for any effusion	– 2D ME bicaval view is best utilized for CW measurement through the septal defect – Figure 24c

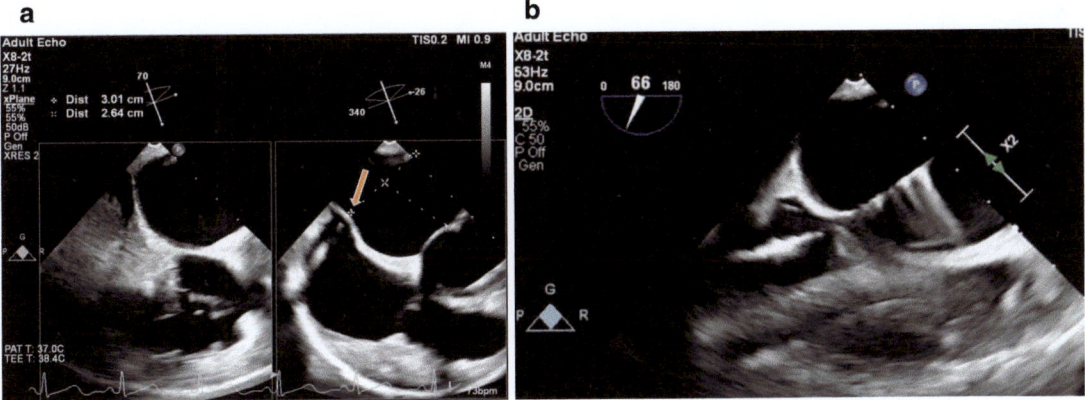

Fig. 22 (**a**) Shows TEE imaging during transeptal puncture positioning (arrow) and imaging confirmation of catheter crossing into the LA (**b**)

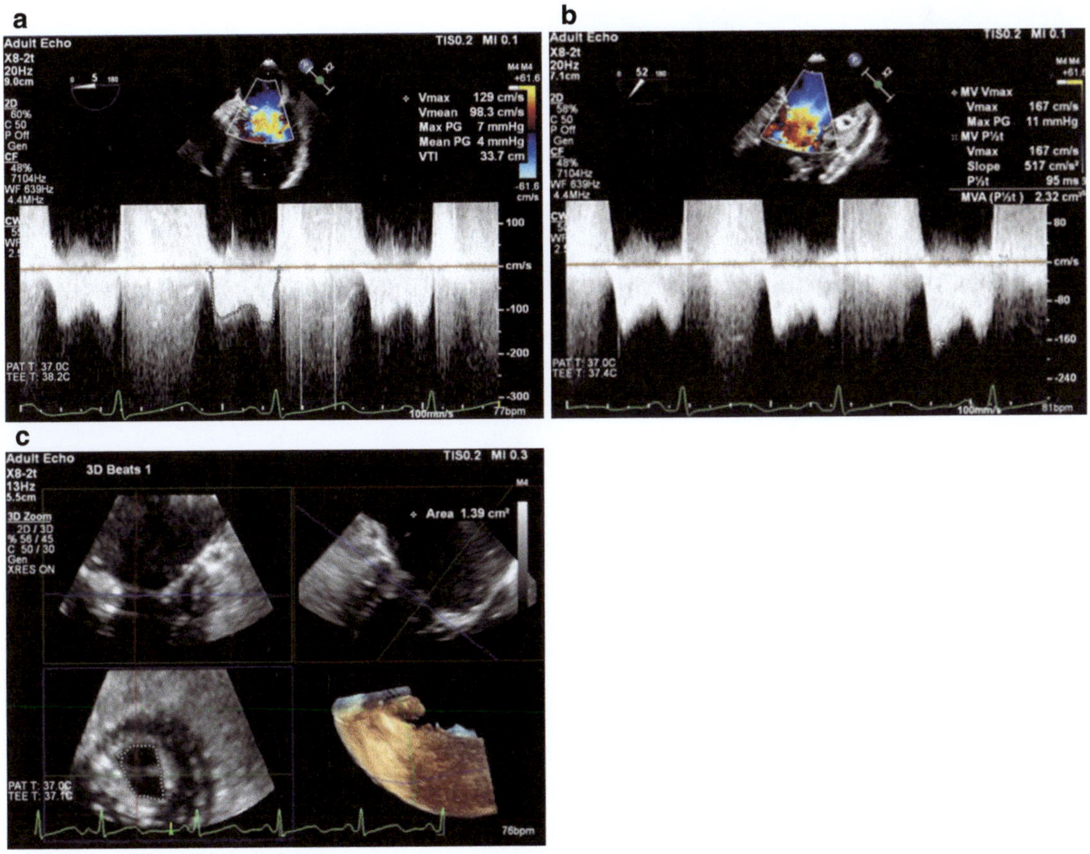

Fig. 23 MS severity measures immediately after first balloon inflation. Both MG and PHT (**a** and **b**) show a significant (>50%) improvement. MVA has also improved significantly to 1.39 cm^2 (**c**)

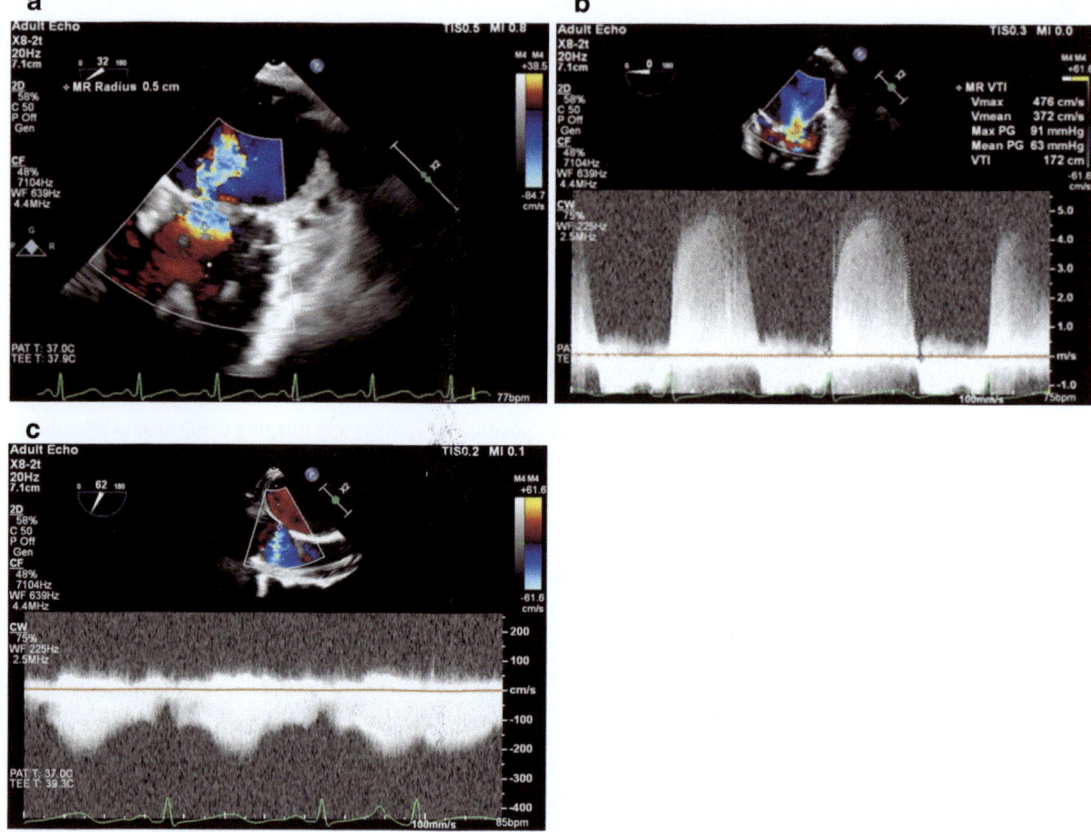

Fig. 24 MR severity measured immediately post balloon inflation. MR PISA (**a**) measurement and CW MR signal (**b**) is shown. (**c**) Residual left to right shunt is noted in the atrial septum

Post procedural Assessment

A TTE is often repeated the next day, typically prior to discharge, to re-assess the MV and to evaluate for any post procedural complications (Table 14). Our patient received her 1 day post procedure TTE which showed a MG of 7 mmHg (HR 72) and a MVA of 1.62 cm² along with moderate MR (Table 15). At 1 month follow up clinic visit, she reported symptomatic improvement as she was able to do more activity without significant dyspnea. TTE should be repeated annually or sooner based on clinical symptoms. At 1 year follow up, our patient continued to do well clinically and TTE findings remained unchanged.

When anatomically favorable patients undergo PBMV, long term outcomes appear to be good. The recurrence of symptomatic MS after a successful PBMV has previously noted to be between 7 to 21% [17]. This case demonstrates the importance of comprehensive evaluation of patients with MS with a specific focus on anatomical favorability for PBMV which can lead to good outcomes for patients.

Multimodality imaging comparison

Table 14 Possible procedural complications to PMBV

Procedural complications
Cardiac chamber perforation
Tamponade
Severe MR
Thromboembolism
Clinically significant left to right shunt

Table 15 Relevant 1 day post procedure MV TTE findings for our patient

Transthoracic echocardiogram parameter	Patient's findings
Mean gradient	7 mmHg (at HR 72)
PHT	173 ms
MVA by planimetry (TTE)	1.62 cm²
Mitral regurgitation	Moderate (EROA 22 m², regurgitant volume 36 mL)

PHT pressure half-time, *MVA* mitral valve area

Modality	Clinical application	Limitations
Transthoracic echocardiography (TTE)	– First line test for assessment of etiology, mechanism and severity of mitral stenosis – Post procedural assessment of mitral stenosis and surveillance of complications	– Lower spatial resolution compared to TEE – Body habitus and artifact may limit adequate assessment of mitral valve
Transesophageal Echocardiography (tee)	– Can aid in the preprocedural evaluation of MS if TTE yields incomplete or discordant findings – Can obtain more precise information about valve anatomy and pathology – Intraprocedural imaging guidance – Immediate post procedure evaluation and evaluation for complications – Rule out LAA thrombus	– Some absolute contraindications include upper GI anatomical considerations, active upper GI bleeding – Requires sedation
Exercise stress echocardiography	– Can aid in pre-procedural planning when discordant findings between clinical symptoms and echocardiographic findings	– Mobility limitations of patient
Cardiac computed tomography (CT)	– Can aid in pre-procedural planning if any concern for atypical anatomy	– No hemodynamic assessment – Radiation exposure
Fluoroscopy	– Intraprocedural guidance	– Limited anatomic assessment – Invasive – Radiation exposure

Clinical Controversies and Clinical Pearls

- The etiology of mitral stenosis (i.e. rheumatic vs. non-rheumatic disease) is key when assessing for possible treatment options as they differ considerably in relation to etiology.
- In patient with severe mitral stenosis due to rheumatic disease, PBMV has shown to be safe and effective when compared to surgery and as such has become the first line treatment when anatomically suitable.
- While the Wilkins Score is a great tool in assessing anatomic suitably for PBMV, it is important to understand its limitations, such as information regarding commissural fusion not being part of the score which can have significant impact on treatment success.
- Exercise stress testing can serve as a valuable tool in assessing patients with MS as it may unmask significant MS with increased cardiac workload.

Key Points
- Echocardiographic imaging, both TTE and TEE, play an integral role in the diagnostic evaluation as well as the pre, intra and post procedural phases of patients with mitral stenosis being considered for PBMV.
- Several studies have established the safety and efficacy of PBMV when compared with surgical techniques and as such PBMV has become the initial procedure of choice in patients with favorable anatomy.
- Clinical and anatomical suitability of patients with mitral stenosis undergoing PBMV and operator expertise are the two most important factors that determine long term success.

Mitral Valve-in-Valve

Case Study

A 75-year-old woman with a past medical history significant for mitral valve endocarditis complicated by an embolic cerebrovascular accident with residual right sided hemiplegia s/p mitral valve replacement (25 mm Edwards Magna bioprosthetic valve) 7 years prior, hypertrophic obstructive cardiomyopathy (HOCM) s/p septal myectomy, non-obstructive coronary artery disease, hypertension and hyperlipidemia who presented to the hospital with a complaint of progressive shortness of breath × 1 week.

Her vital signs were temperature 96.8 °F, heart rate 78 beats/minute, blood pressure 111/63 mmHg and respiratory rate of 20 breaths/minute.

On physical exam she appears alert but anxious, bibasilar rales were noted on lung auscultation with 1+ bilateral lower extremity edema, mildly elevated JVD. Heart exam revealed a regular rate and rhythm with a grade 2/6 systolic murmur at left sternal border. Right sided upper and lower extremity weakness was also noted.

Her electrocardiogram (Fig. 25) showed sinus rhythm with evidence of left atrial enlargement and a chronic left bundle branch block. Chest X-ray obtained was significant for perihilar vascular congestion and interstitial edema suggestive of decompensated heart failure (Fig. 26).

Initial troponin I was <0.045 ng/mL, pro BNP 9626 pg/mL, hemoglobin 16.1 g/dL, and creatinine 0.9 mg/dL.

Her admission diagnosis was acute decompensated heart failure for which she was initiated on IV furosemide diuretic therapy and an urgent 2D echocardiogram was ordered for further evaluation.

2D Echocardiogram demonstrated preserved LV systolic function (Videos 39 and 40) with degeneration of the bioprosthetic valve with restricted leaflet excursion (Fig. 27 with corresponding Video 41) and flow acceleration noted across the bioprosthetic mitral valve on color Doppler (Fig. 28 with corresponding Video 42).

Doppler evaluation of the prosthetic mitral valve noted a peak velocity of 3.4 m/s, mean gradient of 27 mmHg at HR of 84 bpm, PHT: 216 ms, a calculated EOA of 0.70 cm^2 and a DVI of 4.9 (Fig. 29a, b). Findings consistent with severe bioprosthetic stenosis with specific parameters essential to access mitral prosthesis listed in Table 16 [18]. This was also associated with secondary findings of pulmonary hypertension with RVSP calculated at 65 mmHg and left atrial enlargement as shown in Fig. 30a, b.

Given 2D echo findings she was also initiated on metoprolol succinate to reduce her heart rate and improve her diastolic filling period.

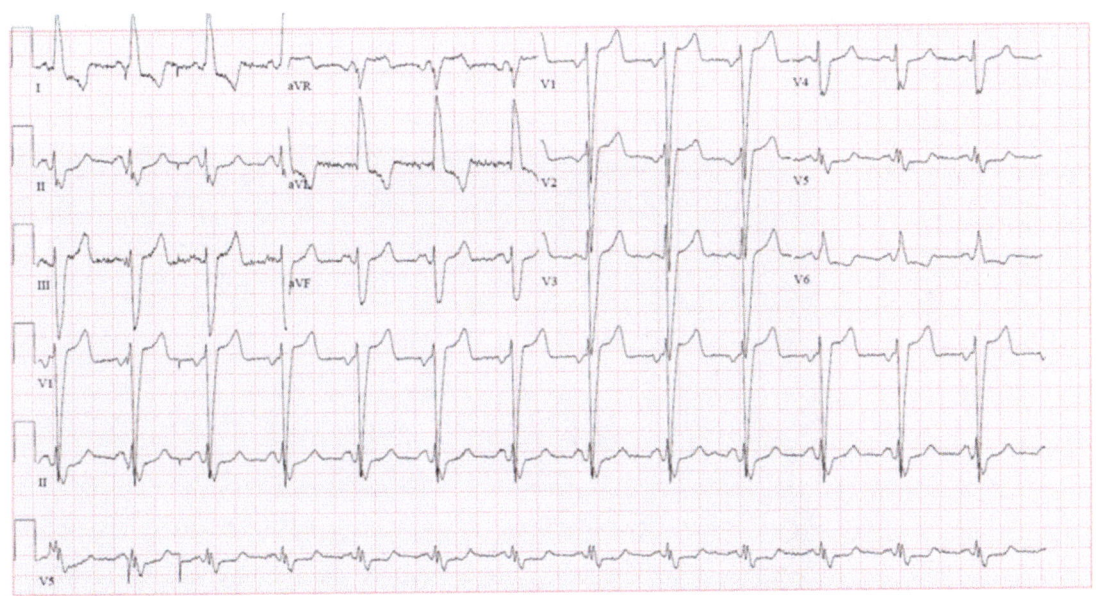

Fig. 25 Electrocardiogram showing sinus rhythm with left bundle branch block and evidence of left atrial enlargement

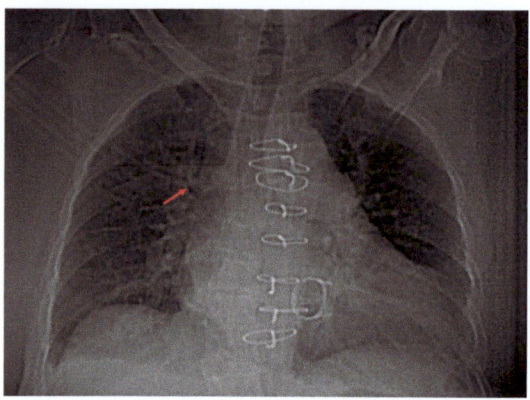

Fig. 26 Posterior-anterior chest X-ray showing perihilar vascular congestion and interstitial edema

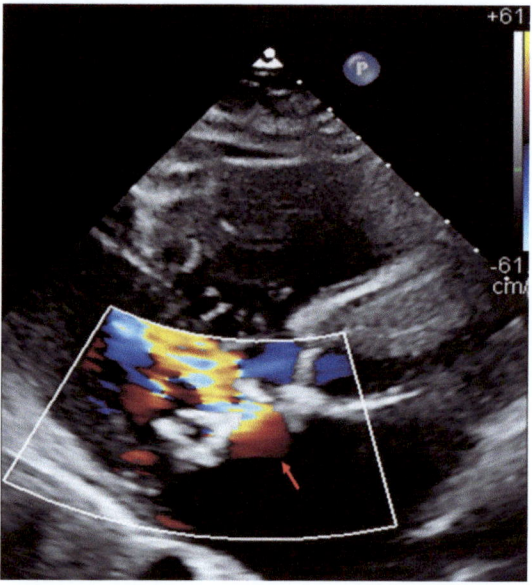

Fig. 28 Color Doppler interrogation shows diastolic flow acceleration across the bioprosthetic mitral valve as indicated by red arrow

Fig. 27 Zoomed PLAX view of the bioprosthetic mitral valve with degeneration and restricted leaflet excursion at end diastole

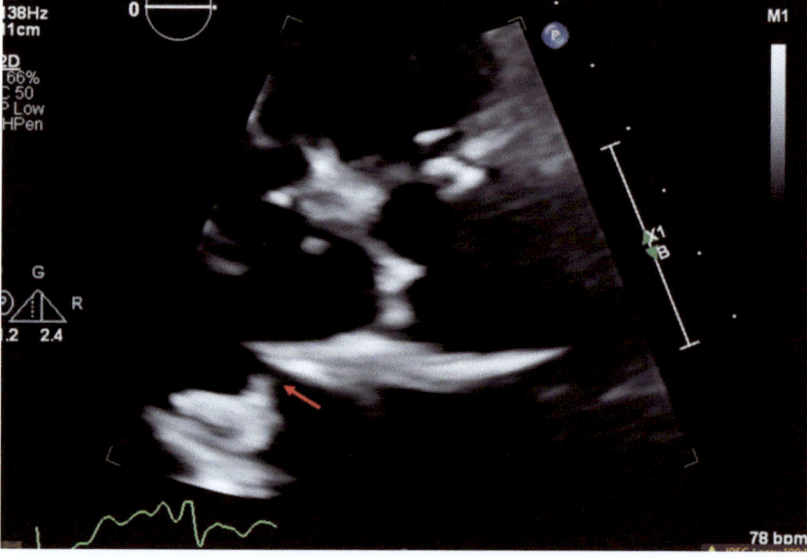

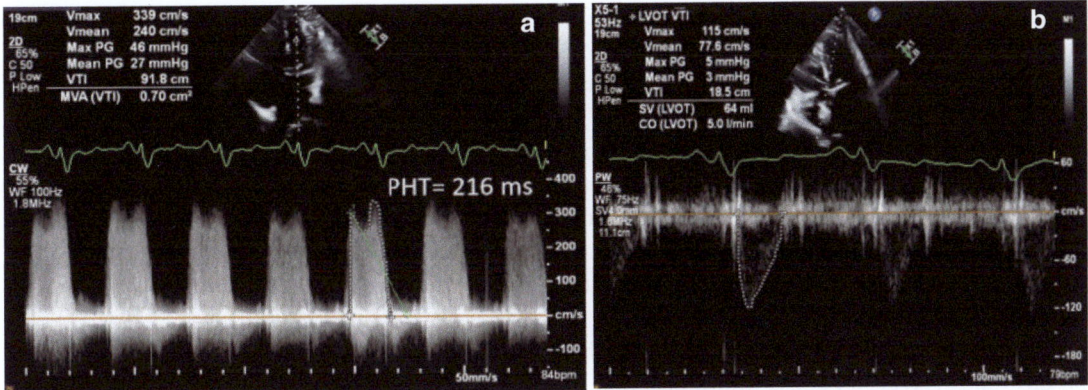

Dimensionless index: VTI prMV/VTI lvot
91.8÷18.5 = 4.9

Fig. 29 (a) Continuous wave Doppler profile across the mitral valve prosthesis. (b) Pulse wave Doppler profile at LVOT

Table 16 Spectral Doppler parameters required for evaluation of mitral prosthetic function

	Normal	Possible stenosis	Significant stenosis
PHT (ms)	<130	130–200	>200
Peak velocity (m/s)	<1.9	1.9–2.5	>2.5
Mean gradient (mmHg)	≤5	6–10	>10
DI:VTI_{prMV}/VTI_{lvot}	<2.2	2.2–2.5	>2.5
EOA (cm^2)	≥2.0	1–2	<1

Adapted from Zoghbi et al. [18]

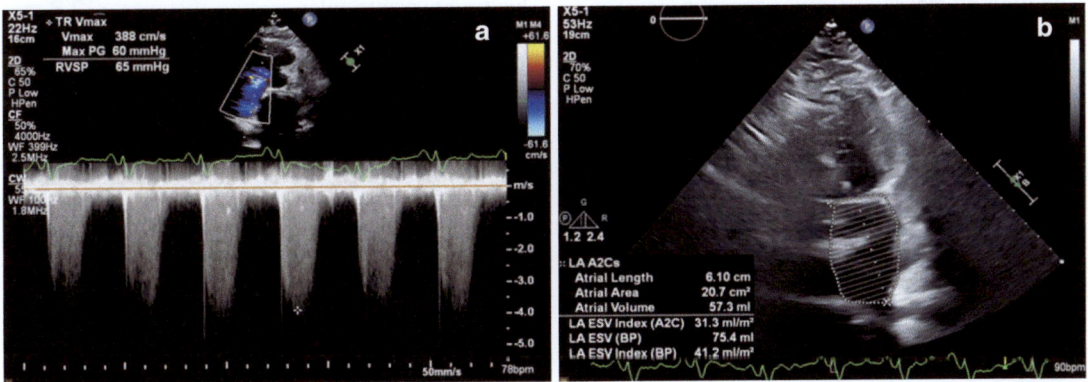

Fig. 30 (a) Continuous wave Doppler profile across the tricuspid valve. (b) 2-CH view of the left atrium showing enlargement

Background and Definitions

Reoperation of failed bioprosthetic valves is associated with significant morbidity and mortality estimated at 3–23% [19–21].

In majority of cases, bioprosthetic mitral valve dysfunction occurs due to cusp calcification resulting in leaflet thickening and stiffening, which may result in valve stenosis with or without concomitant regurgitation. Valve dysfunction can also occur due to pannus overgrowth or thrombus with a 15-year reintervention rate of 40% [22].

Mitral valve in valve (MViV) can be performed by transeptal or transapical approaches under transesophageal echocardiography (TEE) and fluoroscopic guidance.

The Edwards SAPIEN valve (Edwards Lifesciences) is the most used valve for MViV intervention. This is a low-profile, balloon-expandable, bovine pericardial transcatheter valve mounted on a chromium cobalt frame designed for transcatheter aortic valve replacement and is currently used on a compassionate-use basis in the mitral position [23, 24].

Recent outcome studies have shown favorable 30-day and 1-year all-cause mortality rate at 5.4% and 16.7% respectively with excellent technical success and sustained improvement in echo derived mitral valve gradient [24]. Clinical improvement in heart failure at 1 year following intervention has also been reported but there remains a paucity of data on long term outcomes [24, 25].

Inclusion Criteria for MViV Intervention

- Failed bioprosthetic mitral valve disease with mitral stenosis or mitral regurgitation at high or prohibitive risk for redo-operation on evaluation by a cardiovascular surgeon.
- Absence of contraindications to anticoagulation given need for anticoagulation with warfarin post valve implantation.
- Absence of contraindication to transesophageal imaging needed to guide the procedure.
- Not at risk of LVOT obstruction.

Diagnosis and Pre-procedural Evaluation

Pre-procedural evaluation of MViV intervention includes a detailed evaluation of the mechanism of prosthetic valve dysfunction with TTE and TEE. Cardiac computed tomography plays an important role for evaluation of implant valve sizing, optimal fluoroscopic angles, and risk of LVOT obstruction.

The mitral valve anatomy is complex and is near the left ventricular outflow tract (LVOT) which makes preprocedural evaluation crucial.

CT allows for evaluation of the spatial relationship between the aortic and mitral valves to allow appropriate valve and predict whether MViV will result in obstruction of the left ventricular outflow track [26].

The presence of LVOT obstruction is associated with a 34.6% mortality rate and a 19.2% rate of conversion to surgery. Historically, up to 50% of cases rejected for MViV are due to the risk of LVOT obstruction [26–28].

Recent studies have evaluated the risk and predictors of LVOT obstruction in transcatheter mitral valve replacement with use of pre-procedural cardiac CT to identify a threshold of neo-LVOT area to discriminate the risk for LVOT obstruction. The cutoff values of 170–189 mm^2 predict LVOT obstruction with a sensitivity of 96.2–100% respectively in observational studies [27, 29]. The predicted neo-LVOT area is derived using a simulated balloon-expandable transcatheter heart valve in the failed bioprosthetic valve on CT cross sectional imaging at end systole [30].

Other anatomical and device related factors may predispose patients to narrowing of the neo-LVOT dimension including greater device protrusion into the left ventricle, device flaring at its left ventricular outflow tract and a smaller mitral annulus to interventricular septum distance <17.8 mm due to a more pronounced septal bulge [27, 30].

Given findings of severe bioprosthetic mitral valve stenosis on our patient, a TEE was performed for a more detailed evaluation of the mitral valve prosthesis and to evaluate the mechanism of the mitral stenosis and rule out a left atrial appendage thrombus.

On the 4-CH transesophageal view (Fig. 31, Video 43), there is thickening and calcification of the prosthetic valve leaflets with associated restricted diastolic excursion (red arrow) and associated spontaneous echo contrast visualized in the left atrium (yellow arrow).

This restricted diastolic excursion of the leaflets and calcification is also appreciated on 3D imaging (Fig. 32) with no evidence of tissue overgrowth/pannus resulting in obstruction from the atrial or ventricular view as seen in Fig. 33a, b respectively with corresponding Videos 44 and 45.

On color Doppler interrogation, there is flow acceleration noted across the bioprosthetic mitral

Fig. 31 TEE 4-CH view showing thickening and calcification of the prosthetic valve leaflet and spontaneous echo contrast visualized in the left atrium

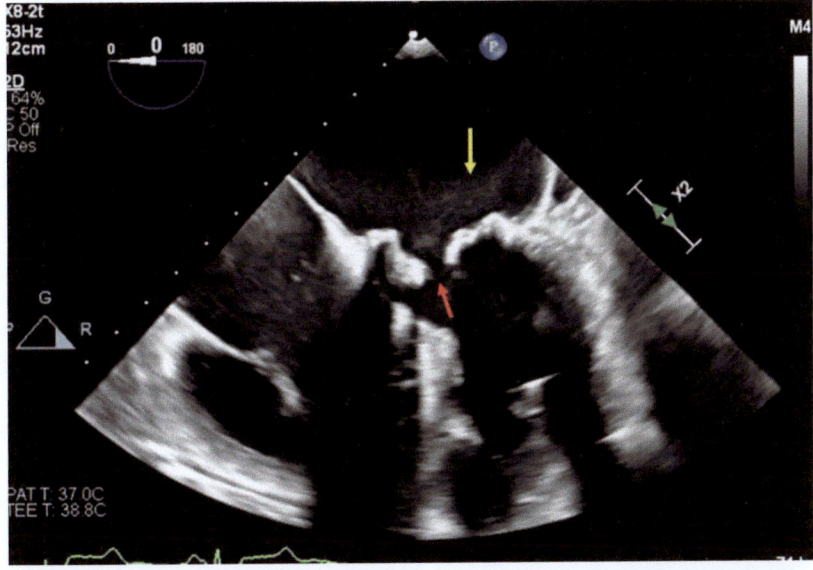

Fig. 32 3D image of the mitral valve prosthesis with restricted diastolic excursion of the leaflets and calcification

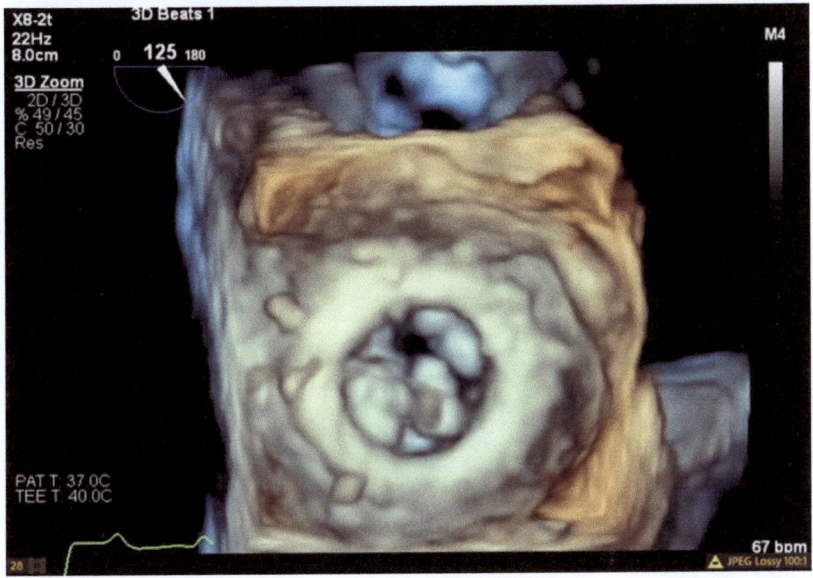

valve (Fig. 34) with mild mitral regurgitation noted (Video 46). Spectral Doppler assessment showed a mean gradient of 18 mmHg at a heart rate of 72 bpm (Fig. 35). Flow in the left ventricular outflow tract (LVOT) was assessed from the deep gastric view and was noted to be normal. The mean gradient was 1 mmHg and peak gradient was 4 mmHg (Fig. 36).

Evaluation of the left atrial appendage showed no evidence of thrombus (Fig. 37).

Given TEE confirmation of structural degeneration of the prosthesis resulting in mitral stenosis, the heart valve team was consulted.

On recommendation by the heart valve team, she underwent a right and left heart catheterization. Angiography showed 40% stenosis of the mid LAD (Fig. 38, yellow arrow) and 70% ostial diagonal branch stenosis (Fig. 38, red arrow) with no significant stenosis seen in the right coronary circulation as seen in Fig. 39 with corresponding Video 48.

Right heart Cath performed showed PCWP 26, PA 72/30, RV 70/12, RA 10, PA sat 67%, Ao

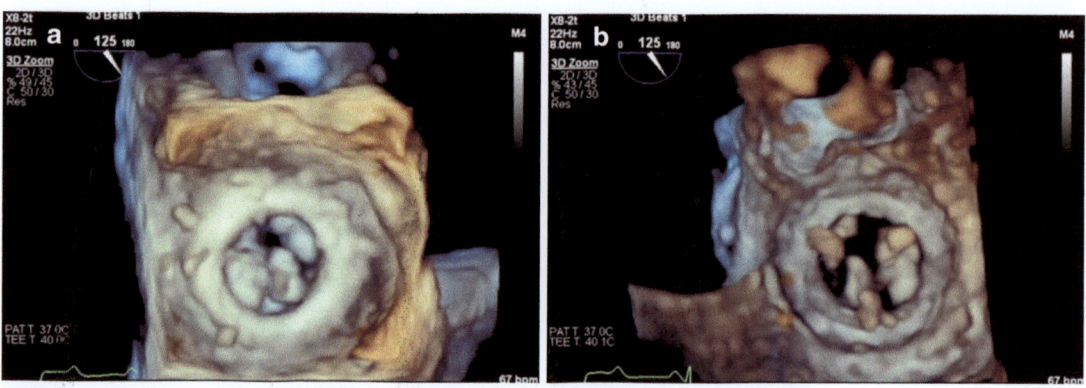

Fig. 33 (a) 3D image of the mitral valve prosthesis from the left atrial perspective. (b) 3D image of the mitral valve prosthesis from the left ventricular perspective

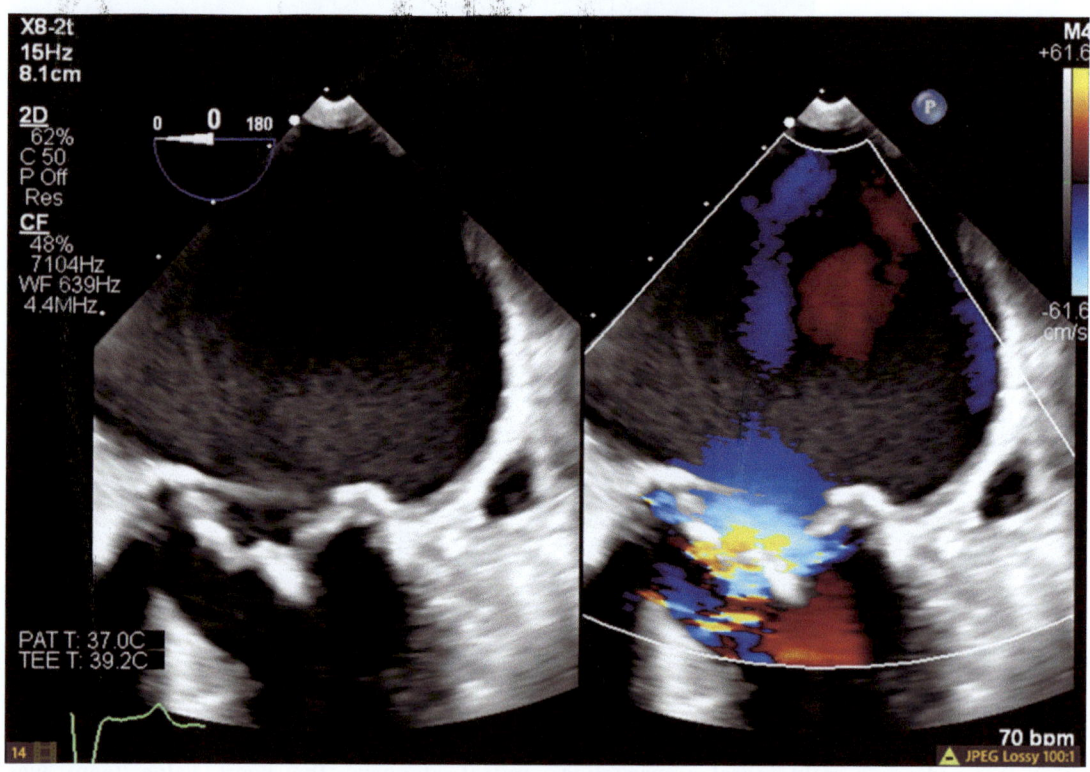

Fig. 34 TEE mid esophageal view with color flow Doppler across the mitral valve prosthesis

sat 89%, cardiac output 5.3 L/min findings consistent with severe post capillary pulmonary hypertension.

She was evaluated by cardiothoracic surgery for redo mitral valve operation but was considered high risk given calculated STS mortality risk score of 15.9% based on the presence of very severe mitral stenosis, acute decompensated heart failure, severe pulmonary hypertension, and history of CVA with residual right sided weakness.

Given her high risk for re-do mitral valve surgery she was evaluated for a transcatheter mitral valve-in-valve intervention and underwent a gated cardiac CT performed for evaluating candidature for TMVR.

CT findings as shown in Fig. 40 depicts a Neo-LVOT area of 180 mm^2, septal-mitral distance of 4.9 mm and an aorto-mitral angle of 58.20°. She was determined to be at high risk for LVOT obstruction given the neo-LVOT area <189 mm^2.

Multimodality Imaging of Mitral Valve Diseases: TEER, Valve in Valve, and Beyond

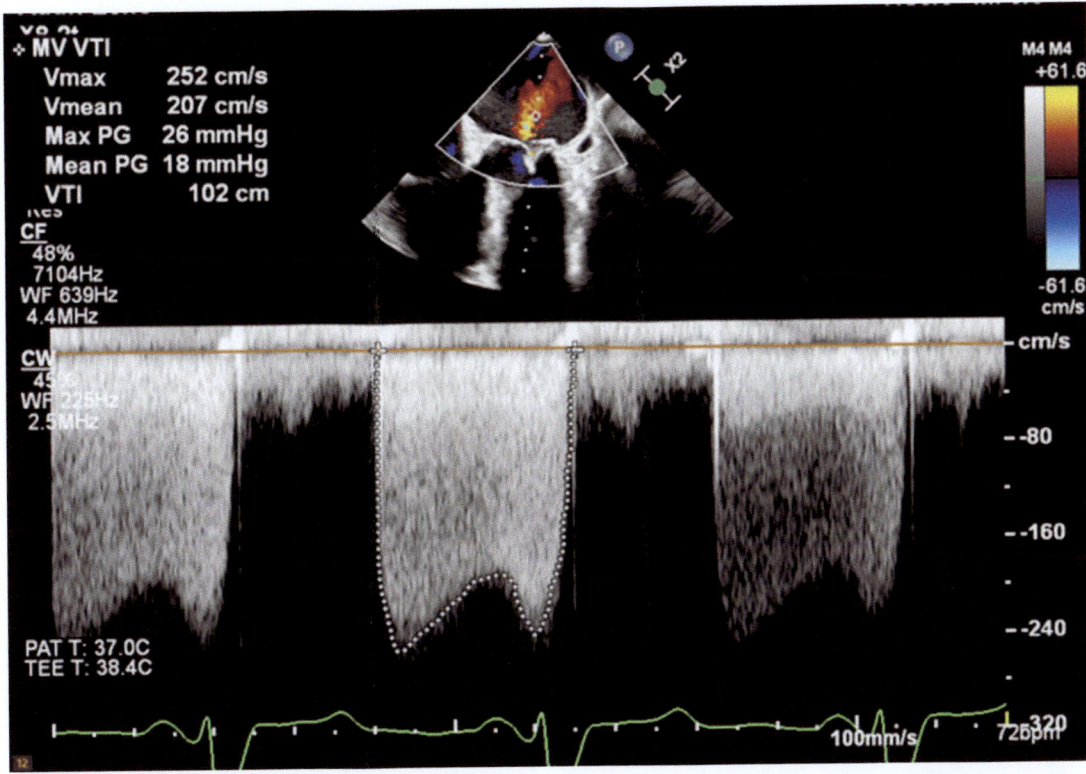

Fig. 35 Continuous wave Doppler profile across the mitral valve prosthesis

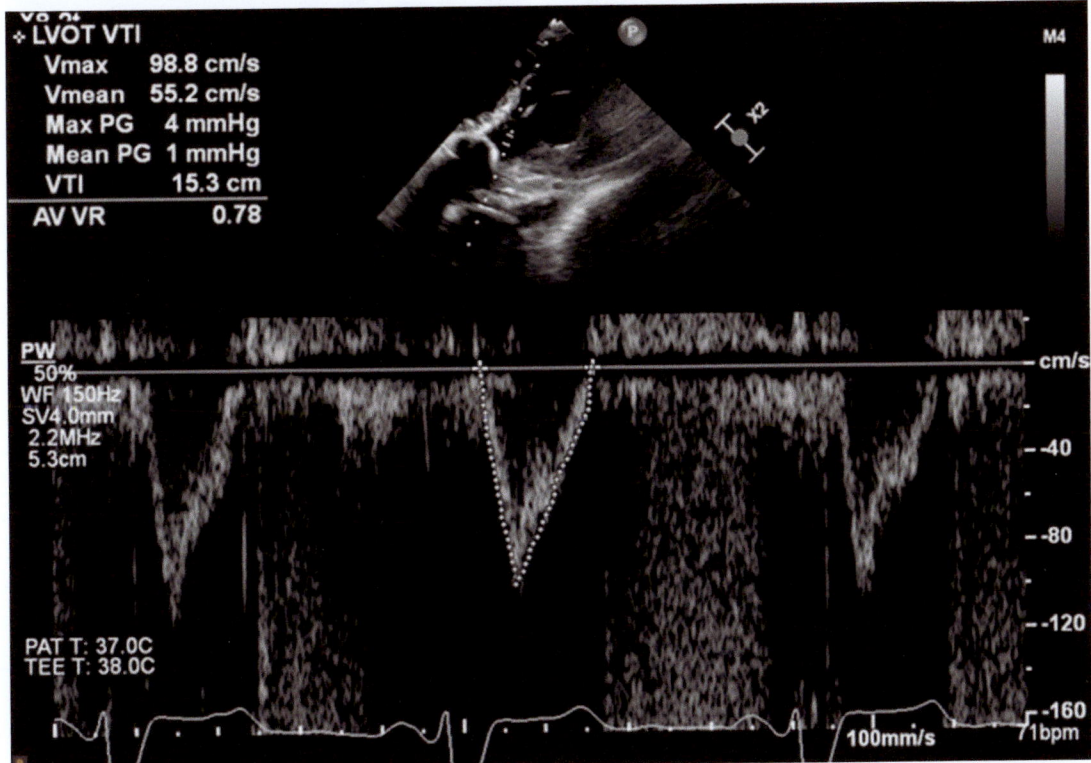

Fig. 36 TEE transgastric view with pulse wave Doppler profile at LVOT

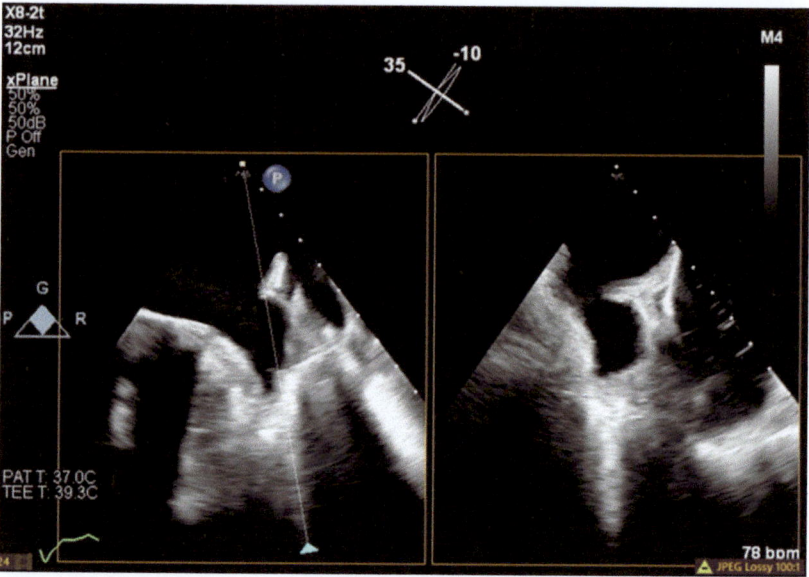

Fig. 37 TEE biplane image of the left atrial appendage shows no evidence of thrombus

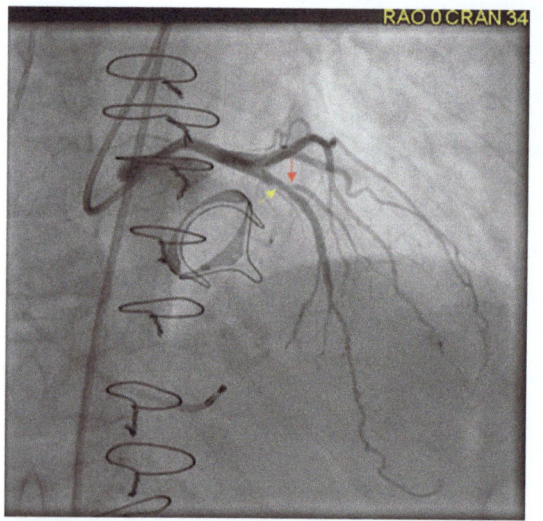

Fig. 38 Coronary angiogram of the left coronary artery with moderate stenosis of the LAD (yellow arrow) and severe stenosis of the ostial diagonal branch (red arrow)

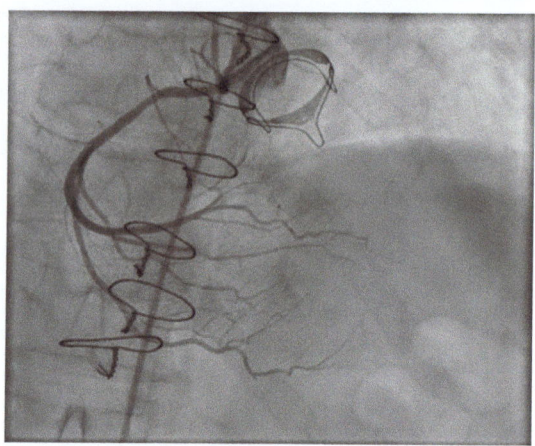

Fig. 39 Coronary angiogram of the right coronary artery

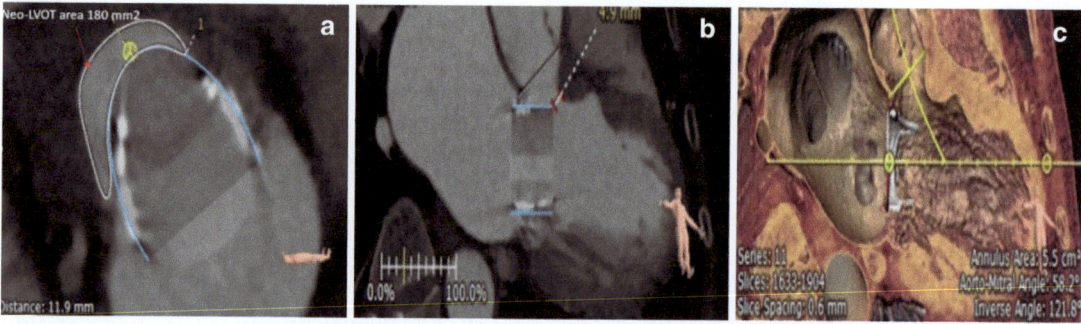

Fig. 40 (**a**) Cardiac CT derived neo-LVOT area. (**b**) 3-CH view showing septal-mitral distance. (**c**) 3D volume rendered CT image showing aorto-mitral angle

Heart Team Approach and Discussion

Given the elevated risk for LVOT obstruction and re-do mitral valve surgery, discussions were had about how best to reduce the risk of obstruction to allow for a successful MViV procedure.

There are two current strategies to reduce the risk of LVOT obstruction prior to TMVR and this includes the Lampoon procedure which is a transcatheter based radiofrequency laceration of the anterior leaflet of the mitral valve via transfemoral retrograde approach as demonstrated allowing blood flow through the open cells of the alloy frame of the prosthesis [31].

Alcohol septal ablation (ASA) has been used as a preemptive strategy to reduce the risk of LVOT obstruction by increasing the neo-LVOT area prior to TMVR or as a bail out strategy in treating LVOT obstruction that occurred following TMVR [32, 33].

The heart team determined that ASA before MViV would be the safest approach for our patient. ASA was performed with selective ablation of the first septal perforator branch as shown in Fig. 41a with corresponding Video 49 with localized septal target region visualized with intracoronary contrast administration as seen in Fig. 41b with no outflow tract obstruction on spectral Doppler evaluation at baseline as seen in Fig. 42.

Procedure was complicated by complete heart block, and she underwent a dual chamber permanent pacemaker placement.

A repeat cardiac CT performed 1 month following alcohol septal ablation showed significant increase in the neo-LVOT area measured at 255 mm² as shown in Fig. 43.

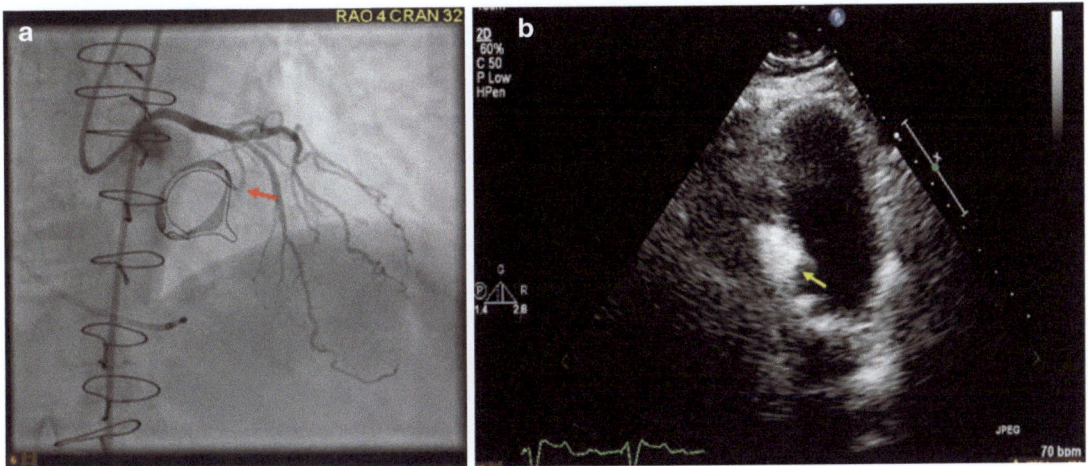

Fig. 41 (a) Selective ablation of the first septal perforator branch (red arrow). (b) 2D echo showing septal target region visualized with intracoronary contrast administration (yellow arrow)

Fig. 42 Continuous wave Doppler profile across the aortic valve shows no evidence of obstruction

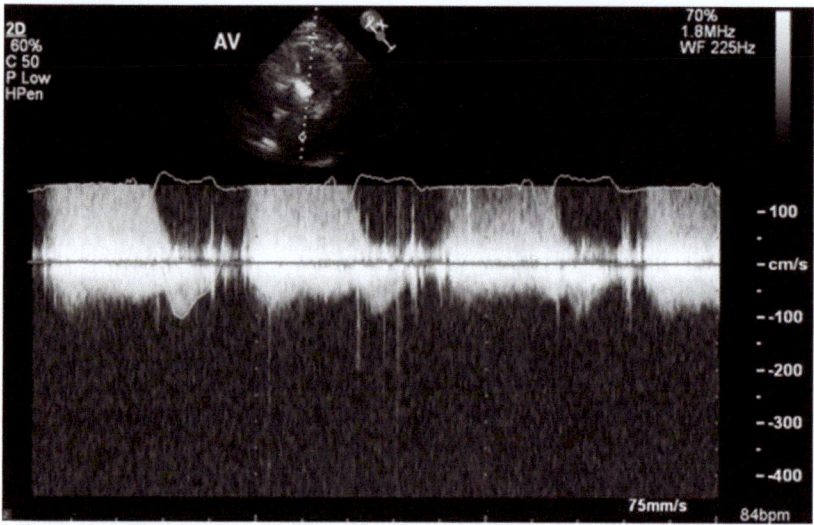

Vmax = 1.04 m/s
Mean gradient = 1.95 mmHg
Peak gradient 4.3 mmHg
VTI = 16 cm

Fig. 43 Cardiac CT derived neo-LVOT area 1 month following alcohol septal ablation

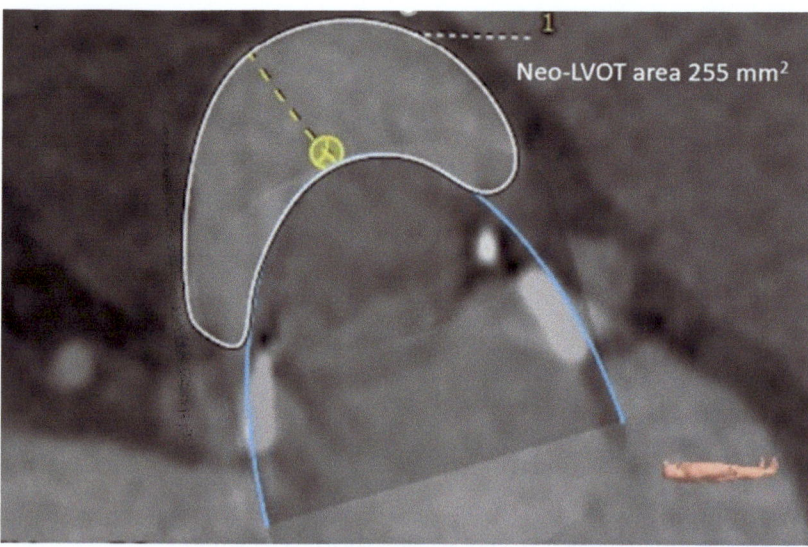

Heart Team Decision

Given improvement in the projected neo-LVOT area, the decision was made by the multidisciplinary heart team to proceed with a MViV procedure 2 months following her alcohol septal ablation.

Intraprocedural Imaging and Assessment

Patient was placed under general anesthesia and baseline intraprocedural TEE showed no significant changes in her prosthetic valve anatomy compared to her prior echo with a mean gradient measured at 22 mmHg at a heart rate of 69 bpm.

Vascular access was obtained in bilateral femoral veins and a 5-F pacing catheter was advanced into the right ventricle via the left femoral vein for rapid pacing during valve deployment. A 14 French sheath was then placed in the right femoral vein over a stiff wire without difficulty. Unfractionated heparin (200 U/kg) was administered to ensure adequate systemic anticoagulation, and the activated clotting time was monitored regularly to maintain a level >300 s.

Under TEE and fluoroscopic guidance, a transseptal puncture was made at the mid fossa using a BRK needle within an SL 1 dilator/sheath with a transeptal height measured at 3.42 cm to the bioprosthetic mitral valve (Fig. 44a) and a guidewire was advanced to the left upper pulmonary vein (Fig. 44b).

The SL 1 dilator/sheath was then exchanged for an NXT small curl steerable guide sheath (Abbott, Chicago, Illinois). A stiff Safari 2 wire (Boston Scientific, Marlborough, Massachusetts) was directed into the left ventricle apex under TEE and fluoroscopic guidance and the atrial septum was sequentially dilated with a 14 mm Mustang (Boston Scientific, Marlborough, Massachusetts) balloon (Fig. 45 with corresponding Video 50).

Following septal dilation, a 26 mm Edwards Sapien 3 Ultra valve was advanced through the interatrial septum and into the 25 mm Edwards Magna bioprosthetic valve.

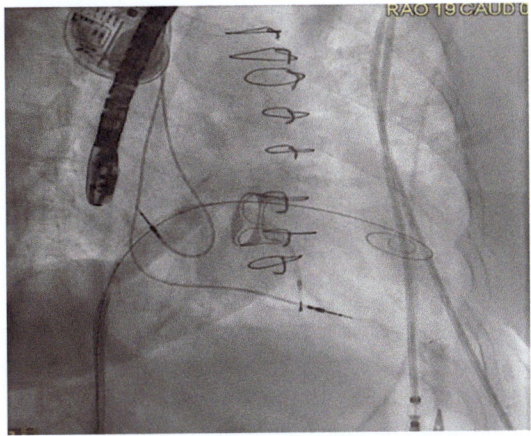

Fig. 45 Fluoroscopic image showing balloon dilation of the interatrial septum

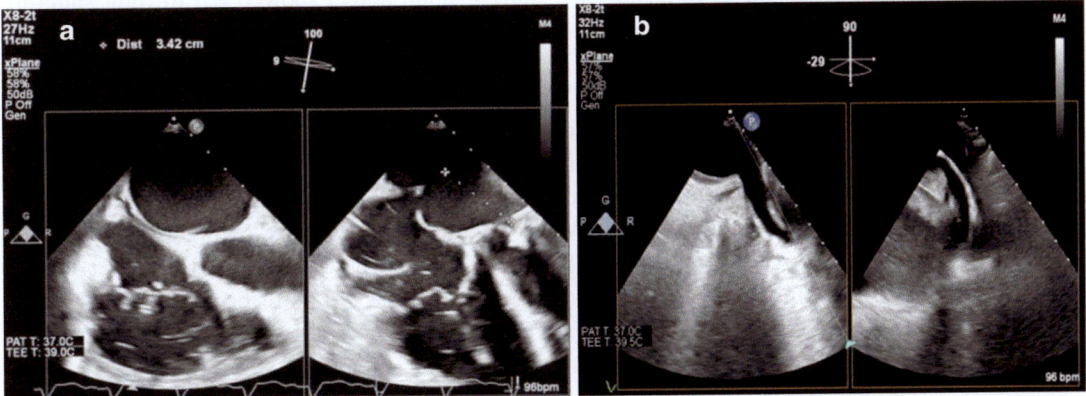

Fig. 44 (**a**) TEE showing point of transeptal puncture with measured distance to mitral valve prosthesis. (**b**) TEE image showing guidewire parked in left upper pulmonary vein

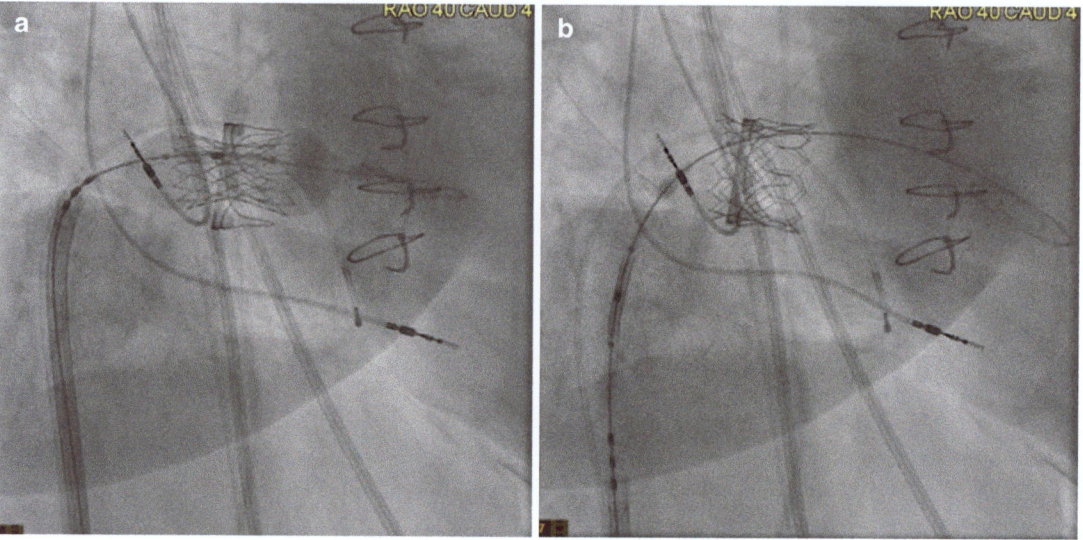

Fig. 46 Fluoroscopic images depicting deployment of the Sapien 3 valve under rapid pacing

Following adequate valve alignment under fluoroscopic imaging, the Sapien 3 valve was successfully deployed under rapid pacing (Fig. 46a, b with corresponding fluoroscopic (Video 51) and TEE (Video 52) videos).

Post procedural Assessment

Post procedural evaluation following valve deployment include:

- Evaluation of the LVOT gradient by TEE from the deep transgastric view.
- 2D evaluation of the prosthesis to ensure the valve is wall seated and leaflets show normal excursion.
- Color Doppler assessment with 2D and 3D imaging for evaluation of transvalvular and perivalvular regurgitation. 3D imaging helps in the localization of the origin of paravalvular regurgitation that can occur following MViV intervention (Fig. 47 with corresponding Video 53) and is useful in guiding transcatheter based closure (Fig. 48 with corresponding Video 54).
- Spectral Doppler evaluation across the prosthesis for assessment of MV gradient.

Following the procedure on our patient, the gradient assessment of the LVOT revealed no evidence of obstruction with a peak gradient of 9 mmHg and mean gradient of 4 mmHg (Fig. 49).

There was significant reduction in the mean gradient across the prosthetic mitral valve from 22 mmHg at HR of 69 bpm to 3 mmHg at 71 bpm with normal diastolic excursion of the valve leaflets post procedure (Fig. 50).

Color Doppler evaluation on 2D and 3D imaging showed trivial transvalvular regurgitation and no paravalvular regurgitation (Fig. 51 with corresponding Videos 55, 56).

Spectral Doppler evaluation of the iatrogenic atrial septal defect showed left to right shunting (Fig. 52) which was not closed.

30 days post intervention, a follow up 2D echocardiogram was obtained with noted preserved biventricular systolic function, a valve-in-valve prosthesis that appears well seated with (Fig. 53 with corresponding Video 57).

There is no valvular regurgitation noted on color Doppler assessment (Video 58) and mean gradient across MV prosthesis was measured at 7.6 mmHg at heart rate of 74 bpm with no LVOT obstruction (Fig. 54a, b) (Table 16).

Multimodality imaging comparison

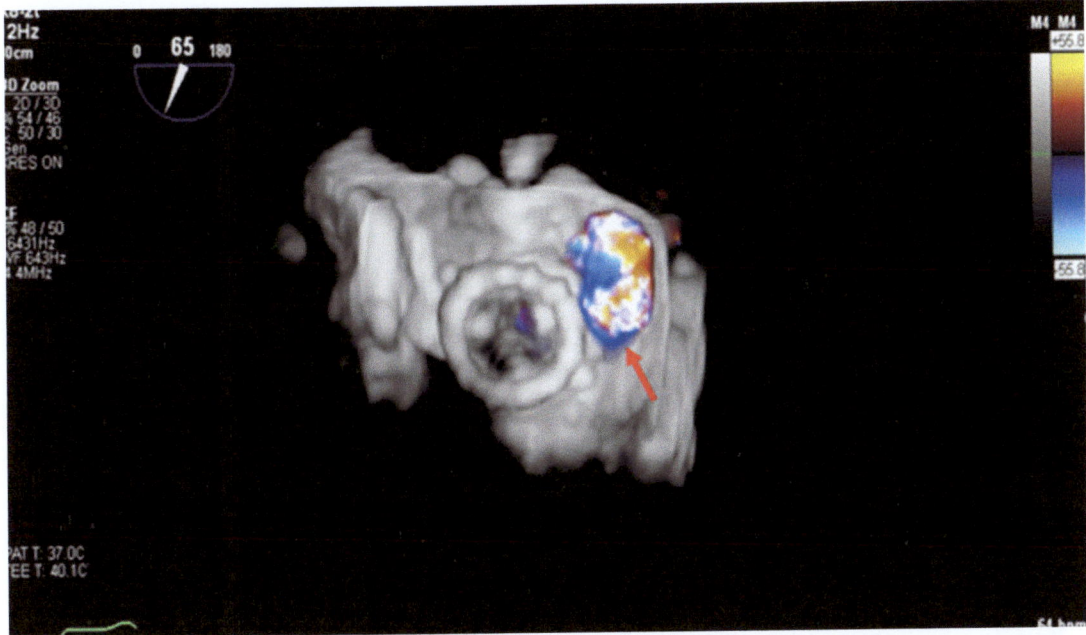

Fig. 47 3D color Doppler image depicting a moderate perivalvular leak lateral to a prosthesis following MViV (red arrow)

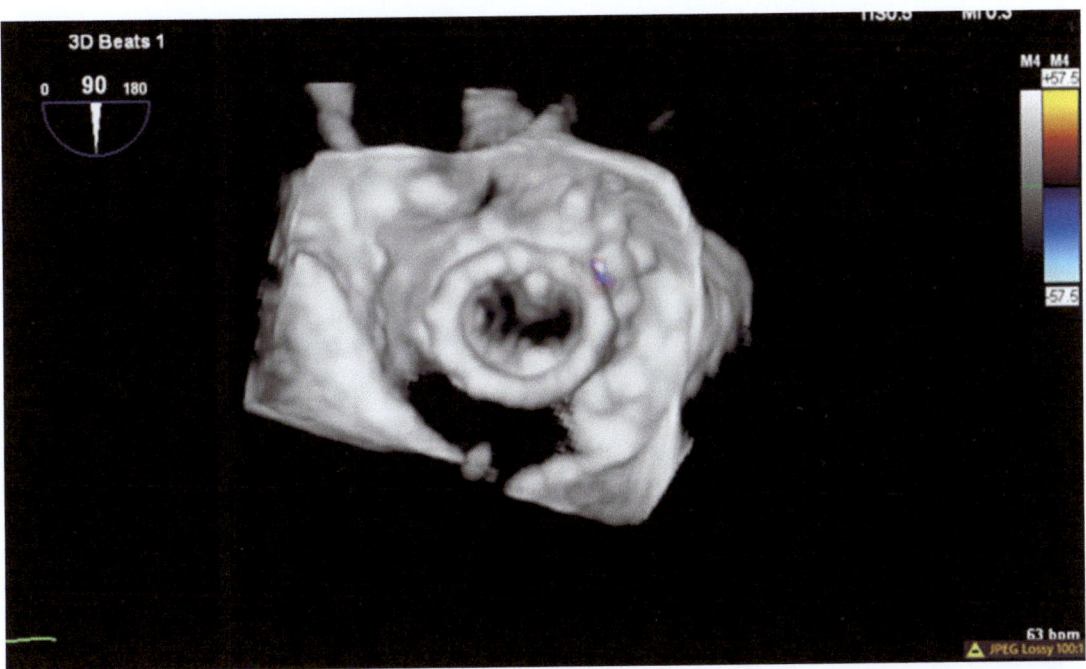

Fig. 48 3D color Doppler image following successful paravalvular leak closure with Amplatzer plugs with trace residual regurgitation

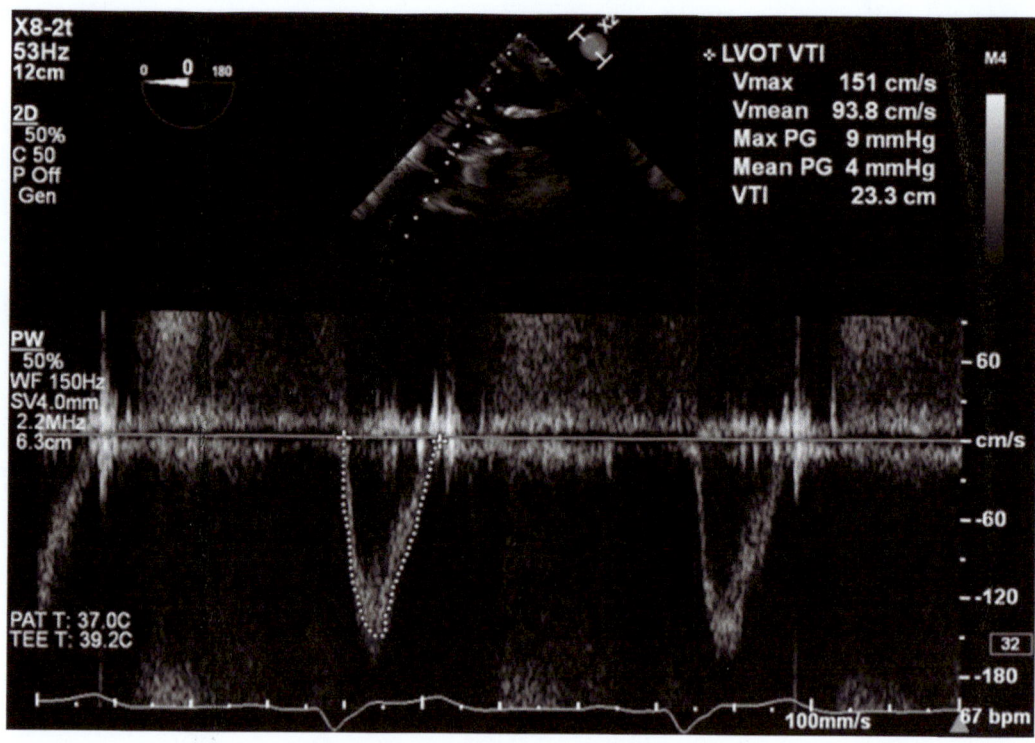

Fig. 49 Pulse wave Doppler profile of the LVOT shows no elevated gradient

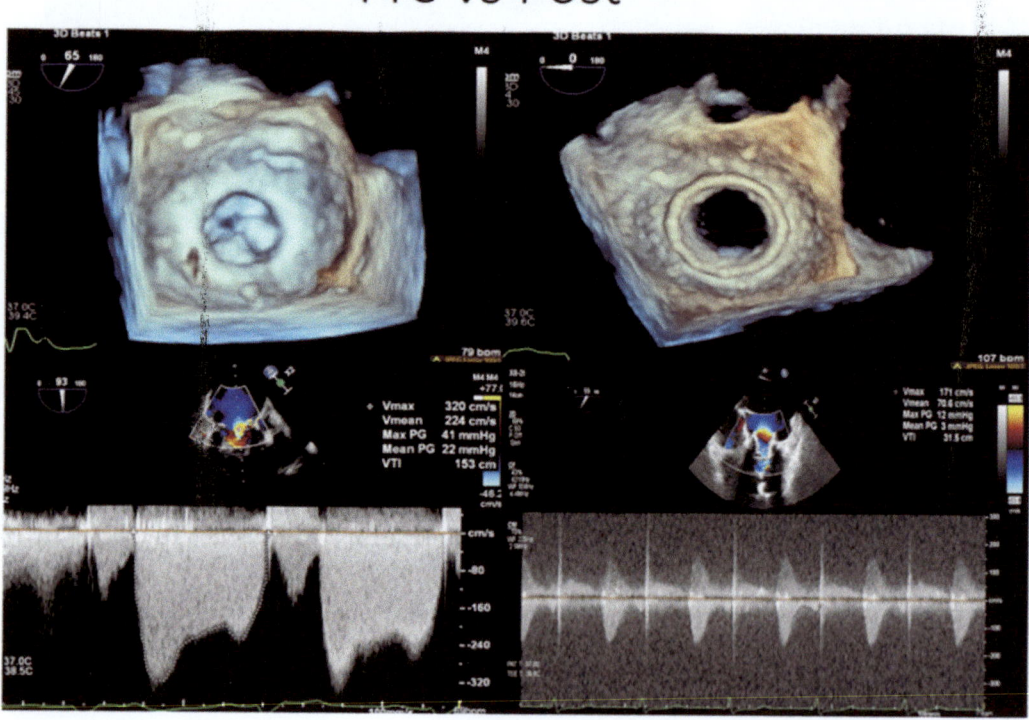

Fig. 50 Continuous wave Doppler across the mitral valve prosthesis pre and post intervention

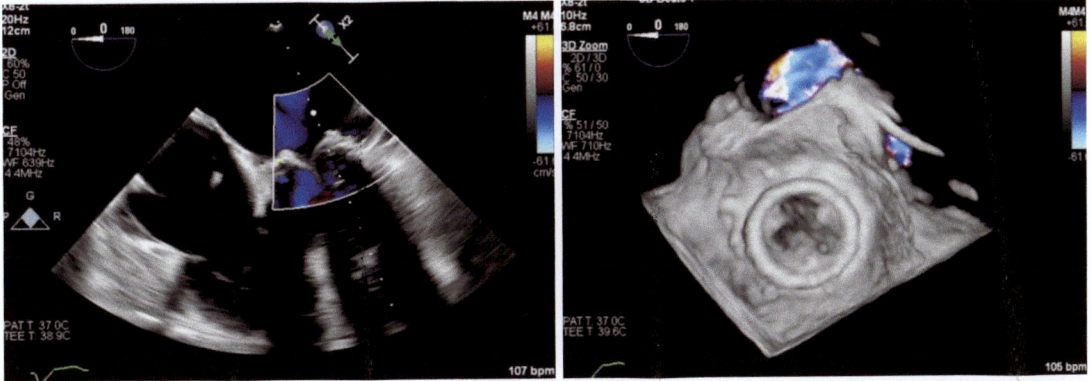

Fig. 51 Color Doppler evaluation on 2D and 3D imaging showing trivial transvalvular regurgitation and no paravalvular regurgitation

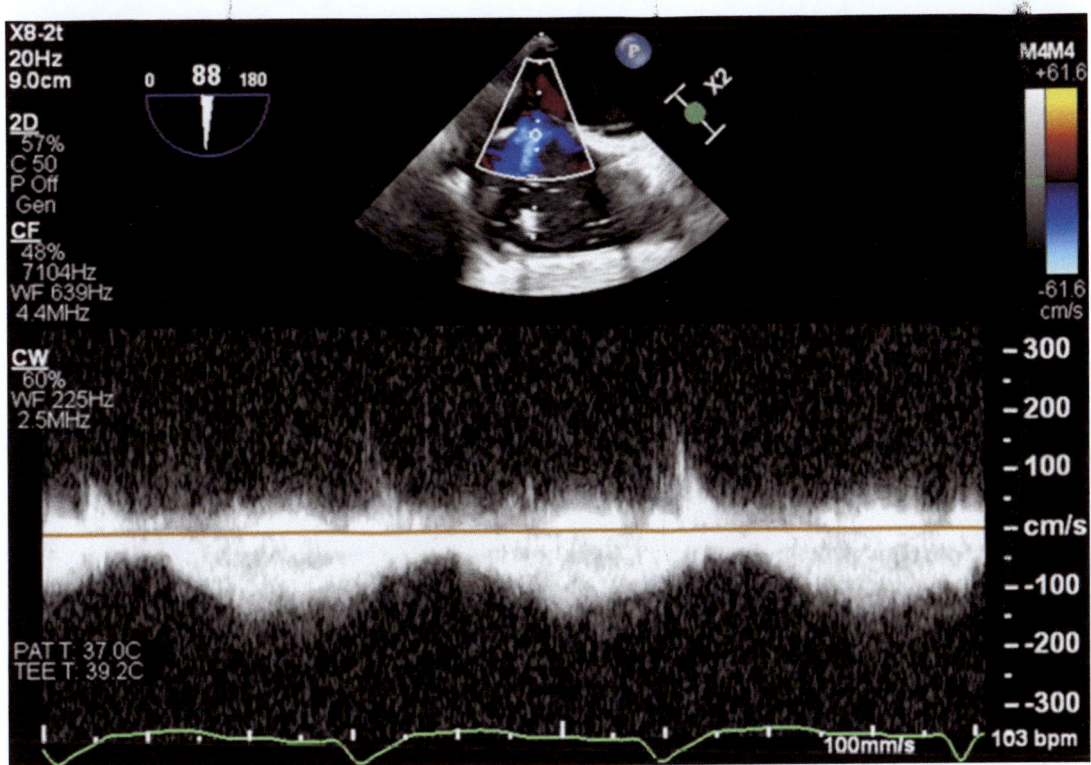

Fig. 52 Continuous wave Doppler across the iatrogenic atrial septal defect with noted left to right shunt

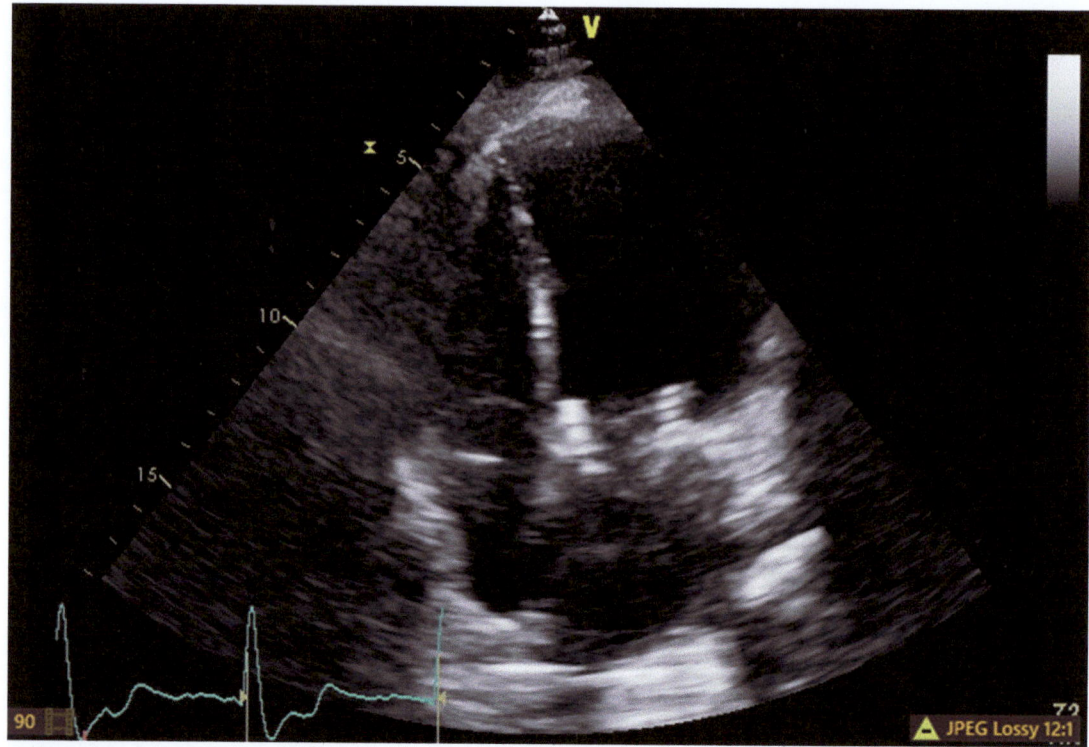

Fig. 53 4-CH view with well seated bioprosthetic mitral valve

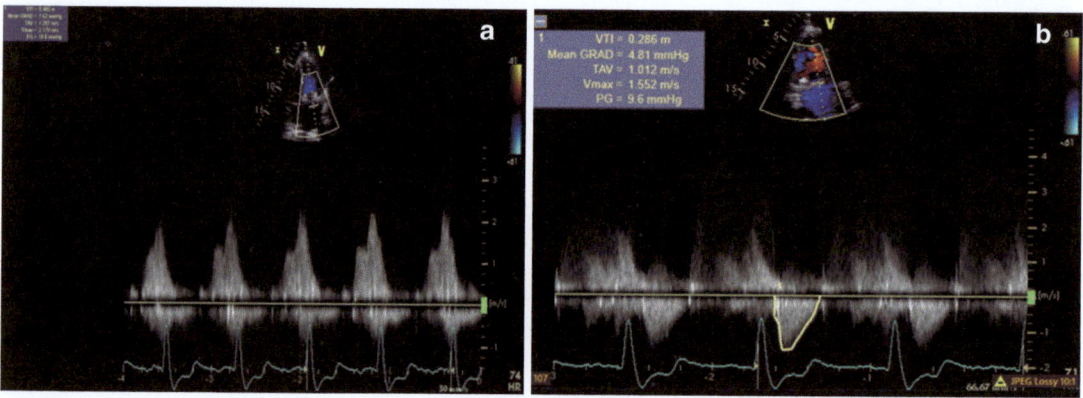

Fig. 54 Continuous wave Doppler profile across mitral valve in valve prosthesis (**a**) and across aortic valve (**b**)

Modality	Clinical application	Limitations
Transthoracic echocardiography (TTE)	− Preprocedural etiology and mechanism of prosthetic valve dysfunction − Assessment of cardiac remodeling and hemodynamic impact of prosthetic dysfunction	− Lower spatial resolution compared to TEE − Shadow artifact may limit adequate assessment of perivalvular regurgitation
Transesophageal Echocardiography (tee)	− Preprocedural evaluation of etiology and mechanism of prosthetic valve dysfunction − Assessment of cardiac remodeling and hemodynamic impact of prosthetic dysfunction − Exclude left atrial appendage thrombus − Intraprocedural imaging guidance − Immediate post procedure evaluation and evaluation for complications	− Absolute contraindicated in patients with esophageal stricture, tumor, active upper GI bleed etc. − Requires sedation
Cardiac computed tomography (CT)	− Pre procedural prosthetic implant sizing − Prediction of risk of LVOT obstruction (neo-LVOT area, septal-mitral distance, aorto-mitral angle)	− No hemodynamic assessment
Fluoroscopy	− Intraprocedural guidance of transseptal puncture − Intraprocedural valve alignment assessment	− Limited anatomic assessment

Clinical Controversies and Clinical Pearls

- Transcatheter valve-in-valve therapy is an excellent strategy for the management of patients with failed bioprosthetic mitral valve disease who are at high or prohibitive risk for redo mitral surgery.
- Echocardiography plays an important role in the diagnosis and intervention of prosthetic valve dysfunction.
- Cardiac CT angiography is important for preprocedural planning given its use in determining implant valve sizing, optimal fluoroscopic angles, and risk of LVOT obstruction.
- Preemptive alcohol septal ablation has been shown to be useful in reducing the risk of LVOT obstruction in patients who are at elevated risk.
- In appropriately selected patients, transcatheter MViV intervention show favorable short-term outcomes including clinical improvement and sustained prosthetic gradient reduction although there remains a paucity of data on long term outcomes.

Key Points

- Transcatheter valve-in-valve therapy is an excellent strategy for the management of patients with failed bioprosthetic mitral valve disease who are at high or prohibitive risk for redo mitral surgery.
- Echocardiography plays an important role in the diagnosis and intervention of prosthetic valve dysfunction.
- Cardiac CT angiography is important for pre-procedural planning given its use in determining implant valve sizing, optimal fluoroscopic angles, and risk of LVOT obstruction.
- Preemptive alcohol septal ablation has been shown to be useful in reducing the risk of LVOT obstruction in patients who are at elevated risk.
- In appropriately selected patients, transcatheter MViV intervention show favorable short-term outcomes including clinical improvement and sustained prosthetic gradient reduction although there remains a paucity of data on long term outcomes.

Disclosures There are no conflicts of interest to disclose.

Chapter Review Questions

1. Which of the following features is unfavorable for a MV transcatheter edge-to-edge repair (TEER)?

    A. Flail width 10 mm
    B. Flail gap 6 mm
    C. Coaptation depth 7 mm
    D. Large leaflet cleft

    Answer: D. Location of MR pathology being present in the leaflet body is an unfavorable characteristic and such a patient is unlikely to benefit from MV TEER. The other choices are all favorable characteristics.

2. What condition must be met prior to a patient qualifying for a MV transcatheter edge-to-edge repair (TEER)?

    A. MR must be primary in nature
    B. MR must be secondary in nature
    C. Patient must be classified as high surgical risk
    D. LVEF <40%

    Answer: C. The current ACC/AHA Practice Guideline for Patients with Valvular Heart Disease recommends MV TEER only for patients at high surgical risk. The other conditions listed are not required for MV TEER eligibility.

3. Which of the following is *not* a contraindication to percutaneous balloon mitral valvuloplasty (PBMV)?

    A. Significant commissural calcification
    B. Commissural fusion
    C. Left atrial appendage thrombus
    D. Severe MR

    Answer: B. Commissural fusion without calcification is the ideal pathology for which PBMV can be very effective. All other choices are contraindications.

4. What is one key characteristic that can help differentiate rheumatic mitral stenosis from non-rheumatic?

    A. Commissural fusion without significant calcification
    B. More common in women
    C. Presents in elderly
    D. Valvular calcification

    Answer: A. While rheumatic MS can present with valvular calcifications, the hallmark of rheumatic MS is commissural fusion without significant valvular calcification which is what differentiates it from non-rheumatic disease.

5. True or False?
    MViV intervention is indicated for the management of patients with failed bioprosthetic mitral valve disease with only mitral stenosis at low risk for redo-operation on evaluation by a cardiovascular surgeon.

    Answer: False. Currently transcatheter MViV intervention should only be considered in the management of failed bioprosthetic mitral valve disease with mitral stenosis or mitral regurgitation at high or prohibitive risk for redo-operation on evaluation by a multidisciplinary heart team.

6. Which of the following factors have been shown to be associated with an increased risk of LVOT obstruction following mitral valve-in-valve intervention?

    A. Neo-LVOT area of 150 mm^2
    B. Large annulus to interventricular septum distance
    C. Neo-LVOT area of 300 mm^2
    D. Large dilated left ventricle

    Answer: A. Pre-procedural cardiac CT identify a threshold of neo-LVOT area to discriminate the risk for LVOT obstruction with cutoff values of 170–189 mm^2 predicting LVOT obstruction with a sensitivity of 96.2–100% respectively in 2 different observational studies.

Other device related factors that may predispose patients to narrowing of the neo-LVOT dimension including greater device protrusion into the left ventricle, device flaring at its left ventricular outflow tract and a smaller mitral annulus to interventricular septum distance <17.8 mm due to a more pronounced septal bulge.

References

1. Otto CM, Nishimura RA, Bonow RO, Carabello BA, Rwin JP, Gentile F, et al. 2020 ACC/AHA guideline for the management of patients with valvular heart disease: a report of the American College of Cardiology/American Heart Association joint committee on clinical practice guidelines. Circulation. 2021;143(5):E72–227.
2. Hahn RT. Transcathether valve replacement and valve repair: review of procedures and intraprocedural echocardiographic imaging. Circ Res. 2016;119(2):341–56. http://circres.ahajournals.org.
3. Feldman T, Foster E, Glower DD, Kar S, Rinaldi MJ, Fail PS, et al. Percutaneous repair or surgery for mitral regurgitation. N Engl J Med. 2011;364(15):1395–406. https://doi.org/10.1056/nejmoa1009355.
4. Stone GW, Lindenfeld J, Abraham WT, Kar S, Lim DS, Mishell JM, et al. Transcatheter mitral-valve repair in patients with heart failure. N Engl J Med. 2018;379(24):2307–18. https://doi.org/10.1056/NEJMoa1806640.
5. Obadia J-F, Messika-Zeitoun D, Leurent G, Iung B, Bonnet G, Piriou N, et al. Percutaneous repair or medical treatment for secondary mitral regurgitation. N Engl J Med. 2018;379(24):2297–306. https://doi.org/10.1056/NEJMoa1805374.
6. Grayburn PA, Sannino A, Packer M. Proportionate and disproportionate functional mitral regurgitation: a new conceptual framework that reconciles the results of the MITRA-FR and COAPT trials. JACC Cardiovasc Imaging. 2019;12(2):353–62. https://doi.org/10.1016/j.jcmg.2018.11.006.
7. Tribouilloy C, Rusinaru D, Grigioni F, Michelena HI, Vanoverschelde JL, Avierinos JF, et al. Long-term mortality associated with left ventricular dysfunction in mitral regurgitation due to flail leaflets: a multicenter analysis. Circ Cardiovasc Imaging. 2014;7(2):363–70. https://doi.org/10.1161/CIRCIMAGING.113.001251/-/DC1.
8. Badhwar V, Bavaria JE, Elmariah S, Hung JW, Lindenfeld J, Morris AA, et al. 2020 Focused update of the 2017 ACC expert consensus decision pathway on the management of mitral regurgitation: a report of the American College of Cardiology Solution Set Oversight Committee. J Am Coll Cardiol. 2020;75:2236–70. https://doi.org/10.1016/j.jacc.2020.02.005.
9. Zoghbi WA, Adams D, Bonow RO, Enriquez-Sarano M, Foster E, Grayburn PA, et al. ASE GUIDELINES AND STANDARDS recommendations for noninvasive evaluation of native valvular regurgitation a report from the American Society of Echocardiography Developed in Collaboration with the Society for Cardiovascular Magnetic Resonance. J Am Soc Echocardiogr. 2017;30:303–71. https://doi.org/10.1016/j.echo.2017.01.007.
10. Yoran C, Yellin EL, Becker RM, Gabbay S, Frater RWM, Sonnenblick EH. Dynamic aspects of acute mitral regurgitation: effects of ventricular volume, pressure and contractility on the effective regurgitant orifice area. Circulation. 2021;60(1):170–6. http://ahajournals.org.
11. Otto CM, Nishimura RA, Bonow RO, Carabello BA, Erwin JP, Gentile F, et al. 2020 ACC/AHA guideline for the management of patients with valvular heart disease: a report of the American College of Cardiology/American Heart Association Joint Committee on Clinical Practice Guidelines. Circulation. 2021;77:E72–227. https://doi.org/10.1161/CIR.0000000000000923.
12. Baumgartner H, Hung J, Bermejo J, Chambers JB, Evangelista A, Griffin BP, et al. Echocardiographic assessment of valve stenosis: EAE/ASE recommendations for clinical practice. J Am Soc Echocardiogr. 2008.; https://www.acc.org/guidelines/hubs/valvular-heart-disease.;10:1–25.
13. Ben FM, Ayari M, Maatouk F, Betbout F, Gamra H, Jarrar M, et al. Percutaneous balloon versus surgical closed and open mitral commissurotomy: 7-year follow-up results of a randomized trial. Circulation. 1998;97(3):245–50. https://pubmed.ncbi.nlm.nih.gov/9462525/.
14. Wilkins GT, Weyman AE, Abascal VM, Block PC, Palacios IF. Percutaneous balloon dilatation of the mitral valve: an analysis of echocardiographic variables related to outcome and the mechanism of dilatation. Br Heart J. 1988;60(4):299–308. https://pubmed.ncbi.nlm.nih.gov/3190958/.
15. Nobuyoshi M, Arita T, Shirai SI, Hamasaki N, Yokoi H, Iwabuchi M, et al. Percutaneous balloon mitral valvuloplasty: a review. Circulation. 2009;119(8):e211. http://circ.ahajournals.org.
16. Lau K-W, Hung J-S. A simple balloon-sizing method in Inoue-balloon percutaneous transvenous mitral commissurotomy. Catheter Cardiovasc Diagn. 1994;33(2):120–9. https://pubmed.ncbi.nlm.nih.gov/7834724/.
17. Kim JB, Ha JW, Kim JS, Shim WH, Kang SM, Ko YG, et al. Comparison of long-term outcome after mitral valve replacement or repeated bal-

loon mitral Valvotomy in patients with restenosis after previous balloon Valvotomy. Am J Cardiol. 2007;99(11):1571–4.
18. Zoghbi WA, Chambers JB, Dumesnil JG, Foster E, Gottdiener JS, Grayburn PA, et al. Recommendations for evaluation of prosthetic valves with echocardiography and Doppler ultrasound: a report from the American Society of Echocardiography's Guidelines and Standards Committee and the Task Force on Prosthetic Valves, developed in conjunction with the American College of Cardiology Cardiovascular Imaging Committee, Cardiac Imaging Committee of the American Heart Association, the European Association of Echocardiography, a registered branch of the European Society of Cardiology. J Am Soc Echocardiogr. 2009;22(9):975–1014. https://pubmed.ncbi.nlm.nih.gov/19733789/.
19. Vemulapalli S, Grau-Sepulveda M, Habib R, Thourani V, Bavaria J, Badhwar V. Patient and hospital characteristics of mitral valve surgery in the United States. JAMA Cardiol. 2019;4(11):1149–55. https://jamanetwork.com/journals/jamacardiology/fullarticle/2752377.
20. Paradis JM, del Trigo M, Puri R, Rodés-Cabau J. Transcatheter valve-in-valve and valve-in-ring for treating aortic and mitral surgical prosthetic dysfunction. J Am Coll Cardiol. 2015;66(18):2019–37.
21. Thourani VH, Weintraub WS, Guyton RA, Jones EL, Williams WH, Elkabbani S, et al. Outcomes and long-term survival for patients undergoing mitral valve repair versus replacement: effect of age and concomitant coronary artery bypass grafting. Circulation. 2003;108(3):298–304. https://doi.org/10.1161/01.CIR.0000079169.15862.13.
22. Ruel M, Kulik A, Rubens FD, Bédard P, Masters RG, Pipe AL, et al. Late incidence and determinants of reoperation in patients with prosthetic heart valves. Eur J Cardiothorac Surg. 2004;25(3):364–70. www.elsevier.com/locate/ejcts.
23. Eleid MF, Cabalka AK, Williams MR, Whisenant BK, Alli OO, Fam N, et al. Percutaneous transvenous transseptal transcatheter valve implantation in failed bioprosthetic mitral valves, ring annuloplasty, and severe mitral annular calcification. J Am Coll Cardiol Interv. 2016;9(11):1161–74. http://www.ubqo.
24. Whisenant B, Kapadia SR, Eleid MF, Kodali SK, Mccabe JM, Krishnaswamy A, et al. One-year outcomes of mitral valve-in-valve using the SAPIEN 3 transcatheter heart valve. JAMA Cardiol. 2020.; https://jamanetwork.com/.;5:1245–52.
25. Eleid MF, Whisenant BK, Cabalka AK, Williams MR, Nejjari M, Attias D, et al. Early outcomes of percutaneous transvenous transseptal transcatheter valve implantation in failed bioprosthetic mitral valves, ring annuloplasty, and severe mitral annular calcification. J Am Coll Cardiol Interv. 2017;10(19):1932–42.
26. Murphy DJ, Ge Y, Don CW, Keraliya A, Aghayev A, Morgan R, et al. Use of cardiac computerized tomography to predict neo-left ventricular outflow tract obstruction before transcatheter mitral valve replacement. J Am Heart Assoc. 2017;6(11):e007353. http://ahajournals.org.
27. Yoon SH, Bleiziffer S, Latib A, Eschenbach L, Ancona M, Vincent F, et al. Predictors of left ventricular outflow tract obstruction after transcatheter mitral valve replacement. JACC Cardiovasc Interv. 2019;12(2):182–93. https://pubmed.ncbi.nlm.nih.gov/30678797/.
28. Leipsic J, Blanke P. Predicting left ventricular outflow tract obstruction after transcatheter mitral valve replacement: from theory to evidence*. J Am Coll Cardiol Interv. 2019;12(2):194–5.
29. Wang DD, Eng MH, Greenbaum AB, Myers E, Forbes M, Karabon P, et al. Validating a prediction modeling tool for left ventricular outflow tract (LVOT) obstruction after transcatheter mitral valve replacement (TMVR). Catheter Cardiovasc Interv. 2018;92(2):379–87.
30. Blanke P, Naoum C, Dvir D, Bapat V, Ong K, Muller D, et al. Predicting LVOT obstruction in transcatheter mitral valve implantation: concept of the neo-LVOT. JACC Cardiovasc Imaging. 2017;10(4):482–5.
31. Babaliaros VC, Greenbaum AB, Khan JM, Rogers T, Wang DD, Eng MH, et al. Intentional percutaneous laceration of the anterior mitral leaflet to prevent outflow obstruction during transcatheter mitral valve replacement: first-in-human experience. J Am Coll Cardiol Interv. 2017;10(8):798–809.
32. Wang DD, Guerrero M, Eng MH, Eleid MF, Meduri CU, Rajagopal V, et al. Alcohol septal ablation to prevent left ventricular outflow tract obstruction during transcatheter mitral valve replacement: first-in-man study. JACC Cardiovasc Interv. 2019;12(13):1268–79. https://pubmed.ncbi.nlm.nih.gov/31272671/.
33. Guerrero M, Wang DD, Himbert D, Urena M, Pursnani A, Kaddissi G, et al. Short-term results of alcohol septal ablation as a bail-out strategy to treat severe left ventricular outflow tract obstruction after transcatheter mitral valve replacement in patients with severe mitral annular calcification. Catheter Cardiovasc Interv. 2017;90(7):1220–6. https://pubmed.ncbi.nlm.nih.gov/28266162/.

Multimodality Imaging of Tricuspid Valve Disease at the Dawn of Transcatheter Intervention

Susheel Kodali and Vratika Agarwal

Abstract

There is growing interest in the impact of tricuspid valve disease. Multiple studies have demonstrated that the presence of tricuspid regurgitation, either in its isolated form or when co-existent with other valvular disease, leads to poor outcomes. Surgical repair or replacement is an option for a limited population fulfilling specific anatomic and clinical criteria. Transcatheter intervention of tricuspid valve disease offers a potentially valuable alternative to surgical treatment. The success and outcomes of the intervention are heavily dependent on understanding the tricuspid valve anatomy and pathophysiology. Multimodality imaging is the cornerstone for pre-procedural, peri-procedural as well as post-procedural assessment and management. This section will discuss the pathophysiology of tricuspid valve disease and the role of different imaging modalities in the diagnosis and preprocedural evaluation of the RV and TV. We will also discuss the role of imaging in guiding the choice of therapeutic intervention and post procedural surveillance and management.

Keywords

Tricuspid regurgitation · Transcatheter tricuspid valve intervention · Right heart disease · Multimodality imaging for tricuspid intervention

Abbreviations

CT	Computed tomography
HF	Heart failure
ICE	Intracardiac echocardiography
IVC	Inferior vena cava
MRI	Magnetic resonance imaging
PA	Pulmonary artery
PVR	Pulmonary vascular resistance
RA	Right atrium
RV	Right ventricle
SVC	Superior vena cava
TA	Tricuspid annulus
TEE	Transesophageal echocardiography
TEER	Transcatheter edge-to-edge repair
TR	Tricuspid regurgitation
TTE	Transthoracic echocardiography
TTVR	Transcatheter tricuspid valve replacement
TV	Tricuspid valve

S. Kodali (✉)
Structural Heart and Valve Center, New York Presbyterian/Columbia University Medical Center, NY, New York, USA
e-mail: sk2427@cumc.columbia.edu

V. Agarwal
Structural and Interventional Imaging, New York Presbyterian/Columbia University Medical Center, NY, New York, USA
e-mail: va2374@cumc.columbia.edu

© The Author(s), under exclusive license to Springer Nature Switzerland AG 2024
A. M. Kelsey et al. (eds.), *Cardiac Imaging in Structural Heart Disease Interventions*,
https://doi.org/10.1007/978-3-031-50740-3_3

Test your learning and check your understanding of this book's contents: use the "Springer Nature Flashcards" app to access questions using ▶ https://sn.pub/ambACS. To use the app, please follow the instructions in the chapter "Transcatheter Aortic Valve Replacement."

Learning Objectives
1. Be able to describe the pathophysiology and natural history of tricuspid valve disease.
2. Be able to describe the most common clinical presentations.
3. Be able to describe use of multimodality imaging for baseline assessment as well as to guide choice of intervention type.
4. Be able to describe the role of pre-, intra-, and post-procedural imaging for optimal patient outcomes.

Case Study
Patient is an 84-year-old male with chronic persistent atrial fibrillation s/p multiple unsuccessful cardioversion attempts, CKD III, HFpEF, who presented to the ED for HF exacerbation. At baseline he is active but lately noticed increased dyspnea on exertion and fatigue. Exam revealed an elevated JVP with prominent V wave and a respirophasic systolic murmur at the right lower sternal border and lower extremity edema. The patient was additionally found to be in atrial fibrillation with rapid ventricular rate. He was admitted for further workup and optimization of his volume status and atrial fibrillation.

Background and Definitions

Introduction

Tricuspid valve disease poses an extraordinary health care burden with age-adjusted prevalence of 0.55% with the highest incidence noted in women over the age of 75 years [1]. Studies suggest that over 1.6 million individuals in the United States are affected by moderate or severe tricuspid regurgitation. TR is associated with a twofold increased cardiac mortality that persists even after adjustment for potential confounders [2]. Historically, TR has been underrecognized and left untreated due (1) an underestimation of the impact of TR on outcomes and (2) due to a lack of evidence in support of treatment options in these patients—many of whom are multimorbid and at high surgical risk. Recent studies associating TR with poor cardiovascular outcomes have shed light on the importance of early recognition and potentially treatment of tricuspid regurgitation [3]. There is growing interest in understanding the pathophysiology, anatomy and etiology of TR in order to effectively treat it with lower risk interventions and reduce the overall healthcare burden imposed by the disease. Recent advances in transcatheter therapies for the treatment of tricuspid regurgitation and a lack of traditional surgical mortality benefit for isolated TV surgery [4, 5] has generated tremendous interest in pursuing early treatment.

Tricuspid Regurgitation

TR is the predominant pathology associated with tricuspid valve. The severity of TR has traditionally been classified via a 3 level grading system encompassing mild, moderate, and severe, as discussed further below. However, more recently, echocardiographic core-lab analyses from clinical trials of percutaneous therapies for TR have suggested a 5 category scheme of mild, moderate, severe, massive, and torrential.

Primary TR is often seen in younger population and is usually in the setting of congenital malformation, endocarditis or trauma.

Secondary TR is encountered far more commonly and is frequently noted in the setting of left-sided valvulopathy and left ventricular systolic or diastolic dysfunction. Left sided disease causes increase in pulmonary pressures which in turn lead to RV remodeling by RV hypertrophy and eventually RV dilatation. The identification of the mechanism of tricuspid regurgitation and the etiology plays a crucial role in determining the appropriate intervention and choosing an optimal device for trans-catheter or surgical intervention.

Classification of TR based on etiology is given below in Table 1.

Tricuspid Stenosis

TS is not commonly seen in native tricuspid valves. Tricuspid stenosis is often diagnosed in the presence of small surgical annuloplasty rings or TV prosthesis. Native TS is often associated with TR and is seen in disease processes such as carcinoid disease (causing thickening and fixation of the TV leaflets) or rheumatic heart disease (thickening and commissural fusion).

Diagnosis and Pre-procedural Assessment

Given the patient's signs and symptoms of right sided heart failure, his murmur, and atrial fibrillation, he underwent transthoracic echocardiography as part of his initial diagnostic testing. TTE revealed preserved LV function with mild to moderate RV dysfunction function, torrential TR and moderate MR. The patient's signs and symptoms of volume overload, dyspnea on exertion, fatigue (likely due to poor cardiac output), and atrial fibrillation are all commonly encountered in severe TR, as listed below.

Clinical Assessment

The clinical presentation mostly depends on etiology of tricuspid regurgitation

- Signs and symptoms of volume overload
- Dyspnea on exertion
- Fatigue due to poor cardiac output
- Congestive hepatopathy
- Arrhythmia (atrial fibrillation is commonly encountered)
- Cardiac cachexia

Similarly, the patient's JVD with V wave prominence, murmur, and lower extremity edema are among the many signs consistent with severe TR, as listed below.

Table 1 Classification of TR based on etiology

Primary tricuspid regurgitation	Secondary tricuspid regurgitation	Prosthetic valve dysfunction
- Myxomatous tricuspid valve disease - Tricuspid valve perforation - Tricuspid valve endocarditis - Tricuspid valve flail (post biopsy) - Carcinoid - Rheumatic - Radiation - Traumatic injury - Congenital abnormality (Ebstein's anomaly) - Tricuspid regurgitation due to pacemaker lead impingement	- Atriogenic tricuspid regurgitation (right atrial dilatation with normal right ventricle) - Ventriculogenic tricuspid regurgitation (RV cardiomyopathy) - Mixed TR (both atrial and ventricular dysfunction) - TR secondary to severe primary pulmonary hypertension - TR due to left sided disease with increased pulmonary pressures and RV remodeling	- Prosthetic annuloplasty dysfunction (TS or TR or both) - Prosthetic valve dysfunction (TS or TR or both)

Physical Examination

Physical findings commonly encountered in tricuspid regurgitation are:

- JVD and systolic thrill
- Prominent C and V waves
- RV lift
- S3 gallop due to RV distension
- S4 due to right ventricular hypertrophy
- Holosystolic murmur right sternal border
- Diastolic rumble with TS
- Murmur may be soft or inaudible if there is torrential or wide-open TR
- Pulsatile hepatomegaly
- Ascites and pedal edema

Cardiac imaging forms the mainstay of diagnostic testing in TR with the goals of:

- Define tricuspid valve anatomy
- Determine the etiology of tricuspid regurgitation
- Assess the severity of tricuspid regurgitation by both qualitative and quantitative methods
- Characterize right ventricular and right atrial anatomy and function
- Assess for other associated valvular pathology and left sided function
- Image extracardiac structures—IVC and SVC
- Evaluate feasibility of tricuspid valve intervention

Transthoracic Echocardiogram (TTE)

TTE is an excellent tool in diagnosing right sided pathology. TTE helps in identifying the etiology and mechanism of tricuspid regurgitation and helps in accurate assessment of degree of tricuspid regurgitation. Tricuspid valve is a complex structure with multiple and sometimes ill-defined leaflets with variable number of chords and papillary muscles [6]. The proximity of the right heart to the chest wall aides in good visualization of the tricuspid valve leaflets as well as the right ventricle. Ideally, both 2D and 3D views should be attained to characterize the tricuspid valve anatomy. Quantification of severity of regurgitation is done using 2D color doppler and 3D color doppler with multi-beat acquisition. The approach to comprehensive assessment of the tricuspid valve and right ventricle are addressed in the American Society of Echocardiography guidelines [7, 8]. The severity of tricuspid regurgitation has traditionally been determined on a 3 grade scale while more recent investigations in the era of transcatheter tricuspid interventions have proposed a 5 grade scale (Table 2). Each of these grading systems is based on integration of a number of quantitative, semi-quantitative, and qualitative factors with the 5 grade scale subdividing the traditional category of "severe" into "severe", "massive," and "torrential" based on quantitative metrics [9].

The key views used for comprehensive assessment of tricuspid valve pathology are (Fig. 1):

- Parasternal RV inflow view with zoomed in view of the tricuspid valve
- Dedicated tricuspid valve view in parasternal short axis at the level of the aortic valve
- Apical RV focused view to assess right ventricular size and function
- Dedicated RV view in apical 4-chamber view for strain assessment and 3D of the RV for assessment of ejection fraction.
- Zoomed in view of the tricuspid valve in 4-chamber view with and without color assessment
- 3D acquisition both with and without color should be done in multiple views (Fig. 2). 2D image should be optimized prior to switching to 3D to allow for better resolution and frame rate.
- Subcostal view for IVC dimension and compressibility and for hepatic vein reversal.

In cases where there are discrepancies between physical exam findings and TTE findings, or clinical history and TTE findings, or TTE findings are conflicting/unclear, or invasive therapies are being considered, further evaluation with either TEE or cardiac MRI should be considered.

Table 2 5 Class Grading Scheme for TR

	Variable	Mild	Moderate	Severe	Massive	Torrential
Qualitative measures	TV morphology	Normal or mildly abnormal leaflets	Moderately abnormal leaflets	Severe valve lesions (flail, severe retraction, large perforation)	Severe valve lesions (flail, severe retraction, large perforation)	Severe valve lesions (flail, severe retraction, large perforation)
	RV and RA size	Usually normal	Normal or mild dilation	Usually dilated	Usually dilated	Usually dilated
	Inferior vena cava diameter	Normal <2 cm	Normal or mildly dilated 2.1–2.5 cm	Dilated >2.5 cm	Dilated >2.5 cm	Dilated >2.5 cm
	Color flow jet area	Small, narrow, central	Moderate central	Large central jet or eccentric wall impinging jet of variable size	Large central jet or eccentric wall impinging jet of variable size	Large central jet or eccentric wall impinging jet of variable size
	Flow convergence zone	Not visible, transient or small	Intermediate in size and duration	Large throughout systole	Large throughout systole	Large throughout systole
	Continuous wave Doppler jet	Faint/partial/parabolic	Dense, parabolic, or triangular	Dense, often triangular	Dense, often triangular	Dense, often triangular
	VC (biplane)	<3 mm	3–6.9 mm	7–13 mm	14–20 mm	≥21 mm
	EROA (PISA)	<20 mm^2	20–39 mm^2	40–59 mm^2	60–79 mm^2	≥80 mm^2
	3D VCA or quantitative EROA	NA	NA	75–94 mm^2	95–114 mm^2	≥115 mm^2

Cardiac Magnetic Resonance (CMR)

CMR provides an adjunctive imaging modality to TTE for the diagnosis and quantification of TR. Similar to echo, it can provide both qualitative and quantitative assessment of regurgitant lesions [10]. Quantitative assessment of TR by CMR can be performed with one of several methods. First, the effective regurgitant orifice area can be directly measured using short axis images through the annular plane. However, this can be challenging in scenarios where the annular plane is difficult to define such as in Ebstein's anomaly or with severe leaflet tethering. An alternative method to estimate TR is to subtract RV stroke calculated from RV cine images from forward stroke volume in the pulmonary artery calculated with the phase contrast sequence (Fig. 3). This will provide regurgitant volume and regurgitant fraction. In addition to quantitating regurgitant volumes, CMR can also be used to estimate pulmonary pressures with its ability to estimate a peak systolic velocity across the tricuspid valve which can then be used to estimate PA pressures. However this calculation may be more accurate with CMR than echo due to its ability to get a perfectly on-axis measurement which can be challenging with TTE in some patients.

Due to its high spatial and temporal resolution, tricuspid valve leaflet anatomy as well as pathology can also be assessed by CMR. Leaflet length, morphology, tenting, prolapse and thickening can all be assessed using sequential thin slice imaging. Presence of arrhythmia often leads to motion artifact. Real time cine imaging without breath hold instructions are used in the patients with arrhythmia however the image resolution in such cases is suboptimal. Shortened free breathing real time acquisition may be used to offset this problem.

CMR also provides accurate and reproducible assessment of RV function, wall motion abnormality, RV volume and tissue characterization. Imaging protocols should account for the dilation of the right ventricle and right atrium and include 4-chamber, RV inflow-outflow and RV short axis images in its entirety. Short-axis cine images are typically used for volumetric measurements by tracing endocardial borders. Right ventricular

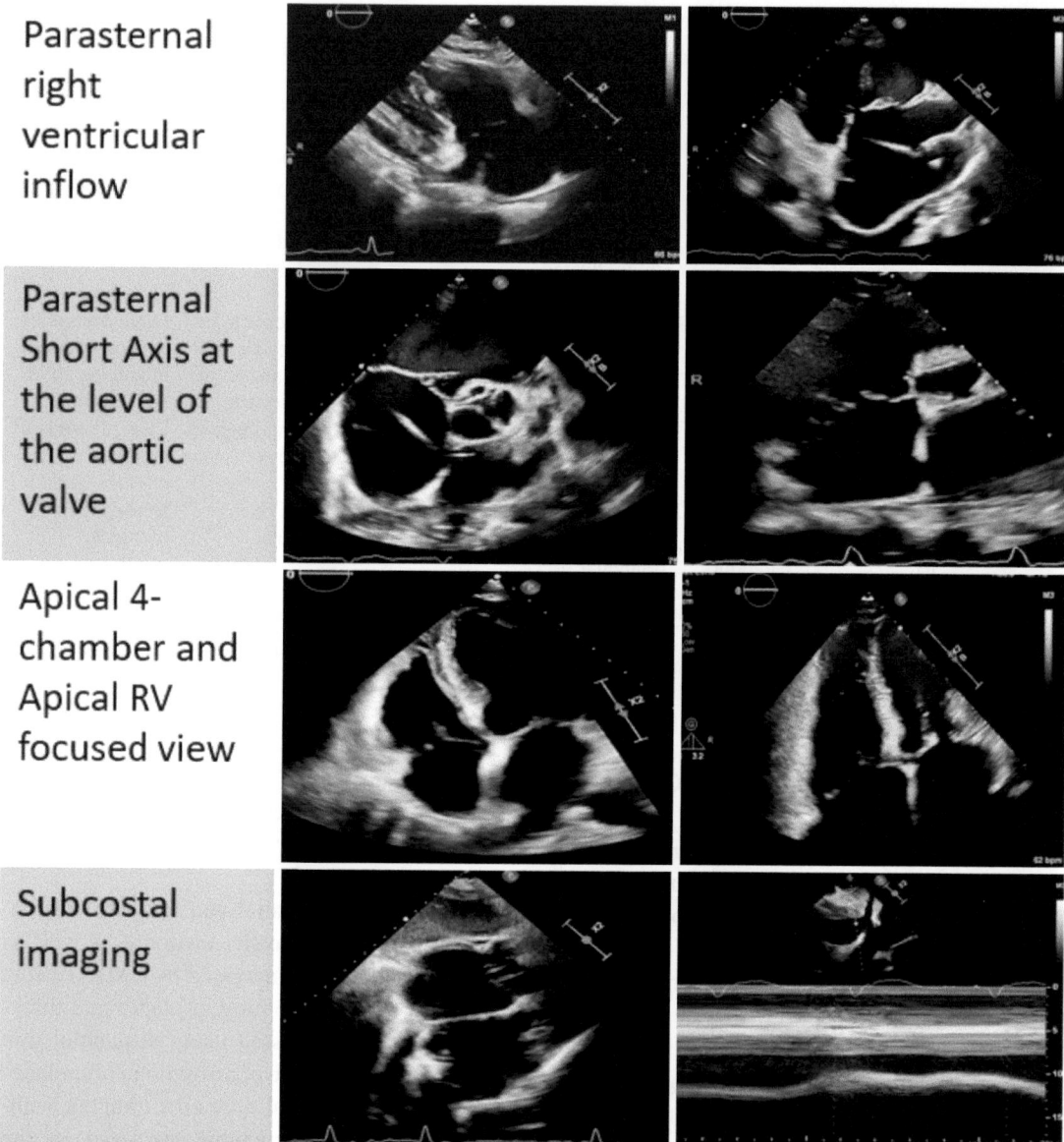

Fig. 1 The key views for comprehensive assessment of tricuspid valve pathology

ejection fraction and stroke volume are derived by using the RV end diastolic and systolic volumes. CMR is considered gold standard in the assessment of RV volumes and function [11, 12]. It has been shown in multiple studies that 2D and 3D echocardiography often underestimates chamber volumes [13, 14]. CMR also plays a unique role in identifying right ventricular pathology without use of ionizing radiation. Right ventricular tissue characterization is possible using native T1 imaging and delayed gadolinium enhancement. Delayed gadolinium enhancement provides assessment of dysfunction in myocarditis, myocardial infarction, infiltrative disease, trauma as well as pulmonary hypertension.

As noted above, CMR is a great tool for qualitative and quantitative assessment of tricuspid regurgitation. However, its clinical application is limited by the complexities of acquiring the scans in elderly patients with multiple comorbidities. The requirement for long scan times with breath holds makes it challenging for some patients.

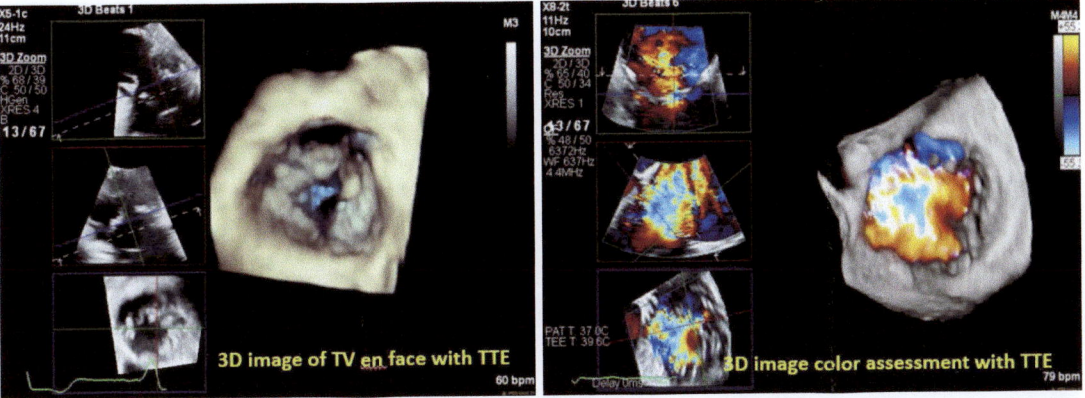

Fig. 2 3-dimensional assessment of tricuspid regurgitation with and without color

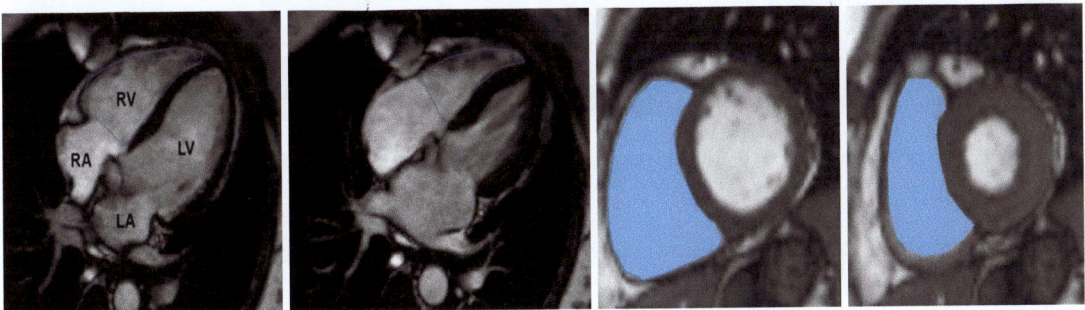

Fig. 3 Assessment of right ventricular volumes in diastole and systole using RV cine imaging to eatimate right ventricular stroke volume

TEE and Computed Tomography: Diagnostic Imaging and Procedural Planning

Transesophageal Echocardiogram (TEE)

Similar to cardiac MRI, TEE can play an important role in the diagnostic evaluation of TR when there are discrepancies between clinical and TTE findings or uncertainty regarding TTE findings. In addition, TEE also allows for careful assessment and quantification of left sided pathology which may be contributing to this disease process [15]. Finally, TEE is crucial in procedural planning. TEE examination of TV should be done at various levels and multiplane angles to allow for complete visualization and assessment of the tricuspid valve apparatus and the right ventricle. Visualization of the TV can be sometimes challenging by TEE in patients with a horizontal heart, left sided prosthesis, lipomatous interatrial septum or atrial septal devices due to acoustic shadowing of the tricuspid valve leaflets as the ultrasound beam crosses these structures. Acoustic shadowing is often encountered in mid-esophageal imaging. Imaging from the distal esophagus and the stomach allows for cleaner views of the TV due to improved proximity between the TV and the imaging probe (Fig. 4). Three-dimensional imaging allows for careful delineation of the TV leaflets, aides in understanding the pathology and allows for planning the interventional procedures.

The key views for comprehensive TEE imaging of the tricuspid valve are:

- Mid-esophageal 4-chamber at 0° rotation and orthogonal biplane view
- Mid-esophageal TV commissural view at 60°–90°
- Deep esophageal 0°/90° orthogonal plane imaging

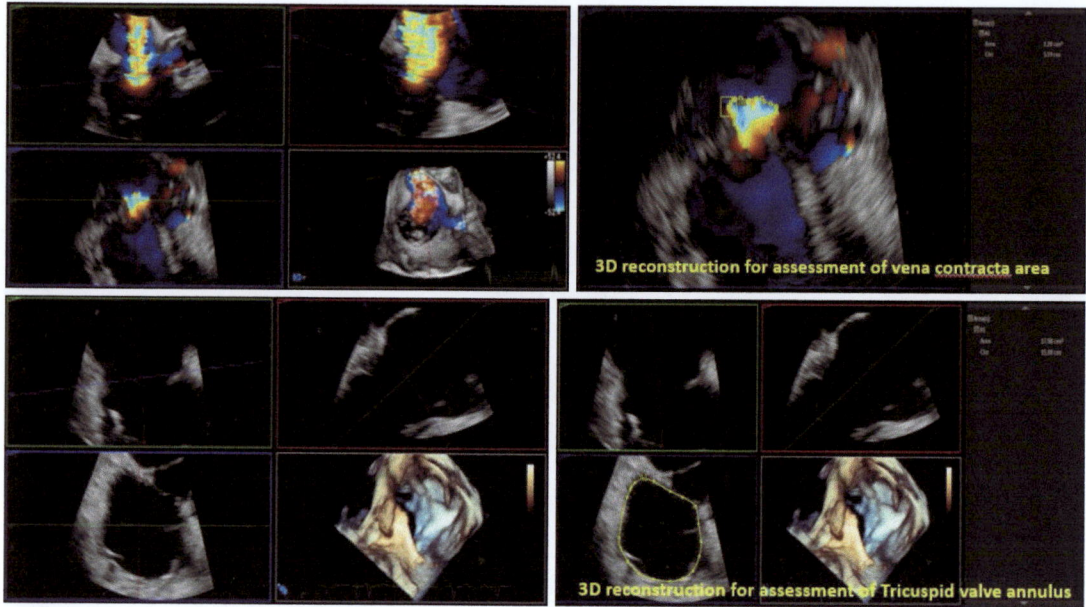

Fig. 4 TEE assessment of the degree of tricupid regurgitation and assessment of annular dimensions using 3-dimensional MPR

- Deep esophageal RV inflow outflow view at 60°–90°
- Trans gastric short axis view of the TV at 20°–60°
- Deep gastric view at 0° and at higher angles of 120°–160° allows for alignment of the doppler beam to the jet.
- 3D assessment should be performed at multiple levels. Deep gastric and transgastric views may often provide cleaner views of the tricuspid valve and hence may be optimal for 3D assessment.

Cardiac Computed Tomography (CT)

Use of cardiac gated CT has become an integral part of evaluating patients with structural heart disease especially prior to transcatheter intervention. Pre-procedural planning with cardiac CTA prior to transcatheter aortic valve replacement has become routine. However, the role in evaluation of the right-sided heart disease is less established but with the emergence of transcatheter therapies for tricuspid regurgitation there is increasing interest. There are several advantages to cardiac CT over echocardiography including reproducibility, ability to image patients with complex cardiac disease including those with pacemakers and relatively short scan times (especially in relation to cardiac MRI). However, the ability to accurately interpret a cardiac CT depends on the quality of the images obtained.

Obtaining a CT scan that allows for accurate interpretation of right sided anatomy requires homogeneous opacification of both the right ventricle and right atrium. In patients with severe tricuspid regurgitation, there are several challenges. To start, the majority of patients are in atrial fibrillation which can result in motion or misregistration artifact. This results in blurring of cardiac structures making accurate interpretations difficult. Care should be taken to optimize scans in these patients by considering the following. First, if tolerated, the use of low dose beta blockers should be considered if patient is tachycardic. Second, capabilities of the scanners should be considered and images should be obtained on the best available machine. The use of a CT with a large detector array (320 slice) will provide the ability to capture the entire region of interest in one acquisition. This will minimize the risk of misregistration artifact. In addition, it will shorten the breath hold required, which can be challenging in elderly patients with heart failure. The use of newer dual source scanners with higher temporal resolution can also minimize this artifact. Finally, although it results in higher radiation, the use of retrospective

ECG gating and low-pitch helical scanning will minimize the risk of artifact in patients with atrial fibrillation. Another challenge often encountered in patients with TR is the presence of concomitant renal dysfunction. The ability to accurately interpret cardiac structures requires the use of contrast which can worsen renal function. In addition, homogenuous opacification of the right side can be challenging. Standard cardiac CT protocols designed for left sided cardiac structures result in heterogenous attenuation of right sided structures resulting in uninterpretable scans. It is critical to develop individualized protocols for patients with TR that focus on obtaining adequate opacification while minimizing contrast [16, 17].

Obtaining a multiphasic CT encompassing the entire cardiac cycle is critical for allowing the selection of the best phases (i.e. those with the least artifact) for analysis of the various structures of interest. In addition, it allows for assessment of changes in RA and RV volumes between systole and diastole. Evaluation of right ventricular function is feasible through a semi-automated segmentation of the RV through 10 phases of the cardiac cycle [16]. Studies have demonstrated good correlation to MRI in assessment of RV function [18].

Evaluation of the CT in patients with TR should be performed in the context of the intervention being planned. The structures of interest will be different depending on whether the intervention planned is transcatheter edge to edge repair, transcatheter annuloplasty or percutaneous valve replacement. Regardless, a careful analysis evaluating all of the key structures should be performed. Tricuspid leaflet morphology including number of leaflets and location of commissures can be seen (Fig. 5). This can be useful when planning edge to edge repair. Dynamic reconstructions throughout the cardiac cycle can demonstrate leaflet tethering and gaps at intended location for the edge to edge repair. This information can supplement the TEE data to provide an assessment of the likelihood of a good quality repair.

In patients intended for transcatheter replacement, analysis of the right sided structures along with the tricuspid valve apparatus is required. Multiplanar reconstructions of the tricuspid annulus are performed allowing measurements of annular dimensions which are necessary for sizing the prosthesis. Multiple measurements should be taken including max and min dimensions, area and perimeter (Fig. 5). Sizing algorithms will vary depending on the prosthesis being chosen. There can be significant changes in size between systole and diastole. Ideally measurements should be taken in diastole which is typically when the largest dimensions are seen. However, care should be taken to review all phases and use the ones with the least artifact. Beyond assessment of the annulus, the entire TV apparatus should be reviewed. Care should be taken to note the location and number of papillary muscles which can interact with the prosthesis or the delivery system. In addition, RA and RV dimensions should be noted to ensure there is room for the delivery catheter to safely deliver the prosthesis. In addition to these measurements, location of pacemaker leads in the RV as well as the trajectory across the tricuspid annulus can be seen nicely in multiplanar reconstructions. Finally, the location and approach of the inferior vena cava into the RA should be evaluated. There is significant variability of this among patients and it can significantly impact the ability of the delivery catheter to reach the tricuspid annulus in a coaxial manner which is critical for most devices [19].

Although transcatheter edge to edge repair and percutaneous tricuspid valve replacement are the primary therapies being evaluated, there are several other approaches being investigated such as transcatheter annuloplasty and heterotopic valve replacement. In patients being considered for annuloplasty, one other important consideration is the location of the right coronary artery which often tracks near the anterior leaflet. Due to this location, it could be injured during annuloplasty. Reconstructions showing the location of the RCA in relation to the TV annulus is useful for preprocedural planning. If annuloplasty is being considered, it is important that the acquisition protocol for the CT ensures adequate contrast opacification on the left side to ensure adequate visualization of the coronary artery. This is the only scenario in which opacification of left sided structures is necessary when evaluating for tricuspid intervention. In patients being considered for heterotopic placement of bioprosthetic valves in the superior and inferior vena cava, careful measurements of these dimensions for appropriate sizing

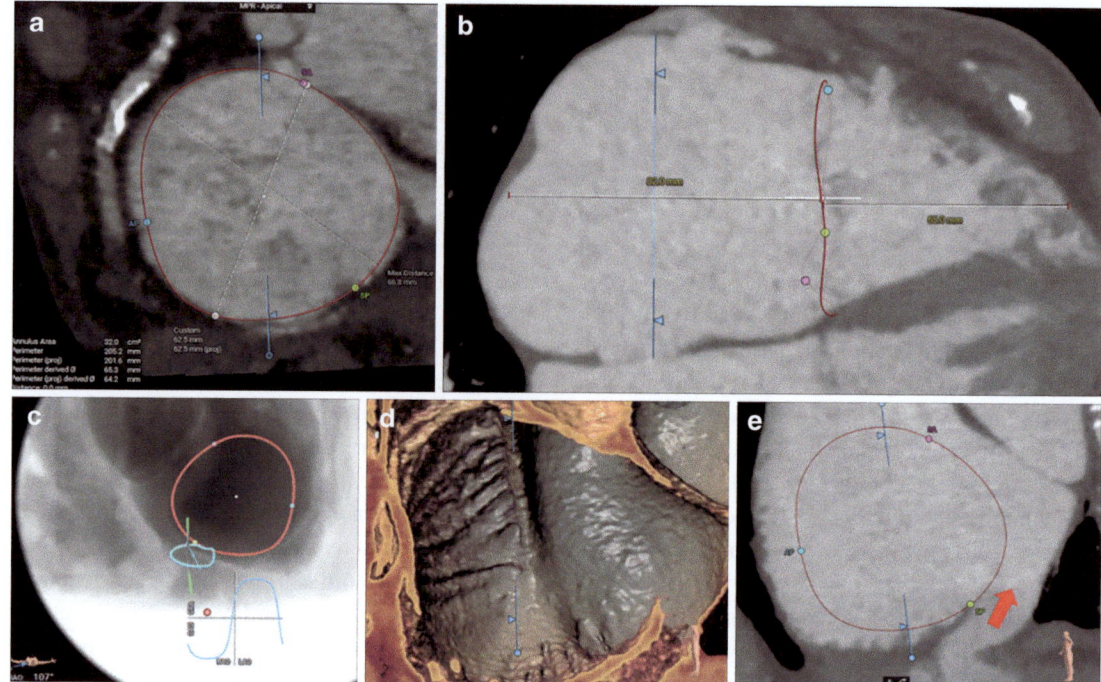

Fig. 5 CT images showing annular assessment (Panel **a**), RV and RA height (Panel **b**), IVC offset to Tricuspid Annulus (Panel **c**), IVC angulation (Panel **d** and **e**). In Panel **e**, red arrow illustrates trajectory of IVC towards septum and away from tricuspid annulus (red circle)

should be performed in multiplanar reconstructions that are coaxial to the structure.

Cardiac Catheterization and Fluoroscopic Evaluation

The evaluation of patients with severe tricuspid regurgitation has typically involved a right and left heart catheterization. Although coronary angiography is standard in patients planned for surgical repair or replacement, the role in patients undergoing transcatheter intervention remains unclear. It is unlikely that coronary revascularization would impact the severity of tricuspid regurgitation. It should be considered primarily in patients where it is clinically indicated for other reasons.

The role of right heart catheterization in patients with TR is critical. First, it may necessary to ensure that patients are medically optimized prior to intervention. It is important to note that TR is dynamic. Optimization of volume status can significantly improve regurgitation and mitigate the need for intervention. Secondly, right heart catheterization to evaluate the presence of pulmonary hypertension is an important consideration. Recent studies have demonstrated that pulmonary hypertension (PAPs >50 mmHg) is a poor prognostic sign in patients with TR even after successful intervention [20]. This same study also demonstrated that non-invasive assessment of pulmonary pressures by echocardiography is poor with a sensitivity of only 55%. Therefore routine right heart catheterization in patients with TR is recommended not only for optimization but also for prognosis.

Fluoroscopy remains an important adjunct to echocardiography during transcatheter intervention. Based on the preoperative CT, fluoroscopic angles that are coaxial to the tricuspid annulus can be calculated. During the procedure, fluoroscopy in these angles can be useful to ensure the device is approaching the tricuspid valve in a coaxial manner, which can be critical for success. In addition, identification of the right coronary artery either by placement or angiography can serve as an important landmark especially in transcatheter annuloplasty procedures.

The present patient underwent TTE with clear delineation of torrential TR and mild to moderate RV dysfunction. Patient underwent a TEE to further assess leaflet morphology. Image quality was sufficient to estimate tricuspid coaptation gaps and annular size. A cardiac CTA was performed to further assess tricuspid valve morphology as well RV size and dimensions. The findings from these studies are outlined in Table 3.

Table 3 Summary of Pertinent Patient Findings

Echocardiogram	- Normal LV function. The ejection fraction = 56% by biplane Simpson's method of discs. - The right ventricular systolic function is mildly to moderately reduced. There is flattening of the interventricular septum only during systole, consistent with RV pressure overload. - Moderate mitral regurgitation - Torrential tricuspid regurgitation with marked tethering of the leaflets, dilatation of the right ventricle and annulus, (>50mm) with marked dilatation of the right atrium. The coaptation gaps measure 4-7 mm.	
Computed tomography	- Severe cardiomegaly with marked enlargement of the right atrium and left atrium - Right ventricular enlargement with mild reduction in function. - Severe calcifications of central coronary arteries.	
Invasive hemodynamics	- RA: Mean 16 mm Hg. A wave 14 and V wave 25 - RV: 31/3 mm Hg. EDP 9 mm Hg - PA: 27/16 mm Hg. Mean 21 mmHg - PW: Mean 14 mm Hg. A wave 15 and V wave 18 - Fick CO 1.86 L/min and CI 1.05 - PVR 3.76 WU	
Coronary Angiogram	- Moderate diffuse CAD, nonobstructive by IVUS in proximal LAD and LM.	

Heart Team Approach and Discussion

All imaging studies, invasive hemodynamic and current treatment regimen were carefully evaluated by the multidisciplinary team that included interventionalists, cardiac surgeons, heart failure specialists as well as cardiac imagers. Management strategies for TR typically revolve on treating underlying conditions (i.e. left sided heart disease) and diuretics. Isolated surgery is rarely recommended except in the setting of symptomatic primary TR with reasonably preserved RV function (Fig. 6). Our patient was thought to have functional TR with a mix of features consistent with both atrial functional (annular dilation) and ventricular functional (leaflet tethering) etiologies. In total, it was felt that the patient's volume overload and symptomatology was due primarily to TR rather than atrial fibrillation and a decision was made to proceed with intervention on the tricuspid valve rather than attempting a rhythm control strategy. The reasons for this approach were several. First, given the severe atrial dilatation, the likelihood of successfully restoring and maintaining sinus rhythm was felt to be low. Second, even if sinus rhythm was restored, it was unlikely that the annular dimensions would decrease enough to improve leaflet coaptation and reduce TR given the baseline torrential TR. Finally, in this patient, there was a component of ventricular functional TR with leaflet tethering that would not improve with restoration of sinus rhythm. For this reason, the decision was made to intervene on the torrential TR as the primary strategy.

Indications for Treatment of TR

Determining procedural risk in isolated surgical tricuspid repair is hampered by the fact that The Society of Thoracic Surgeons (STS) cardiac surgery risk stratification model and the logistic EuroSCORE/EuroSCORE II were not designed to predict outcomes of isolated tricuspid valve surgery. Using the novel TRI-SCORE risk scoring system [21] which factors in age, NYHA class, signs of right heart failure, eGFR, elevated bilirubin, left ventricular function and right ventricular dysfunction, the patient was deemed to be high risk for surgery with a predicted in-hospital mortality of 22%. The patient was subsequently considered for transcatheter tricuspid valve intervention.

Current Targets and Goals of Transcatheter Device Intervention

The potential emergence of transcatheter therapy for tricuspid regurgitation has been welcomed with open arms. This is likely due to the paucity of treatment options for isolated tricuspid regurgitation and the increased morbidity and mortality associated with isolated tricuspid valve surgery [22]. Current transcatheter treatment options however are limited to trials with no commercially approved devices currently available in the United States. Several aspects of the valve are being studied as treatment targets. Figure 7 summarizes the treatment strategies by various devices currently in trials.

It is important to identify the pathology that is being dealt with in order to choose the best treatment strategy. No single device is a fit for all. For example, edge-to-edge repair in someone with large coaptation gap due to severe leaflet tethering from a dilated right ventricle would not yield optimal results. Similarly, current transcatheter tricuspid valve replacement (TTVR) devices are limited by the size of the annulus due to limited number of device sizes available. The advantage of TTVR is complete elimination of tricuspid regurgitation which is usually not possible with edge-to-edge repair technology. Prior to addressing the TR, if appropriate and feasible, the first step is to address the left sided pathology if present. Additionally, patients should undergo optimization of appropriate heart failure GDMT for left sided disease and optimal medical volume management for right sided disease prior to pre-procedural imaging or consideration for tricuspid intervention. Severe right ventricular dysfunction and severe pulmonary hypertension are associated with poor prognosis and have usually been excluded from trials of transcatheter tricuspid intervention and should also be optimized medically.

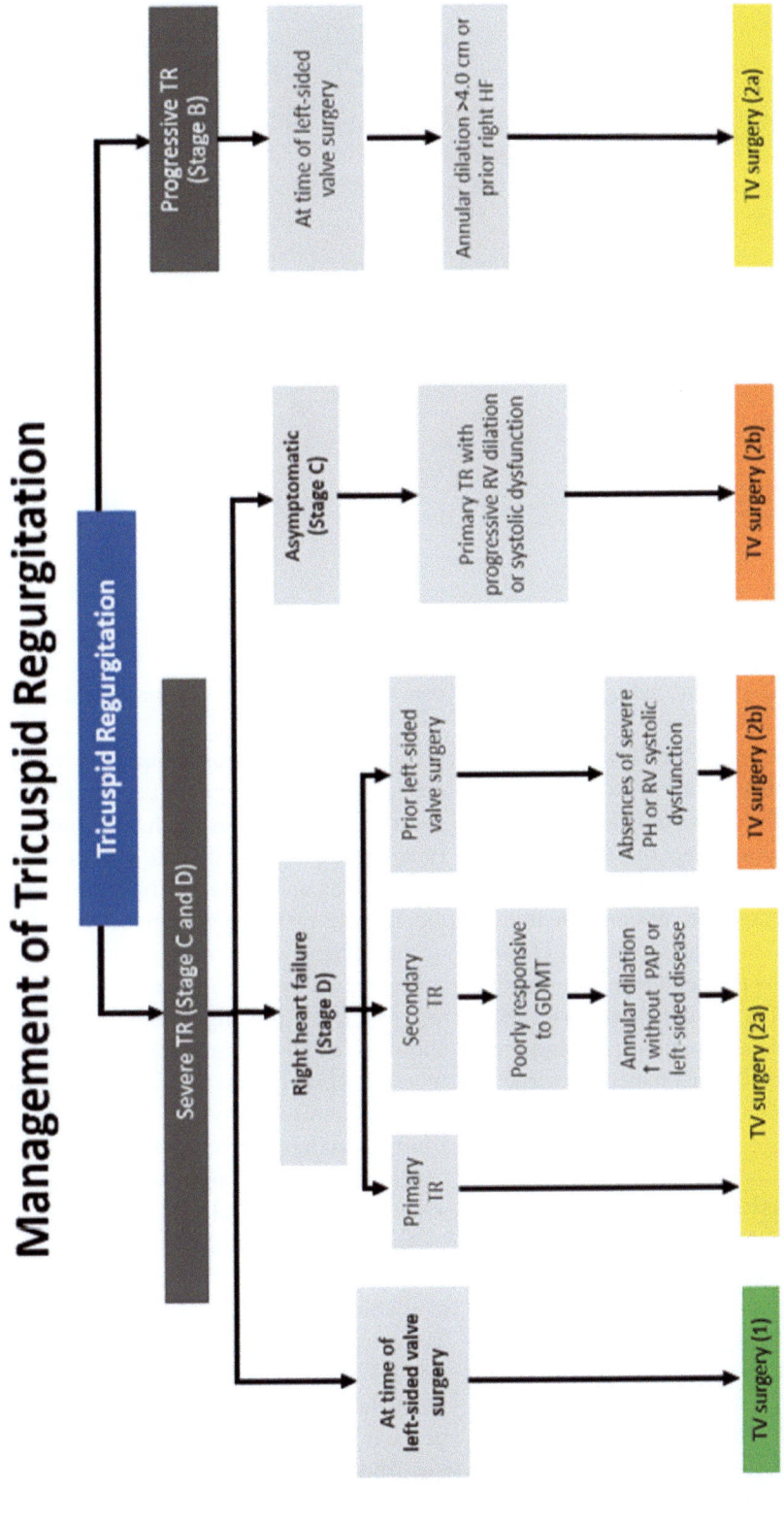

Fig. 6 Current guideline recommendations for management of tricuspid regurgitation

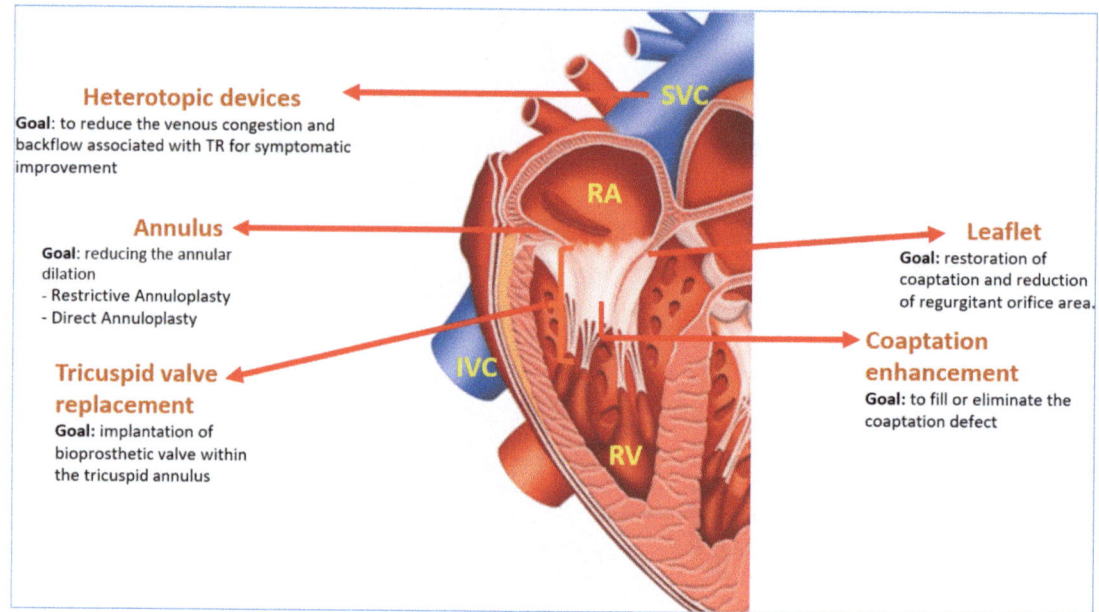

Fig. 7 Treatment targets for transcatheter tricuspid valve intervention

In the case of the present patient, given the baseline torrential TR and broad regurgitant jet, consideration was given for TTVR as that would likely be the best option to eliminate TR. However, annular dimensions (max dimension 58 mm) were too large for the currently approved devices. Therefore consideration was given to other therapeutic options including transcatheter edge to edge repair (TEER). Review of anatomy by the heart team determined that anatomical factors including adequate leaflet length, acceptable coaptation gaps and well visualized leaflets made the patient a suitable candidate for TEER.

Heart Team Decision: Transcatheter Edge-to-Edge Tricuspid Valve Repair

Intraprocedural Imaging Modalities and Measurements

A successful TEER procedure relies on having ideal TEE imaging to verify adequate leaflet tissue in each of the arms. This often requires use of multiple views, usually a deep esophageal view and transgastric short axis. If adequate leaflet insertion cannot be verified, the device cannot be deployed as the likelihood of leaflet detachment is high. In some patients, imaging is difficult due to patient related factors such as horizontal heart or presence of left-sided valve prostheses. Patience is key as often an imaging window can be found where adequate views can be obtained. Certain maneuvers such as placing a role under the right shoulder can help improve imaging. In cases where despite all attempts, acoustic shadowing from the delivery system or patient anatomy limits visualization on TEE, intracardiac echocardiography (ICE) may be necessary and provide incremental value. Intracardiac imaging catheters allow for acquisition of high-quality 2D and 3D images in real-time. The currently available 4D ICE catheters can obtain 2D and 3D volumetric images and cine-videos in real-time (4D). Although currently used to complement the TEE imaging, in the future ICE may be used as a standalone device for imaging during transcatheter intervention of the tricuspid valve.

Although transesophageal echocardiography is the primary imaging modality required for edge to edge repair, fluoroscopy does serve an important adjunctive role that is often overlooked. By adjusting the C-arm to an angle that is coaxial to the tricuspid annulus, the trajectory of the device can be seen to ensure it is approaching the tricuspid annulus in a perpendicular manner. Secondly, in cases where two devices are placed, fluoroscopy is critical to ensuring that the two devices do not interact with each other resulting in dislodgement. Finally, fluoroscopy is necessary to confirm that the device remains closed after locking.

During the TEER procedure, it is important that there is clear communication between the interventional operator and the structural imager. This starts before the case begins with a clear plan agreed to by the team regarding leaflet clipping strategies. Although these strategies almost universally involve clipping the septal leaflet to either the anterior or the posterior leaflet, the location and the orientation of the device will be different depending on the location of the jet. Also the location on the leaflet may be different depending on whether the plan is to place one device or multiple devices. Ideally, the pre-procedural strategy is followed in the case with successful results but often adjustments need to be made interprocedurally. During the procedure, it is critical that the imager and the interventionalist are communicating effectively. Therefore, it is important the imaging is displayed in a manner that is standardized. Typically, the short-axis image is show with the aorta at 4 o'clock. With this as the typical view, it is then easy for the imager and interventionalist to identify the leaflets and the orientation of the device(s). Successful TEER relies on effective communication between the imager and the operator and is truly a team effort.

In our patient, a successful edge-to-edge repair was performed with placement of two PASCAL ACE devices (Edwards Lifesciences, Irvine, CA). The first device was placed between the anterior and septal leaflets with the second device placed posteriorly. It is important to note when placing two devices, the first device should be placed anterior to avoid shadowing of the second device. In our patient, there was a three-grade reduction in TR severity, which was torrential at baseline.

Post procedural Assessment

After successful treatment of TR, it is critical to ensure that optimal medical therapy is continued. The patient was admitted to the floor for an additional 2–3 days of intravenous diuretics to ensure his hemodynamic state was optimized. After transitioning to an oral regiment including diuretics and anticoagulation, patient was discharged home with instructions to monitor his weight closely and follow-up with his heart failure physician within 4 weeks.

At his 30 day follow up appointment, a TTE was obtained revealing that the devices were in place and the TR remained moderate in severity. In addition, RV function remained only mildly depressed. Patients should be followed with TTE at least once a year or sooner if there is a clinical change. Some clinicians have been obtaining follow-up CT scans on patients following tricuspid valve intervention. In patients undergoing TTVR, CT imaging serves an important role to ensure that the valve is in stable position with no obvious injuries to the right ventricle or surrounding anatomy. In addition, the CT scan will reveal whether there is any evidence of leaflet thrombosis. However, in our patient that underwent TEER, the role of post-procedural CT scan is less clear. In cases where there is question regarding RV size or function, both CT and MRI can be used to demonstrate any evidence of RV remodeling or change in RV function.

Multimodality imaging comparison:

Echocardiogram	– Quantification of TR severity – RV size and function – Assessment of pulmonary pressures – Tricuspid valve anatomy and etiology of TR – Intraprocedural guidance – Post procedural assessment	– Acoustic windows may sometimes be challenging for patients with scoliosis, pectus, severe lung disease and rotated anatomy
Intracardiac imaging	– Bailout when compromised TEE windows during intraprocedural imaging – Provides all features of echocardiogram including 3D and doppler	– Invasive – Learning curve involved with maneuvering the ICE catheter – Cost
CT	– Detailed anatomic evaluation – Evaluates degree of annular dilatation and aides in determination of valve choice – RCA course – IVC and SVC measurements – Can help evaluate the right ventricular function	– Challenges with artifact due to arrhythmia and prosthetic material – Less physiological information – Radiation and contrast exposure
MRI	– Provides flow evaluation as well as detailed anatomic evaluation and right ventricular function – No radiation	– Prosthetic material artifact – Can be challenging in patients with atrial fibrillation and frequent ectopy – Cost
Fluoroscopy	– Baseline right heart catheterization for determination of chamber pressures and cardiac output – Intraprocedural imaging – Ability for fusion imaging that provides clarification of landmarks and thereby reduces overall procedure time	– Invasive

Clinical Controversies and Pearls

- Preprocedural planning involving the structural imager and the interventional operator is critical to success.
- Optimization of the patient's hemodynamic state ("pre-hab") prior to assessment and intervention for tricuspid regurgitation improves clinical outcomes.
- 4D intracardiac echo will play an increasingly important role in transcatheter tricuspid intervention, especially with TTEER.

Key Points

- Severe TR is associated with a bleak prognosis with progressive RV dysfunction, renal and hepatic failure, chronic right heart failure requiring increasing doses of diuretics.
- Transcatheter therapies are a less invasive alternative to surgery and may expand the number of patients treated if proven safe and efficacious. However, the outcomes of these trials are still unknown.
- Multimodality imaging plays a crucial role not only in preprocedural assessment and procedural planning but also in intraprocedural guidance as well as post procedural follow up.

Chapter Review Questions

1. 88-year-old man with h/o atrial fibrillation and hypertension presents with worsening lower extremity edema and increased abdominal girth. He had a recent echocardiogram that showed severe tricuspid regurgitation secondary to right atrial and ventricular dysfunction. Left ventricular function was preserved and there was no other valvular dysfunction noted. Stress test done prior to knee surgery 2 years ago showed no evidence of ischemia. What would be the next best step in the management of the patient:
   A. Refer patient to cardiothoracic surgery for risk stratification and consideration for isolated tricuspid valve surgery.
   B. Perform a transesophageal echocardiogram for further assessment of the right ventricle and tricuspid valve
   C. Schedule the patient for right and left heart catheterization for invasive hemodynamics and coronary anatomy.
   D. Review medications and ensure patient is on maximally tolerated goal directed medical therapy (diuretics).

   Answer: D

   Patient has a secondary TR categorized as mixed TR with both atrial and ventricular dysfunction. The next step in management is maximally tolerated medical therapy with diuretics. Although coronary angiography is standard in patients planned for surgical repair or replacement, the role in patients undergoing transcatheter intervention remains unclear. It is unlikely that coronary revascularization would impact the severity of tricuspid regurgitation.

2. Which modality of imaging can be used for intraprocedural guidance when transesophageal imaging yields suboptimal visualization?
   A. Fluoroscopy can be used solely for guiding transcatheter tricuspid valve intervention
   B. Transthoracic echocardiography
   C. Intracardiac echocardiography
   D. Intervention is not possible in this situation and procedure should be aborted

   Answer: C

   Intracardiac echocardiography can be used in cases with compromised TEE windows during procedure.

References

1. Topilsky Y, Maltais S, Medina Inojosa J, Oguz D, Michelena H, Maalouf J, et al. Burden of tricuspid regurgitation in patients diagnosed in the community setting. JACC Cardiovasc Imaging. 2019;12(3):433–42.
2. Messika-Zeitoun D, Verta P, Gregson J, Pocock SJ, Boero I, Feldman TE, et al. Impact of tricuspid regurgitation on survival in patients with heart failure: a large electronic health record patient-level database analysis. Eur J Heart Fail. 2020;22(10):1803–13.
3. Nath J, Foster E, Heidenreich PA. Impact of tricuspid regurgitation on long-term survival. J Am Coll Cardiol. 2004;43(3):405–9.
4. Axtell AL, Bhambhani V, Moonsamy P, Healy EW, Picard MH, Sundt TM 3rd, et al. Surgery does not improve survival in patients with isolated severe tricuspid regurgitation. J Am Coll Cardiol. 2019;74(6):715–25.
5. Alqahtani F, Berzingi CO, Aljohani S, Hijazi M, Al-Hallak A, Alkhouli M. Contemporary trends in the use and outcomes of surgical treatment of tricuspid regurgitation. J Am Heart Assoc. 2017;6(12):e007597.
6. Dahou A, Levin D, Reisman M, Hahn RT. Anatomy and physiology of the tricuspid valve. JACC Cardiovasc Imaging. 2019;12(3):458–68.
7. Rudski LG, Lai WW, Afilalo J, Hua L, Handschumacher MD, Chandrasekaran K, et al. Guidelines for the echocardiographic assessment of the right heart in adults: a report from the American Society of Echocardiography endorsed by the European Association of Echocardiography, a registered branch of the European Society of Cardiology, and the Canadian Society of Echocardiography. J Am Soc Echocardiogr. 2010;23(7):685–713.
8. Lang RM, Badano LP, Tsang W, Adams DH, Agricola E, Buck T, et al. EAE/ASE recommendations for image acquisition and display using three-dimensional echocardiography. Eur Heart J Cardiovasc Imaging. 2012;13(1):1–46.
9. Hahn RT, Zamorano JL. The need for a new tricuspid regurgitation grading scheme. Eur Heart J Cardiovasc Imaging. 2017;18(12):1342–3.

10. Saremi F, Hassani C, Millan-Nunez V, Sanchez-Quintana D. Imaging evaluation of tricuspid valve: analysis of morphology and function with CT and MRI. AJR Am J Roentgenol. 2015;204(5):W531–42.
11. Koch JA, Poll LW, Godehardt E, Korbmacher B, Modder U. Right and left ventricular volume measurements in an animal heart model in vitro: first experiences with cardiac MRI at 1.0 T. Eur Radiol. 2000;10(3):455–8.
12. Jauhiainen T, Jarvinen VM, Hekali PE, Poutanen VP, Penttila A, Kupari M. MR gradient echo volumetric analysis of human cardiac casts: focus on the right ventricle. J Comput Assist Tomogr. 1998;22(6):899–903.
13. Mor-Avi V, Jenkins C, Kuhl HP, Nesser HJ, Marwick T, Franke A, et al. Real-time 3-dimensional echocardiographic quantification of left ventricular volumes: multicenter study for validation with magnetic resonance imaging and investigation of sources of error. JACC Cardiovasc Imaging. 2008;1(4):413–23.
14. Tamborini G, Piazzese C, Lang RM, Muratori M, Chiorino E, Mapelli M, et al. Feasibility and accuracy of automated software for transthoracic three-dimensional left ventricular volume and function analysis: comparisons with two-dimensional echocardiography, three-dimensional transthoracic manual method, and cardiac magnetic resonance imaging. J Am Soc Echocardiogr. 2017;30(11):1049–58.
15. Hahn RT, Abraham T, Adams MS, Bruce CJ, Glas KE, Lang RM, et al. Guidelines for performing a comprehensive transesophageal echocardiographic examination: recommendations from the American Society of Echocardiography and the Society of Cardiovascular Anesthesiologists. J Am Soc Echocardiogr. 2013;26(9):921–64.
16. Ahn Y, Koo HJ, Kang JW, Yang DH. Tricuspid valve imaging and right ventricular function analysis using cardiac CT and MRI. Korean J Radiol. 2021;22(12):1946–63.
17. Khalique OK, Cavalcante JL, Shah D, Guta AC, Zhan Y, Piazza N, et al. Multimodality imaging of the tricuspid valve and right heart anatomy. JACC Cardiovasc Imaging. 2019;12(3):516–31.
18. Raman SV, Shah M, McCarthy B, Garcia A, Ferketich AK. Multi-detector row cardiac computed tomography accurately quantifies right and left ventricular size and function compared with cardiac magnetic resonance. Am Heart J. 2006;151(3):736–44.
19. Ranard LS, Vahl TP, Chung CJ, Sadri S, Khalique OK, Hamid N, et al. Impact of inferior vena cava entry characteristics on tricuspid annular access during transcatheter interventions. Catheter Cardiovasc Interv. 2022;99(4):1268–76.
20. Lurz P, Orban M, Besler C, Braun D, Schlotter F, Noack T, et al. Clinical characteristics, diagnosis, and risk stratification of pulmonary hypertension in severe tricuspid regurgitation and implications for transcatheter tricuspid valve repair. Eur Heart J. 2020;41(29):2785–95.
21. Dreyfus J, Audureau E, Bohbot Y, Coisne A, Lavie-Badie Y, Bouchery M, et al. TRI-SCORE: a new risk score for in-hospital mortality prediction after isolated tricuspid valve surgery. Eur Heart J. 2022;43(7):654–62.
22. Zack CJ, Fender EA, Chandrashekar P, Reddy YNV, Bennett CE, Stulak JM, et al. National trends and outcomes in isolated tricuspid valve surgery. J Am Coll Cardiol. 2017;70(24):2953–60.

Multimodality Imaging of Right Ventricular Outflow Tract Disease in Adults with Congenital Heart Disease

Toi Spates and Richard A. Krasuski

Abstract

As care has advanced for adults with congenital heart disease, interest in assessing right ventricular function, particularly for pathologies affecting right sided structures, has grown. Even for patients with no prior interventions, full assessment of the right ventricle (RV) and right ventricular outflow tract (RVOT) can be challenging. It is even more so in patients with extensive prior surgical and transcatheter interventions. In these patients a multi-modality approach is often indicated to completely assess the cardiac anatomy and quantify RV function.

For patients with RV dysfunction from RVOT and PV pathology, pulmonic valve replacement is an expected long-term consideration. In this chapter, we will review the role of cardiac imaging in patients with pulmonic pathologies, specifically those requiring intervention. We will discuss pathophysiology, review palliative and repair methods, and discuss guideline-based indications for transcatheter pulmonic valve replacement.

Keywords

Right ventricular outflow tract · Right ventricle · Congenital heart disease · Pulmonic valve · Transcatheter pulmonic valve replacement · Cardiac imaging

Abbreviations

ACHD	Adult congenital heart disease
CCT	Cardiovascular computed tomography
CHD	Congenital heart disease
cMRI	Cardiac magnetic resonance imaging
ICE	Intracardiac echocardiography
LVEF	Left ventricular ejection fraction
PA	Pulmonary artery
PR	Pulmonic regurgitation
PS	Pulmonic stenosis
PV	Pulmonic valve
RHC	Right heart catheterization
RV	Right ventricle
RVEF	Right ventricular ejection fraction
RVOT	Right ventricular outflow tract
SSFP	Steady state free precession
TOF	Tetralogy of Fallot
TR	Tricuspid regurgitation
VSD	Ventricular septal defect

Supplementary Information The online version contains supplementary material available at https://doi.org/10.1007/978-3-031-50740-3_4.

T. Spates · R. A. Krasuski (✉)
Duke University Health System, Durham, NC, USA
e-mail: toi.spates@duke.edu; richard.krasuski@duke.edu

Test your learning and check your understanding of this book's contents: use the "Springer Nature Flashcards" app to access questions using ▶ https://sn.pub/ambACS. To use the app, please follow the instructions in the chapter "Transcatheter Aortic Valve Replacement."

Learning Objectives
1. To understand the key features of tetralogy of Fallot and other abnormalities of the right ventricular outflow tract and pulmonic valve.
2. Review the surgical and transcatheter palliative and corrective approaches to managing common lesions.
3. Become familiar with the multi-modality techniques required to adequately visualize the right ventricular outflow tract and pulmonic valve.
4. Recognize the guideline-based indications for transcatheter pulmonic valve replacement.

Case Study
A 58-year-old gentleman has tetralogy of Fallot and a surgical history notable for bilateral Blalock–Taussig–Thomas shunts during infancy, followed by complete surgical repair at 2 years of age. His pulmonic valve was then replaced with a homograft, and he underwent a concomitant tricuspid valve annuloplasty at the age of 35. His post-operative course was complicated by ventricular tachycardia requiring eventual ablation, paroxysmal atrial fibrillation, and a paralyzed right hemidiaphragm resulting in respiratory insufficiency and chronic hypercarbia. The patient now presents with increasing heart failure symptoms secondary to mixed stenosis and regurgitation accompanied by progressive right failure.

Background and Definitions

Abnormalities affecting the right ventricular outflow tract (RVOT) include valvular, sub-valvular, and supravalvular stenoses in addition to multi-faceted lesions. In many patients, the RVOT is difficult to fully visualize with a singular imaging modality, and thus care has evolved to include a multi-modality approach.

Unlike the left ventricle (LV), which is oval-shaped and lies a distance below the sternum, the RV is triangular and lies directly behind the sternum. The RVOT usually wraps itself anteriorly and to the left of the LV outflow tract and abuts the sternum, making it challenging to image, particularly in patients with accompanying congenital lesions and even more so following surgical and transcatheter interventions [1]. Pathologies in which complete imaging of the RVOT is vital for management include isolated valvular and supravalvular pulmonic stenosis, tetralogy of Fallot (TOF), pulmonic atresia with intact ventricular septum, and pulmonic valve (PV) endocarditis.

TOF is the most common cyanotic congenital heart disease. It occurs developmentally because of anterior and superior displacement of the outlet septum. The displacement of the outlet septum onto the right ventricle leads to malalignment of the ventricular septum causing a ventricular septal defect (VSD), an overriding and rightward deviated aorta, and varying levels and degrees of RVOT obstruction with RV hypertrophy [2, 3].

Techniques to palliate and repair TOF have been refined over several decades, resulting in excellent long-term patient survival [4, 5]. Palliation is now reserved for patients with profound cyanosis at birth or poor branch PA arborization that limits an early complete repair. Earlier palliative methods consisted of aorto-pulmonary shunts and subclavian to pulmonary artery shunts to improve cyanosis and encourage PA growth. Subclavian to pulmonary artery shunts are now generally favored due to less resultant congestive heart failure and concern for pulmonary hypertension. Historically as neonates grew and the PAs increased to sufficient size, "complete" repair became possible. This procedure generally includes patch repair of the VSD, resection of the RVOT obstruction, and occasional PA augmentation [4, 6]. Current trends are toward early repair with valve-sparing techniques and a general avoidance of palliative shunting.

The initial technique of "complete" repair included resection of as much tissue as necessary for full relief of RVOT obstruction. RVOT augmentation was then required with a transannular patch. The latter resulted in varying degrees of pulmonic insufficiency, which generally increased over time as the RV and RVOT remodeled. Longstanding and significant pulmonic regurgitation (PR) can lead to RV failure and is a significant source of morbidity and mortality [4, 5]. In the absence of severe pulmonary annular hypoplasia, the surgical approach today is trans-atrial/trans-pulmonary incision with closure of VSD and relief of RVOT obstruction using valve sparing techniques, recognizing residual obstruction is better tolerated (with regression over time) than regurgitation. In other variants of TOF where the pulmonary arterial tree is hypoplastic, valved RV-PA conduits can be used to provide adequate antegrade flow [2, 3, 6]. Patients with pulmonic atresia and intact ventricular septum have a severely atretic pulmonic valve with circulation dependent on the presence of a patent ductus arteriosus and/or an interatrial communication. These patients also have variable degrees of right ventricular and tricuspid valve hypoplasia that complicate the pursuit of complete biventricular repair. During infancy, palliation centers around promotion of pulmonary blood flow. This is achieved via prostaglandin infusions and interventions such as surgical shunts and ductal stents. In the absence of right ventricular dependent coronary flow, decompression is achieved by pulmonary valvotomy with or without transannular repair. For patients who have right ventricular dependent coronary flow or if the right ventricle remains hypoplastic and diminutive despite decompression, a single ventricle surgical repair strategy is often employed. In patients with a sufficient RV and tricuspid valve, the RVOT is reconstructed using a transannular patch, the ASD is closed, and valvotomy is performed. These patients, similar to TOF repaired by transannular patch, undergo repeated PV interventions [2, 3].

In infants with critical isolated pulmonic stenosis (PS), cyanosis is common as the ductus arteriosus begins to close in the first few hours of life and elevated right sided pressures result in right-to-left shunting across the foramen ovale. The anatomy is often described as a dome-shaped valve with commissural fusion, or a dysplastic valve with thickened leaflets [2, 7]. For those infants with severe symptoms, a peak gradient ≥40 mmHg and ductal dependency, catheter based valvuloplasty provides a bridge to definitive surgical intervention later in infancy. While valvuloplasty works well for domed valves, it is less successful for thickened, dysplastic valves, where surgical intervention is usually required [8]. Surgical technique is dependent on the degree of annular hypoplasia. In the absence of severe annular hypoplasia, incision of the commissures may increase valve area; while severe annular hypoplasia and supravalvular stenosis require techniques used in TOF repair, including transannular patching and PA augmentation [2, 6]. Despite good durability, complications like those seen in TOF occur, [5] including RVOT obstruction, PR, and endocarditis.

For patients with PS, follow-up with Adult Congenital Heart Disease (ACHD) providers depends on symptoms and clinical status, with imaging performed as frequently as every 1–5 years depending on lesion severity [9]. Severity in PS is graded similarly to aortic stenosis. Mild PS is identified by a peak velocity <3 m/s and severe PS with a peak velocity >4 m/s. Indications for intervention include at least moderate PS (≥3 m/s velocity) with exertional limitation, cyanosis, or heart failure. RVOT obstruction uses the same velocity criteria and intervention is indicated for patients with at least moderate obstruction of a RV-PA conduit if there is a decline in functional status or increased burden of arrhythmias [9, 10]. For patients with PR, either after management of isolated PS or after repair of TOF, intervention is recommended for at least moderate PR and associated symptoms. If the patient is sedentary, exercise testing can be helpful to uncover functional limitation. Quantitative assessments with imaging can identify a Class IIa indication for valve replacement. Moderate PR associated with significant RV dilation by cardiac magnetic resonance imaging (cMRI) volumes, RV dysfunction or LV dysfunction, or associated moderate or greater tricuspid regurgitation (TR) are indications for PV replacement, as is RVOT obstruction with RVSP ≥2/3 systemic pressure. If there are no additional pathologies that require surgical intervention, a transcatheter approach should be considered [9, 10].

In patients with extensive surgical histories and the presence of bioprosthetic material, limiting the risk of systemic infection is paramount. The ACC/AHA Guidelines recommend antibiotic prophylaxis in patients with prosthetic valves, a prior history of endocarditis, the presence residual shunts at sites of prior repair, history of uncorrected cyanotic heart disease, or recent intervention using prosthetic material in the last 6 months. Should patients present with concerns for systemic infections, blood cultures and dedicated cardiac imaging are required to evaluate for the presence and extent of endocarditis [9, 11].

Surveillance for long-term complications from RVOT pathology is necessary and often utilizes a multi-modality approach. Echocardiography is the first-line tool used to delineate anatomy as justified by appropriate use criteria and is routinely used for the evaluation of structural complications [12, 13]. The AHA/ACC Guidelines recommend the use of additional imaging for more quantitative ventricular assessment or a detailed reconstruction of vascular anatomy [10, 14]. Other imaging modalities include cMRI, CCT, and right heart catheterization (RHC), which can provide hemodynamic, fluoroscopic and intracardiac echo (ICE) evaluation. While imaging modalities like CCT and RHC can provide anatomical detail and hemodynamic assessment, close monitoring of radiation exposure is essential for young adults with CHD. Given concerns regarding lifetime radiation exposure, alternative imaging modalities should be considered whenever possible. cMRI is ideal for patients who require close monitoring of ventricular volumes given the lack of radiation exposure; thereby justifying its Class I recommendation [9–11, 14].

Two-dimensional echocardiography includes transthoracic, transesophageal, and ICE. Chest wall imaging is the main modality used for surveillance in repaired CHD, but can be limited by poor imaging windows (body habitus and lung disease) and artifact from prosthetic material. Sedated intraprocedural transesophageal echo or ICE can eliminate such artifacts. RV dysfunction is defined by echo as a fractional area change <35%, or diminished tricuspid annular excursion as measured by TAPSE and S' velocity [12]. For patients with prior pulmonic interventions or prosthetic PVs, visualization of the RVOT or PV can be challenging. While grading obstruction and stenosis of the RVOT or PV is more direct, quantitative assessment of PR is more challenging. Severity of PR is delineated by jet width, jet density, regurgitant volume and regurgitant fraction. Mild PR is characterized by a regurgitant jet width <20% of annular diameter, an incomplete continuous wave Doppler envelope and a regurgitant fraction <20%. Severe PR is characterized by jet width >40% of annular diameter, dense and complete continuous wave Doppler envelope and regurgitant fraction >40% [12, 15].

Multi-detector CCT with ECG gating can provide vascular, volumetric and structural detail. An advantage of CCT is shorter scan times than cMRI, at the price of ionizing radiation exposure and the need for contrast media administration. While it is possible to create anatomic three-dimensional reconstructions using either CCT or cMRI, CCT is generally favored due to higher spatial resolution. Reconstructions facilitate pre-procedural planning, including the selection of appropriate devices [11, 14, 16] (Fig. 1).

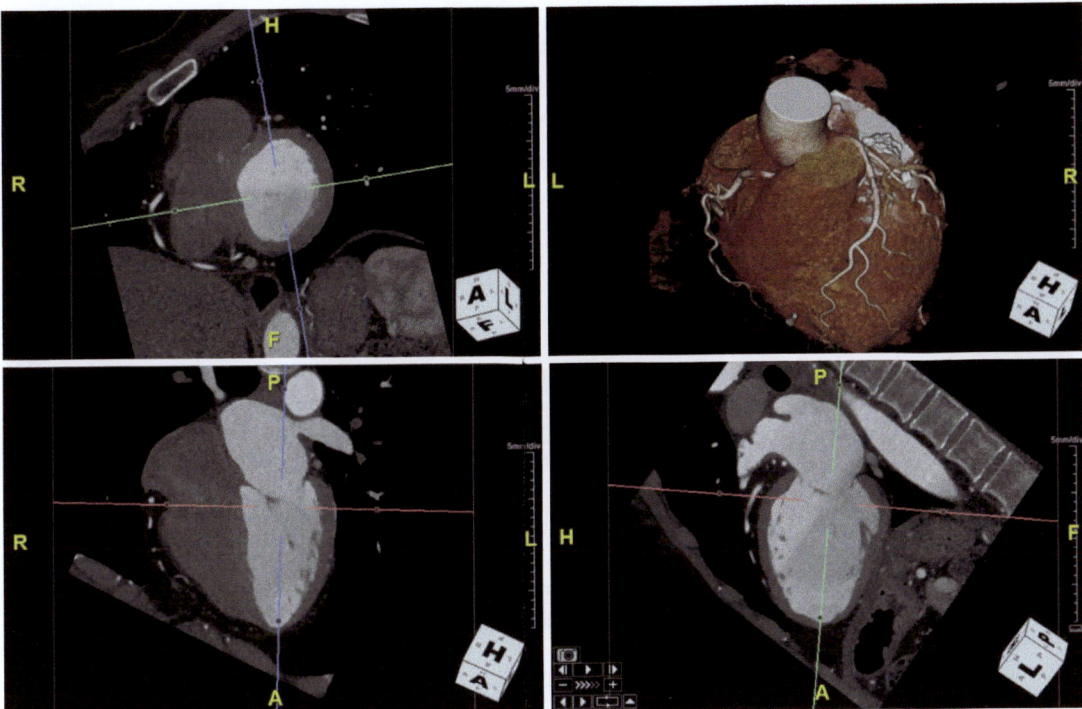

Fig. 1 Cardiac CT of our patient demonstrating a multi-planar reconstruction with short axis, four chamber and 2 chamber view of the left ventricle with volume rendered image

cMRI has emerged as an essential component for the follow-up of patients with congenital heart diseases and is especially valuable in assessing the RV, RVOT and PV. The AHA/ACC Guidelines give a Class I recommendation for cMRI if RV volumes are required to guide management. Quantitative assessment of RVEF can be performed using steady state free precession (SSFP) cine imaging and volumetric calculation, [5] with RV dysfunction defined as an RVEF <50%. Ventricular volumes are indexed to body surface area. Thresholds for intervention in pulmonic regurgitation include an RVEDVI ≥ 160 mL/m^2, RVESVI ≥ 80 mL/m^2, or RVEDV $\geq 2 \times$ LVEDV [9, 10, 14, 17] (Figs. 2, 3 and 4).

Quantification of PS and PR severity can be performed by velocity encoding phase contrast imaging. This sequence assesses the velocity of protons in a particular region in relation to a technician-specified velocity. If that region of interest aliases, it indicates the velocity exceeds that preset parameter. This same modality can not only interrogate stenoses, but also quantify regurgitation by assessing flow during systole and diastole. Velocity encoded imaging is most accurate when interrogating laminar flow. Occasionally velocities can significantly overestimate or underestimate gradients when the regurgitation is eccentric or turbulent. Regurgitant lesions can also be quantified using the volumetric assessments for LV and RV stroke volumes in the absence of any confounding regurgitant lesions [14].

Each imaging modality has inherent limitations. Thus, the use of multiple modalities can provide more complete assessment of anatomy and hemodynamics, more accurately guiding clinical management (Fig. 5).

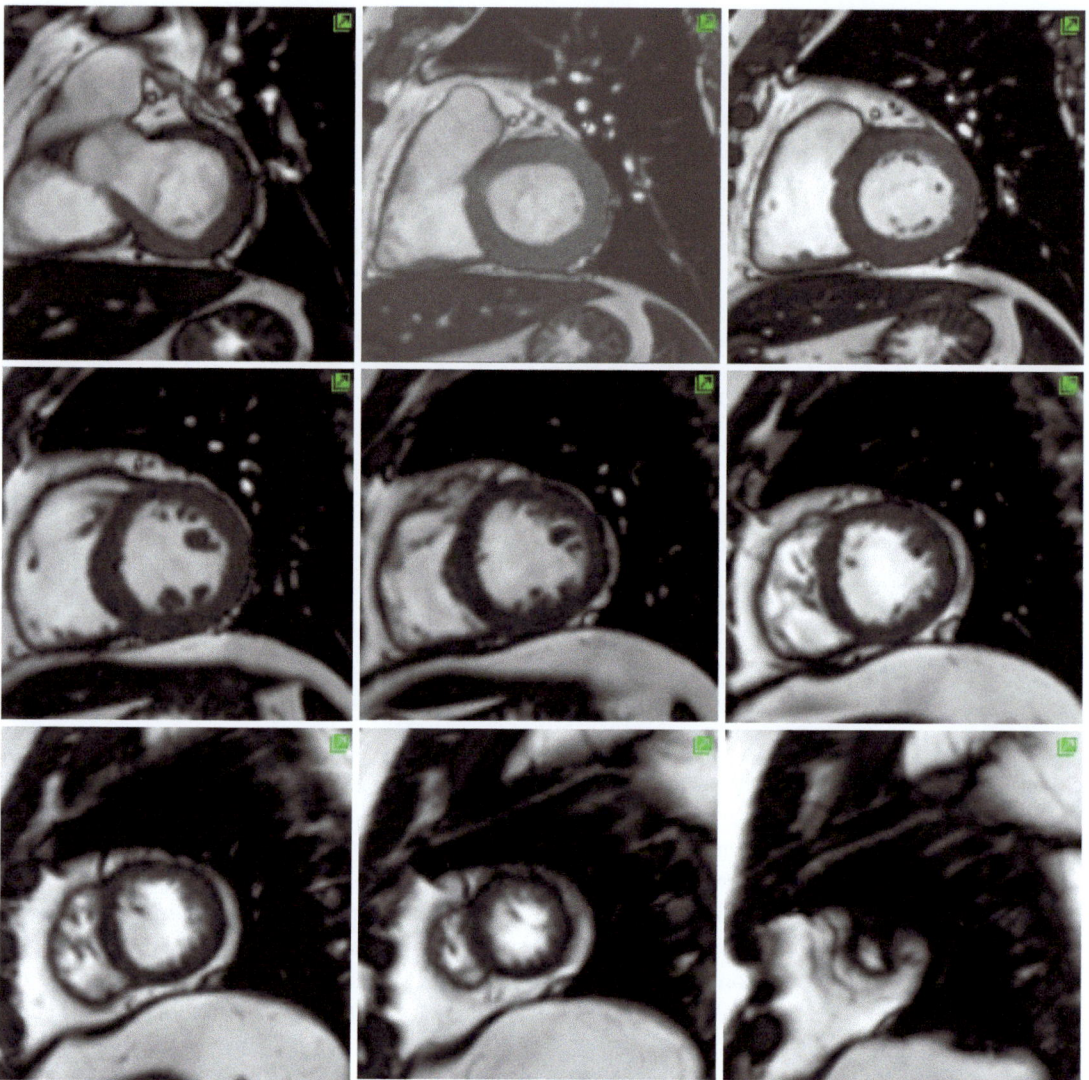

Fig. 2 Short axis slices of the ventricles used for visual assessment and volumetric quantification of ventricular function using SSFP cine imaging

Fig. 3 Dedicated views of the LV using SSFP cine imaging

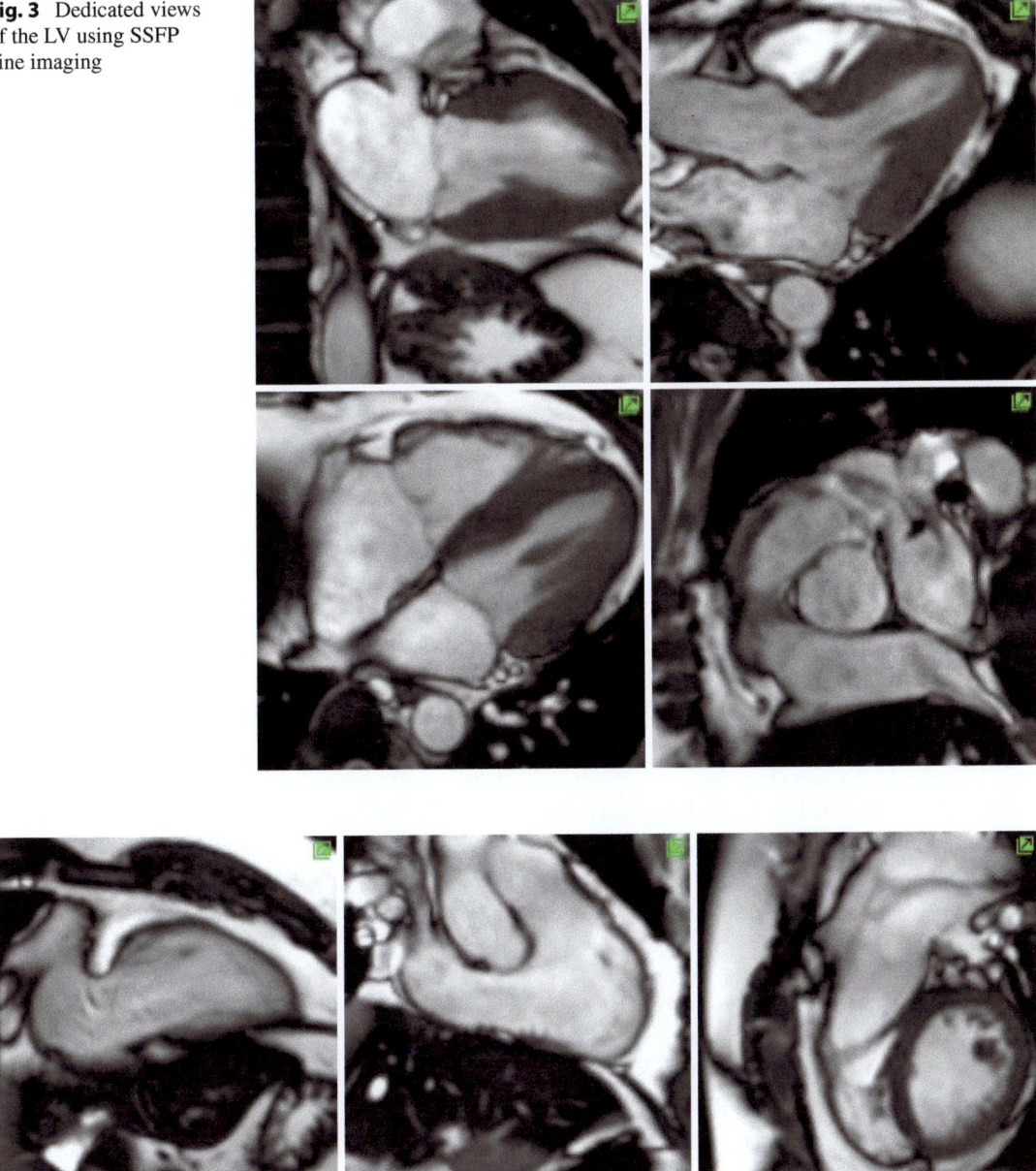

Fig. 4 Dedicated views of the RV using SSFP cine imaging

Fig. 5 Adapted table of appropriate use criteria for multimodality imaging for specific congenital anatomies [13]

Appropriate Use Criteria for Multimodality Imaging in ACHD

Anatomy	Echo (Frequency of imaging)	CMR	CT
Pulmonic Stenosis		1- 3 yrs	May be appropriate prior to procedure or if unable to obtain CMR
mild	3- 5 yrs		
mod-severe	1- 3 yrs		
+ heart failure	3- 12 mths		
Pulmonic Atresia + IVS		1- 3 yrs	May be appropriate prior to procedure or if unable to obtain CMR
mild	2- 3 yrs		
mod-severe	1- 3 yrs		
+ heart failure	3- 12 mths		
Tetralogy of Fallot			May be appropriate if unable to obtain CMR
mild	1 year	2- 3 yrs	
Conduit, RV/LV, valvular dysfunction	6- 12 mths – 2-3 yrs	2- 3 yrs	
+ heart failure	3- 12 mths		

Diagnosis and Pre-procedural Evaluation

The patient had been followed in the Adult Congenital Heart Disease Clinic at ~6-month intervals, with his sole complaint being intermittent lower extremity edema that usually responded well to diuresis. Routine echocardiography revealed grossly normal biventricular function with mild TR, trivial PR and moderate PS with a peak velocity of 3.1 m/s (Fig. 6).

The patient returned to clinic frequently over the course of the next year with complaints of increasing lower extremity edema, shortness of breath, and progressively lower oxygen saturation. His diuretic regimen was increased frequently with intermittent improvement. Given his progressive symptoms, a cMRI was performed.

Calculated LVEF was 67% and RVEF was 45%, with evidence of RV pressure and volume overload. Imaging further demonstrated regional akinesis of the infundibular region with adherence to the sternum. The RVOT patch was stable and there was no evidence of residual VSD. Moderate PR was present, although the regurgitant fraction measured only 19%. The regurgitant jet was turbulent in appearance, with peak velocity measuring 3.2 m/s, consistent with moderate PS. Because the data were largely unchanged from his prior study, routine follow-up at 6 months was planned (Figs. 7 and 8).

At follow-up ~6 months later, the patient was profoundly dyspneic and required direct admission to the cardiovascular intensive care unit for hypoxic respiratory failure, volume overload, and systemic hypotension. A RHC was performed and revealed a transpulmonary peak-to-peak gradient of 31 mmHg at the level of the valve (Fig. 9).

Aggressive diuresis was continued and the need for PV intervention were discussed.

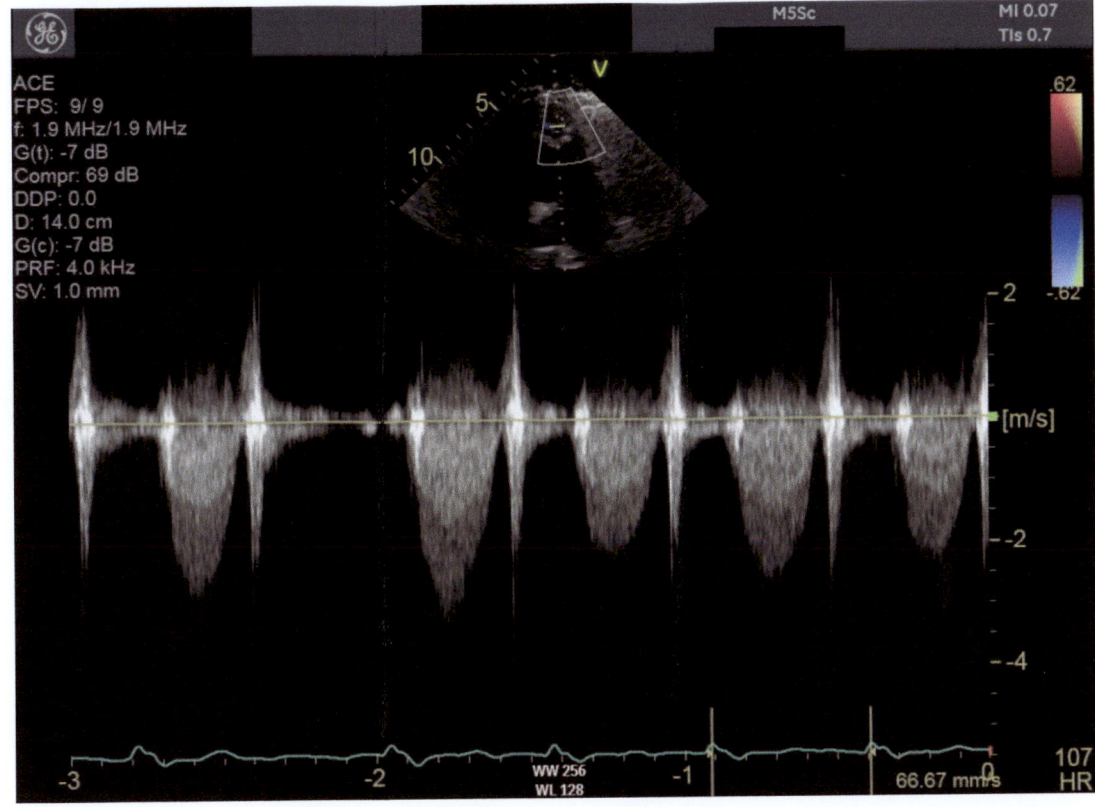

Fig. 6 Peak velocity in the RVOT of 3.1 m/s measured at the level of the PV

Fig. 7 Volumetric assessment to determine LV volumes and function, which were normal. Note the RV stroke volume exceeds that of the LV, consistent with a regurgitant valve and increased RVEDV

Volumetric Analysis	LV	RV
ED Volume (ml)	98.8	193.1
ES Volume (ml)	32.4	106.8
Cardiac Output (L/min)	7.04	9.15
Myocardial Mass (g)	--	--
Stroke Volume (ml)	66.4	86.3
Ejection Fraction (%)	67.2	44.7

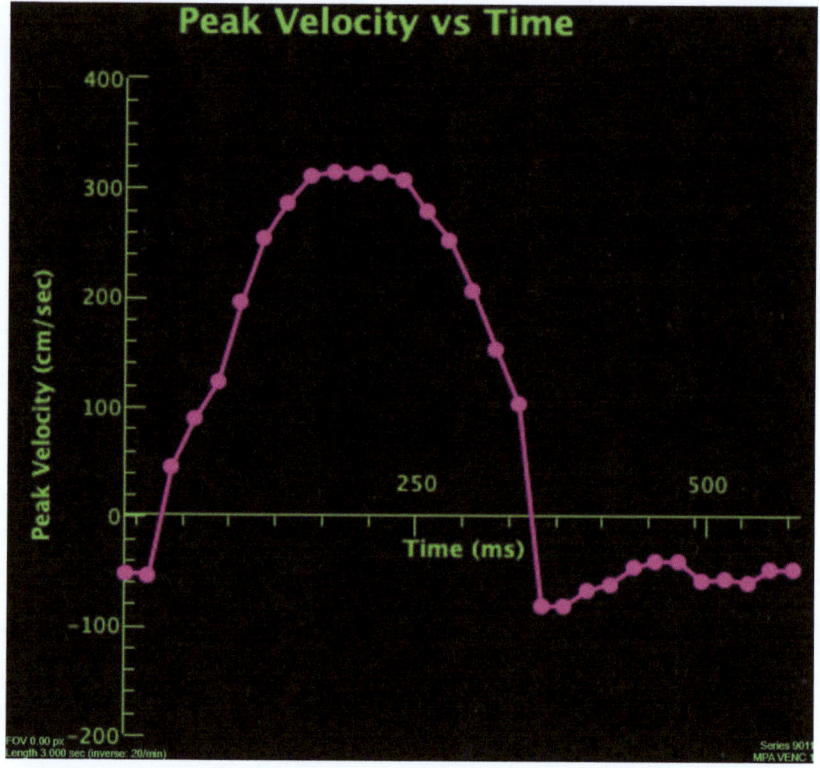

Fig. 8 Velocity encoded phase contrast imaging at the level of main PA revealing a peak velocity of 3.2 m/s. Note the reversal of flow below the baseline, which represents significant regurgitation

Fig. 9 RHC demonstrates a ~31 mmHg peak-to-peak gradient across the pulmonic valve and elevated pulmonary capillary wedge pressure consistent with at least moderate PS and concomitant left ventricular diastolic dysfunction. Of note, the patient was given moderate sedation, which could reduce cardiac output and lead to gradient underestimation

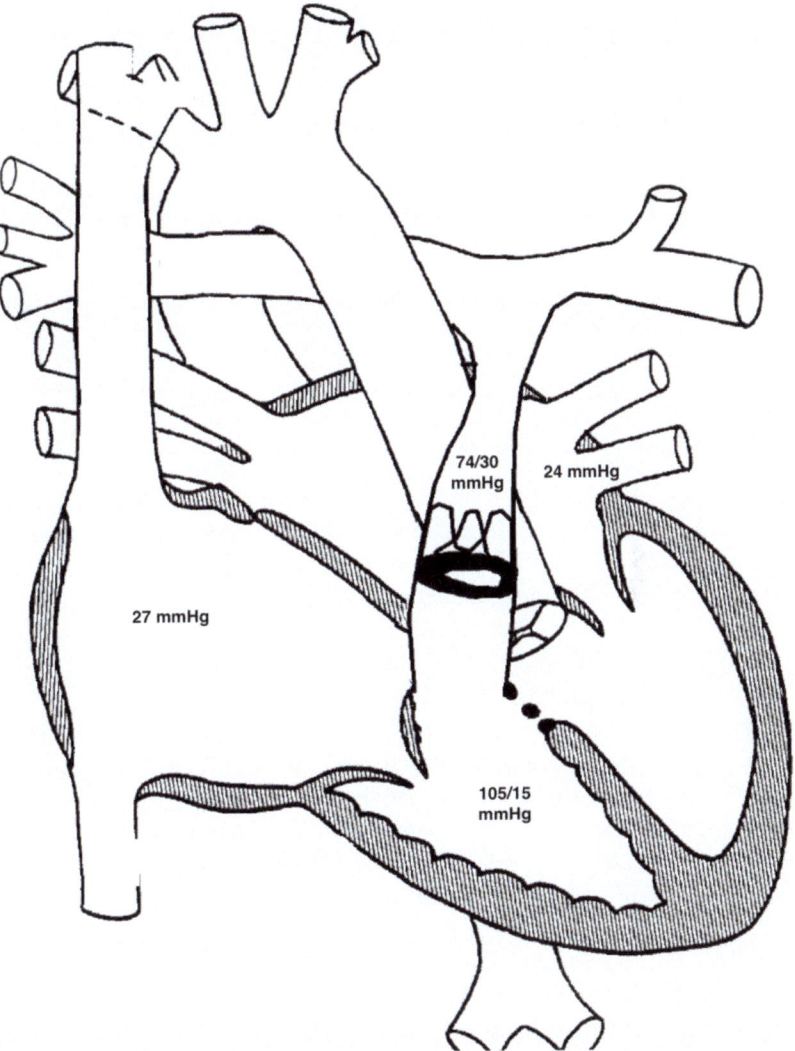

Heart Team Approach and Discussion

Based on admission for decompensated HF and evidence of RV dysfunction with at least moderate PS and/or PR, the patient met a Class I indication for PV intervention based on 2018 AHA/ACC Guidelines for Management of ACHD [9, 10] (Figs. 10 and 11).

Surgical and transcatheter valve replacement options were considered with the patient. Given his respiratory limitation (chronic hypercarbia and hypoxemia), the proximity of RV free wall to sternum, and his advanced clinical status, the decision was made to pursue transcatheter valve implantation.

There are two types of transcatheter pulmonic prostheses currently available, balloon expand-

Fig. 10 Modified table regarding general indications for intervention in PR in repaired TOF [2, 9, 10]

Indications for Pulmonic Valve Replacement
Moderate/Severe RV dysfunction + Symptoms
RV dilation (RVEDVi ≥ 160 ml/m², RVESI ≥ 80 ml/m², RVEDV ≥ 2x LVEDV)
RVSP ≥ $\frac{2}{3}$ systemic pressure
Decreased exercise tolerance
Sustained tachyarrhythmias

Levels of Evidence for Valve Intervention in Repaired TOF
Class I: Moderate - Severe PR + Symptoms
Class IIa: Moderate - Severe PR w/o symptoms + RV dysfunction/enlargement

Fig. 11 Modified table regarding strength of recommendations for intervention in repaired TOF [2, 9, 10, 17]

able and self-expanding platforms/valves. Balloon expandable valves were first developed for delivery into conduits and bioprostheses, which serve as ideal landing zones. The two FDA approved balloon expandable valves are the Melody (Medtronic, Minneapolis, MN) and Sapien (Edwards Lifesciences, Irvine, VA) valves. These valves are generally not able to be delivered into patch-repaired outflow tracts as they are limited in size by the balloon expandable system, with the Melody Valve sized from 18–22 mm and the Sapien Valve from 20–29 mm. Prior to implantation, proper sizing is essential, as is intraprocedural balloon compression testing to ensure no distortion of the aortic or coronary anatomy [18].

Self-expanding devices include the Harmony Valve (Medtronic, Minneapolis, MN) and the Alterra Adaptive Prestent (Edwards Lifesciences, Irvine, VA), the latter of which is used in concert with the 29 mm Sapien S3 Valve (Edwards Lifesciences, Irvine, VA). These devices can expand to much larger sizes without risk for coronary or aortic compression. Neither device by design, however, treats stenosis. For both devices, pre-procedural RVOT assessment is required using a specialized CT scan shared with the respective company to assess candidacy, model the valve implant and determine the ideal landing zone [18].

Intra-procedural Imaging

The patient underwent cardiac catheterization with a plan for RVOT augmentation via stenting followed by placement of a transcatheter pulmonic valve.

Prior to proceeding, the operator ensures absence of coronary artery or aortic compression by inflating a high-pressure balloon across the RVOT/MPA during aortography or selective coronary angiography.

With no coronary artery compression or aortic deformation, the operators proceeded with stent placement [14]. After two stents were deployed (to provide increased radial strength), free PR was present as expected. The stent was further expanded by post-dilatation to ensure an adequately sized delivery zone for the transcatheter valve (Figs. 12 and 13).

A 23 mm Sapien S3 valve was then delivered into the pulmonic position. Mild residual narrowing was still present at the completion of the case, secondary to conduit calcification and external compression, though the transpulmonary gradient was reduced to only 2 mmHg (Fig. 14).

An echocardiogram was performed post-procedurally and revealed no evidence of stenosis or regurgitation (Fig. 15).

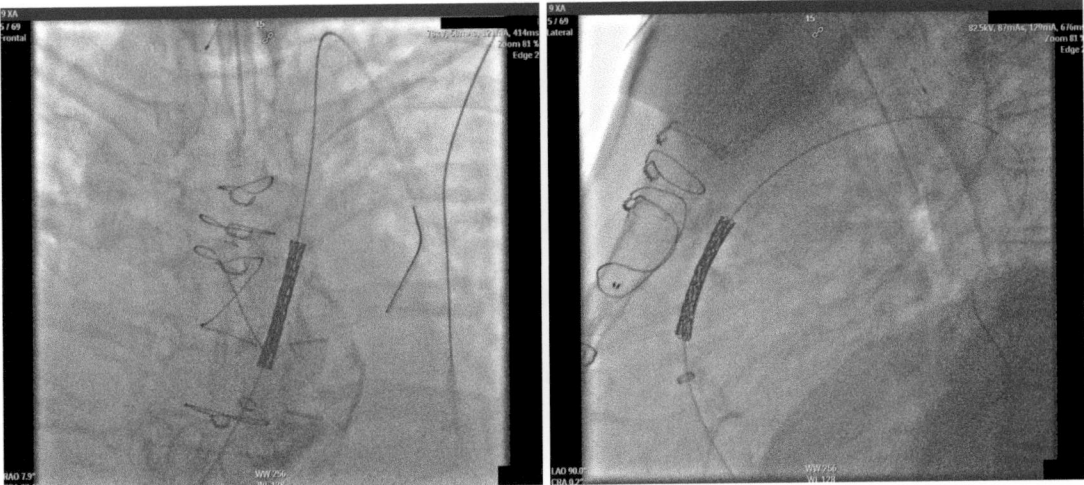

Fig. 12 Fluoroscopic still frame of stent positioning prior to delivery

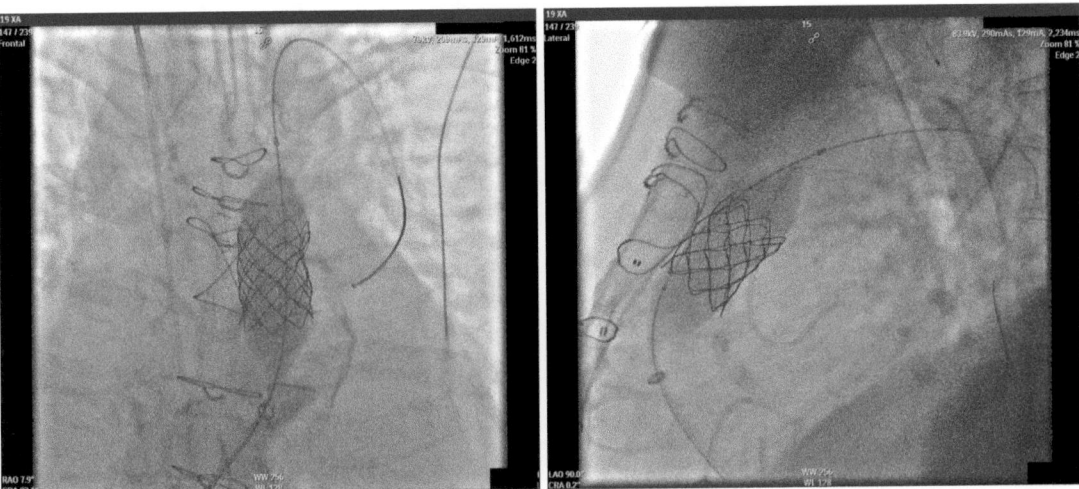

Fig. 13 Fluoroscopic image of stent during high-pressure balloon dilation. Note that a waist is still present, representing external compression due to heavy conduit calcification

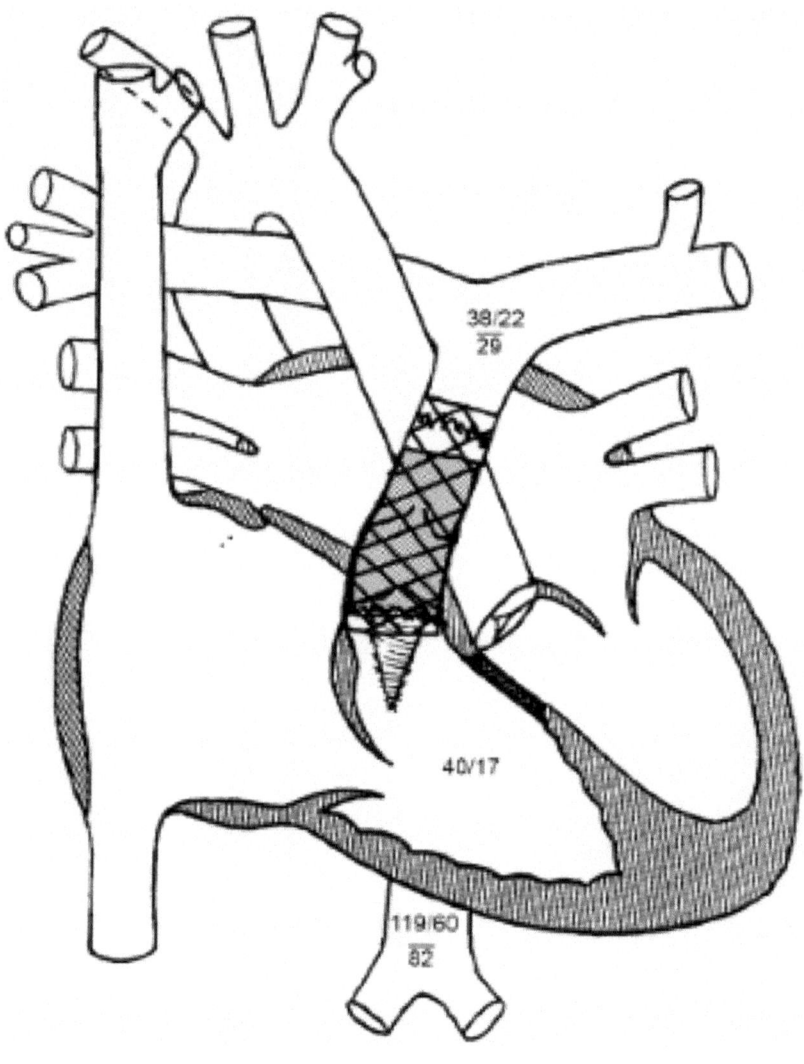

Fig. 14 Post-procedural hemodynamics revealed gradient resolution

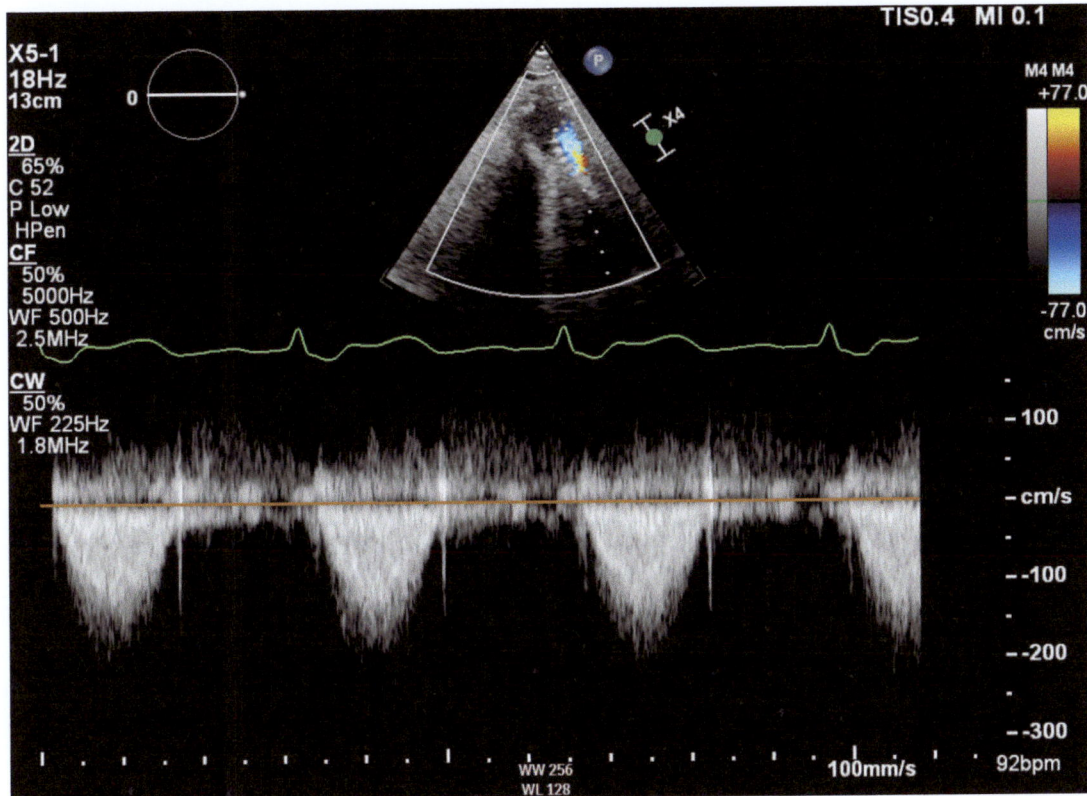

Fig. 15 Doppler gradient showed minimal to no PS

Endocarditis: Prevention and Recognition

One of the most dreaded long-term complications for patients with transcatheter valves is endocarditis. Higher residual gradient after implant appears to be a significant risk factor [19]. In addition to antibiotic prophylaxis with dental procedures, all patients with prosthetic valves (surgical or transcatheter) should also receive a baby aspirin. Early valve failure may be related to leaflet thrombosis and antiplatelet therapy may be preventative.

PV endocarditis is particularly challenging to identify. Symptoms may be indolent and valvular vegetations can be challenging to visualize. An acute increase in outflow murmur intensity or measured transpulmonary gradient should raise the index of suspicion for endocarditis. Blood cultures should be drawn whenever suspicion exists. Transthoracic and transesophageal echocardiographic imaging may not be revealing; and PET CT or cMRI may improve diagnostic sensitivity [20]. ICE can also be diagnostic: the catheter can be delivered across the tricuspid valve and into the right ventricle and images can be taken looking directly into the RVOT and pulmonic valve.

Clinical Controversies and Clinical Pearls

- During transcatheter replacement using balloon expandable prostheses, it is imperative to perform balloon inflation in the RVOT to evaluate for coronary compression or aortic root deformation, as these features generally preclude use of balloon expanding transcatheter valve.
- The use of self-expanding transcatheter devices and the use of pre-stenting allows for more inclusive RVOT anatomies and attenuates the concern for coronary compression.

- An important step to diagnosis of pulmonic valve endocarditis is having a high index of suspicion. An unexplained rise in RVOT gradient is often seen. When transthoracic and transesophageal echo are unrevealing, CT PET, MRI or intracardiac echo should be pursued.

Key Points
- Surgical and transcatheter interventions have improved survival and quality of life in TOF; though long-term follow-up is essential to assess for infectious, structural, and arrhythmogenic sequelae.
- 2D echocardiography is a valuable tool for serially monitoring. ACHD guidelines recommend cMRI be performed when quantitative RV assessment is required to guide management, with appropriate use criteria justifying it at an interval of every 3–5 years or prior to a planned intervention in the absence of acute clinical changes.
- Pulmonic stenosis is graded similar to aortic stenosis, with <3 m/s mild, ≥3 m/s moderate, and ≥4 m/s severe.
- Severe bioprosthetic pulmonic regurgitation is classified as a dense continuous wave Doppler envelope, a jet width: annulus ratio >40%, and regurgitant fraction >40% on echocardiography.
- Pulmonic regurgitation and subsequent RV dysfunction is one of the most common late complications noted in these patients. In the presence of ≥moderate pulmonic valve dysfunction (stenosis or regurgitation) with symptoms of heart failure, decreased exercise tolerance (as demonstrated by cardiopulmonary stress testing), or evidence of RV dilation and enlargement, an intervention should be considered.
- Using cMRI, right ventricular dilation suggesting a need for pulmonic valve replacement for PR includes: RVEDVI ≥160 mL/m^2, RVESVI ≥80 mL/m^2, or RVEDV ≥2 × LVEDV.
- Transcatheter valve replacement should be strongly favored if the patient is a poor surgical candidate, no additional operative interventions are necessary or to limit the number of eventual sternotomies if the patient's anatomy is suitable.

Disclosures Dr. Krasuski serves as a consultant for Actelion/Janssen Pharmaceuticals, Bayer, Gore Medical, Medtronic and Neptune Medical. He receives research funding from the Adult Congenital Heart Association and Actelion/Janssen Pharmaceuticals. He is a principal investigator for trials with Artivion, Corvia, Edwards Lifesciences, and Medtronic.

Chapter Review Questions

1. A 34-year-old gentleman with a history of tetralogy of Fallot presents to clinic for routine evaluation. His history includes surgical bioprosthetic valve placement at the age of 21. He is asymptomatic and had an echocardiogram performed a year ago that demonstrated normal biventricular function and stable bioprosthetic pulmonic valve. The peak velocity was measured at 2.8 m/s with mild pulmonic regurgitation. At what interval should imaging be performed to adequately interrogate valve function?
   A. Every 3–5 years
   B. Every 6 months
   C. Once yearly
   D. Every 2 years
   Answer: C
   For patients with surgical bioprosthetic valves, it is important that a post-operative baseline echocardiogram is performed. The 2020 AHA ACC Guidelines for Valvular Heart Disease states, echocardiograms should then be performed at intervals of 5 years and 10 years following intervention if the patient is without symptoms or clinical exam changes. After 10 years, patients should undergo annual imaging given the increasing concern for progressive valve dysfunction.

2. A 47-year-old woman presents to your clinic for new patient evaluation. She has a history of tetralogy of Fallot repaired by transannular patch with moderate to severe pulmonic

regurgitation. She was closely followed by her previous cardiologist, who performed a cardiac MRI ~8 months ago. This revealed a RVEF 49% with a RVEDVi 133 mL/m^2 and a regurgitant fraction of 37%. She works from home and is fairly sedentary. She notes mild shortness of breath when walking her dog, which she mainly attributes to deconditioning. What is the most appropriate next step?

A. Repeat cardiac MRI
B. Cardiopulmonary stress testing
C. Echocardiogram
D. Right heart catheterization

Answer: B

Cardiopulmonary stress testing to evaluate for exertional intolerance is the most appropriate next step given her moderate to severe regurgitation without significant RV chamber dilation or dysfunction. Should cardiopulmonary stress testing demonstrate cardiovascular limitation, it would be reasonable to consider surgical or transcatheter pulmonic valve replacement with a class I recommendation as per the ACC/AHA Guidelines for Adults with Congenital Heart Disease.

3. A 31-year-old woman presents to clinic for evaluation. She has a history of pulmonary atresia for which she has undergone several right ventricular to pulmonary artery conduit replacements. Her last procedure was a transcatheter pulmonary valve replacement ~7 years ago. She was last seen in clinic ~2 years ago. At that time, she had an echocardiogram revealing normal biventricular systolic function and stable pulmonary valve function. On exam today, there is a prominent grade 3/6 systolic ejection murmur at the LUSB with a grade 2 diastolic murmur. The patient reports no exertional limitations, but has experienced mild malaise, fatigue, and lack of appetite over the last few weeks that she attributes to "work stress." What is the most reasonable clinical approach?

A. Return to clinic in 1 year with echocardiogram
B. Echocardiogram at the next available appointment
C. Echocardiogram and draw 2 sets of blood cultures today
D. Arrange for stat heart catheterization

Answer: C

Her physical exam is concerning for a significant change in bioprosthetic valve function. While simple device degeneration is possible, her symptoms of fatigue and malaise raise concern for a possible subacute infectious process. Given these concerns, it is most reasonable to perform both an echocardiogram to assess bioprosthetic function and to draw blood cultures to evaluate for systemic infection. It is important to note that the imaging recommendations for patients with transcatheter pulmonic valves suggest an echocardiogram be performed yearly.

References

1. Wang JMH, Rai R, Carrasco M, Sam-Odusina T, Salandy S, Gielecki J, et al. An anatomical review of the right ventricle. Transl Res Anat. 2019;17:100049.
2. Gatzoulis MA, Webb GD, Daubeney PEF. Diagnosis and management of adult congenital heart disease, vol. 14. 3rd ed. Philadelphia: Elsevier; 2018. p. 721.
3. Karl TR. Tetralogy of Fallot: current surgical perspective. Ann Pediatr Cardiol. 2008;1(2):93–100.
4. Murphy JG, Gersh BJ, Mair DD, Fuster V, McGoon MD, Ilstrup DM, et al. Long-term outcome in patients undergoing surgical repair of tetralogy of Fallot. N Engl J Med. 1993;329(9):593–9.
5. Nollert G, Fischlein T, Bouterwek S, Bohmer C, Klinner W, Reichart B. Long-term survival in patients with repair of tetralogy of Fallot: 36-year follow-up of 490 survivors of the first year after surgical repair. J Am Coll Cardiol. 1997;30(5):1374–83.
6. Mavroudis C, Backer CL. Atlas of pediatric cardiac surgery. 1st ed. London: Springer; 2015.
7. Cuypers JA, Witsenburg M, van der Linde D, Roos-Hesselink JW. Pulmonary stenosis: update on diagnosis and therapeutic options. Heart. 2013;99(5):339–47.
8. Feltes TF, Bacha E, Beekman RH 3rd, Cheatham JP, Feinstein JA, Gomes AS, et al. Indications for cardiac catheterization and intervention in pediatric cardiac disease: a scientific statement from the American Heart Association. Circulation. 2011;123(22):2607–52.
9. Stout KK, Daniels CJ, Aboulhosn JA, Bozkurt B, Broberg CS, Colman JM, et al. 2018 AHA/ACC guideline for the management of adults with congenital heart disease: executive summary: a report of the American College of Cardiology/American Heart

Association task force on clinical practice guidelines. Circulation. 2019;139(14):e637–e97.
10. Baumgartner H, De Backer J. The ESC clinical practice guidelines for the Management of Adult Congenital Heart Disease 2020. Eur Heart J. 2020;41(43):4153–4.
11. Wiant A, Nyberg E, Gilkeson RC. CT evaluation of congenital heart disease in adults. Am J Roentgenol. 2009;193(2):388–96.
12. Rudski LG, Lai WW, Afilalo J, Hua L, Handschumacher MD, Chandrasekaran K, et al. Guidelines for the echocardiographic assessment of the right heart in adults: a report from the American Society of Echocardiography endorsed by the European Association of Echocardiography, a registered branch of the European Society of Cardiology, and the Canadian Society of Echocardiography. J Am Soc Echocardiogr. 2010;23(7):685–713.
13. Sachdeva R, Valente AM, Armstrong AK, Cook SC, Han BK, Lopez L, et al. ACC/AHA/ASE/HRS/ISACHD/SCAI/SCCT/SCMR/SOPE 2020 appropriate use criteria for multimodality imaging during the follow-up Care of Patients with Congenital Heart Disease: a report of the American College of Cardiology Solution set Oversight Committee and Appropriate use Criteria Task Force, American Heart Association, American Society of Echocardiography, Heart Rhythm Society, International Society for Adult Congenital Heart Disease, Society for Cardiovascular Angiography and Interventions, Society of Cardiovascular Computed Tomography, Society for Cardiovascular Magnetic Resonance, and Society of Pediatric Echocardiography. J Am Coll Cardiol. 2020;75(6):657–703.
14. Saremi F, Gera A, Ho SY, Hijazi ZM, Sanchez-Quintana D. CT and MR imaging of the pulmonary valve. Radiographics. 2014;34(1):51–71.
15. Zoghbi WA, Chambers JB, Dumesnil JG, Foster E, Gottdiener JS, Grayburn PA, et al. Recommendations for evaluation of prosthetic valves with echocardiography and doppler ultrasound: a report From the American Society of Echocardiography's Guidelines and Standards Committee and the Task Force on Prosthetic Valves, developed in conjunction with the American College of Cardiology Cardiovascular Imaging Committee, Cardiac Imaging Committee of the American Heart Association, the European Association of Echocardiography, a registered branch of the European Society of Cardiology, the Japanese Society of Echocardiography and the Canadian Society of Echocardiography, endorsed by the American College of Cardiology Foundation, American Heart Association, European Association of Echocardiography, a registered branch of the European Society of Cardiology, the Japanese Society of Echocardiography, and Canadian Society of Echocardiography. J Am Soc Echocardiogr. 2009;22(9):975–1014.
16. Yoo SJ, Hussein N, Peel B, Coles J, van Arsdell GS, Honjo O, et al. 3D modeling and printing in congenital heart surgery: entering the stage of maturation. Front Pediatr. 2021;9:621672.
17. Sanchez Ramirez CJ, Perez de Isla L. Tetralogy of Fallot: cardiac imaging evaluation. Ann Transl Med. 2020;8(15):966.
18. Gales J, Krasuski RA, Fleming GA. Transcatheter valve replacement for right-sided valve disease in congenital heart patients. Prog Cardiovasc Dis. 2018;61(3–4):347–59.
19. McElhinney DB, Sondergaard L, Armstrong AK, Bergersen L, Padera RF, Balzer DT, et al. Endocarditis after transcatheter pulmonary valve replacement. J Am Coll Cardiol. 2018;72(22):2717–28.
20. Corey KM, Campbell MJ, Hill KD, Hornik CP, Krasuski R, Barker PC, et al. Pulmonary valve endocarditis: the potential utility of multimodal imaging prior to surgery. World J Pediatr Congenit Heart Surg. 2020;11(2):192–7.

Pre- and Intraprocedural Imaging Considerations in Paravalvular Leak Closure

Adriana Postolache, Simona Sperlongano, Mathieu Lempereur, Raluca Dulgheru, François Damas, Nils Demarneffe, and Patrizio Lancellotti

Abstract

Paravalvular regurgitation or leak (PVL) is not an uncommon complication of prosthetic valve disease and can be associated with severe heart failure, hemolytic anemia, or both. The management of these patients often having multiple comorbidities is challenging and the choice between surgical intervention, transcatheter closure and medical treatment should be decided by the Heart Team on a case-by-case basis. Transcatheter PVL closure has emerged as an attractive and efficient treatment option for these patients and the success of the procedure relies on a careful pre-procedural evaluation, for selecting the patients suitable for a transcatheter intervention, and expert imaging guidance during the procedure. Pre-procedural evaluation should determine the location and the number of the jets and the severity of the PVL. Echocardiography holds a central role in the pre-procedural evaluation of patients with PVLs, but other imaging modalities, such as cardiac magnetic resonance imaging (CMR) and cardiac computed tomography (CT) can offer useful adjunctive information for grading the severity of the regurgitation and for selecting the type and the size of the prosthesis. The intervention is performed under fluoroscopic and transesophageal/intra-cardiac echocardiographic guidance. The use of fusion imaging can facilitate the delivery of the device. Echocardiography has an important role on the procedural guidance, being especially useful for selecting the size of the device(s), confirming the correct location of the device(s) and its lack of interference with the prosthetic valve function or adjacent structures (such as the coronary arteries for aortic PVLs) and for evaluating the presence of complications. A good communication between the echocardiographer and the interventional cardiologist, at every step of the procedure, is essential for the success of the intervention.

A. Postolache · M. Lempereur · R. Dulgheru · F. Damas · N. Demarneffe · P. Lancellotti (✉)
Department of Cardiology, University of Liège Hospital, Liège, Belgium
e-mail: adriana.postolache@chuliege.be; mathieu.lempereur@chuliege.be; redulgheru@chuliege.be; fdamas@chuliege.be; ndemarneffe@chuliege.be; plancellotti@chuliege.be

S. Sperlongano
Division of Cardiology, Department of Translational Medical Sciences, University of Campania Luigi Vanvitelli, Naples, Italy
e-mail: simona.sperlongano@unicampania.it

Keywords

Paravalvular leak · Pre-procedural planning · Intra-procedural guidance · Transcatheter mitral paravalvular leak closure · Transcatheter aortic paravalvular leak closure · Transcatheter tricuspid paravalvular leak closure

© The Author(s), under exclusive license to Springer Nature Switzerland AG 2024
A. M. Kelsey et al. (eds.), *Cardiac Imaging in Structural Heart Disease Interventions*,
https://doi.org/10.1007/978-3-031-50740-3_5

Test your learning and check your understanding of this book's contents: use the "Springer Nature Flashcards" app to access questions using ▶ https://sn.pub/ambACS. To use the app, please follow the instructions in the chapter "Transcatheter Aortic Valve Replacement."

Learning Objectives
1. Describe the indications and the contraindications for transcatheter paravalvular leak closure;
2. Describe how to evaluate the severity of PVLs by using an integrative multiparametric and multimodality approach;
3. Describe the principles of the procedural guidance during percutaneous paravalvular leak closure;
4. Describe the key points of pre- and intra-procedural evaluation for mitral, aortic and tricuspid PVL closure.

Case Study on Transcatheter Mitral PVL Closure

A 67-year-old female comes to our attention during a follow-up outpatient visit reporting worsening of dyspnea over the last few months. She is affected by type 2 diabetes mellitus on insulin therapy, permanent atrial fibrillation, and stage IIIA chronic kidney disease. Her mobility is poor due to a recent femur fracture with endoprosthesis implantation. She had a previous mitral valve surgical replacement (1991) with a Carbomedics 25 mm bileaflet mechanical prosthetic valve. Blood tests show chronic severe hemolytic anaemia (which is partially responsible for the symptoms) and no evidence of infection. Transthoracic echocardiography (TTE) is performed as the initial imaging test. On TTE, left ventricle is not enlarged and its systolic contractility is preserved, left atrium is severely dilated, and moderate aortic regurgitation and severe tricuspid regurgitation are found. TTE also reveals the presence of a mitral prosthesis paravalvular leak (PVL), which appears significant on color Doppler analysis.

The TTE evaluation of our patient suggested the presence of mitral prosthesis regurgitation, limited by acoustic artifacts of the mechanical valve, so a transesophageal echocardiography (TEE) was performed to confirm the diagnosis. A TEE showed normal functioning of the 2 mitral leaflets, with a mild (non-significant) intraprosthetic washout. Multiple PVLs were detected, the larger located anteriormedially. The "en face" view (surgical view) of the mitral prosthesis on 3-dimensional (3D) TEE displays a large antero-medial echo dropout area outside the sewing ring, confirmed by color Doppler, due to a calcified and fibrotic annulus, resulting in disruption of the sutures. The jet density and turbulence, the wide vena contracta, the large proximal isovelocity surface area (PISA) shell, and the systolic retrograde flow into the pulmonary veins support the severity of the mitral paravalvular regurgitation.

Background and Definitions

Prosthetic paravalvular regurgitation or paravalvular leak (PVL) is an abnormal communication between the ring of a surgical or transcatheter prosthesis, and the native valve annulus. A few cases of PVL have also been described in patients with mitral valve repair.

It is not an uncommon complication of prosthetic valve disease, occurring in 7–17% of patients with mitral and 2–10% of patients with surgical aortic prostheses [1, 2]. The incidence of PVL is higher in transcatheter prosthetic valves, even though the incidence of significant aortic regurgitation in patients undergoing transcatheter aortic valve implantation (TAVI) has significantly decreased in the last 20 years, with 0.6–5.3% of patients undergoing TAVI having at least moderate PVL, in more recent trials [3–6]. Taking into consideration the increase in transcatheter valvular replacements, the incidence of PVL is likely to increase in coming years.

Paravalvular regurgitation may result from an interaction of factors related to the intervention (poor technique, use of sutures without pledgets, use of continuous sutures for the mitral prostheses, supra-annular prostheses, inappropriate size of a transcatheter valve) and factors related to the local tissue (important annular calcifications, tissue friability, the presence of infection).

The clinical presentation is highly variable, ranging from an incidental finding on the follow-up echocardiographic study to severe heart failure, hemolytic anemia, or infective endocarditis. The vast majority of PVLs are mild and are considered benign, in the absence of infective endocarditis, with only a few cases being associated with hemolysis. Approximately 2–5% of PVLs on surgical valves are clinically relevant, being associated with heart failure, hemolytic anemia, or both [7].

The diagnosis, in particular, estimating the severity of PVL, and the management of these patients are challenging. Figure 1 presents a proposed management plan for patients with PVL. The choice between redo-surgery, transcatheter closure and medical palliative treatment should be made by the Heart Team, on a case-by-case basis. According to the latest ESC and ACC/AHA guidelines on valvular heart disease, surgical reintervention remains the first treatment option for patients with PVL associated with heart failure or severe hemolytic anemia needing repeated blood transfusions, whereas transcatheter intervention can be considered in patients at high or prohibitive cardiac risk, with anatomically suitable PVLs for a percutaneous closure [8, 9].

Transcatheter PVL closure has emerged as an attractive treatment option in these patients who often have many comorbidities and are at high

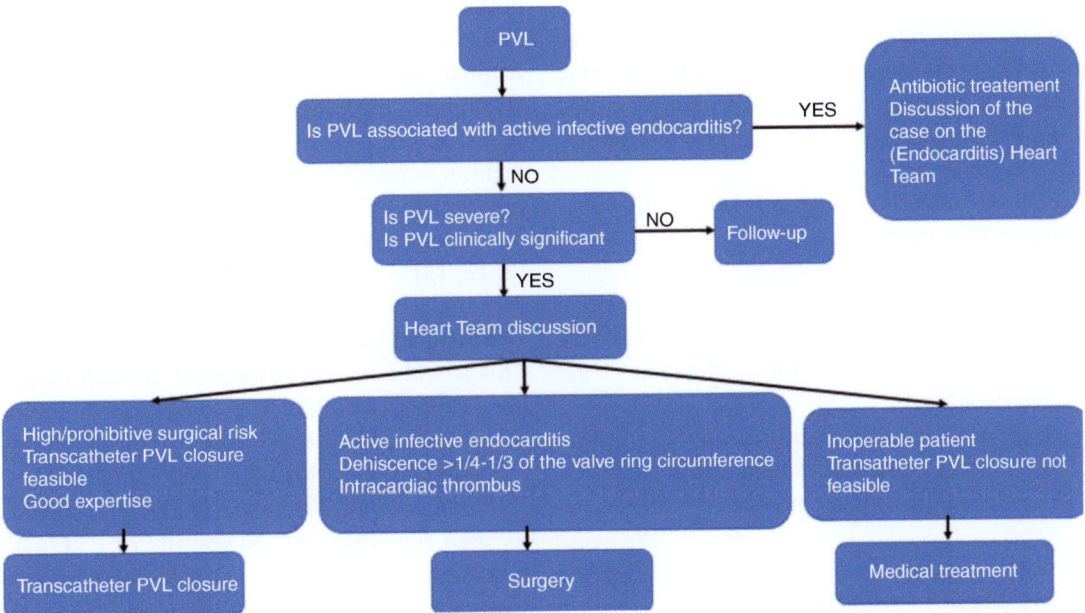

Fig. 1 Proposed management plan for patients with paravalvular regurgitation. The detection of paravalvular leak (PVL) on an echocardiogram should prompt for the search of infective endocarditis. In the absence of infective endocarditis, non-severe PVLs usually do not need and intervention as only few cases can be associated with severe hemolytic anemia. Patients with severe, clinically significant PVLs should be discussed in the Heart Team meeting, and the choice between surgical (re)intervention, transcatheter closure and medical treatment should be made on a case-by-case basis

surgical risk. In centers with good expertise, transcatheter PVL closure has a high feasibility rate (>90%), a good success rate (reduction in PVL to <mild in >70% of cases), which is associated with an improvement in heart failure symptoms, mid- and long-term survival and, in most cases, a decrease in hemolytic anemia severity [10, 11]. Although the success rate for the surgical reintervention is higher than for transcatheter closure (<mild residual regurgitation in >90% of cases), this comes with the price of a higher peri-procedural mortality and complications risk, and a risk of PVL recurrence, without an advantage on long-term survival [10]. Nowadays, many high-volume centers consider the transcatheter intervention as the first treatment option in feasible patients, with surgical reintervention being reconsidered afterwards in case of failure of the transcatheter procedure [10].

Based on current knowledge, transcatheter closure is contraindicated in patients with active infective endocarditis, in patients with a significant dehiscence of the prosthetic valve ring, involving >1/4–1/3 of the circumference, and in patients with intracardiac thrombus [7]. It can however be considered, after the resolution of the infectious process and the disappearance of the thrombus, in patients that are judged to be inoperable by the Heart Team.

The key steps for having a successful transcatheter PVL closure are:

- Careful pre-procedural evaluation for selecting the patients suitable for transcatheter intervention and for planning the intervention;
- Expert imaging guidance during the procedure, with constant communication between the operator(s) and the imager.

Principles of Pre-procedural Assessment Before Transcatheter PVL Intervention

The evaluation of para-valvular regurgitation is difficult and should try to determine the following points:

- The location and the number of the jet(s);
- Estimate the severity of PVL.

Pre-procedural evaluation is helpful for planning the procedure, by selecting the best approach for delivering the device(s) in the individual patient, and it offers an estimation of the type and size of the device(s) that would best close the defect.

Location and Number of the Jet(s)

Echocardiography is the first and main imaging modality for the diagnosis of prosthetic valve dysfunction, and transthoracic (TTE) and transesophageal echocardiography (TEE) are usually used together, as complementary exams. With regards to the location of the regurgitant jets, TTE is limited for the evaluation of mechanical mitral PVLs, when often, the jet can only be visualized in an off-axis view (such as the sub-costal view), and TEE is key for diagnosis. On the other hand, for aortic PVLs, TTE and TEE are more complementary, with TTE being useful for the visualization of anteriorly located jets, whereas posterior jets are better visualized by TEE [12]. 3D echocardiography, in particular 3D TEE, facilitates a more precise location of PVLs [12]. To improve the communication between the different actors involved in the patient's management, it is recommended that the location of the regurgitant jet(s) should be described on a clock face or on anatomical criteria, as shown in Fig. 2 [7, 12, 13].

Grading the Severity of PVL

This is without a doubt the most difficult part of the evaluation of PVLs and an integrative, multiparametric, and, in many cases, a multimodality imaging approach should be used [7, 12, 13].

Echocardiography is the main imaging modality used for estimating the severity of PVL and, in a similar way to native valve regurgitation, an integrated approach, which takes into consideration qualitative, semi-quantitative and quantitative parameters, from all echocardiographic methods (2D, color, PW, CW Doppler, 3D echocardiography) is recommended for determining the severity of PVLs [7, 12, 13]. We outline some of the important points in the evaluation of PVLs:

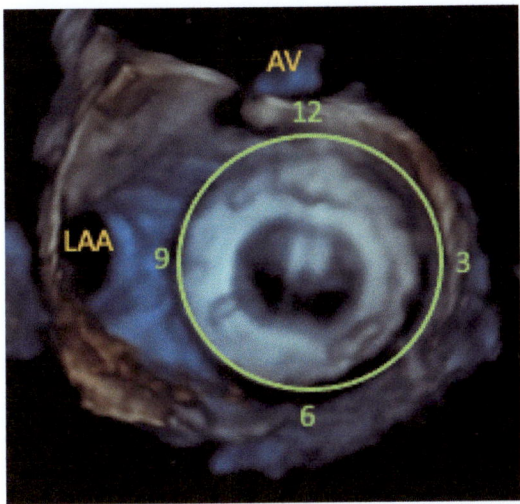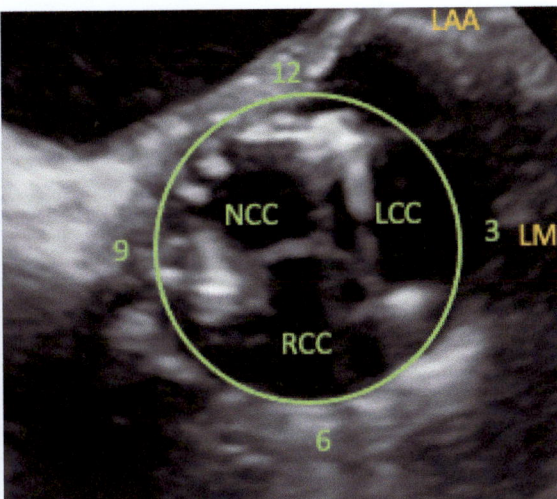

Fig. 2 Localization of paravalvular regurgitant jets. To improve the communication between the Heart Team members it is recommended that the location of the regurgitant jet(s) should be described on a clock face or on anatomical criteria. For the mitral position, the 3D surgical-en face view of the mitral prosthesis should be viewed as a clock face, with the aortic valve located at 12 o'clock, the interventricular septum at 3 o'clock at the left atrium auriculum at 9 o'clock position. Most mitral PVLs are found between 10 and 2 o'clock and between 6 and 7 o'clock. For the aortic prosthesis, most centers prefer to describe the location of the jets in relation to the corresponding "aortic cusps" or on an "en face" clock way, similar to the mitral location, with the right coronary cusp located at 6 o'clock and the left main origin at 3 o'clock. Most aortic PVLs are located around the non-coronary and the left-coronary cusp. *AV* aortic valve, *LAA* left atrial auriculum, *LM* left main coronary artery

- The presence of excessive rocking motion of a mitral prosthesis (>15° from the annulus), or the presence of discordant motion of an aortic prosthesis in comparison to the aortic annulus, indicate severe mitral and, respectively, aortic PVL [7, 12].
- A semi-quantitative evaluation based on the circumferential extent of the regurgitant jet(s) is useful, in particular in the case of multiple leaks, with a value >30%, being in favor of severe paravalvular regurgitation [7, 12, 13].
- The vena contracta method can be used, in case of a single leak, provided that the proximal area can be visualized.
- As the jets are often multiple and their shape is non-circular, the PISA method is, in most cases, not applicable [7, 12].
- The volumetric method can be performed but is cumbersome and its reproducibility is rather low [7, 12].
- The presence of parameters with a high specificity for severe regurgitation, such as systolic retrograde venous reflow in mitral and tricuspid PVL(s), diastolic flow reversal in the aorta, in aortic PVL, can be very useful for grading the severity of prosthetic regurgitation.
- The development or aggravation of preexistent ventricular dilatation or dysfunction (in the absence of another cause), or an increase in pulmonary artery pressure suggests the presence of a significant regurgitation [7, 12, 13].

The PVL Academic Research Consortium recommends the use of a 5-grade system for defining the severity of PVL: trace, mild, moderate, moderate-to severe and severe [7, 13].

Cardiac magnetic resonance imaging (CMR) can measure the regurgitant volume and the regurgitant fraction, even in the case of multiple jets, and should be considered in particular when the echocardiographic grading of PVL severity is discordant to the patient's symptoms or the degree of LV dilatation/dysfunction [7, 12, 13].

Cardiac computer tomography (CT) angiography with 3D/4D reconstruction can be used in cases where TTE and TEE are unable to clearly delineate the extent and the location of PVL, as can be the case for mechanical valves with significant shadowing during sonographic imaging [7, 12, 13]. CT can identify not only the leak location and the size of the defect, but can also evaluate the tract trajectory, the presence of calcification within the tract and the surrounding structures. The information obtained from CT can also be used for fusion imaging, facilitating the wiring and the cannulation during the procedure [14]. Also, in more recent years, 3D printing on CT data can help to understand the defect and can help in selecting the devices(s) [15, 16].

Fluoroscopy can show the presence of excessive prosthetic motion, indicating severe PVL.

Our patient's clinical case was discussed by the Heart Team and an interventional treatment was chosen because of the patient's symptoms and the severe anaemia, refractory to medical therapy. The patient was deemed at too high surgical risk, considering her clinical condition (NYHA class III), her comorbidities, and the previous surgery (EuroSCORE II >8% for a single elective procedure on the mitral valve and >13% for 2 procedures on both the mitral and the tricuspid valve). Therefore, the patient was scheduled for percutaneous closure of the main mitral PVL.

Intra-procedural Guiding of Transcatheter PVL Closure

Transcatheter PVL closure is performed under fluoroscopic and echocardiographic guidance.

Fluoroscopy is superior to echocardiography at visualizing the catheters, the wires, the prostheses, but, except for calcified and metallic structures, it does not allow for the visualization of cardiac structures. On the other hand, echocardiography offers the possibility for visualizing the intra-cardiac structures in multiple planes. While 3D TEE is the echocardiographic modality used in most centers, intracardiac echocardiography (ICE) can be used, depending on local availability and expertise, in aortic PVLs [17]. 3D TEE guided procedures are performed under general anesthesia, which can also pose a risk in these high-risk, often old and frail patients, whereas ICE-guided procedures can be performed under conscious sedation. The combination of the TEE and ICE is also possible, with ICE used at the beginning of the procedure, for guiding transseptal puncture, and 3D TEE used for guiding the implantation of the device. Fusion imaging, superimposing the live 2D/3D echocardiographic images, or the pre-procedural 3D CT data, on the fluoroscopic image, can facilitate the passage of the guide wire through the defect and thus improve the success rate, while decreasing procedure time and radiation exposure [14, 18, 19].

Approach

The approach used for passing the wires and delivering the prostheses is chosen prior to the intervention, based on the location of the paravalvular leak and certain patient characteristics. The approach can be retro-grade or antero-grade, trans-septal, trans-aortic or trans-apical and is described in more detail on the following sections on mitral, aortic and tricuspid PVL closure.

Type and Sizing of the Prostheses/Devices

The type of device(s) chosen for closing a PVL depends on the local availability and the size and shape of the defect.

There is no specifically designed device for PVL closure approved by the FDA. As such, in the USA, different self-expander occluder devices are used in an off-label fashion, the most used being the Amplatzer family of plugs:

- the Amplatzer vascular plugs (AVP II and IV)
- the Amplatzer duct occluder (ADO I and II)
- the Amplatzer atrial septal occluder (ASO)
- the Amplatzer muscular ventricular septal defect occluder (AMVSDO) [20].

Of these, the AVP II and IV, which can be recaptured after deployment, are the most often used devices in the US.

In Europe, the AVP III device, which has an oblong shape, and the Occlutech device, specifically designed for PVL closure and which comes on a rectangular- or a square-shape, are also available [20]. Although there are a few comparative data, the AVP III and the Occlutech devices seem to have a somewhat higher technical and clinical success rate (>90%), and a lower risk of complications than the other devices [21–23].

The size of the device(s) is based on the echocardiographic measurement of the 2D and, preferably 3D, dimensions of the jet at the vena contracta. With the exception of the Occlutech device, the chosen device(s) should be larger than the dimensions of the defect, in order to avoid embolization, but not so large as to interfere with valve function, particularly in the case of mechanical prostheses PVL [20]. Pre-procedural CT data can also be used for selecting the right size of the device, in particular in aortic PVLs [15, 16, 20]. Table 1 presents a comparison of the different imaging modalities used for the pre-procedural and intraprocedural evaluation of trans-catheter PVL closure.

After selecting the size of the device, careful 2D and 3D imaging throughout the procedure is necessary for:

- Evaluating the position of the catheter and the device(s);
- Confirming the correct, full deployment of the device(s) in the intended position;
- Confirming the lack of interference of the device with the prosthetic valve function or adjacent anatomical structures (such as the coronary arteries for the aortic position);
- Confirming a stable device deployment;
- Evaluating for the presence of residual regurgitation and the need for further intervention;
- Confirming the safe removal of catheters and imaging of the transseptal shunt in case of transseptal approach;
- Evaluating the presence of complications (see Table 2) [7].

Table 1 Multimodality imaging comparison of patients with paravalvular leak

Imaging modalities	Advantages	Limitations
Transthoracic echocardiography (TTE)	Evaluates prosthetic function, LV size and function, pulmonary pressure Better than TEE for visualizing the anteriorly located aortic PVLs	Acoustic shadowing can limit the evaluation of mitral PVLs and posteriorly located aortic PVLs
Transesophageal echocardiography (TEE)	Extremely useful for diagnosis in patients with mitral PVL and in patients with posterior aortic PVL The most used imaging modality for procedural guidance	Acoustic shadowing can limit the evaluation of anteriorly located aortic PVL Need for general anesthesia
3D echocardiography	Improves the localization of PVLs Useful for selecting the size of the device and guiding the passage of the guidewires and device deployment	Image resolution can be limited by the lower frame rates
Intracardiac echocardiography (ICE)	Allows procedural guidance under conscious sedation	Limited in mitral PVL closure
Fluoroscopy	Very useful for procedural guidance A rocking motion of the prosthesis indicates severe PVL	Does not visualize anatomical structures unless calcified
Cardiac magnetic resonance imaging	Useful in patient with discordant clinical and echocardiographic evaluation Can quantify regurgitation severity in patients with multiple jets	Artifacts from metallic structures Dependent on patient compliance
Cardiac computer tomography	Can be useful in patients with mechanical prostheses and significant acoustic shadowing on echocardiographic images Can be very useful for planning the procedure and selecting the size of the devices Through the use of fusion imaging, can be useful for guiding the device delivery	Artifacts can limit image resolution Radiation exposure and use of contrast agents

Table 2 Complications of transcatheter PVL closure

Access site related complications:
- Femorale venous/arterial approach: dissection, stenosis, perforation, rupture, arteriovenous fistula, pseudoaneurysm, hematoma, irreversible nerve injury, compartment syndrome, distal emolization causing limb ischemia;
- Apical approach: Hemothorax, pericardial effusion, coronary laceration

Complications of transseptal crossing: intracardiac shunt

Bleeding complications

New or worsening of hemolytic anemia (may also resolve after several months, after the endothelization of the device)

Stroke (hemorrhagic or ischemic) and transient ischemic attack

Acute kidney injury

Coronary obstruction:
- Aortic PVL closure may cause left main or right coronary artery obstruction
- Postero-lateral mitral PVL closure may occasionally cause left circumflex occlusion

Device interference with the prosthetic valve function after device release:
- On fluoroscopy, evidence of mechanical valve obstruction
- On echocardiography, a sudden increase in prosthetic valve regurgitation or in trans-prosthetic gradients

Device or valve thrombosis that interferes with valve function

Device erosion

Device or prosthetic valve endocarditis

Device embolization:
- From the aortic position, may travel anywhere, most often being lodged at the aortic bifurcation or in the iliac arteries and can be removed percutaneously
- From the mitral position, small devices can pass the aortic valve and then be removed percutaneously, but larger devices may need surgical intervention for removal

Heart block (antero-medial tricuspid PVL closure)

Conversion to open surgery

Mortality: immediate (<72 h) and 30 days procedure-related mortality

A good communication between the echocardiographer and the interventional cardiologist, at every step of the procedure, is essential for the success of the procedure.

Percutaneous Closure of Mitral PVL

PVL is present in 7–17% of patients with mitral prostheses [1, 2]. As mitral surgical reintervention is associated with an increased risk of death in these patients, often associating multiple comorbidities, transcatheter closure represents a valuable treatment option in suitable patients with mitral PVL and heart failure or severe hemolytic anemia.

Diagnosis and Pre-procedural Assessment of Mitral PVL

The main aspects of the pre-procedural evaluation of patients with mitral PVLs are:

- TTE can show indirect signs of a significant prosthetic regurgitation (increase in trans-prosthetic gradients, LV dilatation or dysfunction), while the jet can be visualized only from off-axis transthoracic images, such as the sub-costal view.
- TEE is the imaging of choice for the evaluation of mitral PVLs, offering important information about the location, the shape, the size and the severity of PVL.
- The addition of 3D echo to the transesophageal images, offers a more precise localization of the regurgitant jet(s) around the ring of the prosthetic valve. When using the recommended clock face description for the location of the regurgitant jets (see Fig. 2), most mitral PVLs are found between 10 and 2 o'clock and between 6 and 7 o'clock [24, 25].
- The evaluation of the severity of mitral PVL follows the same principles described earlier and a multiparametric approach is recommended, with emphasis on those parameters with a high specificity for severe regurgitation. According to the Paravalvular Leak Academic Research Consortium, the parameters in favour of a severe mitral PVL are:
  – An excessive rocking motion of the sewing ring;

- The presence of LV dilatation or the increase in pulmonary artery pressure, in the absence of another cause;
- An increase in pressure gradients (mean gradient >5 mmHg);
- A dense, holosystolic or triangular CW Doppler envelope of the regurgitant jet;
- The ration between the mitral prosthetic flow and the sub-aortic flow on PW Doppler ≥2.5;
- A large, visible proximal convergence;
- a large vena contracta ≥7 mm;
- the presence of systolic flow reversal in the pulmonary veins, which is specific for severe PVL;
- the circumferential extent of the regurgitant jet(s) on color Doppler ≥30%
- a regurgitant volume ≥60 mL, a regurgitant orifice area ≥40 mm² and a regurgitant fraction ≥50%, according to the volumetric method [7].
* CMR should be considered when the echocardiographic grading of PVL severity is discordant to the patient's symptoms or the degree of LV dilatation/dysfunction [7, 12].
* Cardiac CT is seldom necessary for the characterisation of mitral PVLs.

Intraprocedural Imaging Modalities and Measurements During Transcatheter Mitral PVL Closure

Transcatheter closure of mitral PVLs is, in general, performed under general anesthesia, with real-time 3D TEE and fluoroscopic guidance. ICE is often limited for guiding mitral PVLs closure. The use of fusion imaging, can facilitate the passage of the guide wire through the defect and improve the success rate.

There are 3 main approaches for delivering the prosthesis: the antegrade transseptal, the most commonly used, the retrograde transaortic and the retrograde transapical. The choice between the 3 approaches is made depending on the location of the jet and on patient characteristics:

* the antegrade transseptal approach is not applicable in patients with prior PFO/ASD transcatheter closure;
* the retrograde transaortic approach is not applicable in patients with associated aortic prosthesis or in patients with prior interatrial septal closure;
* the retrograde transapical approach, has the highest technical success rate but is associated with a higher risk of complications (hemothorax, pericardial effusion, coronary laceration); it is reserved to patients with prior interatrial septal closure or those with medially located defects.

The size of the device(s) is based on the shape of the defect and the 3D dimensions of the jet(s) at the vena contracta, as described earlier.

Once the device is in place, it should not be released before making sure that it doesn't impede on prosthetic function, and careful evaluation for the presence of complications (see Table 2) is recommended.

Post-procedural Assessment

Post-procedural assessment is usually performed at 30 days and should include a clinical evaluation for heart failure symptoms, a biological evaluation for the presence of hemolytic anemia, and an echocardiographic evaluation. The transthoracic echocardiogram can evaluate the function of the prosthetic valve, the dimensions and the function of the left ventricle and pulmonary artery pressure, but for mitral prosthesis, transesophageal echocardiogram is necessary for confirming that the device is in place and for evaluating the importance of residual regurgitation (Table 1). The timing of the transesophageal echocardiogram is variable in different centers, between 1 and 3 months after the intervention. Based on the results of this evaluation, in patients with persistent symptomatic significant PVL, the choice between another percutaneous PVL closure attempt and surgical intervention should be discussed.

Percutaneous Closure of Aortic PVL

Aortic PVL in present in 2–10% of patients with surgical aortic prostheses [1, 2]. Although the incidence of at least moderate aortic PVL in patients undergoing TAVI has significantly decreased in the last 20 years, some studies showing rates similar to the ones seen in SAVR patients, the incidence of mild PVL remains higher in TAVI than in SAVR patients [3–6].

The approaches to PVL after SAVR and TAVI are different. In patients with PVL after SAVR, the choice between surgical reintervention and transcatheter PVL closure should be decided by the Heart Team on a case-by-case basis. In TAVI patients, the approach depends on the cause/mechanism of the PVL:

- In case of a PVL due to a low implantation of the prosthesis, a valve-in-valve procedure is the best way to close the leak;
- In case of a mal apposition of the valve to the annulus or valve under-expansion, post-dilatation of the valve can improve the leak;
- In the case of a large calcification pushing against the frame of the prosthesis, post-dilatation carries the risk of annular rupture and percutaneous PVL can be considered, but is more difficult than in SAVR patients owing to significant annular and valvular calcifications, the presence of sealing skirts, and the, generally, smaller sized defects [20, 26–28].

Diagnosis and Pre-procedural Assessment of Aortic PVLs

The main aspects of the pre-procedural evaluation of patients with aortic PVLs are:

- Echocardiography is the imaging technique of choice to identify and quantify aortic PVLs, TTE and TEE being used together and offering complementary information. Due to the acoustic shadowing of the prosthesis, posterior PVLs are more difficult to visualize on TTE, whereas anterior PVLs may be under-detected or under-estimated on TEE [29]. Sometimes, on both TTE and TEE, off-axis and intermediary views are needed to reveal lateral and medial paravalvular jets.
- 3D imaging, especially when performed during TEE, is ideal for PVL evaluation, allowing a better definition of the jet location, trajectory and shape. Most aortic PVLs are located around the non-coronary and the left-coronary cusp [25, 30]. Also, TTE and, in particular TEE, can be used for determining the origin of the coronary arteries, an important aspect of the pre-procedural evaluation of patients with aortic PVL, as a low implantation of the coronary arteries poses a risk of coronary ostia obstruction after the device(s) deployment.
- The evaluation of the severity of aortic PVL follows the same principles described earlier, and a multiparametric approach is recommended, with emphasis on those parameters with a high specificity for severe regurgitation. According to the Paravalvular Leak Academic Research Consortium and the Valve Academic Research Consortium 3, the parameters in favour of a severe aortic PVL are:
  - the presence of discordant motion of an aortic prosthesis in comparison to the aortic annulus
  - the presence of LV dilatation in the absence of another cause;
  - a short deceleration time (<200 ms);
  - A dense CW Doppler envelope of the regurgitant jet and often multiple jets;
  - An E/A ratio >1.5;
  - A large visible proximal convergence and a large jet width at its origin;
  - a large vena contracta ≥6 mm;
  - the presence of holodiastolic flow reversal in the proximal descending aorta with an end-diastolic velocity ≥30 cm/s;
  - the (sum of the) circumferential extent of the regurgitant jet(s) on color Doppler ≥30%;
  - a regurgitant volume ≥60 mL, a regurgitant orifice area ≥40 mm^2 and a regurgitant fraction ≥50% according to the volumetric method [7, 13].

- CMR is particularly useful in patients with multiple jets but can be limited by the presence of metal artefacts.
- Cardiac CT is a very useful adjunctive test to echocardiography for pre-procedural planning in aortic PVLs. It allows a detailed visualization of the size, the location and path of aortic PVLs and is very useful for determining the origin of coronary arteries.

Intraprocedural Imaging Modalities and Measurements During Transcatheter Aortic PVL Closure

Transcatheter closure of aortic PVLs can be performed under general anesthesia, with real-time 3D TEE and fluoroscopic guidance, or under conscious sedation with ICE and fluoroscopic guidance. ICE imaging from the right ventricular outflow tract may improve the identification of leaks located anteriorly, which are frequently challenging to identify at TEE due to the prosthesis' acoustic shadowing. The use of fusion imaging, by superimposing the real-time 2D/3D echocardiographic image or the 3D reconstruction of the pre-procedural cardiac CT data on the fluoroscopic image, can facilitate the passage of the guide wire through the defect and improve the success rate, with a decrease in procedure time [14, 18, 19].

Aortic PVLs are usually corrected with a retrograde trans-aortic approach and 3 techniques can be used for delivering the device:

- A catheter-only technique, can be used in small defects which can be closed with a single device;
- An "anchor wire" technique, in which a wire is placed in the left ventricle, allows for sequential deployment of multiple devices if needed.
- An arterio-arterial rail can be used, when a more stable support for device(s) delivery is needed. The Glide wire crosses the defect, then is advanced in the left ventricle and then through the aortic prosthesis into the descending aorta and from there it can be snared and exteriorized to the contralateral femoral artery. It is rarely necessary and is not recommended in patients with mechanical aortic PVLs, in which cases, for more stability, the snaring of the catheter through a transseptal or a transapical approach can be used [31].

The size of the device(s) is based on the shape and the size of the defect as determined mainly based on the 2D and 3D dimensions of the jet at the level of the vena contracta, although, in the case of aortic PVLs, the information obtained from the pre-procedural CT can also be very useful [15, 16, 20].

An important step of the procedure is checking for the normal functioning of the aortic prosthesis, the mitral valve apparatus (in particular for leaks located around the "non-coronary" cusp) and ruling out coronary ostia obstruction after the device(s) deployment. In this respect, coronary angiography may be necessary to confirm coronary flow once the device has been positioned.

In our patient, the procedure was performed on general anesthesia, under fluoroscopic and transesophageal guidance, and an anterograde transseptal approach was chosen by the interventional cardiologist. At the beginning of the procedure, the presence of intracardiac thrombi was excluded by conventional TEE. 3D TEE identified the position of the main PVL, located anterior-medially, between 1 and 3 o'clock on the "en face" view of the mitral valve. 3D TEE also defined the anatomy and the size of the defect, helping the selection of the most appropriate closure device, in this case the Amplatzer Vascular Plug II of 10 mm. Figure 3a, b both conventional and 3D TEE were used to assist the interventional cardiologist in the transseptal puncture and in guiding the wire and the catheter through the defect. Once the position of the catheter was considered adequate, the device was deployed under ultrasound guidance. Immediately after the device deployment, its proper seating was ensured by TEE and a residual, no more than mild paravalvular regurgitation was detected by

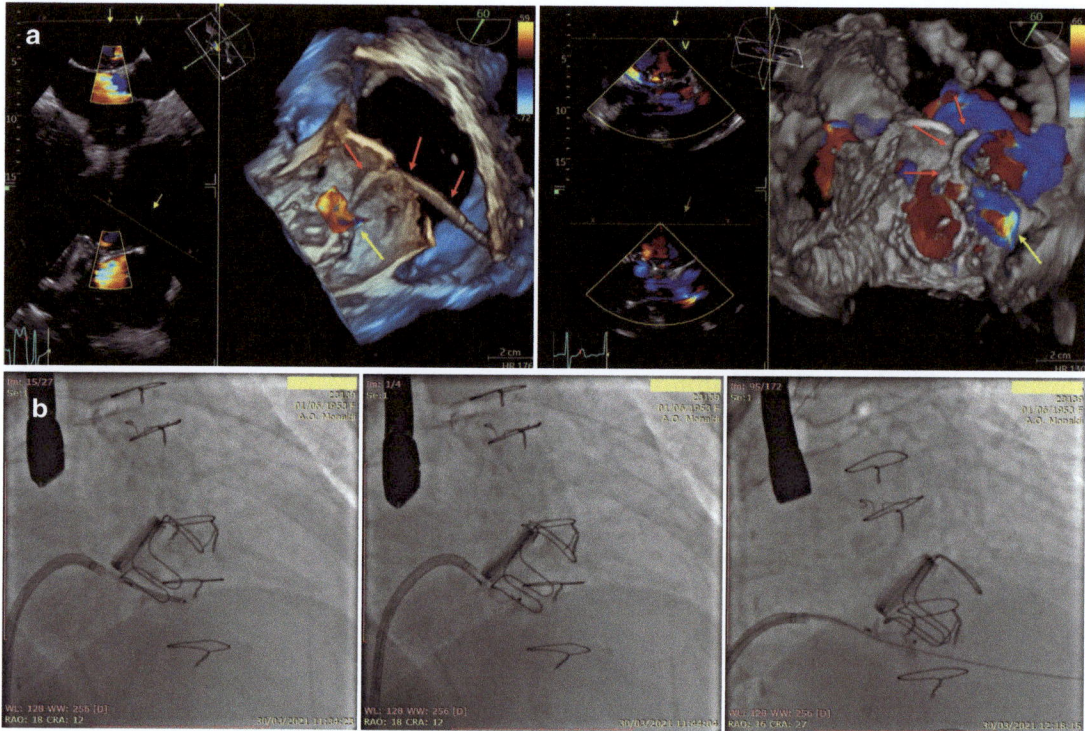

Fig. 3 (**a**) Intra-procedural 3D TEE imaging to guide mitral PVL closure. In this "en face" view of the mitral valve, PVL appears as a large echo dropout area outside of the sewing ring, located anterior-medially (between 1 and 3 o'clock), confirmed by color Doppler (yellow arrows). 3D TEE images assist the interventional cardiologist in guiding the device release system through the defect (red arrows). (**b**) Intra-procedural fluoroscopic imaging to guide mitral PVL closure. After transseptal puncture, the catheter is guided through the mitral PVL and the Vascular Plug is released, allowing an almost complete obliteration of the defect. [*Images courtesy of professor Paolo Golino, head of Cardiology Unit of University of Campania "Luigi Vanvitelli", Monaldi Hospital, Naples (interventional cardiologist: prof. Paolo Golino, echocardiographer: dr. Gemma Salerno)*]

color Doppler. The 30-day follow-up evaluation showed, mild paravalvular regurgitation and improvement of heart failure symptoms.

Post procedural Assessment

The goals of the post-procedural assessment of aortic PVL closure are similar to those of mitral PVL closure. The transthoracic echocardiogram can evaluate the function of the prosthetic valve, the dimensions and the function of the left ventricle, estimate filling and pulmonary pressures and can be sufficient for evaluating the presence of residual regurgitation. Transesophageal echocardiogram can however be necessary in patients with suspected significant paravalvular regurgitation, in particular in the case of posteriorly located jets. In our patient, the 30-day follow-up evaluation was good, with mild paravalvular regurgitation and improvement of heart failure symptoms.

A Second Case Study of Transcatheter Aortic PVL Closure

A 76-year-old female patient with symptomatic severe aortic stenosis and at low surgical risk, underwent, according to the Heart Team decision, a surgical aortic valve replacement. The surgeon opted for a mini-invasive aortic valve replacement via right anterior thoracotomy and implantation of a sutureless Perceval M valve. The valve needed repositioning due to malposition near the non-coronary sinus leaflet, due to heavy calcifications. The pre-procedural transesophageal echocardiogram (TEE) described a mild para-valvular aortic regurgitation and the hemodynamic status was good at the end of the surgical intervention.

She was then transferred to the intensive care unit where, the next day, her condition deteriorated, and she developed cardiogenic shock. Transthoracic echocardiographic images were difficult. Control TEE showed severe paravalvular aortic regurgitation with a jet located around the non-coronary leaflet (the region where the most important calcifications were described on the surgical protocol) (Fig. 4a).

The case of the patient was once more discussed in the Heart Team meeting and, given the high risk associated with a surgical reintervention on a patient on cardiogenic shock, it was decided to proceed with percutaneous PVL closure.

The procedure was performed under general anesthesia with transesophageal and fluoroscopic guidance. The 2D vena contracta was 4.7 mm (Fig. 4b). Using a 6F femoral access, the PVL orifice was crossed with an Aquatrack® (Cordis) wire using a JR4 guiding

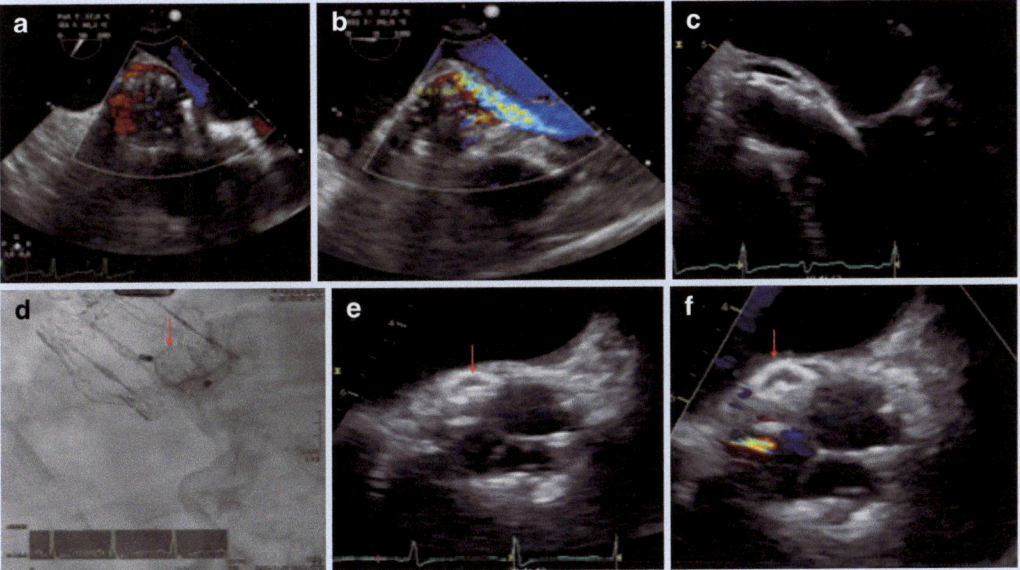

Fig. 4 (**a–f**) (**a**) and (**b**) present the pre-procedural TEE examination showing the presence of a regurgitant jet all around the cusp located in the non-coronary sinus (**a**), with a 2D vena contracta measured at 4.7 mm (**b**). The resolution of the 3D images was low in this patient. Based on the crescent shape of the regurgitant orifice and the dimension of the vena contracta, an Amplatzer vascular Plug III 12/5 mm was considered to be the best device for closing the leak. The delivery catheter is seen passing through the defect (**c**) and the device is then delivered after assuring the correct location of the device, without interference with the prosthetic valve function. The device (red arrow) is then released, as seen on the fluoroscopic (**d**) and echocardiographic short-axis images (**e**), with mild residual paravalvular regurgitation on color Doppler (**f**)

catheter (Fig. 4c). After exchange with an Amplatz Super Stiff™ (Boston Scientific) wire, the delivery catheter was advanced and an *Amplatzer*™ *Vascular Plug III* (12 mm long axis × 5 mm short axis) (Abbott) was implanted (Fig. 4d, e) with a mild residual paravalvular regurgitation and no evidence of interference of the device with the prosthetic valve function (Fig. 4f).

The clinical evolution was good, and the patient was transferred on the flour the next day following the percutaneous paravalvular leak closure. She, however developed a pseudo-aneurysm at the femoral artery puncture site, which was resolved with an ultrasound-guided thrombin injection. The patient left the hospital 6 days after the percutaneous PVL closure.

The 30-day follow-up transthoracic echocardiographic evaluation showed a good functioning aortic prosthesis, with a mild paravalvular regurgitation.

Percutaneous Closure of Tricuspid PVLs

Percutaneous closure of tricuspid PVLs has not been as well described as mitral or aortic PVL closure, probably because hemodynamically significant tricuspid PVL, leading to severe heart failure, liver dysfunction or severe hemolysis, is rare. A few cases of transcatheter PVL closure have been reported in literature, particularly in patients with underlying congenital heart disease [32–34]. A right internal jugular or femoral vein approach is used and the procedure is usually performed under fluoroscopic and TEE guidance, although TTE can also be used [32–34]. The sizing of the device(s) is based on the size of the defect determined from the echocardiographic images and the procedure is performed in a similar way to mitral PVL closure. A particular possible complication of antero-medial tricuspid PVL, due to its proximity to the nodal tissue, is the occurrence of heart block [34].

Echocardiography plays a pivotal role in the pre-procedural diagnosis and patient selection as well as peri-procedural interventional guidance. Other imaging technologies can offer important information for pre-procedural evaluation and, with the use of fusion imaging, can also facilitate the implantation of the devices(s).

Key Points
- The presence of active infective endocarditis, of intracardiac thrombus or of a significant prosthetic valve dehiscence are contraindications for percutaneous paravalvular leak closure.
- Pre-procedural evaluation is extremely important for evaluating the feasibility of a transcatheter approach and for planning the procedure.
- The device should not be released before confirming its correct location, and its lack of interference with prosthetic valve function or surrounding structures.

Conclusions

Paravalvular leak is not an uncommon complication of surgical or transcatheter prostheses and can be associated with severe heart failure or severe hemolytic anemia. Percutaneous PVL closure is a useful and safe alternative to conventional surgery for the treatment of these patients.

Chapter Review Questions

1. Which of the following affirmations related to transcatheter paravalvular leak (PVL) closure is FALSE? (choose all correct answers)
    A. It is an effective treatment option for reducing hemolytic anemia.

B. The presence of intracardiac thrombus is an absolute contraindication for performing transcatheter PVL closure.
C. It should be considered in suitable patients with moderate PVL;
D. According to the latest guidelines, surgery is the first treatment option for patients with clinically significant PVL.

Answer: A, B, C

The effectiveness of transcatheter PVL closure for treating hemolytic anemia is less straightforward than for heart failure treatment. Although, in most cases, hemolytic anemia is reduced after transcatheter PVL closure, there are also a few cases of aggravated hemolytic anemia after transcatheter closure.

The presence of intra-cardiac thrombus represents a RELATIVE contraindication for performing transcatheter closure, related to the risk of embolism, but transcatheter PVL closure can be performed afterwards, once the thrombus has disappeared under anticoagulant treatment.

In general, non-severe PVL has a good prognosis and does not require treatment, although some studies suggest its presence is associated with a higher risk of infective endocarditis.

A 75 years-old patient with a history of mechanical mitral valve replacement for infective endocarditis performed 8 years prior to the actual presentation, was hospitalized for heart failure in the context of atrial fibrillation. The transthoracic echocardiogram showed a mildly reduced ejection fraction with diffuse hypokinesia and increased mitral prosthesis gradients (mean gradient of 7 mmHg but for a heart rate of 110 bpm), whereas the disks mobility was normal. The patient was referred for electrical cardioversion and transesophageal echocardiogram was performed for excluding intracardiac thrombus. The exam showed the presence of a posteriorly located paravalvular leak (PVL) whose evaluation can be seen in the following image.

2. Which of the following affirmations is true (choose all correct answers)
  A. The patient has moderate PVL
  B. PVL is severe
  C. The patient should be discussed in the Heart Team meeting, but transcatheter PVL closure using a transseptal approach can be performed
  D. the exclusion of infective endocarditis is necessary.

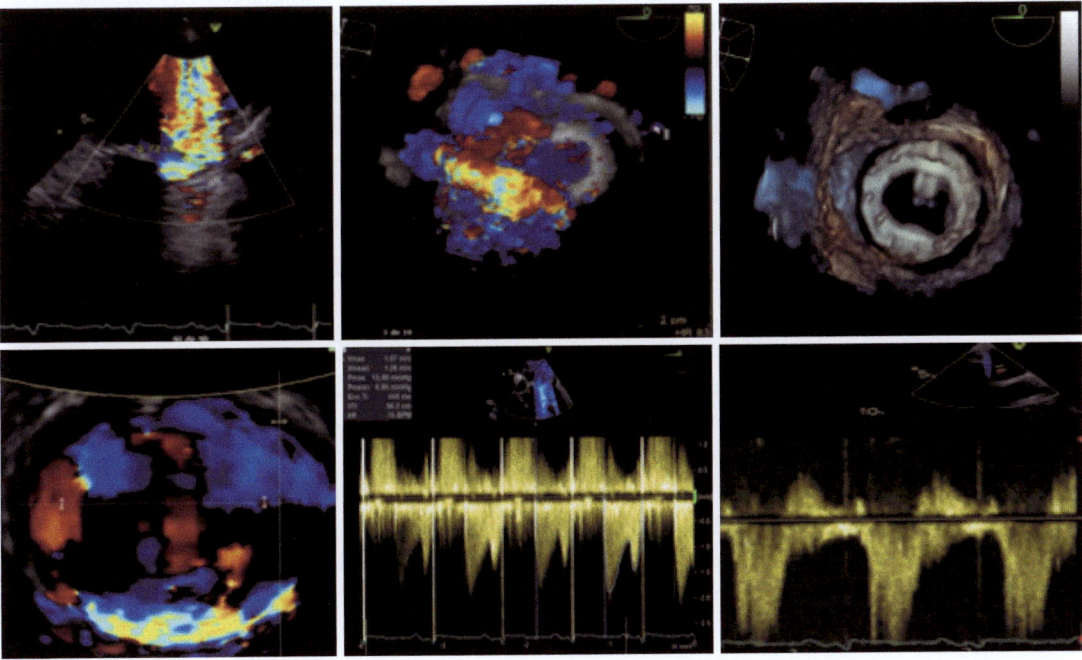

Answer: B and D

The transesophageal images show the presence of a posteriorly located paravalvular regurgitation with several echocardiographic parameters in favor of a severe PVL: the 2D vena contracta is >7 mm, the circumferential extent represents 30% of the annular circumference, there is an increase in trans-prosthetic gradients, but the mobility of the disks is normal and there is a systolic flow reversal in the pulmonary veins. The patient had systolic flow reversal in all pulmonary veins, a sign which is specific for severe mitral regurgitation.

The evaluation for the presence of infective endocarditis is necessary in all patients diagnosed with a previously unknown paravalvular regurgitation. Our patient had already been operated on for infective endocarditis and, as such, he is at higher risk for infective endocarditis recurrence. The lab tests in our patient showed the presence of a hemolytic anemia and an inflammatory syndrome. Blood cultures were negative (the patient had been prescribed an antibiotic 2 weeks prior, for a suspected pulmonary infection). On the transesophageal echocardiogram, there was no image suspected of a vegetation, but the PET-CT was positive with an intense fixation of the tracer all around the mitral prosthesis. The patient was diagnosed with culture negative active infective endocarditis, which is a contraindication for transcatheter PVL closure. His case was discussed on the Endocarditis Heart Team meeting and surgical reintervention was performed.

3. Select the correct affirmations about aortic paravalvular leak (PVL) (choose all correct answers):
   A. Posteriorly located jets are easily visualized on the transthoracic echocardiogram
   B. A vena contracta >6 mm suggests severe PVL
   C. Holodiastolic flow reversal with an end-diastolic velocity in the descending thoracic aorta >20 cm/s, is highly suggestive of severe aortic PVL
   D. Left ventricular dilatation can be a sign of severe aortic PVL.

Answer: B, D

Posteriorly located aortic PVLs are more difficult to visualize and can be missed on the transthoracic images, but they are better visualized on the transesophageal images.

The vena contracta >6 mm and the development or an increase of left ventricular dilatation in the absence of another cause, indicate the presence of a severe aortic PVL. The end-diastolic velocity in the descending thoracic aorta >20 cm/s suggests moderate-to severe aortic regurgitation, whereas a velocity >30 cm/s suggests severe aortic prosthetic valve regurgitation.

4. Which of the following aspects about percutaneous mitral PVL closure is INCORRECT:
   A. It can be performed under fluoroscopic and intracardiac echocardiography imaging guidance
   B. Fusion imaging can facilitate the passage of the catheters through the leak and decrease procedure time and radiation exposure
   C. Transesophageal echocardiography is essential for confirming the correct location of the guiding catheter and the device inside the leak
   D. Before releasing the device, careful evaluation is necessary for confirming the lack of interference of the device with the prosthetic valve function

Answer: A

Percutaneous mitral PVL is performed under transesophageal and fluoroscopic guidance, and the use of fusion imaging can facilitate the passage of the catheters through the leak and decrease procedure time and radiation exposure. Intracardiac echocardiography is limited for guiding the delivery of the device in the mitral position. Confirming a correct location of the device and its lack of interference with the prosthetic valve function are essential steps of the procedural evaluation.

5. The following aspects about percutaneous aortic paravalvular leak (PVL) closure are true (choose all correct answers):
   A. Careful echocardiographic and angiographic evaluation is necessary for ruling out coronary ostia obstruction after device deployment
   B. It is always performed on general anesthesia, under fluoroscopic and transesophageal imaging guidance
   C. In patients with PVL after TAVI related to a low implantation of the prosthesis, transcatheter PVL is the best way for closing the leak
   D. A retrograde transfemoral approach is used.

   Answer: A, D

   Transcatheter aortic PVL closure can be performed under general anesthesia, on fluoroscopic and transesophageal guidance, or under conscious sedation, on fluoroscopic and intracardiac echocardiography guidance. A retrograde transfemoral approach is used. An important step in the procedural evaluation is ruling out coronary ostia obstruction after device deployment, a possible complication of aortic PVL closure. In patients with paravalvular leak after TAVI related to a low implantation of the prosthesis, a valve-in-valve is usually the best choice for treating paravalvular regurgitation.

References

1. Ionescu A, Fraser AG, Butchart EG. Prevalence and clinical significance of incidental paraprosthetic valvar regurgitation: a prospective study using transoesophageal echocardiography. Heart. 2003;89(11):1316–21. https://doi.org/10.1136/heart.89.11.1316.
2. Hammermeister K, Sethi GK, Henderson WG, Grover FL, Oprian C, Rahimtoola SH. Outcomes 15 years after valve replacement with a mechanical versus a bioprosthetic valve: final report of the veterans affairs randomized trial. J Am Coll Cardiol. 2000;36(4):1152–8. https://doi.org/10.1016/s0735-1097(00)00834-2.
3. Leon MB, Smith CR, Mack MJ, Makkar RR, Svensson LG, Kodali SK, Thourani VH, Tuzcu EM, Miller DC, Herrmann HC, Doshi D, Cohen DJ, Pichard AD, Kapadia S, Dewey T, Babaliaros V, Szeto WY, Williams MR, Kereiakes D, Zajarias A, Greason KL, Whisenant BK, Hodson RW, Moses JW, Trento A, Brown DL, Fearon WF, Pibarot P, Hahn RT, Jaber WA, Anderson WN, Alu MC, Webb JG, PARTNER 2 Investigators. Transcatheter or surgical aortic-valve replacement in intermediate-risk patients. N Engl J Med. 2016;374(17):1609–20. https://doi.org/10.1056/NEJMoa1514616.
4. Reardon MJ, Van Mieghem NM, Popma JJ, Kleiman NS, Søndergaard L, Mumtaz M, Adams DH, Deeb GM, Maini B, Gada H, Chetcuti S, Gleason T, Heiser J, Lange R, Merhi W, Oh JK, Olsen PS, Piazza N, Williams M, Windecker S, Yakubov SJ, Grube E, Makkar R, Lee JS, Conte J, Vang E, Nguyen H, Chang Y, Mugglin AS, Serruys PW, Kappetein AP, SURTAVI Investigators. Surgical or transcatheter aortic-valve replacement in intermediate-risk patients. N Engl J Med. 2017;376(14):1321–31. https://doi.org/10.1056/NEJMoa1700456. Epub 2017 Mar 17.
5. Popma JJ, Deeb GM, Yakubov SJ, Mumtaz M, Gada H, O'Hair D, Bajwa T, Heiser JC, Merhi W, Kleiman NS, Askew J, Sorajja P, Rovin J, Chetcuti SJ, Adams DH, Teirstein PS, Zorn GL 3rd, Forrest JK, Tchétché D, Resar J, Walton A, Piazza N, Ramlawi B, Robinson N, Petrossian G, Gleason TG, Oh JK, Boulware MJ, Qiao H, Mugglin AS, Reardon MJ, Evolut Low Risk Trial Investigators. Transcatheter aortic-valve replacement with a self-expanding valve in low-risk patients. N Engl J Med. 2019;380(18):1706–15. https://doi.org/10.1056/NEJMoa1816885.
6. Mack MJ, Leon MB, Thourani VH, Makkar R, Kodali SK, Russo M, Kapadia SR, Malaisrie SC, Cohen DJ, Pibarot P, Leipsic J, Hahn RT, Blanke P, Williams MR, McCabe JM, Brown DL, Babaliaros V, Goldman S, Szeto WY, Genereux P, Pershad A, Pocock SJ, Alu MC, Webb JG, Smith CR, PARTNER 3 Investigators. Transcatheter aortic-valve replacement with a balloon-expandable valve in low-risk patients. N Engl J Med. 2019;380(18):1695–705. https://doi.org/10.1056/NEJMoa1814052. Epub 2019 Mar 16.
7. Ruiz CE, Hahn RT, Berrebi A, Borer JS, Cutlip DE, Fontana G, Gerosa G, Ibrahim R, Jelnin V, Jilaihawi H, Jolicoeur EM, Kliger C, Kronzon I, Leipsic J, Maisano F, Millan X, Nataf P, O'Gara PT, Pibarot P, Ramee SR, Rihal CS, Rodes-Cabau J, Sorajja P, Suri R, Swain JA, Turi ZG, Tuzcu EM, Weissman NJ, Zamorano JL, Serruys PW, Leon MB, Paravalvular Leak Academic Research Consortium. Clinical trial principles and endpoint definitions for paravalvular leaks in surgical prosthesis: an expert statement. J Am Coll Cardiol. 2017;69(16):2067–87. https://doi.org/10.1016/j.jacc.2017.02.038.
8. Otto CM, Nishimura RA, Bonow RO, Carabello BA, Erwin JP 3rd, Gentile F, Jneid H, Krieger EV, Mack M, McLeod C, O'Gara PT, Rigolin VH, Sundt TM 3rd, Thompson A, Toly C. 2020 ACC/AHA guideline for the management of patients with valvular heart disease: executive summary: a report of the American College of Cardiology/American Heart Association Joint Committee on Clinical Practice Guidelines

[Erratum in: Circulation. 2021 Feb 2;143(5):e228. Erratum in: Circulation. 2021 Mar 9;143(10):e784.]. Circulation. 2021;143(5):e35–71. https://doi.org/10.1161/CIR.0000000000000932. Epub 2020 Dec 17.
9. Vahanian A, Beyersdorf F, Praz F, Milojevic M, Baldus S, Bauersachs J, Capodanno D, Conradi L, De Bonis M, De Paulis R, Delgado V, Freemantle N, Gilard M, Haugaa KH, Jeppsson A, Jüni P, Pierard L, Prendergast BD, Sádaba JR, Tribouilloy C, Wojakowski W, ESC/EACTS Scientific Document Group. 2021 ESC/EACTS guidelines for the management of valvular heart disease [Erratum in: Eur Heart J. 2022 Feb 18]. Eur Heart J. 2022;43(7):561–632. https://doi.org/10.1093/eurheartj/ehab395.
10. Alkhouli M, Rihal CS, Zack CJ, Eleid MF, Maor E, Sarraf M, Cabalka AK, Reeder GS, Hagler DJ, Maalouf JF, Nkomo VT, Schaff HV, Said SM. Transcatheter and surgical management of mitral paravalvular leak: long-term outcomes. JACC Cardiovasc Interv. 2017;10(19):1946–56. https://doi.org/10.1016/j.jcin.2017.07.046.
11. Wells JA 4th, Condado JF, Kamioka N, Dong A, Ritter A, Lerakis S, Clements S, Stewart J, Leshnower B, Guyton R, Forcillo J, Patel A, Thourani VH, Block PC, Babaliaros V. Outcomes after paravalvular leak closure: transcatheter versus surgical approaches. JACC Cardiovasc Interv. 2017;10(5):500–7. https://doi.org/10.1016/j.jcin.2016.11.043.
12. Lancellotti P, Pibarot P, Chambers J, Edvardsen T, Delgado V, Dulgheru R, Pepi M, Cosyns B, Dweck MR, Garbi M, Magne J, Nieman K, Rosenhek R, Bernard A, Lowenstein J, Vieira ML, Rabischoffsky A, Vyhmeister RH, Zhou X, Zhang Y, Zamorano JL, Habib G. Recommendations for the imaging assessment of prosthetic heart valves: a report from the European Association of Cardiovascular Imaging endorsed by the Chinese Society of Echocardiography, the inter-American Society of Echocardiography, and the Brazilian Department of Cardiovascular Imaging. Eur Heart J Cardiovasc Imaging. 2016;17(6):589–90. https://doi.org/10.1093/ehjci/jew025. Epub 2016 May 3.
13. VARC-3 WRITING COMMITTEE, Généreux P, Piazza N, Alu MC, Nazif T, Hahn RT, Pibarot P, Bax JJ, Leipsic JA, Blanke P, Blackstone EH, Finn MT, Kapadia S, Linke A, Mack MJ, Makkar R, Mehran R, Popma JJ, Reardon M, Rodes-Cabau J, Van Mieghem NM, Webb JG, Cohen DJ, Leon MB. Valve Academic Research Consortium 3: updated endpoint definitions for aortic valve clinical research. Eur Heart J. 2021;42(19):1825–57. https://doi.org/10.1093/eurheartj/ehaa799.
14. Krishnaswamy A, Tuzcu EM, Kapadia SR. Integration of MDCT and fluoroscopy using C-arm computed tomography to guide structural cardiac interventions in the cardiac catheterization laboratory. Catheter Cardiovasc Interv. 2015;85(1):139–47. https://doi.org/10.1002/ccd.25392. Epub 2014 Jan 29.
15. Cruz-González I, Barreiro-Pérez M, Valverde I. 3D-printing in preprocedural planning of paravalvular leak closure: feasibility/proof-of-concept. Rev Esp Cardiol (Engl Ed). 2019;72(4):342. https://doi.org/10.1016/j.rec.2018.04.008. Epub 2018 May 7.
16. Espinoza Rueda MA, Alcántara Meléndez MA, González RM, Jiménez Valverde AS, García García JF, Rivas Gálvez RE, Esparza TH, Rodríguez G, Sandoval Castillo LD, Merino Rajme JA. Successful closure of paravalvular leak using computed tomography image fusion and planning with 3-dimensional printing. JACC Case Rep. 2021;4(1):36–41. https://doi.org/10.1016/j.jaccas.2021.08.017.
17. Ruparelia N, Cao J, Newton JD, Wilson N, Daniels MJ, Ormerod OJ. Paravalvular leak closure under intracardiac echocardiographic guidance. Catheter Cardiovasc Interv. 2018;91(5):958–65. https://doi.org/10.1002/ccd.27318. Epub 2017 Oct 10.
18. Balzer J, Zeus T, Hellhammer K, Veulemans V, Eschenhagen S, Kehmeier E, Meyer C, Rassaf T, Kelm M. Initial clinical experience using the EchoNavigator®-system during structural heart disease interventions. World J Cardiol. 2015;7(9):562–70. https://doi.org/10.4330/wjc.v7.i9.562.
19. Bartel T, Müller S. Intraprocedural guidance: which imaging technique ranks highest and which one is complementary for closing paravalvular leaks? Cardiovasc Diagn Ther. 2014;4(4):277–8. https://doi.org/10.3978/j.issn.2223-3652.2014.08.04.
20. Bernard S, Yucel E. Paravalvular leaks-from diagnosis to management. Curr Treat Options Cardiovasc Med. 2019;21(11):67. https://doi.org/10.1007/s11936-019-0776-6.
21. Cruz-Gonzalez I, Rama-Merchan JC, Arribas-Jimenez A, Rodriguez-Collado J, Martin-Moreiras J, Cascon-Bueno M, Luengo CM. Paravalvular leak closure with the Amplatzer vascular plug III device: immediate and short-term results. Rev Esp Cardiol (Engl Ed). 2014;67(8):608–14. https://doi.org/10.1016/j.rec.2013.09.031. Epub 2014 Feb 11.
22. Yildirim A, Goktekin O, Gorgulu S, Norgaz T, Akkaya E, Aydin U, Unal Aksu H, Bakir I. A new specific device in transcatheter prosthetic paravalvular leak closure: a prospective two-center trial. Catheter Cardiovasc Interv. 2016;88(4):618–24. https://doi.org/10.1002/ccd.26439. Epub 2016 Feb 23.
23. Onorato EM, Muratori M, Smolka G, Malczewska M, Zorinas A, Zakarkaite D, Mussayev A, Christos CP, Bauer F, Gandet T, Martinelli GL, Costante AM, Bartorelli AL. Midterm procedural and clinical outcomes of percutaneous paravalvular leak closure with the Occlutech Paravalvular Leak device. EuroIntervention. 2020;15(14):1251–9. https://doi.org/10.4244/EIJ-D-19-00517.
24. Gafoor S, Franke J, Bertog S, Lam S, Vaskelyte L, Hofmann I, Sievert H, Matic P. A quick guide to Paravalvular Leak closure. Interv Cardiol. 2015;10(2):112–7. https://doi.org/10.15420/ICR.2015.10.2.112.

25. Krishnaswamy A, Kapadia SR, Tuzcu EM. Percutaneous paravalvular leak closure-imaging, techniques and outcomes. Circ J. 2013;77(1):19–27. https://doi.org/10.1253/circj.cj-12-1433. Epub 2012 Dec 15.
26. Nietlispach F, Maisano F, Sorajja P, Leon MB, Rihal C, Feldman T. Percutaneous paravalvular leak closure: chasing the chameleon. Eur Heart J. 2016;37(47):3495–502. https://doi.org/10.1093/eurheartj/ehw165. Epub 2016 May 8.
27. Hahn RT, Pibarot P, Webb J, Rodes-Cabau J, Herrmann HC, Williams M, Makkar R, Szeto WY, Main ML, Thourani VH, Tuzcu EM, Kapadia S, Akin J, McAndrew T, Xu K, Leon MB, Kodali SK. Outcomes with post-dilation following transcatheter aortic valve replacement: the PARTNER I trial (placement of aortic transcatheter valve). JACC Cardiovasc Interv. 2014;7:781–9.
28. Okuyama K, Jilaihawi H, Kashif M, Soni V, Matsumoto T, Yeow WL, Nakamura M, Cheng W, Kar S, Makkar RR. Percutaneous paravalvular leak closure for balloon-expandable transcatheter aortic valve replacement: a comparison with surgical aortic valve replacement paravalvular leak closure. J Invasive Cardiol. 2015;27(6):284–90.
29. Lázaro C, Hinojar R, Zamorano JL. Cardiac imaging in prosthetic paravalvular leaks. Cardiovasc Diagn Ther. 2014;4(4):307–13. https://doi.org/10.3978/j.issn.2223-3652.2014.07.01.
30. Ruiz CE, Jelnin V, Kronzon I, Dudiy Y, Del Valle-Fernandez R, Einhorn BN, Chiam PT, Martinez C, Eiros R, Roubin G, Cohen HA. Clinical outcomes in patients undergoing percutaneous closure of periprosthetic paravalvular leaks. J Am Coll Cardiol. 2011;58(21):2210–7. https://doi.org/10.1016/j.jacc.2011.03.074.
31. Alkhouli M, Sarraf M, Maor E, Sanon S, Cabalka A, Eleid MF, Hagler DJ, Pollak P, Reeder G, Rihal CS. Techniques and outcomes of percutaneous aortic paravalvular leak closure. JACC Cardiovasc Interv. 2016;9(23):2416–26. https://doi.org/10.1016/j.jcin.2016.08.038.
32. Turner ME, Lai WW, Vincent JA. Percutaneous closure of tricuspid paravalvular leak. Catheter Cardiovasc Interv. 2013;82(4):E511–5. https://doi.org/10.1002/ccd.24808. Epub 2013 Apr 18.
33. Heo YH, Kim SJ, Lee SY, Baek JS. A case demonstrating a percutaneous closure using the amplatzer duct occluder for paravalvular leakage after tricuspid valve replacement. Korean Circ J. 2013;43(4):273–6. https://doi.org/10.4070/kcj.2013.43.4.273. Epub 2013 Apr 30.
34. Mukherji A, Anantharaman R, Subramanyan R. Percutaneous closure of symptomatic large tricuspid paravalvular regurgitation using two muscular VSD occluders. Indian Heart J. 2017;69(3):334–7. https://doi.org/10.1016/j.ihj.2016.10.009. Epub 2016 Nov 3.

Part II

Percutaneous Therapeutic Intervention in Non-valvular, Non-congenital Structural Heart Diseases

Left Atrial Appendage Closure Periprocedural Imaging

Mesfer Alfadhel and Jacqueline Saw

Abstract

Percutaneous left atrial appendage closure (LAAC) has become an important tool for stroke prevention in patients with nonvalvular atrial fibrillation (AF). LAAC is an alternative to oral anticoagulation (OAC) and, thus, is a desirable option for patients at high risk for bleeding. In the early days of LAAC, concerns were raised about the procedure's safety and long-term efficacy. However, operator technique improvements, pre-, and periprocedural imaging advancements, and device development have improved safety and technical success rates. This chapter reviews the periprocedural multimodality imaging in percutaneous LAAC when using the 2 FDA-approved devices, Watchman FLX (Boston Scientific Corporation) and Amulet (St. Jude Medical, Minneapolis, MN).

Keywords

Amulet · Atrial fibrillation · CCTA · Left atrial appendage closure · TEE · Watchman · Echocardiography

Abbreviations

CCTA	Cardiac computer tomography angiography
DOAC	Direct oral anticoagulation
IAS	Interatrial septum
ICE	Intracardiac echocardiography
LA	Left atrium
LAAC	Left atrial appendage closure
LV	Left ventricle
MPR	Multiplanar reconstruction
OAC	Oral anticoagulation
PFO	Patent foramen ovalis
TEE	Transoesophageal echocardiography
TTE	Transthoracic echocardiography

Test your learning and check your understanding of this book's contents: use the "Springer Nature Flashcards" app to access questions using ▶ https://sn.pub/ambACS. To use the app, please follow the instructions in the chapter "Transcatheter Aortic Valve Replacement."

Learning Objectives
- The main tasks for periprocedural imaging are to provide high-quality images of the LAA and its surrounding structures to:

M. Alfadhel · J. Saw (✉)
Division of Cardiology, Vancouver General Hospital, University of British Columbia, Vancouver, BC, Canada
e-mail: jsaw@mail.ubc.ca

1. Rule out pre-existing thrombus
2. Provide adequate LAA measurements for device-sizing
3. Guide the position and technique of TS puncture
4. Guide placement of the delivery sheath
5. Optimize positioning and guide deployment of the device
6. Visualize peri-device leaks and uncovered proximal lobes
7. Assess device stability to minimize the risk of embolization

> **Case**
> 86-year-old man with atrial fibrillation and a CHADVASC score of 3 (age and hypertension) had recurrent hemarthrosis on Rivaroxaban. He was changed to low-dose apixaban with no improvement. He continued to have small to medium knee effusion, affecting his mobility and quality of life. There were no reversible mechanical causes found after consultation with orthopedic surgery. He was deemed unsuitable for chronic oral anticoagulation and was referred for left atrial appendage closure.

Background

Atrial fibrillation (AF) is the most common cardiac arrhythmia, with an estimated lifetime prevalence of 25% after 40 years of age [1]. In the Global Burden of Disease study, the worldwide prevalence of AF in 2010 was estimated at 0.5%, equating to 33.5 million patients, with a projected dramatic increase in prevalence over the next few decades [2]. AF increases the risk for stroke by fivefold, is responsible for >20% of all strokes, and leads to more disabling symptoms, with higher mortality and healthcare costs than other causes of stroke [3, 4].

The Watchman 2.5 device was the first FDA-approved left atrial appendage closure (LAAC) dedicated device after the two landmark trials PROTECT-AF [5] (Watchman Left Atrial Appendage System for Embolic Protection in Patients With Atrial Fibrillation) and PREVAIL (Prospective Randomized Evaluation of the WATCHMAN LAA Closure Device in Patients With Atrial Fibrillation vs. Long-Term Warfarin Therapy) [6] confirmed the safety and efficacy of warfarin in patients who were eligible for long-term anticoagulation. The 2020 ESC guidelines for the management of AF recommended that LAAC with current devices may be considered in patients with a high risk of stroke and contraindication to long-term oral anticoagulation (OAC) (class IIb, level of evidence B) [7]. The 2019 AHA/ACC/HRS AF guidelines focused update made a similar recommendation [8].

Watchman FLX

The Watchman FLX (Boston Scientific Corporation) is the latest iteration of the Watchman device (Fig. 1a). It includes several modifications that are aimed at improving both safety and efficacy. Compared to Watchman 2.5, the FLX has a closed distal end to lessen the likelihood of perforation and is fully recapturable. It covers a wider size range (five device sizes ranging from 20–35 mm) and more overlap between sizes, allowing for deployment in LAA ostia ranging from 14 to 31.5 mm. The FLX device has 50% more anchors, which are now J-shaped rather than straight, resulting in three times greater holding strength. In addition, the new FLX is less tapered distally, allowing greater apposition with the LAA wall, and has reduced metal exposure that may potentially minimize the risk of DRT.

The PINNACLE FLX study enrolled 400 patients prospectively at 29 sites implanted with the FLX device [9]. Antithrombotic therapy con-

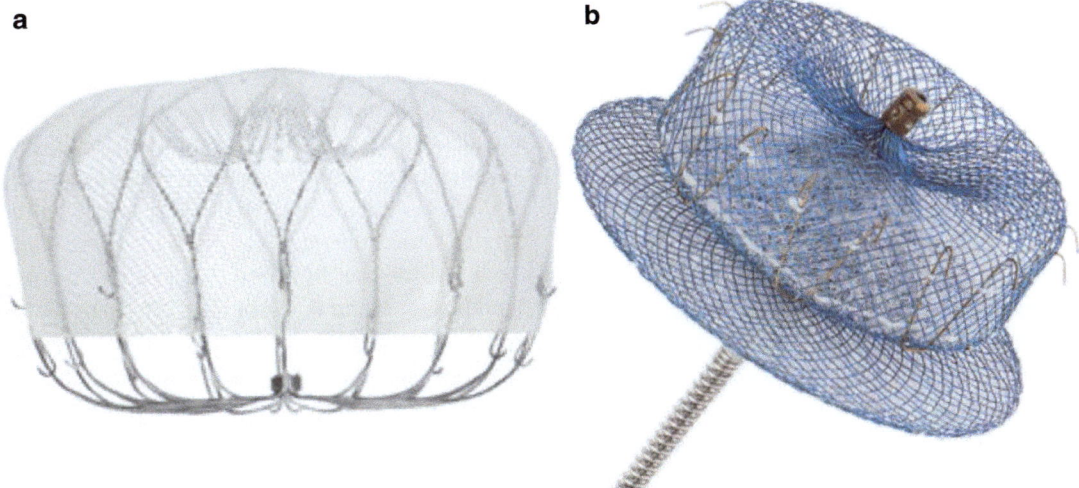

Fig. 1 (**a**) Watchman FLX device, (**b**) Amulet device

sisted of a DOAC plus aspirin for 45 days, followed by clopidogrel plus aspirin through 6 months, and then aspirin indefinitely. Device deployment was successful in 98.8% of cases, with 100% having effective closure at 1 year. The rate of all-cause death, ischemic stroke, systemic embolism, or device/procedure-related events requiring open cardiac surgery or major endovascular intervention between implantation and either 7 days or discharge was as low as 0.5%, and the rate of pericardial effusion was 1%. There was no device embolization. At 1 year, there was a 6.6% rate of all-cause death and a 2.6% rate of stroke.

Amulet

The Amulet is a second-generation Amplatzer LAAC device (Figs. 1b). Compared to the first-generation Amplatzer Cardiac Plug (ACP), the Amulet device has more anchoring hooks, wider lobe, larger disc, longer waist, and recessed end-screw to reduce exposed metal in the left atrium. The device consists of a lobe (ranging from 16 to 34 mm) and a disc to cover the ostium of the LAA, with the 34 mm device having the largest disc at 41 mm. The Amulet IDE study (Amplatzer Amulet Left Atrial Appendage Occluder Versus Watchman Device for Stroke Prophylaxis, was a randomized controlled trial comparing the Amulet device to the Watchman 2.5 device, enrolling ~1900 patients. The study showed Amulet to be non-inferior for safety and effectiveness of stroke prevention for nonvalvular AF compared with the Watchman device, and superiority in terms of appendage seal (lower peri-device leak) [12].

Pre-procedural Imaging

Several imaging modalities are utilized to plan and determine the patient's anatomical suitability for LAAC. This usually includes baseline transthoracic echocardiography (TTE), TEE, and CCTA.

Transthoracic Echocardiography

Baseline TTE is important to evaluate left atrium (LA) dimensions, volumes, and left ventricular (LV) function for patients considered for LAAC. Transoesophageal echocardiography (TEE) can exclude contraindications for LAAC, such as valvular AF (severe mitral stenosis), other significant structural abnormalities requiring surgery, or an LV thrombus requiring Oral anticoagulants (OAC).

Our patient had a transthoracic echocardiogram which showed normal LV/RV size and function, moderately dilated Left atrium, and no significant valvular disease.

Transesophageal Echocardiography

LAAC imaging with TEE requires an echocardiographer with experience in structural imaging, including measuring device sizing and selection. First, TEE is used to rule out LAA thrombus, a contraindication to LAAC. Secondly, it provides anatomical details of the LAA, including bends (location, angulation), lobes and bifurcations, and details of the pectinate muscle, ridge, and trabeculations. Thirdly, it allows measurements of the LAA ostium, device landing zone, and the depth of the appendage, as well as envisioning the LAA device fit. Lastly, assessing the surrounding structures (septum, LA, pulmonary veins, pulmonary artery, etc.) is important, as the left upper pulmonary vein and mitral annulus are in close proximity to the LAA; and the LAA can be adjacent to the pulmonary artery. TEE is currently the most widely accepted imaging tool for LAAC. It has high a sensitivity and specificity (92% and 98%, respectively) for detecting LAA thrombi, and high negative and positive predictive values (100% and 86%, respectively) [13]. Figure 2 shows LAAC clot with the use of echocardiography contrast for better sensitivity.

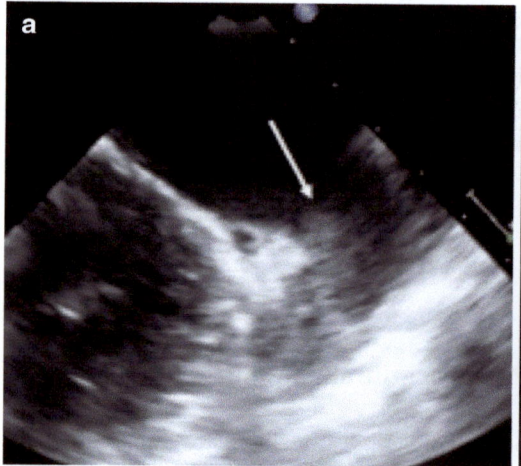
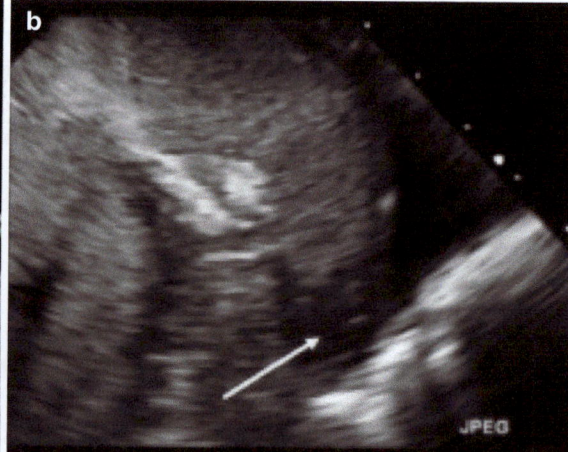

Fig. 2 (**a**) Two-dimensional TEE showing spontaneous echocardiographic contrast (arrow) in the LAA. (**b**) Two-dimensional TEE with use of ultrasound contrast revealing thrombus (filling defect) in the distal portion of LAA (arrow). (with permission) [10]

Device Sizing Using TEE

Proper sizing enables optimal device selection and is paramount to procedural safety and efficacy. LAA sizing requires that two measurements be ascertained; (1) the orifice/landing zone diameter and (2) LAA length/depth; both are primary prerequisites for device choice and sizing. With the TEE probe at the level of the mid-esophagus, multiple TEE imaging planes can be obtained by changing the Omniplane angulation. First, a full 0°–135° sweep should be performed to assess the LAA shape, size, number of lobes, and location of lobes. The LAA orifice diameter is typically obtained at 0°, 45°, 90°, and 135°, together with measurements of the usable LAA length. Broadly, the long-axis view of the LAA enables measurement of maximum LAA depth, whereas the short-axis view typically enables measurement of the maximal LAA orifice diameter. The long axis of the LAA can be found at 0°, 45°, or 90°, depending on the orientation of the LAA. Measuring the depth of the LAA from this axis of view allows for ascertaining the maximum LAA usable length, which is particularly important for the Watchman FLX device. The short axis of the LAA is typically obtained at 135° imaging plane. This angle usually provides imaging of the widest diameter of the LAA orifice.

For the Amulet device, the landing zone determines the size and position of the device. It is measured at 12 mm inside the echocardiographic orifice (the line connecting the circumflex artery and PV ridge). The echocardiographic orifice from the pulmonary vein ridge to the inferior origin of the LAA should be measured to gauge the size of the appropriate Amulet disc. For the Watchman FLX, the anatomic orifice (line from circumflex artery inferiorly to a point 1–2 cm inside the tip of the PV ridge superiorly) is measured. Device sizing is typically upsized by 2–4 mm for Amulet at the landing zone, and 10–30% for Watchman FLX at the anatomic orifice to allow adequate compression. LAA depth also needs to be considered to ensure enough depth to accommodate the delivery system/device, which is especially important with the Watchman FLX device, although a significantly less required depth compared to the Watchman 2.5 generation. The Amulet device does not require as much LAA depth (only 10–12 mm minimum depth) than the Watchman devices.

The Interatrial Septum

Assessment of the interatrial septum (IAS) on TEE is also essential to optimize the location for transseptal puncture. The IAS should be evaluated for its thickness, the presence of a concomitant atrial septal aneurysm, patent foramen ovalis (PFO), or atrial septal defects. The complexity of the transseptal puncture increases if the IAS is thick or aneurysmal. Various technical alterations may be considered in such cases, including using a radiofrequency needle for a transseptal puncture and creating larger curves on the standard transseptal needles to 'reach' the IAS, especially if the atrial chambers are enlarged. In the presence of PFO, it is generally recommended not to utilize the PFO to cross into the LA but instead to perform a standard transseptal puncture to optimize the angle for the sheath approach into the LAA. More details are in the next section below.

Three-Dimensional TEE

Three-dimensional TEE (3D-TEE) has become widely available in recent years. Technical advancements, including software upgrades and higher resolution probes, have substantially improved imaging support of complex interventional procedures, including LAAC, with more reliable measurements than two-dimensional (2D) and better orientation to neighboring structures. 3D TEE measurements better correlate with multidetector computer tomography [14, 15]. It helps additionally in the differentiation between thrombus and pectinate muscle [16]. Furthermore, the potential of having 2D biplane imaging is valuable for difficult LAA angles.

Cardiac Computer Tomography Angiography

Multislice cardiac computer tomography angiography (CTA) provides superior spatial resolution and 3D volumetric data to assess the complex LAA anatomy and surrounding structures comprehensively. Pre-procedural CTA is an excellent choice for planning a successful LAAC. Similar to TEE, CTA can rule out LAA thrombus (especially when a delayed scan is incorporated for better specificity), examine the LAA anatomy in more detail, precise details on surrounding structures, and as well as guide device and equipment selection, and anticipate potential obstacles, which collectively can reduce procedural time, contrast dose, and complications (Fig. 3). Many studies have shown that the measurements of LAA dimensions are larger on CTA than TEE. In a 50-patient cohort study, Saw [17] showed the maximal LAA diameter was significantly larger for CTA (24.1 ± 4.7 mm) versus TEE (22.3 ± 4.9 mm) ($p < 0.001$). Wang [18] also showed that CTA LAA sizing was consistently larger than 2D and 3D TEE (2–3 mm). 3D-TEE correlated better with CTA measurements but was still undersized ($p = 0.022$). Depth dimensions by 2D-TEE were similarly smaller than 3D TEE, and both of which were smaller than CTA [17].

For assessing the orifice, multiplanar reconstruction (MPR) is required, and this can be easily obtained by manipulating the cross-sectional orthogonal views in the imaging software. First, an oblique view of the LAA ostium is delineated

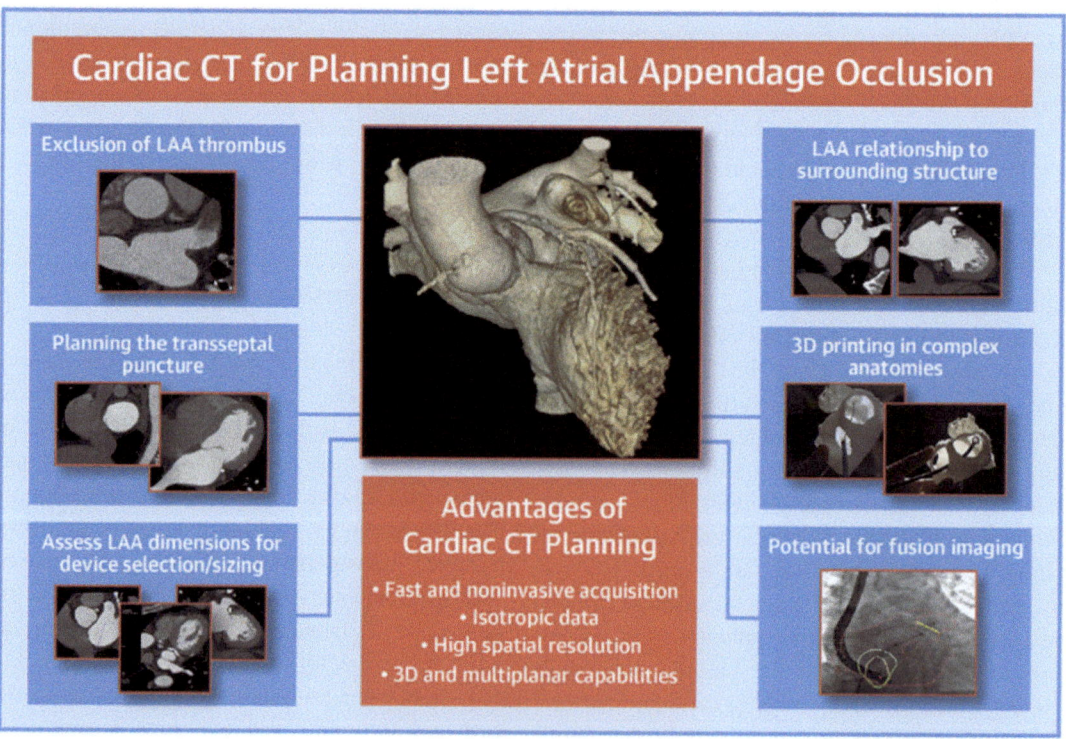

Fig. 3 The utility of pre-procedural with baseline cardiac CTA (with permission) [11]

on MPR, selecting a plane where the circumflex artery, the pulmonary vein ridge, and the LAA can be depicted. An orthogonal cross-section of this plane is then obtained to ensure an appropriate coaxial plane. Then the orthogonal "end-on" view is utilized to measure this ostium's maximum and minimum dimensions. Once the LAA orifice diameters have been measured, the depth of the LAA must also be ascertained. The Watchman FLX requires that the depth be measured from the anatomical orifice to the most distal tip of the selected lobe (Fig. 4).

The shape of the LAA can be ascertained by viewing the volume rendered (VR) three-dimensional images obtained by CTA (Fig. 5). The classification involving four distinct shapes

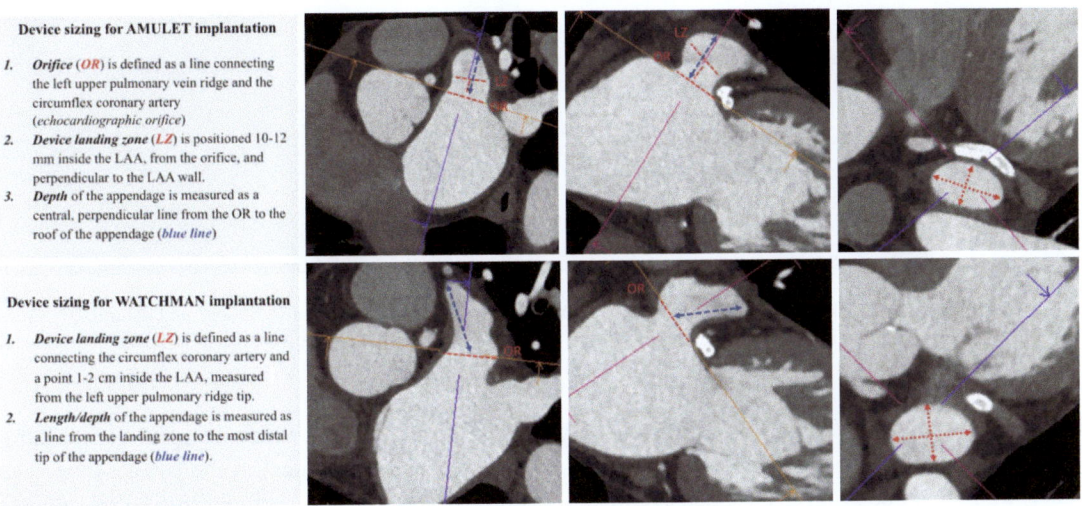

Fig. 4 Illustration of device sizing for the Amulet and Watchman devices on cardiac CTA [11]

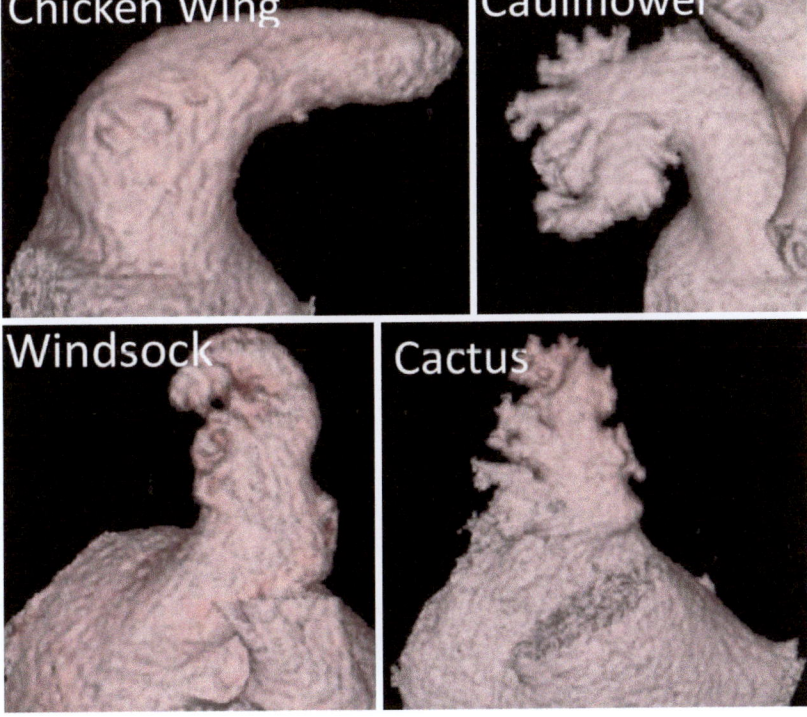

Fig. 5 Volume rendering of three-dimensional images of common LAA shapes

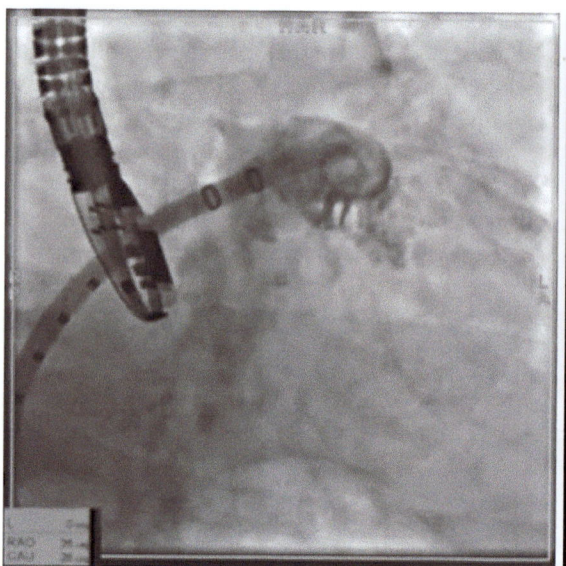 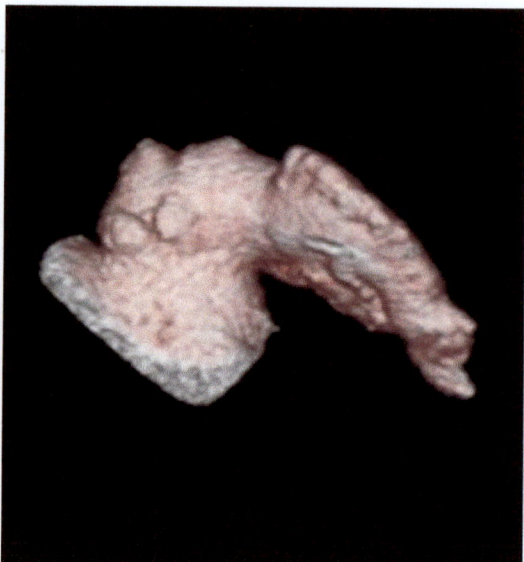

Fig. 6 Volume rendering three-dimensional cardiac CTA correlation to fluoroscopic images in a patient with inferiorly oriented chicken-wing shaped LAA: (**a**) corresponding fluoroscopy image in RAO 26° and caudal 26° view, (**b**) CTA volume rendered image in RAO 26° and caudal 26° view

described by DiBiase et al. has been widely adopted, which include the windsock (single primary lobe without significant bend), chicken-wing (pronounced bend in the body of LAA), cactus (major central lobe with multiple secondary lobes), and cauliflower (short LAA body that branches into several lobes) shapes [19]. Ascertainment of the LAA shape can be informative to the operator from a technical and procedural complexity point of view. For example, the "windsock" shape is often thought to be the least challenging for implantation compared to the "chicken-wing" shape, with a proximal and sharp bend that may increase the complexity of the device implantation. The "cactus" and "cauliflower" shapes are often shallow, which may pose a challenge for device implantation.

Manipulation of the VR images can assist in determining the best corresponding fluoroscopic views to guide device placement during the procedure. For example, the right anterior oblique view with cranial projection shows the orifice and proximal segment of the LAA well, which is useful when implanting the disc of the Amulet device. On the other hand, an RAO/Caudal view allows visualization of the body and distal segment of the LAA, which is ideal for guiding access sheath placement in the correct lobe. The pre-procedural CTA 3-dimensional VR images can be rotated to select the precise fluoroscopic angles that best visualize the implant angle for the selected device (Fig. 6).

Device Sizing on CTA

Careful assessment of the shape and dimensions of the LAA is essential before selecting the optimal device. Using multiplanar reconstruction, a view is identified where the LCX artery, the PV ridge, and the LAA ostium are seen. For Amulet implantation, the LAA ostium cross-section is obtained at right-angle projections to this plane to improve the coaxial measurement of the orifice. Then the widest diameter of the landing zone, 12 mm inside the orifice for Amulet device is measured, making sure that the measurement is coaxial. For Watchman FLX, the cross-section of the right-angle projection to the anatomic LAA ostium is used for device sizing. For the Amulet device, a minimum depth of 10–12 mm measured from the LAA orifice to the back wall of the LAA is required. For the Watchman FLX, the depth is measured from the LAA ostium to the most distal tip of the distal lobe, which must be as deep as half the size of the ostium in general as a minimum (i.e., for a 24 mm device in a 20 mm ostium, a minimum of 10 mm depth is required). Therefore, preselecting the lobe of choice also facilitates the selection of the appropriate access sheath (double-curve, single-curve, anterior curve) to achieve coaxial engagement into that lobe.

Our patient underwent a CTA, which (1) ruled out an LAA thrombus, (2) provided anatomical details of the LAA including size and shape, and (3) provided anatomical details of the adjacent structures and pre-procedural planning information, which we will discuss below. The anatomy was deemed suitable for percutaneous closure with either device. Procedural imaging with TEE or ICE is performed to guide placement of the device.

Device Selection

The CTA analysis of our patient using MPR is shown in Fig. 7.

Details of the LAA anatomy were as follows:

- Ostium diameter: 34.3 by 27.2 mm and a depth of 17 mm
- Landing zone diameter: 20.1 by 19.7 mm
- LAA shape: Cactus
- Lobes and bifurcation: 2 lobes with a distal bifurcation
- Other: it had a wide ostium, a short body with slight inferior angulation before dividing into lobes. With a wider orifice compared to the body of the LAA.

The selected device option was an Amulet 28 mm (disc size 35 mm). A Watchman FLX device was considered, however, the larger size of the ostium

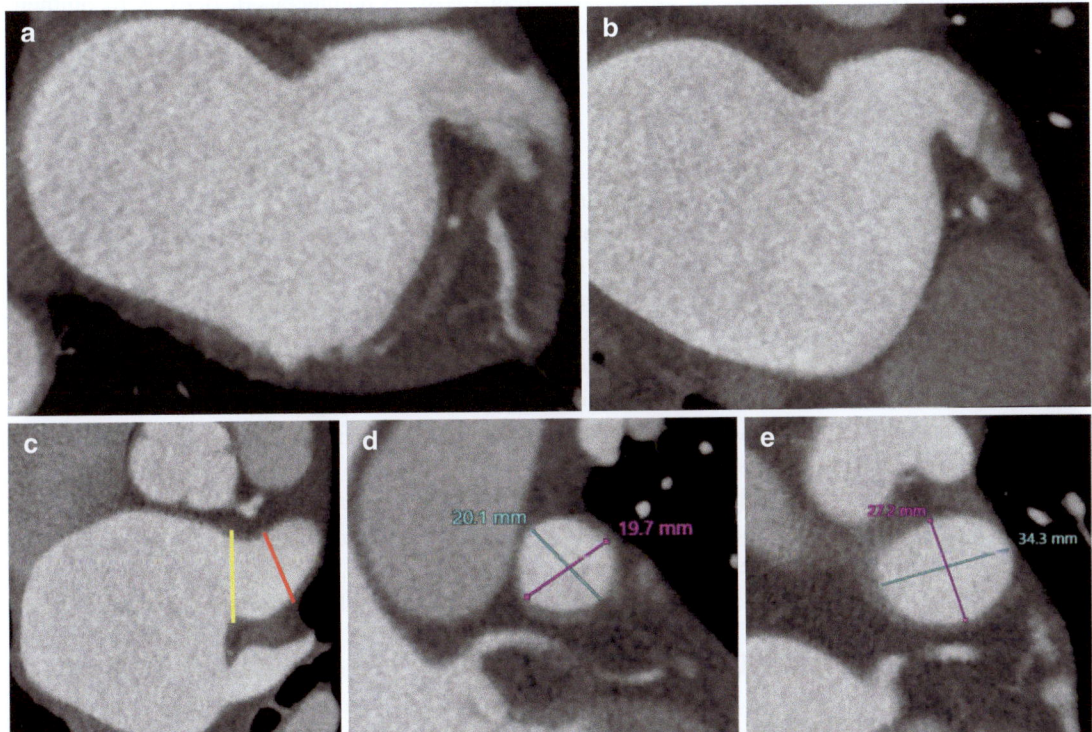

Fig. 7 (**a**, **b**) CTA MPR of the LAA, with (**c**) cross-sectional diameter measurements of the landing zone (red line) measured on (**d**), and the echocardiographic ostium (yellow line) measured on (**e**)

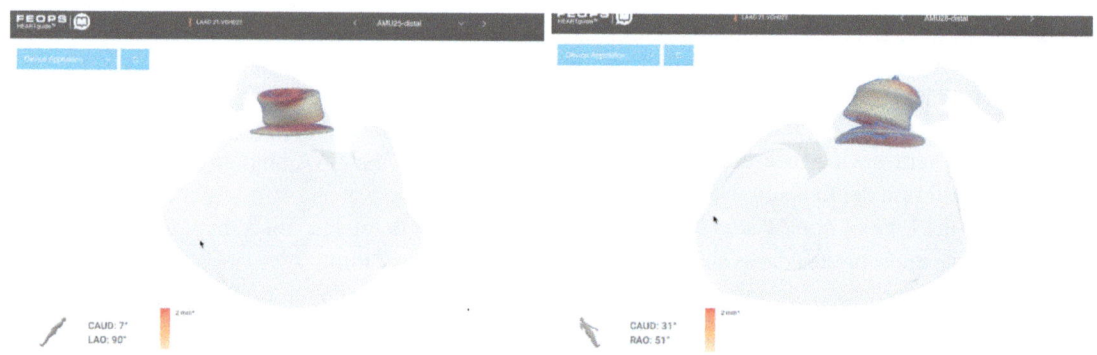

Fig. 8 Pre-procedural computer simulations based on cardiac CTA (FEops HEARTguide™). Panel left shows Amulet 25 mm device simulation, with red color indicating suboptimal contact with the LAA wall. Panel right shows a simulated Amulet 28 mm device with a good contact against LAA wall and compression of lobe

and slight angulation inferiorly of the appendage favored the Amulet device, since the disc can cover the entire LAA orifice. Whereas with the Watchman FLX device, there may be a proximal superior shoulder left uncovered, and there may be protrusion of the inferior shoulder of the device into the LA.

FEops HEARTguide Computer Simulations

The FEops (FEops HEARTguide™) software simulates device deployments into patient-specific LAA anatomies, allowing visualization of different device compressions and contacts at different positions within the LAA. This provides the operator with several choices of different sizes and positions of the closure device within the specific anatomy. In our case, the computer simulation provided simulations of the 25 mm and 28 mm Amulet devices with corresponding predicted position/seal (Fig. 8 show both simulations, favoring the 28 mm device).

Heart Team Decision and Discussion

Our heart team discussed the case for clinical and anatomical suitability. As this is a structural heart procedure to prevent stroke and such patients are suffering from bleeding conditions, our heart team includes neurologists, hematologists, and cardiologists with imaging and device implantation expertise. The patient was considered at high risk of stroke given his CHADVASC score, and OAC was considered harmful given his recurrent bleeding episodes. His LAA imaging modalities were reviewed and were deemed suitable for current LAAC percutaneous devices. A recommendation was made to proceed to percutaneous LAAC.

Procedural Imaging

The procedure was performed under general anesthesia. TEE was then performed with the interrogation of the LAA for (1) exclusion of LAA thrombus, (2) sizing confirmation of the LAA, (3) re-assessment of the other cardiac structures, including chamber size and function, as well as assessing for pericardial effusion peri procedurally, and (4) to guide the procedure.

Venous access is preferred through the right femoral vein for more direct route to the heart for transseptal access. The subcutaneous tissue at the access site should be well separated and dilated with a scalpel and forceps to ease the advancement of the large (in our case, 14 Fr) sheath. Manual compression, "figure-of-8" suture, and pre-closing with 6 Fr Perclose-ProGlide suture-mediated closure are various approaches for venous hemostasis; we prefer the Perclose method.

The optimal location for transseptal puncture for LAA closure is usually inferior and posterior at the fossa ovalis. This position is well-visualized with the bi-caval and short-axis TEE views, respectively. A PFO should not be used for sheath access as the resulting transseptal angle is not optimal for a coaxial approach to the LAA. Instead, performing a separate transseptal puncture inferoposteriorly is advised to provide a more direct vector orientation to access the LAA, which arises anteriorly and superiorly. Intravenous heparin is administered before or immediately following transseptal puncture to maintain ACT >250 s. Adequate mean left atrial pressure (>12 mmHg) should be attained with fluid bolus for accurate LAA measurements. We used the VersaCross radiofrequency (RF) system (Baylis Medical), an RF-tipped pigtail wire-based TSP system, to perform the TS puncture in an inferior posterior location (Fig. 9).

Over the VersaCross wire, a steerable 14 F delivery sheath was advanced to the LA; a 5F pigtail catheter was inserted into the LAA. Using the overlay system (CT)–fluoroscopy (EP navigator®, Philips Medical Systems, Best, The Netherlands), fusion imaging was used to guide the fluoroscopy angles better and display the appendage's anatomical landmarks for enhanced fluoroscopic visualization (Fig. 10). This technology may reduce radiation dosage, contrast volume and procedural time during LAAC.

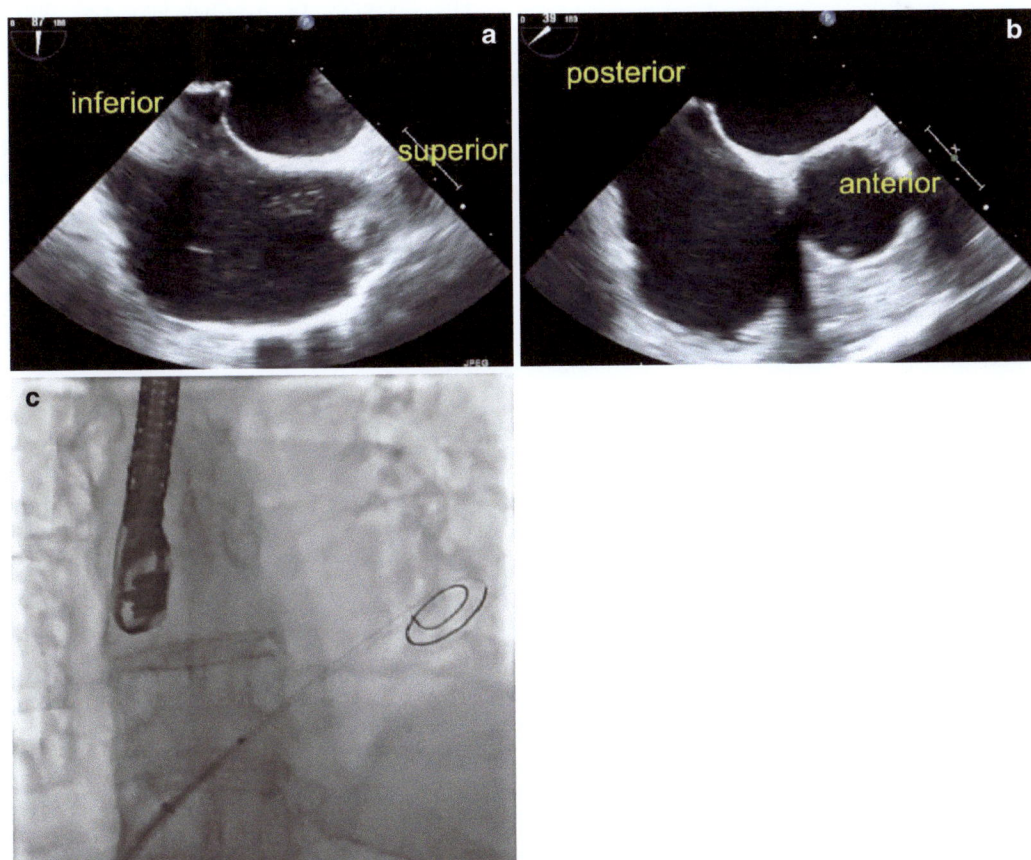

Fig. 9 (a) Transseptal tenting inferiorly in the bicaval view (which showed superior and inferior positioning on the fossa ovalis), (b) transseptal tenting posteriorly in the short-axis view (which showed anterior and posterior positioning on the fossa ovalis), and (c) VersaCross radiofrequency wire used for transseptal puncture and advanced into the left atrium

The prepped Amulet device was then advanced to the tip of the delivery sheath, which is positioned at the landing zone of the LAA (12 mm for the ostium). The first step of the Amulet deployment is unsheathing by withdrawing the delivery sheath to deploy the "ball" (Fig. 11). Once the "ball" is formed, the system can be advanced or withdrawn relatively safely within the LAA to achieve optimal position. The remainder of the lobe was then deployed by a "push-pull" maneuver, which often requires concomitant counterclock rotation of the sheath to allow coaxial positioning of the lobe for complete contact against the LAA neck. The lobe was then assessed for good positioning on cine angiogram and TEE. The disc was then deployed in the left atrium to cover the LAA orifice (Fig. 11). There are five criteria for good deployment that should be met before releasing the ACP/Amulet device: (1) tire-shaped lobe (ensures adequate compression of the lobe and engagement of stabilizing wires), (2) separation of the lobe and disc (ensures that the disc is pulled in against the LAA orifice with a good seal), (3) concavity of the disc (indicating traction of the disc against the lobe with a good seal), (4) axis of the lobe perpendicular to the neck axis at the landing zone (ensures proper contact of lobe and stabilizing wires against the LAA), and (5) lobe is ≥2/3 within the circumflex artery TEE (provides that the device is deep enough).

The presence of residual leak (>5 mm in width) was assessed on TEE with the Nyquist limit lowered to 50 cm/s, and contrast injection was performed through the delivery sheath to evaluate for optimal positioning and appendage opacification. Once good placement was confirmed, the device was released with counterclock rotation of the delivery cable. The delivery sheath was then withdrawn to the IVC, a right to left shunt was excluded by TEE, the sheath was removed, and the puncture was closed with Proglide.

The patient had a TTE later on the day to rule out effusion and confirm the device position; he was discharged the next day.

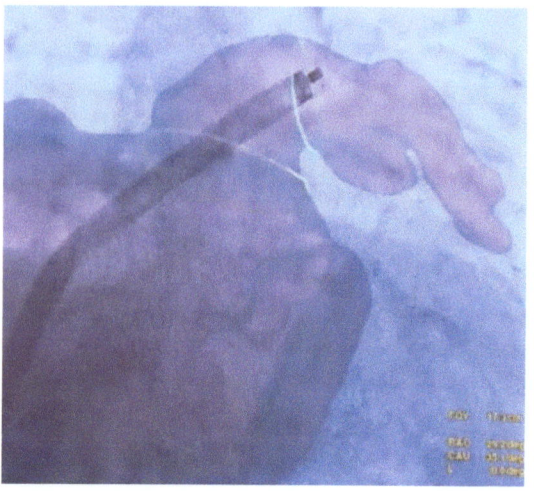

Fig. 10 X-ray fluoroscopy with CT overlay showing the overlying anatomy of the LAA

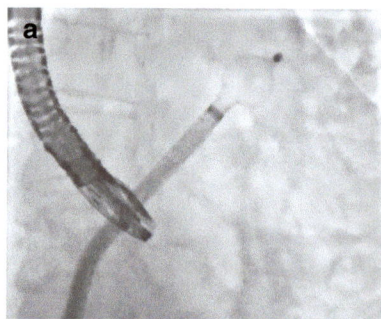 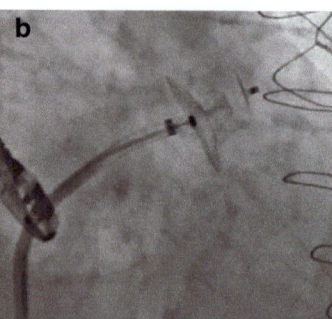 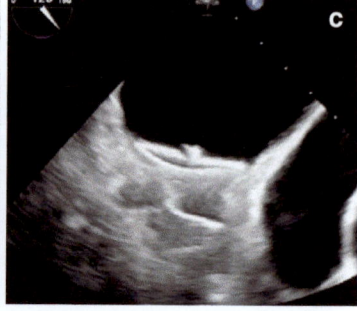

Fig. 11 (**a**) The Amulet device in a "ball" configuration, allows for safe atraumatic advancement prior to unsheathing, (**b**) the Amulet lobe and disc deployed before release of the cable, and (**c**) TEE showing the released Amulet device

Intracardiac Echocardiography

Intracardiac echocardiography (ICE) is emerging as a novel imaging tool for procedural guidance for percutaneous LAA closure. ICE utilization for structural intervention allows procedures to be performed safely under local anesthesia, avoiding the need for general anesthesia. Importantly, ICE utilization has also been shown to reduce overall procedural time [20]. Nevertheless, there is a significant learning curve for ICE LAA imaging, with subsequent improvement in procedural time, contrast load, and fluoroscopic time with experience.

The Viewflex Xtra (St. Jude Medical) and the AcuNav (BioSense Webster) are two commercially available ICE catheters. Both catheters are 90 cm in length with diameters ranging between 8 and 10 F. At the tip of each catheter is an ultrasound transducer with 64 phased-array elements. The catheters are inserted from the femoral vein via large venous sheaths (9–10 F) and passed superiorly from the inferior vena cava to its starting position in the right atrium. The 'home view' is obtained at this location. ICE imaging is performed by a combination of the operator's catheter rotation (clock-counter clock motion) and manipulation of two separate knobs on the catheter handle. Each of the knobs allows for anteroposterior tilt or right-left tilt. A combination of rotation, tilt and catheter position allows different intracardiac structures to be visualized. Imaging the LAA with ICE can be achieved from multiple positions. The more straightforward right atrial approach does not require accessing the LA with the ICE probe; however, the LAA images may be suboptimal. Viewing the LAA from the coronary sinus, para-coronary sinus, and pulmonary artery has been described but may be challenging to obtain. Nevertheless, the technical success rate of LAA closure with right atrial-based ICE guidance was shown to be as high as 97.5% with experienced operators [20].

Alternatively, accessing the LA with the ICE probe can be performed, dramatically improving imaging of the LAA since the ICE probe can be adjacent to the structure. This can be done through a double-transseptal approach (separate transseptal puncture for the ICE probe) or through a single-transseptal approach (by accessing the same transseptal puncture for both access sheath and ICE probe). For the later approach, the ICE probe can be advanced through the same transseptal puncture utilized for the access sheath. Although this approach may be more straightforward, the risk of persistent iatrogenic atrial septal defect may be higher than the double-transseptal approach [20]. Three key views can be obtained from with ICE catheter from the LA side: (1) left upper pulmonary vein view (similar to a TEE 0° view), providing good visualization of the LAA long axis view; (2) mid-atrial view (similar to a TEE 45° view), which is preferred for landing the LAA device; and (3) supra-mitral view provides good visualization of the LAA short axis view (similar to a TEE 135° view) (Fig. 12).

Post procedural Imaging

Cardiac CTA can also be utilized for postprocedural device surveillance. This can be performed within 1–6 months of device implantation. The roles of CTA in this context is to assess for device-associated thrombus and in detecting peri-device leak. CTA can detect thrombus on the device or adjacent LA wall [22]. The CT linear attenuation coefficient (Hounsfield unit) measurement enables the detection of residual flow into the LAA. CCTA is much more sensitive compared to TEE for this purpose. CCTA also identifies the mechanism of a residual leak, such as off-axis device implantation, gaps in the LAA orifice not covered by the device, and persistent fabric leak (likely due to incomplete endothelialization) [22]. However, the clinical significance of CCTA detected persistent contrast opacification of the LAA (patency) remains unknown.

The patient returned for post-procedural CCTA, which showed good device position and no DRT or PLD.

In conclusion, periprocedural imaging is paramount to the success of LAAC. It provides anatomical assessment for the suitability of LAAC and the precise procedural technique and optimal device selection. Intraprocedural guidance with multimodality imaging is utilised for the safety and efficacy of the device implant.

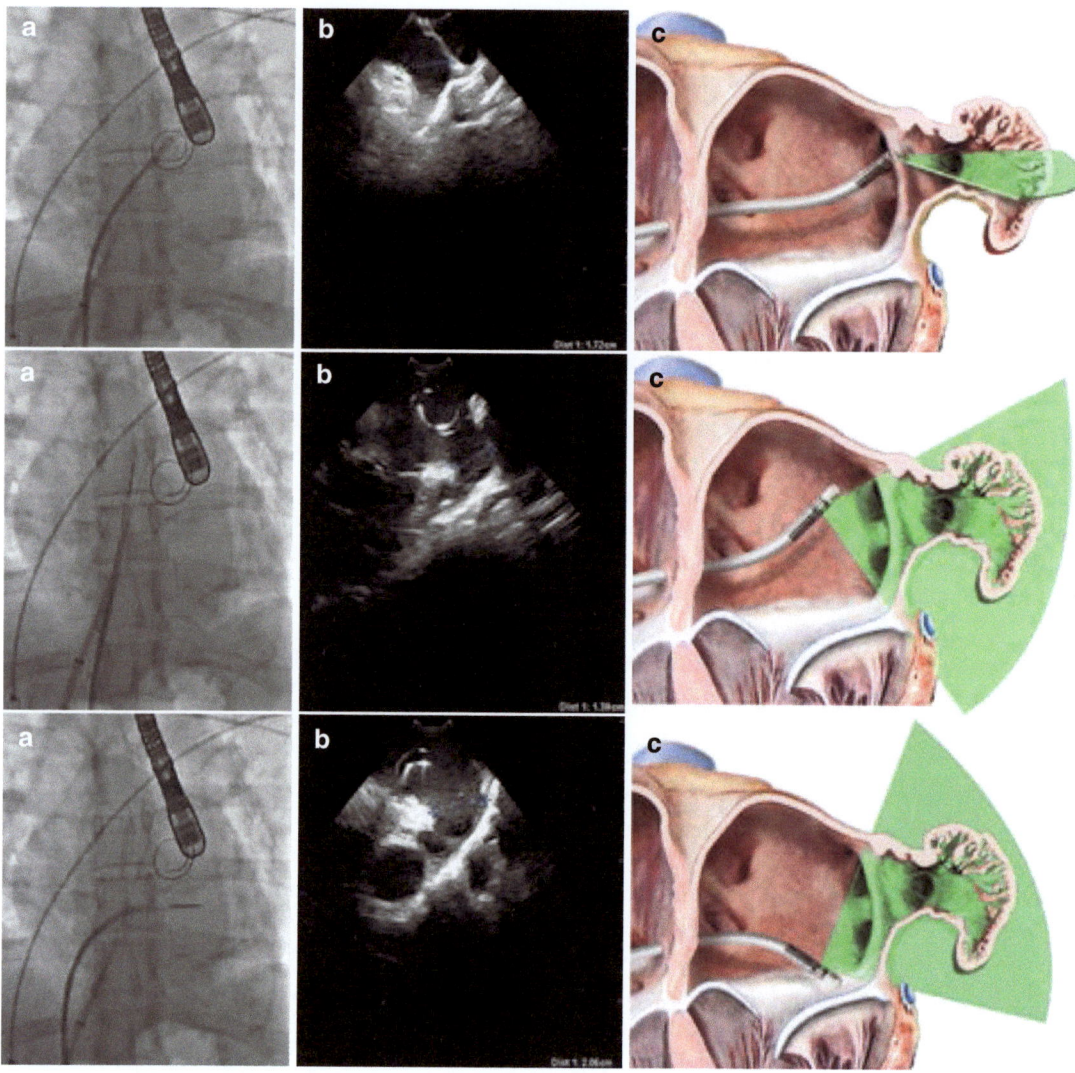

Fig. 12 Fluoroscopy, ICE and color images panel (1) LUPV view, (2) mid-LA view (3) supra-mitral view (with permission ICE LAA consensus 2021) [21]

Key Points

- LAAC with two FDA-approved devices: Watchman FLX and Amulet are alternatives to oral anticoagulation (OAC) for patients at high risk for bleeding
- Periprocedural evaluation with TEE or CTA is needed for a successful LAAC to
  - Rule out pre-existing thrombus
  - Provide adequate LAA measurements for device-sizing
  - Guide the position and technique of TS puncture
  - Guide placement of the delivery sheath
  - Optimize positioning and guide deployment of the device
  - Visualize peri-device leaks and uncovered proximal lobes
  - Assess device stability to minimize the risk of embolization
- Intracardiac Echocardiography (ICE) is emerging as a novel imaging tool for procedural guidance for percutaneous LAA closure
- Post-procedural monitoring for device-related thrombus and peri-device leakage can be done with TEE or cardiac CTA.

Imaging study	Benefits	Disadvantages
Echocardiogram	**TTE:** Baseline TTE provides important information regarding LA and LV dimensions, volumes, and function and assessing contraindications for LAAC, such as valvular AF (severe mitral stenosis), LV thrombosis or other significant structural abnormalities **TEE:** 1. Widely accepted method with high accuracy for ruling out LAA or LA thrombosis 2. It provides anatomical details of the LAA, including measurements of the LAA ostium, device landing zone, and the depth of the appendage, as well as envisioning the LAA device fit 3. Assessing the surrounding structures (septum, LA, pulmonary veins, pulmonary artery, etc.) **3D TEE (three-dimensional TEE):** Provides more reliable measurements than two-dimensional (2D) TEE with better correlation with CTA	TTE has limited value for LAA evaluation TEE is a semi-invasive method and commonly required general anesthesia or IV sedation
CT	- Multislice cardiac computer tomography angiography (CTA) provides superior spatial resolution and 3D volumetric data to assess the complex LAA anatomy and surrounding structures comprehensively - Pre-procedural CTA is an excellent choice for planning a successful LAAC, rule out LAA thrombus, examine the LAA anatomy and surrounding anatomy in more detail	- Radiation exposure - Risk of contrast induced nephropathy
Intra cardiac echocardiogram	- ICE can be done safely during procedure with local anesthesia, and obviating the need for TEE and general anesthesia - ICE utilization can reduce overall procedural time	- Needs learning curve for ICE LAA imaging

Disclosure Dr. Saw has received unrestricted research grant support (from the Canadian Institutes of Health Research, Heart and Stroke Foundation of Canada, National Institutes of Health, University of British Columbia Division of Cardiology, AstraZeneca, Abbott Vascular, St Jude Medical, Boston Scientific, and Servier), salary support (Michael Smith Foundation of Health Research), speaker honoraria (AstraZeneca, Abbott Vascular, Boston Scientific, and Sunovion), consultancy and advisory board honoraria (AstraZeneca, St Jude Medical, Abbott Vascular, Boston Scientific, Baylis, Gore, FEops), and proctorship honoraria (Abbott Vascular, St Jude Medical and Boston Scientific), all outside the submitted work. Dr. Alfadhel has no disclosures.

Chapter Review Questions

An 80-year-old man with AF rhythm and high risk for internal bleeding, and candidate for percutaneous LAA closure:

1. In the pre-procedural evaluation of the interatrial septum (IAS) by TEE which of the following is INCORRECT?
    A. In the presence of a large PFO, utilizing PFO to cross the septum is recommended to avoid iatrogenic ASD.
    B. Presence of a thick or aneurysmal IAS can be challenging for septostomy.
    C. The optimal location for transseptal puncture for LAA closure is inferior and posterior of IAS.
    D. The best TEE view during transseptal puncture is bi-caval and short axis views.
    Answer: A
    A PFO should not be used for sheath access as the resulting transseptal angle is not optimal for a coaxial approach to the LAA. Instead, performing a separate transseptal puncture inferoposteriorly is advised to provide a more direct vector orientation to access the LAA, which arises anteriorly and superiorly.

2. The morphology of LAA is described as a short LAA body that branches into several lobes. Which of the following shape is matched this definition:
    A. Windsock
    B. Chicken-wing
    C. Cauliflower
    D. Cactus
    Answer: C
    The cauliflower morphology has a short LAA body that branches into several lobes.

3. Which TEE views commonly provide the widest diameter of the LAA orifice?
    A. 0°
    B. 45°
    C. 90°
    D. 135°

Answer: D The short axis of the LAA is typically obtained at 135° imaging plane. This angle usually provides imaging of the widest diameter of the LAA orifice.

4. In the percutaneous LAA closure pre-procedural evaluation by cardiac CT
    A. LAA dimensions by cardiac CT are larger than LAA dimensions by TEE
    B. LAA dimensions by cardiac CT are smaller than LAA dimensions by TEE
    C. LAA dimensions by cardiac CT are comparable to LAA dimensions by TEE
    D. Cardiac CTA is not recommended for pre-procedural evaluation
    Answer: A
    Many studies have shown that the measurements of LAA dimensions are larger on CTA than TEE. Depth dimensions by 2D-TEE were similarly smaller than 3D TEE, and both were smaller than CTA.

References

1. Lloyd-Jones DM, Wang TJ, Leip EP, et al. Lifetime risk for development of atrial fibrillation: the Framingham heart study. Circulation. 2004;110(9):1042–6. https://doi.org/10.1161/01.CIR.0000140263.20897.42.
2. Chugh SS, Havmoeller R, Narayanan K, et al. Worldwide epidemiology of atrial fibrillation: a global burden of disease 2010 study. Circulation. 2014;129(8):837–47. https://doi.org/10.1161/CIRCULATIONAHA.113.005119.
3. Alkhouli M, Alqahtani F, Aljohani S, Alvi M, Holmes DR. Burden of atrial fibrillation–associated ischemic stroke in the United States. JACC Clin Electrophysiol.

2018;4(5):618–25. https://doi.org/10.1016/j.jacep.2018.02.021.
4. January CT, Wann LS, Calkins H, et al. 2019 AHA/ACC/HRS focused update of the 2014 AHA/ACC/HRS guideline for the management of patients with atrial fibrillation: a report of the American College of Cardiology/American Heart Association task force on clinical practice guidelines and the Heart Rhythm Society. J Am Coll Cardiol. 2019;74(1):104–32. https://doi.org/10.1016/j.jacc.2019.01.011.
5. Reddy VY, Holmes D, Doshi SK, Neuzil P, Kar S. Safety of percutaneous left atrial appendage closure: results from the watchman left atrial appendage system for embolic protection in patients with AF (PROTECT AF) clinical trial and the continued access registry. Circulation. 2011;123(4):417–24. https://doi.org/10.1161/CIRCULATIONAHA.110.976449.
6. Holmes DR Jr, Kar S, Price MJ, et al. Prospective randomized evaluation of the Watchman Left Atrial Appendage Closure device in patients with atrial fibrillation versus long-term warfarin therapy: the PREVAIL trial. J Am Coll Cardiol. 2014;64:1–12.
7. Hindricks G, Potpara T, Dagres N, et al. 2020 ESC guidelines for the diagnosis and management of atrial fibrillation developed in collaboration with the European Association for Cardio-Thoracic Surgery (EACTS). Eur Heart J. 2021;42(5):373–498. https://doi.org/10.1093/eurheartj/ehaa612.
8. January CT, Wann LS, Calkins H, et al. 2019 AHA/ACC/HRS focused update of the 2014 AHA/ACC/HRS guideline for the management of patients with atrial fibrillation: a report of the American College of Cardiology/American Heart Association task force on clinical practice guidelines and the Heart Rhythm Society in collaboration with the Society of Thoracic Surgeons. Circulation. 2019;140(2):e125–51. https://doi.org/10.1161/CIR.0000000000000665.
9. Kar S, Doshi SK, Sadhu A, et al. Primary outcome evaluation of a next generation left atrial appendage closure device: results from the PINNACLE FLX trial. Circulation. 2021;4:1754–62. https://doi.org/10.1161/circulationaha.120.050117.
10. Gilhofer TS, Saw J. Periprocedural imaging for left atrial appendage closure: computed tomography, transesophageal echocardiography, and intracardiac echocardiography. Card Electrophysiol Clin. 2020;12(1):55–65. https://doi.org/10.1016/j.ccep.2019.11.007.
11. Korsholm K, Berti S, Iriart X, et al. Expert recommendations on cardiac computed tomography for planning transcatheter left atrial appendage occlusion. JACC Cardiovasc Interv. 2020;13(3):277–92. https://doi.org/10.1016/j.jcin.2019.08.054.
12. Lakkireddy D, Thaler D, Ellis CR, et al. AMPLATZER™ AMULET™ left atrial appendage occluder versus WATCHMAN™ device for stroke prophylaxis (AMULET IDE): a randomized controlled trial. Circulation. 2021;144:1543–52. https://doi.org/10.1161/CIRCULATIONAHA.121.057063.
13. Manning WJ, Weintraub RM, Waksmonski CA, et al. Accuracy of transesophageal echocardiography for identifying left atrial thrombi. A prospective, intraoperative study. Ann Intern Med. 1995;123(11):817–22. https://doi.org/10.7326/0003-4819-123-11-199512010-00001.
14. Nucifora G, Faletra FF, Regoli F, et al. Evaluation of the left atrial appendage with real-time 3-dimensional transesophageal echocardiography: implications for catheter-based left atrial appendage closure. Circ Cardiovasc Imaging. 2011;4(5):514–23. https://doi.org/10.1161/CIRCIMAGING.111.963892.
15. Perk G, Biner S, Kronzon I, et al. Catheter-based left atrial appendage occlusion procedure: role of echocardiography. Eur Heart J Cardiovasc Imaging. 2012;13(2):132–8. https://doi.org/10.1093/ejechocard/jer158.
16. Marek D, Vindis D, Kocianova E. Real time 3-dimensional transesophageal echocardiography is more specific than 2-dimensional TEE in the assessment of left atrial appendage thrombosis. Biomed Pap Med Fac Univ Palacky Olomouc Czech Repub. 2013;157(1):22–6. https://doi.org/10.5507/bp.2012.012.
17. Saw J, Fahmy P, Spencer R, et al. Comparing measurements of CT angiography, TEE, and fluoroscopy of the left atrial appendage for percutaneous closure. J Cardiovasc Electrophysiol. 2016;27(4):414–22. https://doi.org/10.1111/jce.12909.
18. Wang Y, di Biase L, Horton RP, Nguyen T, Morhanty P, Natale A. Left atrial appendage studied by computed tomography to help planning for appendage closure device placement. J Cardiovasc Electrophysiol. 2010;21(9):973–82. https://doi.org/10.1111/j.1540-8167.2010.01814.x.
19. di Biase L, Santangeli P, Anselmino M, et al. Does the left atrial appendage morphology correlate with the risk of stroke in patients with atrial fibrillation? Results from a multicenter study. J Am Coll Cardiol. 2012;60(6):531–8. https://doi.org/10.1016/j.jacc.2012.04.032.
20. Berti S, Paradossi U, Meucci F, et al. Periprocedural intracardiac echocardiography for left atrial appendage closure: a dual-center experience. JACC Cardiovasc Interv. 2014;7(9):1036–44. https://doi.org/10.1016/j.jcin.2014.04.014.
21. Berti S, Pastormerlo LE, Korsholm K, et al. Intracardiac echocardiography for guidance of transcatheter left atrial appendage occlusion: an expert consensus document. Catheter Cardiovasc Interv. 2021;98(4):815–25. https://doi.org/10.1002/ccd.29791.
22. Saw J, Fahmy P, DeJong P, et al. Cardiac CT angiography for device surveillance after endovascular left atrial appendage closure. Eur Heart J Cardiovasc Imaging. 2015;16(11):1198–206. https://doi.org/10.1093/ehjci/jev067.

Alcohol Septal Ablation in the Management of Hypertrophic Obstructive Cardiomyopathy (HOCM)

Daniel B. Loriaux, Andrew Wang, and Todd L. Kiefer

Abstract

Hypertrophic cardiomyopathy (HCM) is the most common monogenic heart disease and often associated with symptoms that impair functional status and quality of life. Alcohol septal ablation is a proven interventional treatment for patients with symptomatic, obstructive HCM, with success rates surpassing 95% and procedural mortality less than 1% at experienced centers. This chapter will discuss the clinical presentation of HCM, available diagnostic modalities, and the cardiovascular imaging features that guide candidacy for septal reduction therapies such as alcohol septal ablation or surgical myectomy. Beginning with a case presentation, the authors aim to highlight the imaging considerations involved in the Heart Team's approach to the patient with HCM and severe left ventricular outflow tract obstruction and selection for septal reduction therapy with a focus on procedural guidance for alcohol septal ablation.

Supplementary Information The online version contains supplementary material available at https://doi.org/10.1007/978-3-031-50740-3_7.

D. B. Loriaux · A. Wang · T. L. Kiefer (✉)
Division of Cardiology, Department of Medicine, Duke University Medical Center, Durham, NC, USA
e-mail: daniel.loriaux@duke.edu; a.wang@duke.edu; todd.kiefer@duke.edu

Keywords

Hypertrophic cardiomyopathy · Septal reduction therapy · Alcohol septal ablation · Surgical myectomy

Test your learning and check your understanding of this book's contents: use the "Springer Nature Flashcards" app to access questions using ▶ https://sn.pub/ambACS.
To use the app, please follow the instructions in the chapter "Transcatheter Aortic Valve Replacement."

Learning Objectives

At the conclusion of this chapter, the reader will have improved understanding of:

1. The cardiovascular imaging modalities indicated for establishing a diagnosis of HCM.
2. The role of cardiovascular imaging in determining patient candidacy for septal reduction therapies.
3. The key intraprocedural echocardiography findings to guide alcohol septal ablation.
4. Recommendations for imaging follow up.

> **Case Study**
> A 72-year-old female with past medical history of hypertension and hyperlipidemia presents to the Emergency Department for further evaluation of progressive shortness of breath, chest discomfort, exercise intolerance, and recent syncopal episodes. Her physical examination is notable for a grade III, crescendo-decrescendo murmur, which is heard best over the left lower sternal border and augments with Valsalva maneuver. Initial laboratory studies are remarkable for an elevated serum NT-proBNP and high sensitivity troponin. Her electrocardiogram shows normal sinus rhythm with normal axis, normal intervals, and no evidence of acute ischemia. A chest radiograph shows normal lung fields with an enlarged cardiac silhouette.

Background and Definitions

Hypertrophic Cardiomyopathy (HCM) is a heritable cardiomyopathy characterized by thickened myocardium, defined as an absolute increase in LV wall thickness of 15 mm or more in any region, and in the absence of another cardiac or systemic condition capable of producing a similar magnitude of LVH [1]. HCM with outflow tract obstruction (HOCM) is present in approximately 60–70% of patients with HCM, and is defined as a resting or provoked pressure gradient of 30 mmHg or more, typically due to systolic anterior motion (SAM) of the mitral valve.

The clinical presentation of HOCM is highly variable, with presentations ranging from asymptomatic persons to patients with advanced heart failure symptoms, syncope, or sudden cardiac death. Patients with HOCM are more likely to develop advanced heart failure symptoms over time compared with patients with non-obstructive HCM. Medical therapy to reduce contractility may reduce dynamic outflow tract obstruction, thereby reducing symptoms of HCM, but without reducing left ventricular hypertrophy.

Septal Reduction Therapy (SRT) with either surgical septal myectomy (SM) or selective alcohol septal ablation (ASA) is recommended for symptomatic HOCM refractory to medical management. Although there are no randomized studies comparing these two treatment strategies, surgical myectomy is regarded as the preferred option for patients with significant LVOTO (>50 mmHg), NYHA III or IV symptoms despite optimal medical management, and acceptable operative risk.

Percutaneous Alcohol Septal Ablation (ASA), which entails injection of 1–2 mL absolute ethanol into a proximal septal perforator branch of the LAD to cause a limited myocardial infarction of the hypertrophied, basal left ventricular septum, is an alternative to myectomy in selected patients with advanced age, increased surgical risk, or strong preference against surgical myectomy. Creation of a transmural infarct within the area of LVOTO leads to akinesis and progressive thinning of the basal septum, alleviating the obstruction and improving HCM morbidity to a degree that is comparable to surgery.

Selection Criteria for ASA include anatomic features and patient characteristics. Anatomically, the LVOT gradient must be attributable to a region of the basal septum that is perfused by a major septal perforator. The absence of a perforating vessel perfusing the region of obstruction, the septal perforator perfuses other cardiac structures (RV free wall, papillary muscle) in addition to the basal septum, the presence of extensive collateral circulation to the basal interventricular septum, significant contribution to the LVOTO due to mitral valve pathology, septal wall thickness less than 18 mm or greater than 30 mm are all features that favor SM over ASA. Similarly, SM should be favored in patients with other concomitant surgical indications (CABG, MVR, etc) and in younger patients. ASA is not recommended in patients younger than the age of 40 and carries a Class III indication for those under the age of 21.

Diagnosis and Pre-procedural Assessment

In patients with suspected HCM, transthoracic echocardiography is an essential component of the initial diagnostic assessment (Table 1).

The patient's TTE demonstrated normal chamber dimensions, hyperdynamic left ventricular function with no wall motion abnormalities, severe asymmetric septal hypertrophy with basal septal wall thickness measuring 18 mm, systolic anterior motion of the mitral valve with mild mitral regurgitation, and dynamic left ventricular outflow tract obstruction with a peak gradient of 170 mmHg at rest.

To further evaluate this patient's chest pain and to assess her candidacy for potential septal reduction therapies, diagnostic coronary angiography was performed. Note that as an alternative to coronary angiography, cardiac CTA also receives a Class I recommendation in the 2020 AHA/ACC guidelines for the diagnosis and treatment of patients with hypertrophic cardiomyopathy. While CTA is useful to exclude concomitant obstructive coronary artery disease, septal perforator anatomy is not well-defined with CTA and invasive angiography is preferred in patient under consideration for potential ASA. Pertinent guidelines for diagnostic angiography in patients with HCM are shown in Table 2.

Cardiac catheterization confirmed normal epicardial coronary arteries with a prominent first septal perforator branch, resting LVOTG 150 mmHg, and LVEDP 42 mmHg. The patient was referred to the Heart Team to discuss management options for newly diagnosed HOCM.

Table 1 Diagnostic echocardiography guidelines in suspected HCM [2]

COR	LOE	Guideline recommendation
1	B-NR	In patients with suspected hypertrophic cardiomyopathy (HCM), a transthoracic echocardiogram (TTE) is recommended in the initial evaluation
1	B-NR	For patients with HCM and resting left ventricular outflow tract gradient <50 mmHg, a TTE with provocative maneuvers is recommended
1	B-NR	For symptomatic patients with HCM who do not have a resting or provocable outflow tract gradient ≥50 mmHg on TTE, exercise TTE is recommended for the detection and quantification of dynamic left ventricular outflow tract obstruction (LVOTO)

Selection or recommendations pertaining to diagnostic transthoracic echocardiography (TTE) from the 2020 AHA/ACC Guidelines for the Diagnosis and Treatment of Patients with Hypertrophic Cardiomyopathy. Class of Recommendation (COR) 1 indicates a strong recommendation with benefits greatly outweighing risks. Level of Evidence (LOE) B-NR indicates moderate-quality evidence from one or more well-designed, well-executed nonrandomized studies, observational studies, or registry studies

Table 2 Diagnostic angiography guidelines in HCM [2]

COR	LOE	Guideline recommendation
1	B-NR	In patients with HCM with symptoms or evidence of myocardial ischemia, coronary angiography (CT or invasive) is recommended
1	B NR	For patients with HCM who are candidates for SRT and for whom there is uncertainty regarding the presence or severity of LVOTO on noninvasive imaging studies, invasive hemodynamic assessment with cardiac catheterization is recommended
1	B-NR	In patients with HCM who are at risk of coronary atherosclerosis, coronary angiography (CT or invasive) is recommended before surgical myectomy

Selection of recommendations pertaining to diagnostic angiography from the 2020 AHA/ACC Guidelines for the Diagnosis and Treatment of Patients with Hypertrophic Cardiomyopathy. Class of Recommendation (COR) 1 indicates a strong recommendation with benefits greatly outweighing risks. Level of Evidence (LOE) B-NR indicates moderate-quality evidence from one or more well-designed, well-executed nonrandomized studies, observational studies, or registry studies

Heart Team Approach and Discussion

The patient discussed in this case presented to the Emergency Department with several cardinal features of HOCM: dyspnea, palpitations, and syncope. Her physical examination was notable for the classic dynamic outflow tract murmur of HOCM. The transthoracic echocardiogram acquired on admission demonstrated multiple features of HOCM (Fig. 1). Given the severity of her symptoms and LVOT gradient, septal reduction therapy was recommended. The patient opted for a trial of conservative management prior to pursing SRT. After 1 year of conservative management with metoprolol and disopyramide, she returned to Cardiology clinic with NYHA Class III symptoms. In this setting of progressive symptoms despite optimal medical management, the patient was now in agreement with the recommendation to undergo SRT (Table 3).

The options of septal myectomy and alcohol septal ablation were discussed in detail with the patient and Heart Team for a shared-decision making approach. The patient's age (>40 years), imaging features (maximal wall thickness of 1.8 cm at the basal septum, LVOT gradient 170 mmHg due to systolic anterior motion of the mitral valve), favorable coronary anatomy, absence of any concomitant indications for cardiovascular surgery (no significant coronary or valvular heart disease), and preference to avoid surgical intervention favored ASA over SM.

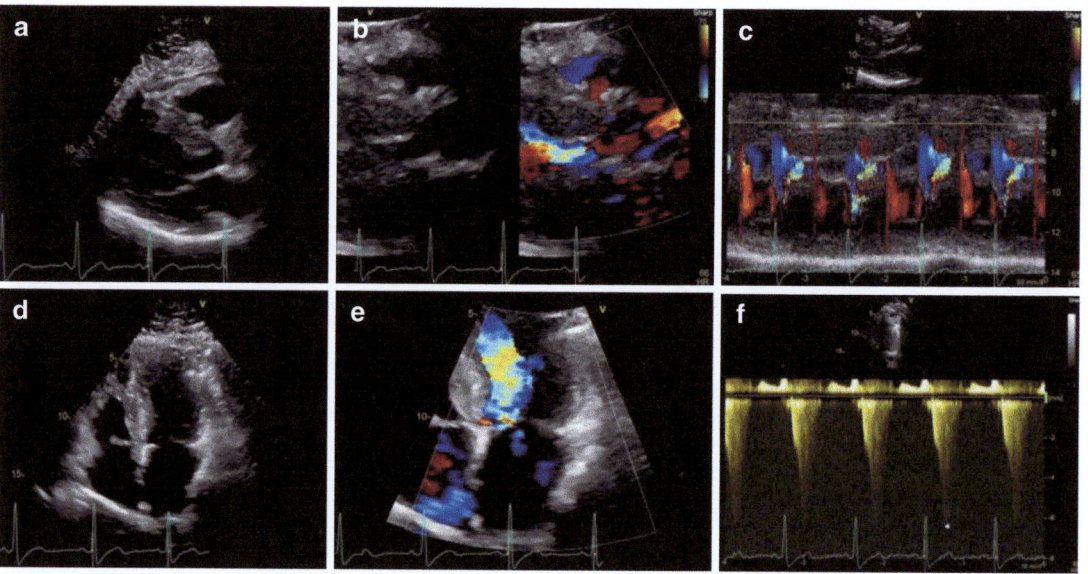

Fig. 1 Initial diagnostic transthoracic echocardiogram. (**a**) parasternal long axis view showing severe (18 mm) septal hypertrophy. (**b**) Narrowed left ventricular outflow tract with turbulent flow across left ventricular outflow tract obstruction. (**c**) M-Mode demonstrating systolic anterior motion of the mitral valve and dynamic left ventricular outflow tract obstruction. (**d**) Apical four-chamber view demonstrating severe septal hypertrophy. (**e**) Apical four chamber view illustrating turbulent flow across left ventricular outflow tract. (**f**) Continuous wave doppler across left ventricular outflow tract acquired from an apical three-chamber view showing a peak velocity of 6.52 m/s, corresponding to a resting gradient of 170 mmHg

Table 3 Recommendations for invasive management of patients with symptomatic HOCM [2]

COR	LOE	Guideline recommendation
1	B-NR	In patients with HCM who remain severely symptomatic despite GDMT, SRT in eligible patients, performed at experienced centers, is recommended for relieving LVOTO
1	B-NR	In symptomatic patients with obstructive HCM who have associated cardiac disease requiring surgical treatment (e.g., associated anomalous papillary muscle, markedly elongated anterior mitral leaflet, intrinsic mitral valve disease, multivessel CAD, valvular aortic stenosis), surgical myectomy, performed at experienced centers, is recommended
1	C-LD	In adult patients with obstructive HCM who remain severely symptomatic, despite GDMT and in whom surgery is contraindicated or the risk is considered unacceptable because of serious comorbidities or advanced age, alcohol septal ablation in eligible patients, performed at experienced centers, is recommended

2b	B-NR	In patients with obstructive HCM, earlier (NYHA class II) surgical myectomy performed at comprehensive HCM centers may be reasonable in the presence of additional clinical factors, including
		  a. Severe and progressive pulmonary hypertension thought to be attributable to LVOTO or associated MR
		  b. Left atrial enlargement with ≥1 episodes of symptomatic AF
		  c. Poor functional capacity attributable to LVOTO as documented on treadmill exercise testing
		  d. Children and young adults with very high resting LVOT gradients (>100 mmHg)

2b	C-LD	For severely symptomatic patients with obstructive HCM, SRT in eligible patients, performed at experienced centers, may be considered as an alternative to escalation of medical therapy after shared decision making including risks and benefits of all treatment options
3: Harm	C-LD	For patients with HCM who are asymptomatic and have normal exercise capacity, SRT is not recommended
3: Harm	B-NR	For symptomatic patients with obstructive HCM in whom SRT is an option, mitral valve replacement should not be performed for the sole purpose of relief of LVOTO

Selection of recommendations pertaining to the invasive management of patients with symptomatic HOCM from the 2020 AHA/ACC Guidelines for the Diagnosis and Treatment of Patients with Hypertrophic Cardiomyopathy. Class of Recommendation (COR) 1 indicates a strong recommendation with benefits greatly outweighing risks. COR 2b indicates a recommendation with weak evidence and uncertain effectiveness that may be reasonable to consider in certain clinical settings. COR 3 indicates harmful interventions that should not be performed due to evidence that risk significantly outweighs benefit. Level of Evidence (LOE) B-NR indicates moderate-quality evidence from one or more well-designed, well-executed nonrandomized studies, observational studies, or registry studies. LOE C-LD indicates limited evidence from randomized or nonrandomized observational studies with limitations of design or execution

Heart Team Decision

The patient's age, imaging, and hemodynamics satisfied criteria for ASA: (1) age >21 years, (2) septal wall thickness between 18 and 30 mm, (3) LVOT gradient greater than 50 mmHg at rest, (4) the dynamic LVOT gradient was not attributable to the primary pathology of the mitral valve or papillary muscles, (5) coronary angiography confirmed the presence of a large septal perforator artery supplying the region of maximal LVOT obstruction, and (6) her imaging revealed no concomitant surgical indication (i.e. she did not have multivessel coronary artery disease or surgical valve disease). As a candidate for either septal myectomy or alcohol septal ablation, strong patient preference to avoid median sternotomy at her advanced age was the primary reason for choosing to pursue ASA in shared-decision making.

Intraprocedural Imaging Modalities and Measurements

The patient was brought to the catheterization laboratory for elective ASA. A temporary pacing wire was inserted into the apex of the right ventricle with capture at 0.4 mA from a right internal jugular vein approach under direct ultrasound guidance. Access was acquired via the right radial artery and the left main coronary artery was engaged using an XB 3.0 guide catheter. After confirming therapeutic anticoagulation (ACT >250), a coronary wire was advanced into the first septal branch (Supplementary Fig. 1, Fig. 2).

A 2.0 × 6 mm balloon was advanced into the septal over the coronary wire and inflated to a pressure of 8–10 atmospheres (Fig. 3). A balloon diameter equal to the septal vessel diameter is selected so that when inflated to nominal pressure it will prevent reflux of alcohol delivered via the over-the-wire balloon out of the septal branch into the left anterior descending coronary artery (LAD).

The coronary wire was removed and a test injection of angiography contrast after balloon inflation was delivered to confirm occlusion of the septal perforator (no competitive flow from or reflux into the parent LAD artery) (Supplementary Fig. 2).

Injection of echocardiography contrast (5 cc perflutren lipid microspheres diluted 1:1 with normal saline) was then performed. The transthoracic echocardiography images demonstrated contrast enhancement of the basal septum at the site of LVOTO without other LV or RV opacification (Fig. 4).

Absolute ethanol (1 cc) was then injected slowly over a period of 10 min. A repeat intraprocedural echocardiogram was performed and demonstrated focal akinesis of the basal septum

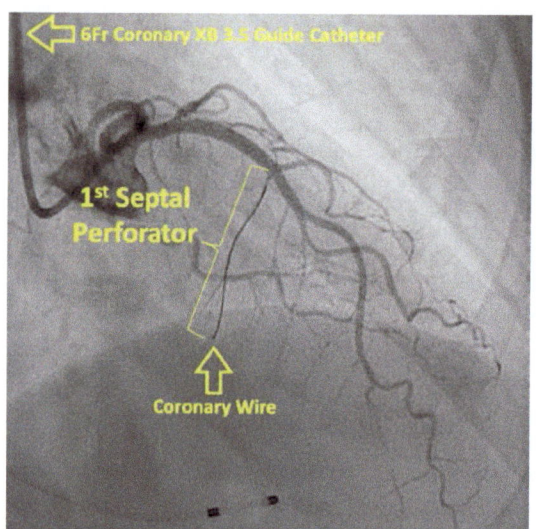

Fig. 2 Coronary wire advanced into first septal perforator. RAO cranial projection showing coronary wire advanced into the first septal perforator artery

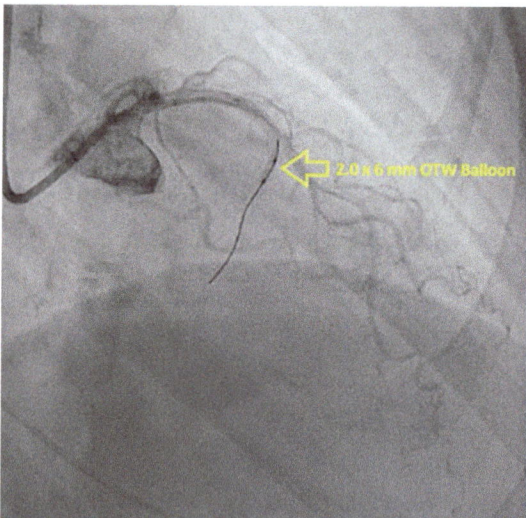

Fig. 3 OTW balloon inflation. RAO cranial projection showing inflation of the over-the-wire (OTW) balloon within the first septal perforator artery

but otherwise normal wall motion in LAD territory—apex and anterior wall. Repeat Doppler echocardiographic measurement of the LVOT peak gradient showed improvement from a baseline of 158–18 mmHg post-ablation at the conclusion of the procedure (Fig. 5).

The coronary balloon was flushed slowly with 0.5 cc of normal saline, deflated, and removed. Post-ablation angiography confirmed 100% occlusion of the septal perforator with intact and an unchanged parent LAD artery (Supplementary Fig. 3, Fig. 6).

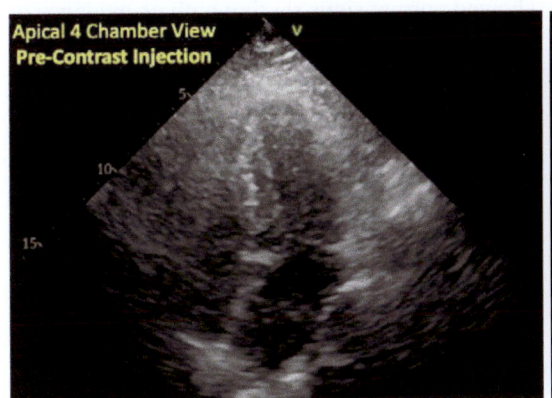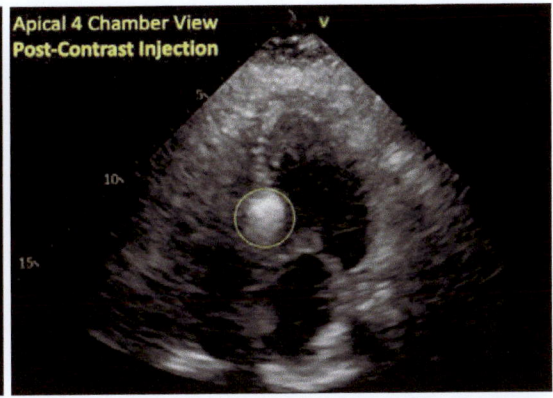

Fig. 4 Contrast enhancement of basilar septum. Apical four-chamber window with injection of echocardiography contrast demonstrating selective enhancement of basal septum at the site of left ventricular outflow tract obstruction (LVOTO) without accompanying left ventricular or right ventricular contrast enhancement. *FW* left ventricular free wall, *LA* left atrium, *LV* left ventricle, *MV* mitral valve, *RA* right atrium, *RV* right ventricle, *VS* ventricular septum

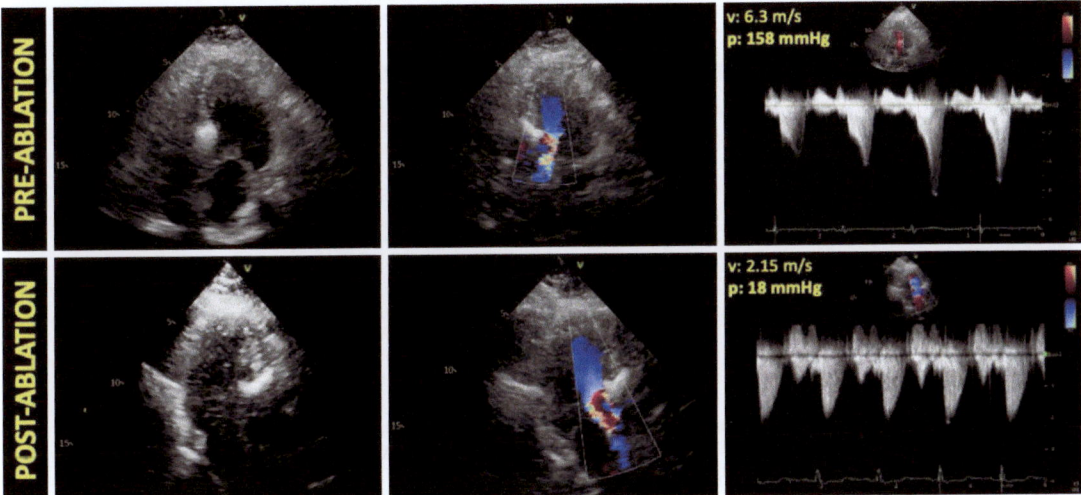

Fig. 5 Pre and post-ablation intraprocedural echocardiography. (Top panel) Pre-ablation apical four chamber view showing selective contrast enhancement of the basal septum at the site of left ventricular outflow tract obstruction (LVOTO). Continuous wave Doppler with peak pre-ablation resting velocity 6.3 m/s, corresponding to peak resting gradient 158 mmHg. (Bottom panel) Post-ablation apical three-chamber view showing effective reduction of LVOTO to peak velocity 2.15 m/s, peak gradient 18 mmHg. *P* peak pressure, *V* peak velocity

The procedure was completed without complication and with resolution of the patient's symptoms (NYHA Class I).

Post procedural Assessment

The patient was transferred to the Cardiovascular Intensive Care Unit for continued overnight monitoring for potential development of new atrioventricular block with the transvenous temporary pacing wire in place. Review of her telemetry showed normal sinus rhythm with no evidence of high-grade block. Her post-ablation electrocardiogram showed new right bundle branch block (Fig. 7).

Note that although 12-lead ECG abnormalities such as localized or widespread repolarization changes, prominent precordial voltages, left axis deviation, or deep inferior and lateral Q-waves may be present on the baseline ECG for patients with HCM, these changes are neither sensitive nor specific. None of these abnormalities were present on the pre-ablation ECG for this patient with chronic and severely elevated LVOT gradient. On her post-ablation ECG a new right bundle branch block (RBBB) is seen, which occurs in 60% of patients undergoing ASA [3, 4]. RBBB develops because the septal branches supplying the region of hypertrophied septum also

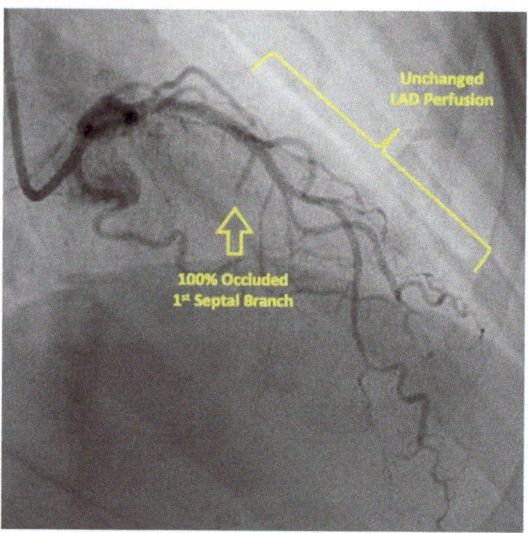

Fig. 6 Post-ablation angiography showing 100% occlusion of septal branch. Post-ablation angiography in RAO cranial projection showing 100% occlusion of first septal perforator artery with unchanged left anterior descending artery (LAD) perfusion

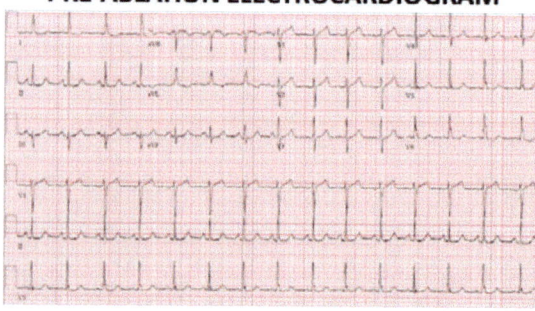 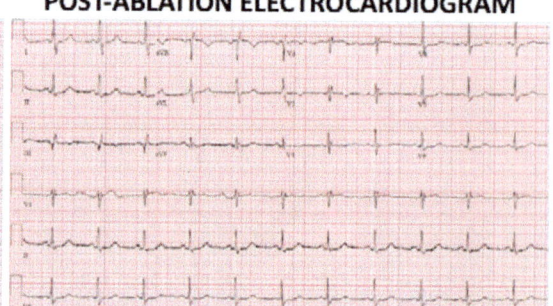

Fig. 7 Pre and post-ablation electrocardiograms. (Left panel) Pre-ablation electrocardiogram showing normal sinus rhythm with narrow QRS complexes. (Right panel) Post-ablation electrocardiogram showing normal sinus rhythm with new right bundle branch block

provide perfusion to the right bundle branch. The development of new RBBB following ASA has not been shown to adversely affect clinical outcomes [5].

On postoperative day 1, the temporary pacing wire was removed and the patient was transferred to the cardiology stepdown unit. She was discharged home on postoperative day 3.

At the patient's 1-week post-ablation follow-up visit, she continued to report significantly improved symptoms (NYHA Class I). Follow-up echocardiography performed 3-months post-ablation showed persistent normalization of her LVOT gradient.

Key Points
- Transthoracic echocardiography is the diagnostic study of choice for HCM.
- Alcohol septal ablation offers a safe, effective, and minimally invasive treatment strategy for HCM.
- With less invasive nature, accelerated recovery, and similar symptomatic improvement compared with surgical myectomy, alcohol septal ablation is currently the most commonly performed septal reduction therapy for obstructive HCM.

Introduction

Hypertrophic cardiomyopathy (HCM) is the most common heritable cardiac disorder, affecting 0.2–0.5% of the general population, and a leading cause of sudden cardiac death (SCD) in younger patients [20, 21]. HCM is inherited in an autosomal dominant pattern from pathogenic variants in multiple genes encoding sarcomere proteins [2, 22]. Sporadic cases without a family history of HCM also occur. Partially due to considerable heterogeneity in genotypic and phenotypic presentation, HCM remains significantly underdiagnosed. It is estimated that up to 85% of all HCM cases phenotypic expression remain undiagnosed [3]. The significant gap that continues to exist between confirmed and undiagnosed HCM highlights the need for improved understanding of its presentation, diagnosis, and widely available treatments. This chapter will focus on interventional therapy for HCM, percutaneous alcohol septal ablation (ASA), including the history of HCM and ASA, recommended approach to diagnosis, evolution of available treatment strategies, complex management considerations, and the central role of cardiovascular imaging in each stage of HCM diagnosis and treatment.

Section 1—History

History of HCM and ASA: The Groundwork for Modern Diagnosis and Treatment

The current understanding and management of HCM has been shaped by the historic work of anatomists, pathologists, geneticists, surgeons, and clinicians whose shared efforts have made it possible to understand, diagnose, and treat the complex pathophysiology that defines the disease.

The modern description of HCM is credited to the English forensic pathologist Dr. Robert Teare. In 1958, while working at St. George's Hospital in London, Teare published a landmark description of asymmetrical myocardial hypertrophy identified at the time of autopsy in eight patients [23]. Massive cardiomegaly with disproportionate enlargement of the interventricular septum was found on post-mortem examination of each sudden death victim [24]. In his report, Teare described the cardinal clinical and histopathological features of HCM: chest discomfort, palpitations, exertional dyspnea, and syncope in patients with pathologic Q-waves on electrocardiogram and "myocyte disarray" with fibre hypertrophy on autopsy (Fig. 8) [23]. In an addendum to this paper, Teare was also the first to suggest a hereditary cause when he reported the sudden death of the 16-year-old brother of one of the original eight cases. In a single communication, Teare united many unanswered pieces of medical history into a single disease entity [25]. Building upon Teare's description of HCM in the British Heart Journal, the stage was set for discovery of an effective treatment for HCM, including the focus of this chapter: alcohol septal ablation.

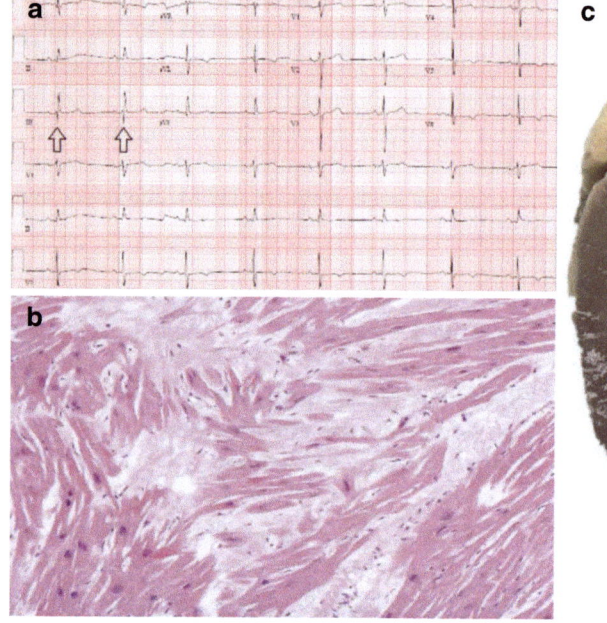
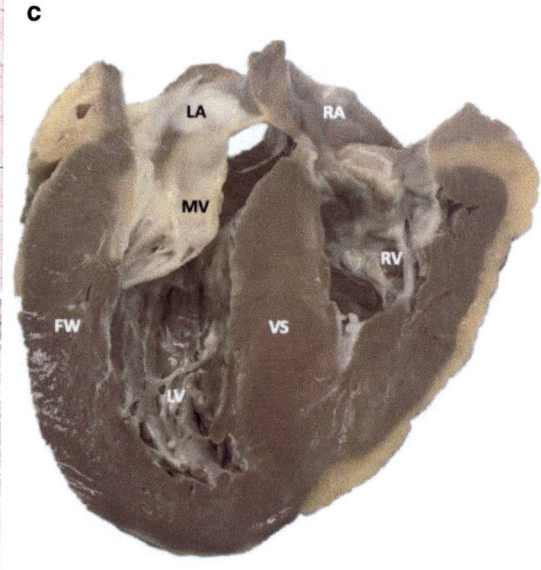

Fig. 8 Electrocardiographic, histopathologic, and anatomic features of HCM. (**a**) Classic electrocardiographic features in hypertrophic cardiomyopathy (HCM) including sharp, "dagger" Q-waves (arrows), which may be seen in the lateral (I, aVL, V5, V6) and/or inferior (II, III, aVF) leads. (**b**) HCM histopathology demonstrating architectural disarray of hypertrophied myocytes. (**c**) Characteristic gross pathology for a patient with sudden cardiac death who was diagnosed with HCM at the time of autopsy. A cross section of the heart is shown with severe, asymmetric left ventricular hypertrophy

In the early 1960s at the National Institutes of Health, Dr. Glenn Morrow pioneered transaortic ventricular septal myectomy (Morrow procedure) as a method for relieving LV outflow tract obstruction. A small portion of myocardium (3–10 g) was resected from the proximal ventricular septum. His experience with this technique was published in a report of 25 patients [26]. For over 30 years, myectomy remained the only proven septal reduction therapy for HCM.

It was not until the mid-1990s that alcohol septal ablation (ASA) was introduced by Dr. Ulrich Sigwart at the Royal Brompton Hospital in the United Kingdom as a minimally invasive alternative to surgical myomectomy [27, 28]. The idea of producing septal infarction by catheter-based techniques as a treatment for HCM, Sigwart states, "Was suggested by observations that systolic and diastolic myocardial function of selected areas in the left ventricle can be selectively suppressed by balloon occlusion of the supplying artery during coronary angioplasty" [27]. In this original description of the procedure, Sigwart reported three patients with advanced hypertrophic obstructive cardiomyopathy, all between the ages of 60 and 70 years, who underwent injection of "absolute alcohol into the first major septal coronary vessel" to produce septal infarction. All three patients tolerated the procedure well and achieved striking symptomatic improvement on the first day after treatment [27]. As stated by Dr. Sigwart, "The attraction of the procedure resides in its simplicity, minimal morbidity, and the fact that the outcome of the definite ablation can be estimated by temporary occlusion of the target vessel" [27].

In the decades that have passed since the first septal ablation was performed by Sigwart, percutaneous procedures have revolutionized the management of structural heart disease. ASA has proven to significantly improve morbidity in patients with HCM by decreasing the left ventricular outflow tract (LVOT) gradient, reducing mitral regurgitation, and alleviating heart failure symptoms through a minimally invasive approach with substantially shorter recovery times than surgery [29]. The efficacy and safety of alcohol septal ablation is now well established, with greater than 95% of patients free of recurrent CV events at 15 years. The EURO-ASA registry, which includes acute and long-term data from 1000 patients treated with ASA in 10 tertiary centers from 7 European countries, confirms the safety and durable relief of LVOT obstruction in patients with HCM who are treated with ASA [30]. All consensus and guideline panels regard ASA as an effective alternative treatment strategy to SM in patients with obstructive HCM who are sub-optimal surgical candidates (i.e. those with extensive comorbidities, advanced age, multiple prior sternotomies, or a strong aversion to surgery) [2]. The number of ASA procedures performed worldwide now greatly exceeds the number of surgical myectomies each year [4]. Following the introduction and widespread utilization of ASA, novel percutaneous options for SRT in HOCM have been described including coil embolization, radiofrequency ablation, and transcatheter electrosurgical myotomy [31, 32]. However, these alternative SRT methods have been studied in a limited number of patients and without long-term outcomes.

The success of ASA as a treatment for HCM is contingent upon careful preprocedural evaluation and assessment of patient candidacy involving a multidisciplinary heart team evaluation including a cardiac surgeon experienced in surgical myomectomy. The focus of the remaining sections of this chapter will be on the cardiovascular imaging modalities that play a central role in guiding ASA patient selection, procedural intervention, and post-procedural monitoring.

Section 2: Pre-procedural Assessment of HCM

Clinical Presentation and Diagnosis of HCM

HCM has potential for clinical presentation in all phases of life, from infancy to old age [1]. Early diagnosis and accurate risk stratification promotes timely intervention and a significant reduction in disease related morbidity and mortality [33]. With efficient diagnosis and treatment, a new diagnosis of HCM is compatible with normal life expectancy and little or no disability for the majority of patients [2]. Effective clinical screening for HCM must include a three-generation family history, comprehensive physical examination, and electrocardiogram [1]. When the clinical features of HCM are present, further evaluation with comprehensive 2D echocardiography is indicated. Echocardiography is the cornerstone of screening, diagnosis, and prognostication for HCM [13, 34]. A comparison of imaging modalities for the assessment of HCM is shown in Table 4. The diagnostic features of HCM on 2D echocardiography are summarized in Table 5.

Table 4 Multimodality imaging comparison

Modality	HCM application	Advantages	Limitations
TTE	• For patients undergoing ASA, TTE or intraoperative TEE with intracoronary ultrasound-enhancing contrast injection of the candidate's septal perforator is recommended (class I, LOE B-NR) [2] • Recommended 3–6 months following SRT to evaluate procedural results (class I, LOE B-NR) [2] • Myocardial contrast echo enhances endocardial definition and defines myocardial perfusion territories to guide alcohol septal ablation	• Availability and cost • Preferred method for assessment of diastolic function • Superior to CMR in quantification of outflow tract gradient • Able to provoke physiological gradients with exercise in patients who have a resting LVOT gradient less than 30 mmHg at rest • Contrast echocardiography is able to reliably delineate location and extent of septal perfusion territory prior to ASA	• Doppler-specific angle dependence in assessing LVOTG • Less precise differentiation of endocardial borders and blood pool relative to CMR • Less reliable in distinguishing epicardial fat, pericardium, and trabeculations relative to CMR • More likely to underestimate magnitude of hypertrophy [6]

(continued)

Table 4 (continued)

Modality	HCM application	Advantages	Limitations
TEE	• Can be considered in patients with inconclusive TTE or as an alternative or complementary investigation to CMR • Can be useful in excluding subaortic membrane or mitral regurgitation secondary to structural abnormalities of the mitral valve apparatus, or in the assessment of the feasibility of ASA (class 2a, LOE B-NR) [2] • Used perioperatively for surgical myectomy to guide surgical approach, monitor for complications, and assess residual gradient (class I, LOE B-NR) [2]	• Particularly useful for assessing mitral valve apparatus in patients with significant LVOTO and unclear mechanism of obstruction • Superior endocardial visualization relative to TTE • Enhanced spatial resolution relative to TTE • In patients undergoing SM, TEE should be used to guide surgical intervention and monitor for intraoperative surgical complications (i.e. VSD, acute aortic regurgitation, residual LVOTO) • Following SM, TEE can confirm adequacy of myectomy [7]	• Doppler-specific angle dependence in assessing LVOTG • Invasive procedure • Less precise differentiation of endocardial borders and blood pool relative to CMR • Less reliable in distinguishing epicardial fat, pericardium, and trabeculations relative to CMR • More likely to underestimate magnitude of hypertrophy [6] • Unable to provoke physiological gradients with exercise in patients who have a resting LVOT gradient less than 50 mmHg
CMR	• CMR is indicated for diagnostic clarification in cases of suspected HCM when echocardiography is inconclusive (class I, LOE B-NR) [2] • CMR is indicated to inform selection and planning of SRT for patients with HOCM in whom the anatomic mechanism of obstruction is inconclusive on echocardiography (class I, LOE B-NR) [2] • CMR is useful for patients with LVH in whom there is a suspicion of alternative diagnoses such as infiltrative or glycogen storage diseases, athlete's heart, etc. (class I, LOE B-NR) [2] • For patients who are not identified as high-risk for SCD, CMR is beneficial to assess for maximum LV wall thickness, LVEF, LV apical aneurysm, and extent of fibrosis with LGE (class I, LOE B-NR) [2]	• Superior endocardial visualization with excellent demarcation between myocardium and blood pool [8] • Enhanced spatial resolution and image quality, enabling identification of morphologic HCM variants that are more likely to be missed on TTE [8–10] • Superior to 2D echo in measurement of LV mass, detection of myocardial crypts, papillary muscle pathology, LV apical and anterolateral hypertrophy, aneurysms, and thrombi [11, 12] • Reproducibility; less inter-user variability relative to echocardiography • Particularly helpful for treatment planning in the setting of multiple areas of LV obstruction and/or accompanying RV obstruction • Enables quantification of septal fibrosis [13] • Prognostication value; the presence of LGE has been correlated to increased CV mortality, heart failure, and arrythmias [14–19]	• Higher cost • Less widely available • Longer duration study • Institutional differences in magnetic resonance hardware and software, inconsistent optimization of inversion times, improperly nulled LV myocardium, different types and dosage protocols for gadolinium contrast, and diverse LGE protocols may all significantly impact study interpretation [6] • Unable to provoke physiological gradients with exercise in patients who have a resting LVOT gradient less than 50 mmHg • CMR is less reliable than TTE in assessing LVOT hemodynamics • Turbulent LVOT flow can result in significant CMR artifacts

Comparison of the clinical applications, advantages, and disadvantages of common diagnostic imaging modalities for hypertrophic cardiomyopathy

ASA alcohol septal ablation, *CMR* cardiac magnetic resonance imaging, *HCM* hypertrophic cardiomyopathy, *LV* left ventricle, *LVOT* left ventricular outflow tract, *LVOTG* left ventricular outflow tract gradient, *SCD* sudden cardiac death, *TEE* transesophageal echocardiography, *TTE* transthoracic echocardiography, *VSD* ventricular septal defect

Table 5 Diagnostic features of HCM on echocardiography

Variable	HCM features and significance	Sample imaging
LVH	• Unexplained maximal wall thickness >1.4 cm in any myocardial segment at end-diastole [35] • Maximal wall thickness >1.2 in patients with family history of HCM or positive genetic testing [35] • Measurement in M-mode should be avoided to prevent overestimation by oblique cut • Maximal LV wall thickness 3.0 cm or greater (right) is associated with increased risk for SCD	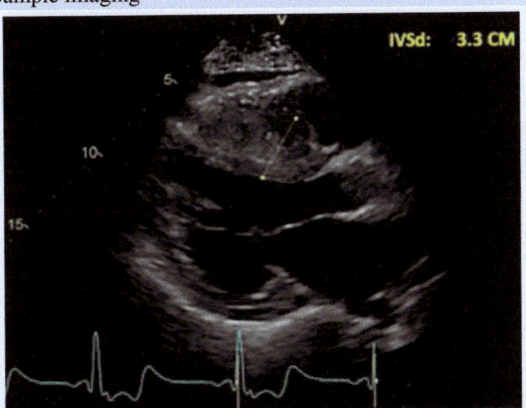
SAM	• 33% prevalence of SAM in HCM on rest images [13] • Additional 30–40% prevalence of provocable LVOT gradient >30 mmHg with maneuvers that alter loading conditions and contractility [13, 36] • SAM nearly always results in failure of normal leaflet coaptation and MR • SAM-related MR is inherently dynamic in nature; its severity varies with degree of LVOTO • MR jet appears in mid-late systole and has posterior orientation – Note that a central or anteriorly oriented jet raises suspicion for intrinsic mitral valve pathology and should prompt further assessment with TEE • M-mode (right) is frequently used to confirm SAM	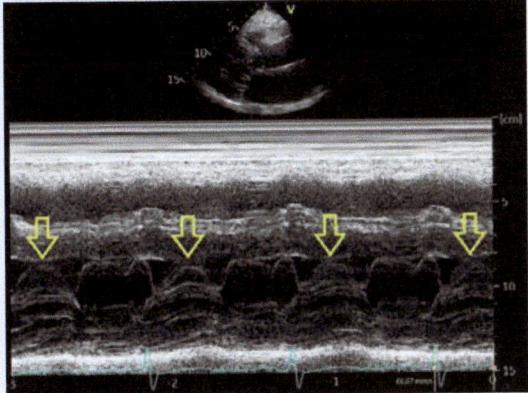
BBM	• Echocardiographic analogue of the Brockenbrough–Braunwald–Morrow Sign: a paradoxical decrease in arterial pulse pressure during the post-PVC beat seen in patients with HCM [37, 38] • Severe AS can also translate to significantly increased CW Doppler gradient following a PVC. To carry diagnostic value in HCM, this finding must occur in the absence of severe AS	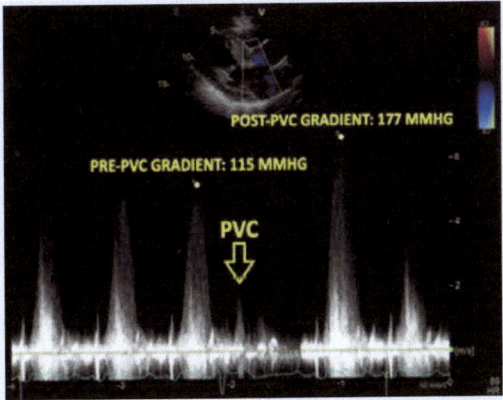

(continued)

Table 5 (continued)

Variable	HCM features and significance	Sample imaging

LVOTO	• Defined as a peak instantaneous gradient ³30 mmHg [2]
	  – 70% of patients with HCM have LVOTO ³30 mmHg either at rest or with provocation [39]
	• Late peaking "dagger shape" Doppler profile
	• Pulse wave Doppler is recommended to localize obstruction (apical, mid-cavitary, or outflow tract)
	• Doppler of MR jet for direct comparison with LVOT doppler waveform is recommended to ensure that MR is not mistaken for LVOT velocity
	  – Doppler should be performed in multiple views (especially apical 5 and apical 3) to align Doppler signal and avoid MR
	• Treatment threshold (SRT) ³50 mmHg [2, 40]
	  – Peak instantaneous LVOT gradient, not mean gradient, dictates treatment decisions
	  – When resting gradient is <50 mmHg in a patient with suspected HCM, it is essential to perform provocative maneuvers (Valsalva, squat-to-stand, upright exercise) to uncover a significant LVOTO [41]
	• Exercise stress echo is recommended in *symptomatic* patients when bedside maneuvers fail to induce LVOTO ³50 mmHg
	  – Pharmacologic provocation with dobutamine is not recommended unless the patient is unable to exercise
		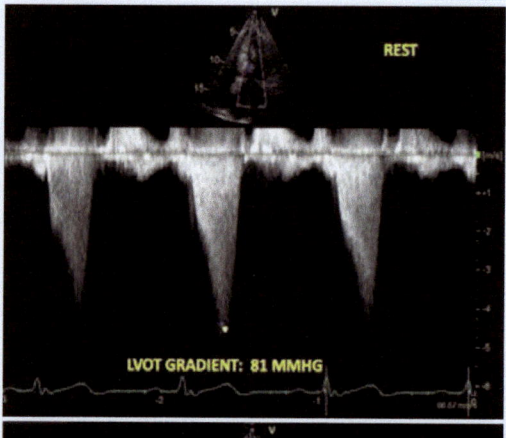
		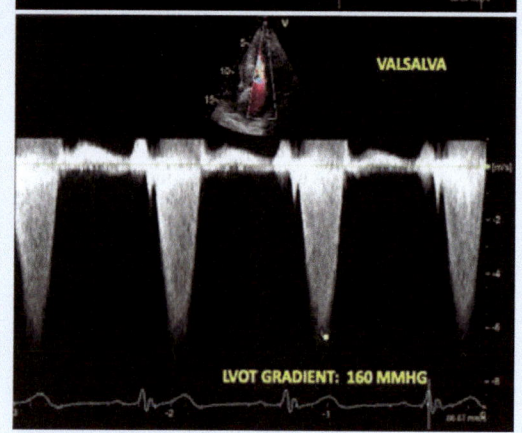

Diagnostic features of hypertrophic cardiomyopathy by transthoracic echocardiography. (Top panel) Severe left ventricular hypertrophy (LVH) involving the basilar interventricular septum (3.3 cm). (Second panel) M-mode showing systolic anterior motion (SAM) of the anterior mitral leaflet (yellow arrows). (Third panel) Echocardiography equivalent of the Brockenbrough–Braunwald–Morrow (BBM) Sign: increased left ventricular outflow tract gradient corresponding to a decreased arterial pulse pressure following a premature ventricular contraction (yellow arrow). (Bottom panel) Left ventricular outflow tract obstruction shown at rest and with valsalva in an apical three-chamber window

IVSd interventricular septal diameter, *LV* left ventricle, *LVOTO* left ventricular outflow tract obstruction, *MR* mitral regurgitation, *PVC* premature ventricular contraction, *SCD* sudden cardiac death, *SRT* septal reduction therapy

If a segment of the LV cannot be adequately visualized using chest wall echocardiography, it is recommended that enhanced imaging with ultrasound contrast agents, transesophageal echocardiography, and/or cardiovascular magnetic resonance imaging (CMR) be considered [13, 42]. CMR provides detailed information about cardiac morphology, function, and myocardial characteristics in an infinite number of planes with high-resolution images that enable precise quantification of myocardial thickening, flow, and extent of fibrosis [43–45]. Data acquired from CMR is often complementary to echocardiography. The diagnostic features of HCM using CMR are presented in Table 6.

The presence of LVH and significant LVOTO on echocardiography or CMR is not pathognomonic for HCM. A diagnosis of HCM relies on these findings in the absence of another cardiac or systemic disease capable of producing the magnitude of hypertrophy characteristic of HCM [2]. As there are many systemic disorders

Table 6 Diagnostic features of HCM on CMR

Variable	HCM features and significance	Sample imaging
HCM anatomy	• Basal asymmetric hypertrophy accounts for 60–70% HCM cases (Panel A) • CMR particularly useful for detecting less common patterns of hypertrophy: apical HCM variants (Panel B) or obstruction arising secondary to thickened chordal apparatus and/or abnormal papillary muscles (Panel C)	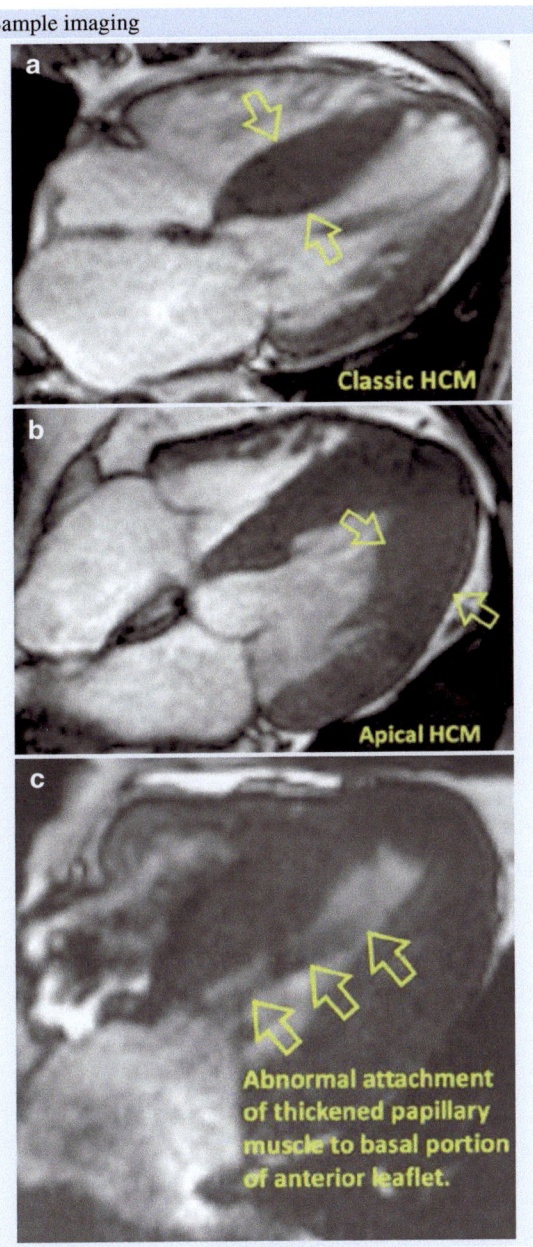

(continued)

Table 6 (continued)

Variable	HCM features and significance	Sample imaging
LVOTG and Mechanism of Obstruction	• Cine phase contrast MR imaging can be used to quantify blood flow through the LVOT • CMR planimetry-derived LVOT area of 2.7 cm² or less identifies significant LVOT obstruction in patients with HCM with 100% accuracy [46] • LVOT/Ao diameter ratio less than 0.45 is an accurate and reproducible method for predicting severity of LVOT obstruction [47] • Identification of atypical mechanisms for LVOT obstruction (i.e. papillary muscle hypertrophy, mitral valve apparatus) is essential in determining candidacy for ASA	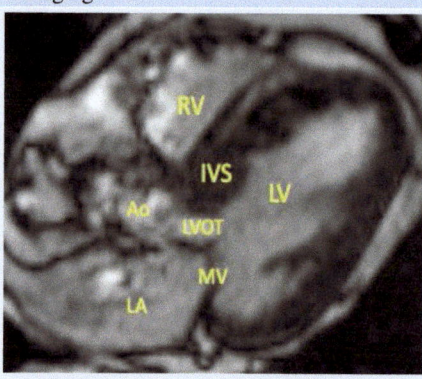
T1 and T2 mapping	• T1 and T2 mapping enables identification of myocardial injury without gadolinium-based contrast agents • T1 mapping identifies regions of myocardial scarring as well as interstitial fibrosis • T2 mapping serves as a marker of myocardial edema or inflammation • Native T1 values in segments of severe hypertrophy (highlighted region, top panel) demonstrate significantly higher T1 values than segments of mild or moderate hypertrophy [48] • Mean T2 values of segments with moderate or severe hypertrophy (highlighted region, bottom panel) are significantly higher than those of mild hypertrophy [48] • In patients with HCM, T1 and T2 remodeling precedes morphological and functional remodeling in HCM [48]	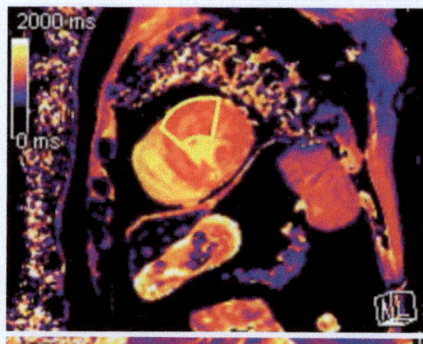 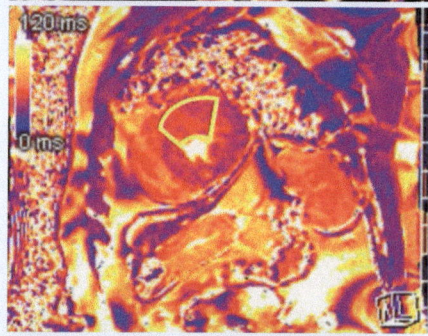
LGE	• Marker of myocardial fibrosis • Valuable indicator for risk stratification of SCD (HCM patients with ≥15% LGE relative to LV mass have been found to have increased risk of sudden cardiac death events) • Usually identified at hypertrophied insertion points of the interventricular septum • LGE valuable in identifying end-stage HCM: reduced LVEF (<50%), coexistence of myocardial hypertrophy and thinning, and extensive LGE reflecting diffuse myocardial scarring	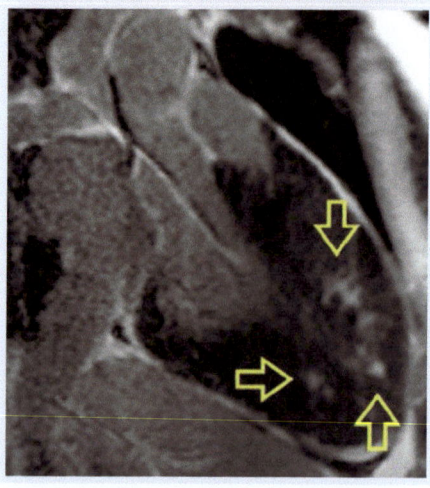

Table 6 (continued)

Variable	HCM features and significance	Sample imaging
Assessment of ASA	• LGE identifies region of ablated hypertrophied septum • Location and extent of LGE induced by ASA is predictive of success rate [49] • CMR is useful both in planning and in follow-up for ASA; infarction size and location correlates with total septal mass reduction and LVOTG alleviation [49]	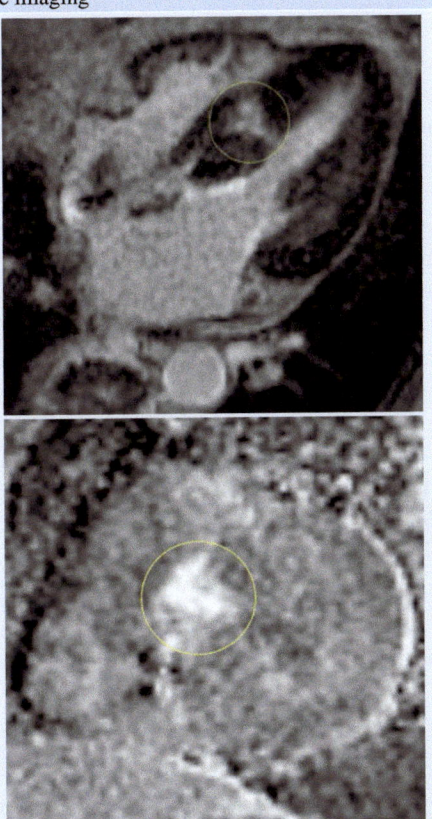

Diagnostic features of hypertrophic cardiomyopathy (HCM) on cardiac magnetic resonance imaging (CMR). Features highlighted include patterns of hypertrophy (top panel), mechanisms for left ventricular outflow tract obstruction (second panel), T1 and T2 mapping to identify areas of myocardial fibrosis or edema without the use of gadolinium contrast agents (third panel), patterns of late gadolinium enhancement (LGE) pre-ablation (fourth panel) and post-ablation (bottom panel)

Ao aorta, *ASA* alcohol septal ablation, *IVS* interventricular septum, *LA* left atrium, *LV* left ventricle, *LVOT* left ventricular outflow tract, *LVOTG* left ventricular outflow tract gradient, *MV* mitral valve, *RV* right ventricle

and secondary causes of LVH, it is crucially important to consider a full differential including glycogen or lysosomal storage diseases, mitochondrial myopathies, infiltrative processes, amyloid, sarcoid, and other heritable cardiomyopathies [2]. Carefully differentiating the unique etiologies for LVH and LVOTO using diagnostic criteria and appropriate cardiovascular imaging is essential as management varies significantly with each of these cardiovascular conditions [2, 35].

Dynamic outflow tract obstruction in HCM is most commonly related to systolic anterior motion (SAM) of the mitral valve [50, 51]. SAM in HCM is a result of narrowing of the LVOT causing increased flow velocity and decreased pressure above the anterior mitral leaflet (Venturi effect) [51]. In addition to the Venturi effect, patients with SAM have primary structural abnormalities of the mitral apparatus including anterior displacement of the papillary muscles, inward displacement of the papillary muscles toward one another, and mitral leaflet elongation [52, 53]. These primary structural changes in the mitral valve apparatus, even in the absence of significant septal hypertrophy, can result in SAM and LVOTO [51]. There is a small number of HOCM patients who have minimal LVH but severe LVOTO due to prominent SAM from leaflet elongation, papillary muscle displacement, or a combination of both. Surgical plication of an elongated MV leaflet or trans-aortic Alfieri stich placement are feasible interventions that may be used to reduce SAM and alleviate the obstruction [54, 55]. Differentiating the mechanism of LVOTO is essential in guiding therapy, as patients with severe LVOTO attributed predominantly to these mitral valve abnormalities may not have adequate LVOTO reduction with ASA alone [56, 57].

Mitral valve regurgitation in patients with HOCM must be carefully evaluated to determine whether the MR is attributable predominantly to SAM or other intrinsic MV pathologies. Intrinsic MV pathologies might include leaflet prolapse, degeneration, chordal rupture, or stenosis. For these patients, SRT alone is unlikely to be effective and surgical intervention is indicated [2]. For the majority of patients with HOCM, intrinsic mitral valve pathology is not present and reduction in LVOTG will alleviate MR due to SAM. A retrospective analysis of over 2100 septal myectomies performed at the Mayo Clinic between 1993 and 2014 found that less than 5% of patients undergoing myectomy required concomitant MV repair or replacement and the percentage of patients with MR grade ≥3 decreased from 54.3 to 1.7% [58]. For patients who have primary MV disease and require MV intervention during surgical myectomy, survival is superior for those who undergo repair rather than replacement of the mitral valve [58].

The recommended diagnostic algorithm for HCM, adapted from the 2020 AHA/ACC Guideline for the Diagnosis and Treatment of Patients With Hypertrophic Cardiomyopathy, is shown in Fig. 9.

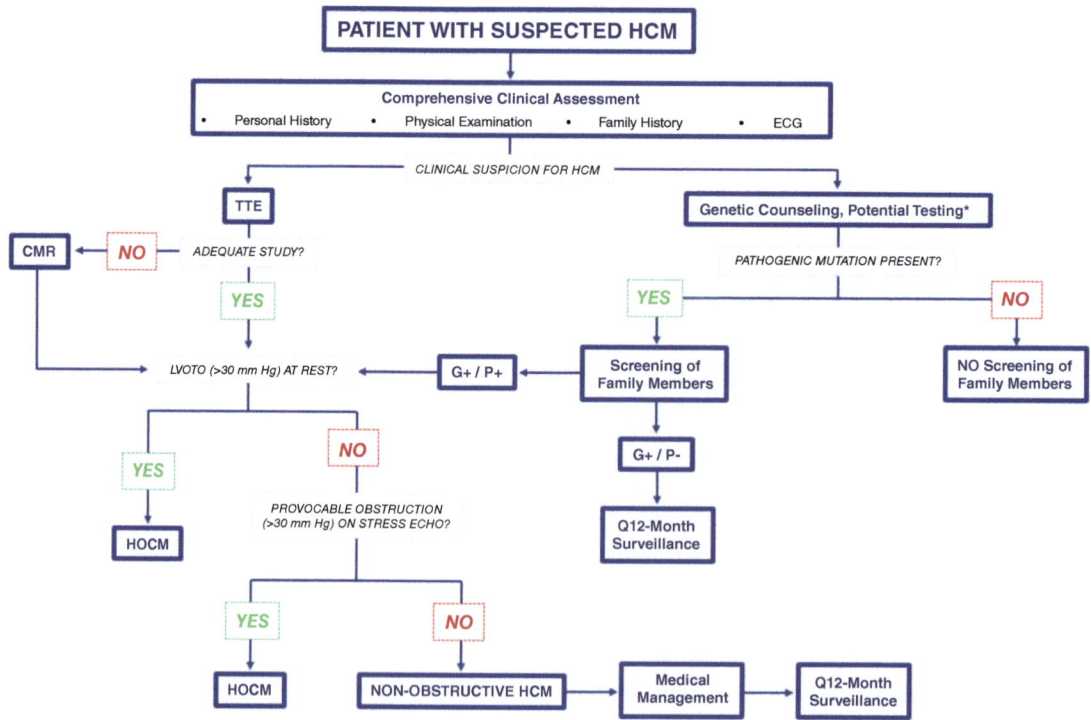

Fig. 9 HCM diagnostic algorithm [2, 21]. Recommended screening algorithm for patients with suspected hypertrophic obstructive cardiomyopathy (HOCM) including electrocardiography (ECG), transthoracic echocardiography (TTE), cardiac magnetic resonance imaging (CMR), and genetic testing. *G+* presence of pathogenic genetic variants, *P+* phenotype positive HOCM, *P−* phenotype negative HOCM, *Q12* every 12 months

Section 3: Pre-procedural Management of HCM

Early HCM Management

Selection of appropriate therapy for HCM is dictated by two factors: (1) the presence or absence of symptoms; and (2) the presence and severity of LVOTO measured on echocardiography, CMR, or by invasive hemodynamic monitoring. It is estimated that approximately two-thirds of patients with newly diagnosed HCM will have evidence of obstructive disease on initial diagnostic imaging [39, 59]. The management algorithm for HCM leading into septal reduction therapy (Fig. 10) will be the focus of this section.

As highlighted in the HCM management algorithm above, SRT is reserved for patients whose symptoms remain refractory to pharmacologic therapies. Negative inotropic agents (beta blockers, calcium channel blockers, and disopyramide) are the centerpiece of medical management for symptomatic HCM [60]. Tailoring medical management of HCM should also include elimination of vasodilating medications (decreased systemic vascular resistance may lead to increased outflow obstruction) and diuretics (decreased preload may lead to decreased LV dimensions and greater obstruction). Optimal medical management of HCM augments LV preload and prolongs diastole, thereby reducing LVOTO, minimizing microvascular ischemia, decreasing MR severity, and reducing left atrial pressures.

In the six decades that have passed since Braunwald and Morrow sparked the earliest attempts to treat HCM with beta blockade, fewer than 50 pharmacologic studies enrolling slightly more than 2000 patients have been performed [39, 61, 62]. Beta-blockers continue to remain the first-line agent for patients with obstructive HCM [2]. For patients who do not respond to

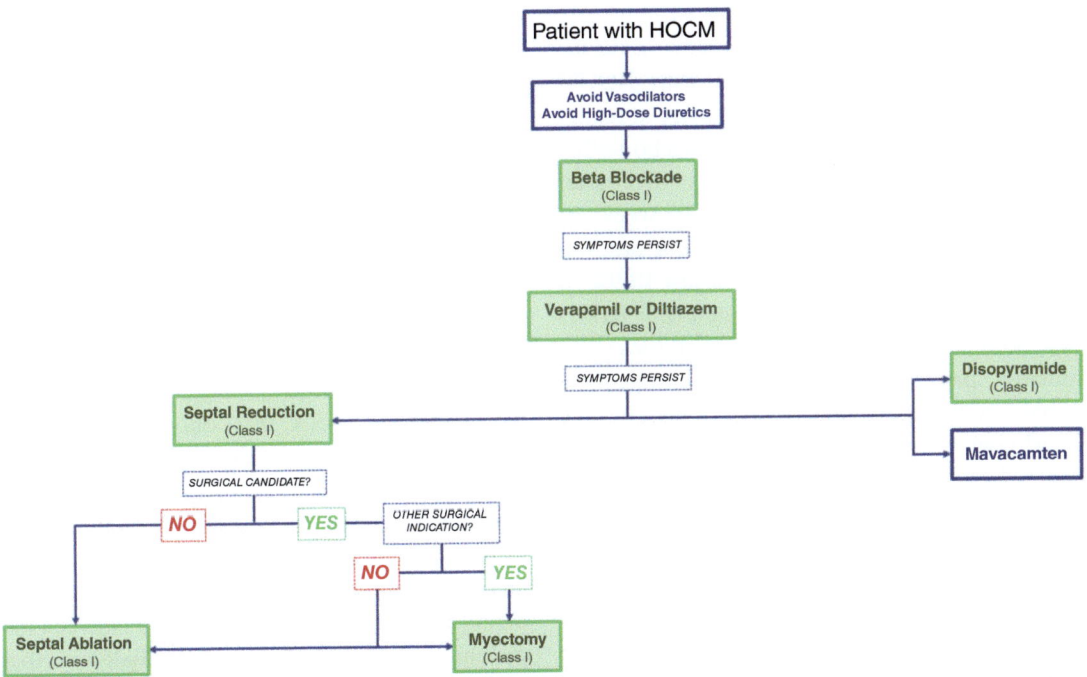

Fig. 10 Hypertrophic obstructive cardiomyopathy treatment algorithm. Colors correspond to Class of Recommendation from 2020 AHA/ACC Guideline for the Diagnosis and Treatment of Patients with Hypertrophic Cardiomyopathy. Mavacamten, FDA approved in April 2022, is included in algorithm as an alternative to disopyramide. *GDMT* guideline directed medical therapy, *HCM* hypertrophic cardiomyopathy, *HFrEF* heart failure with reduced ejection fraction, *LVEF* left ventricular ejection fraction

beta blockade, calcium channel blockers may be considered. Although several studies have demonstrated that non-dihydropyridine calcium channel blockers are efficacious in alleviating the symptoms of HCM, these agents must be used with some caution due to the potential to rarely worsen LVOTO by promoting peripheral vasodilation and decreasing LV preload [2, 40]. Finally, in patients who have not responded to first-line or second-line therapies, disopyramide may be considered [40]. Disopyramide, a class 1A antiarrhythmic, possesses negative inotropic properties and is an important therapeutic option (particularly in patients who are not candidates for SRT). As disopyramide has the potential to enhance conduction across the atrioventricular node, it must be given in combination with atrioventricular nodal blockade [40]. Mavacamten, a small molecule modulator of beta-cardiac myosin that reversibly binds to myosin and reduces myocardial contractility, is an alternative to disopyramide in highly symptomatic patients with HOCM [63]. A Study to Evaluate Mavacamten in Adults with Symptomatic Obstructive HCM Who Are Eligible for Septal Reduction Therapy (VALOR-HCM) randomized 112 patients with HOCM (defined as LVOT gradient ≥50 mmHg at rest or with exertion) to mavacamten or placebo with a primary endpoint of eligibility for SRT after 16 weeks of treatment [63]. After 16 weeks of therapy, 76.8% of patients in the placebo arm satisfied criteria for SRT compared to just 17.9% of patients randomized to mavacamten ($p < 0.001$) [63]. Longer term freedom from SRT for symptomatic patients treated with mavacamten remains to be determined.

Although the majority of patients with HCM can achieve adequate symptom control using medical treatment alone, responsiveness to pharmacotherapy for HCM can be highly variable [1]. When symptoms remain refractory to optimal medical management, involvement of the Heart Team for consideration of septal reduction strategies (surgical myectomy or alcohol septal ablation) should be considered. Invasive management of HCM with septal reduction therapy will be the focus of the next section.

Section 4: Procedural Management of HCM

Overview of Septal Reduction Therapies

It has been less than 70 years since the first septal reduction procedure was performed and less than 30 years since the first septal ablation. Over this relatively short timeframe, the utilization of septal reduction therapies has grown exponentially. Thousands of septal reduction procedures are now performed each year worldwide. Surgical septal myectomy continues to be regarded as the gold standard treatment for symptomatic HCM refractory to medical management [64]. However, annual rate of ASA is increasing while that of SM is slowly decreasing [65]. The use of ASA as an alternative to surgery has continued to rise and ASA has now become the primary septal reduction strategy in many parts of the world [64].

There are no randomized clinical trials comparing the efficacy and safety of septal ablation relative to surgical myectomy. Current guideline statements continue to rely solely on expert opinion and observational data, which have demonstrated similar short-term and long-term outcomes between ASA and SM (Table 7) [66]. The Hypertrophic Cardiomyopathy Guideline Statements published in 2011 and 2014 differed significantly with respect to recommendations for septal reduction therapy [57]. In 2011, surgical myectomy (receiving a Class IIa recommendation) was decisively favored over alcohol septal ablation (Class IIb) [57]. In the 2011 version of the guidelines, ASA was only recommended when surgery was either deemed to be contraindicated or high risk [57]. In the 2014 and 2020 guidelines, equal Class I status is given to each strategy for the management of adult patients with symptoms refractory to medical management [2, 3]. Shared decision-making between the patient and Heart Team with dialogue that includes full disclosure of all available treatment options, risks, benefits, and patient goals is essential in choosing the most appropriate management strategy for HCM.

Table 7 Clinical comparison of ASA vs SM [3, 4, 66–68]

Procedure	First case	US prevalence	Estimated healthcare costs	Mass of myocardium affected	Primary ECG change	Permanent pacemaker placement	LOS	Any procedural complication	Reoperation rate	Operative mortality	Long term mortality
Alcohol septal ablation	1994	40–50% annual SRT cases	15–20 k	16 +/− 7 g	RBBB (60%)	15–20%	3 days	20–30%	15–20%	<1–5%	Equal to general population
Surgical myectomy	1958	50–60% annual SRT cases	40–50 k	6 +/− 4 g	LBBB (50%)	5–10%	5–7 days	20–30%	1–2%	<1–5%	Equal to general population

Clinical comparison of alcohol septal ablation (ASA) versus surgical myectomy (SM) including history, prevalence, cost, mass of myocardium affected by the procedure, percent procedural complications including complete heart block requiring permanent device placement, average hospital length of stay (LOS) following the procedure, reoperation rate, and mortality (in-hospital and long-term)

ASA Technical Considerations

Alcohol septal ablation entails injecting 1–2 mL of 96% ethanol into a septal perforator artery supplying the hypertrophied ventricular septum to produce a myocardial infarction, induce septal thinning, and alleviate outflow obstruction [64]. Studies evaluating lower (1–2 mL) versus higher (>2 mL) doses of ethanol have shown no difference in ASA safety and efficacy [69]. Candidacy for ASA must be carefully considered. Factors favoring ASA include advanced age, extensive comorbidities, high surgical risk, prior sternotomy, and patient preference. Septal myectomy is recommended in patients who have other indications for surgery (CABG, MVR, etc), severe septal hypertrophy (>3 cm), or coronary anatomy that does not allow for successful ablation. The interventricular septum is the most heavily vascularized area of the left ventricle, receiving blood supply from all perforator branches as well as the posterior descending artery.

Successful ASA is contingent upon several factors: the injected volume of ethanol must be able to reach the area of obstruction within the LVOT, cause a focal infarct, resulting in a myocardial scar with subsequent thinning of this territory [64, 66]. When assessing patient candidacy for ASA, septal hypertrophy should be within the range of 18–30 mm. Patients with less than 18 mm of septal hypertrophy are at risk of excessive wall thinning, and those with greater than 30 mm hypertrophy are unlikely to achieve adequate reduction in septal wall thickness and outflow tract gradient [70]. Significant abnormalities within the mitral valve apparatus contributing to the outflow gradient, such as elongated leaflets and anomalous insertion of papillary muscles, should be absent in patients undergoing ASA [64] to achieve optimal reduction in LVOT obstruction. Patients less than 21 years of age should not undergo ASA (Class III indication) and the procedure is discouraged in patients younger than 40 [2, 3]. The anatomic, pathophysiologic, and clinical profiles that warrant consideration when assessing candidacy for ASA are outlined in Fig. 11.

For patients with medication refractory HCM who satisfy the above selection criteria, ASA is a safe and effective treatment strategy. Echocardiography guided ASA has greatly improved procedural success, decreased intervention time, and minimized complication rates [2, 13]. Utilizing echocardiography guidance and a perflutren lipid microsphere contrast agent or agitated saline via an over the wire coronary bal-

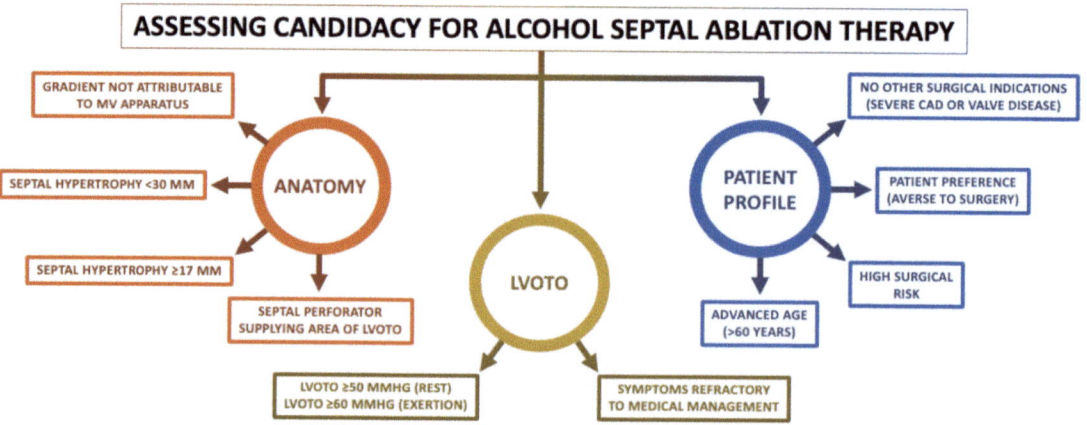

Fig. 11 Clinical features to guide selection of septal reduction therapy. Overview of variables impacting candidacy for alcohol septal ablation versus surgical myectomy. *LVOTO* left ventricular outflow tract obstruction

loon selectively placed in the septal perforator of interest, the septal artery supplying the portion of the basal septum can be confirmed prior to injection of ethanol [40]. Contrast opacification occurs from epicardium to endocardium, so slow injection of contrast with imaging over several minutes may be needed to fully assess septal perfusion. When perfusion of the basal septum endocardium is deemed inadequate, the contrast agent appears predominantly in the right ventricular endocardium, or another cardiac structure such as the RV free wall or a papillary muscle is opacified, the procedure is aborted (Supplementary Fig. 4).

When the contrast agent confirms perfusion of the basal septum (particularly endocardium of septum) at the site of SAM-septal contact (Supplementary Fig. 5), ASA is performed using approximately 1 cc of absolute ethanol per 1 cm septal thickness [3]. The ethanol is slowly administered via the over the inflated wire balloon over 10 min. During this time, the cardiac rhythm is closely monitored, and infusion slowed with the development of frequent premature ventricular contractions and/or with PR prolongation or transient AV block. In addition, frequent evaluation of the endoflator is performed to ensure that the baseline atmospheres of pressure that inflated the coronary balloon in the septal perforator are maintained. Similarly, periodic fluoroscopy to ensure the balloon remains inflated and in the correct position is performed.

A full overview of the ASA procedure is provided in Table 8.

It cannot be overstated that optimization of the interventional management of HCM requires a dedicated multidisciplinary team working at a comprehensive HCM center of excellence where a high volume of septal reduction therapies are performed annually [2]. In this setting, the outcomes of septal reduction therapies are excellent. A summary of outcomes and complications of ASA in comparison to SM is provided in Table 9.

Table 8 Procedural overview of ASA

Step	Description

Consent	• **Candidacy:**
	  – Septal thickness >16 mm, <30 mm [13, 57]
	  – Advanced age, extensive comorbidities, or patient preference
	  – High operative risk with no concomitant surgical indications
	• **Risks:**
	  – Vascular access complications
	  – Contrast dye reactions
	  – Extravasation of alcohol beyond target vessel
	  – Guide catheter complications (dissection, CVA)
	  – Heart block requiring permanent pacemaker placement (10–20% general risk, up to 50% in those with baseline LBBB) [2, 3, 71]
	  – Need for repeat ablation or surgical myectomy (10–20%) [2, 3, 71]
	• **Benefits:**
	  – Reduction of LVOTO and alleviation of symptoms
	  – Improved long-term mortality free of cardiac events
	  – Shorter duration recovery relative to surgical myectomy

(continued)

Table 8 (continued)

Step	Description

TVP placement 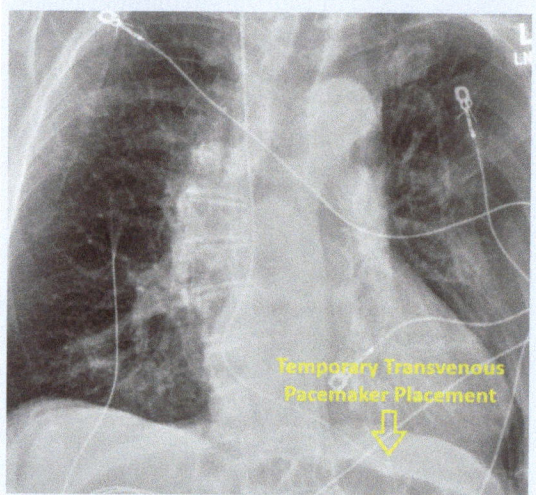	• **_Transvenous pacemaker placement:_**
	  – Required in the absence of PPM or transvenous ICD in situ
	  – Preferably via IJ access
	  – Capture threshold <1.0 mA
	  – Confirmation of placement in RV apex by fluoroscopy, CXR
	  – Placement maintained for 24–48 h post-procedure

Identification of septal perforator 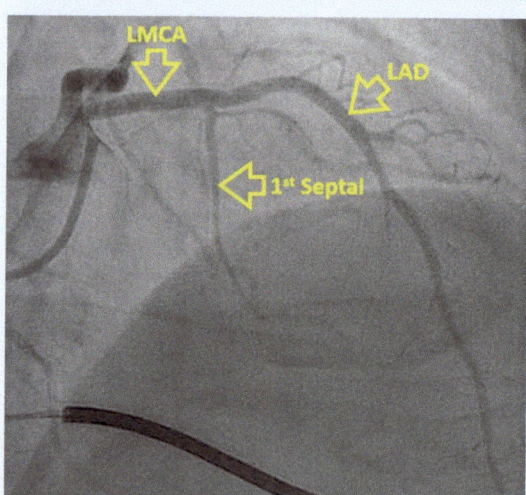	• Preferably right radial arterial access • 6 Fr guide catheter introduced into left main coronary artery • Baseline angiogram in the RAO 30° and cranial 30° projection for optimal visualization of the septal perforator branches • 0.014 inch coronary guidewire (300 cm) is advanced via the guide catheter into first septal perforator – Unfractionated heparin given for ACT >250–300 prior to advancing guidewire

Table 8 (continued)

Step	Description
Balloon positioning	• Over-the-wire (OTW) coronary balloon (slightly larger in diameter than septal branch) is advanced into the proximal portion of the vessel over the coronary guidewire • Balloon positioned to ensure placement entirely within the septal branch without encroachment on LAD • Inflate OTW balloon to nominal pressure per specific balloon ATM chart • Test injection of angiographic contrast dye with OTW balloon inflated to confirm absence of contrast reflux into native LAD while balloon is inflated • Injection of definity echo contrast to confirm opacification of basal septum without other LV or RV opacification

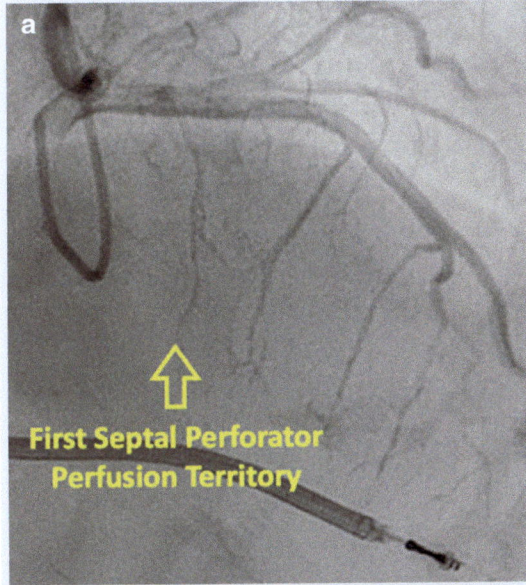

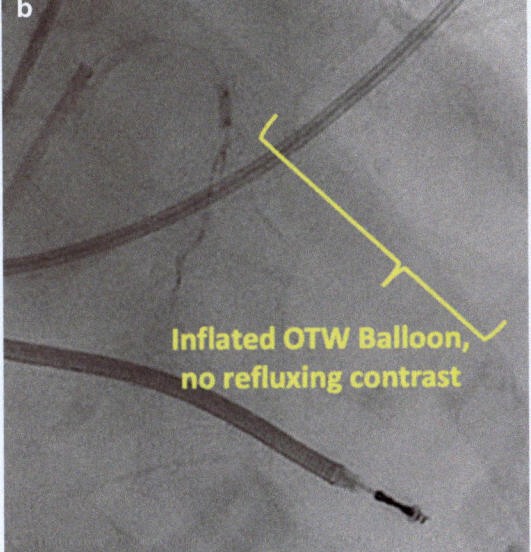

(continued)

Table 8 (continued)

Step	Description
Echocardiography guidance 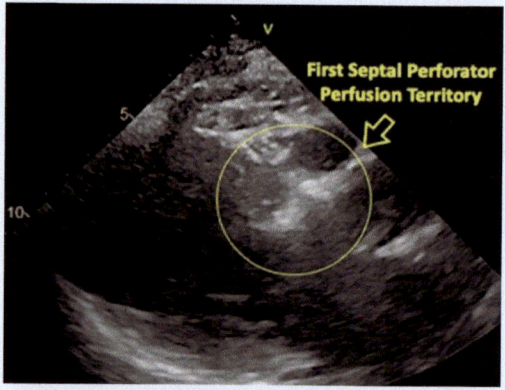 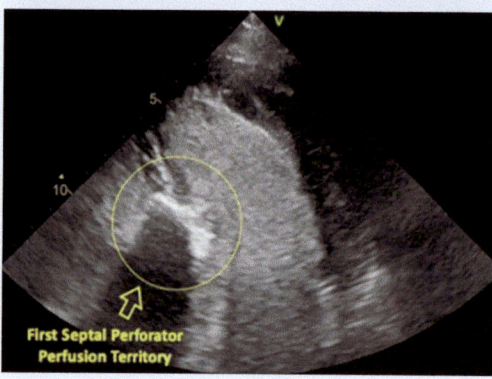	• TTE performed to assess baseline wall motion, LVOT gradient, SAM, and MR • Coronary wire is removed, balloon inflated, and small volume of echocardiographic contrast dye is injected via the OTW balloon to highlight area of myocardium subtended by septal branch • Echocardiographic images are acquired in the short axis, parasternal long axis, and apical 3-chamber views to confirm the presence of contrast-enhancement of the basal septum at the location of SAM • If the region supplied by septal branch does not correspond to area of obstruction on chest wall echo, another septal branch should be evaluated, or the procedure aborted
Ethanol injection 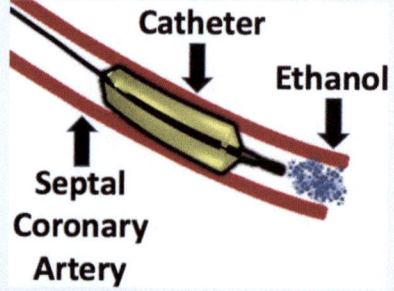 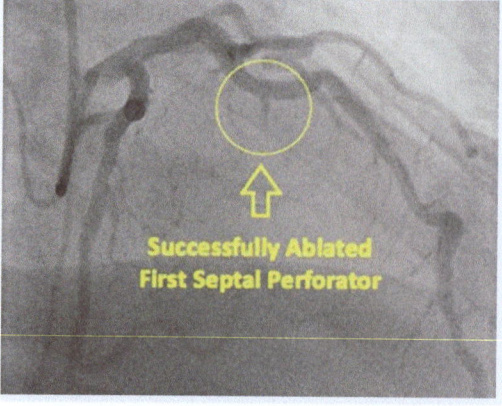	• 1–2 cc 100% ethanol injected slowly over 10 min • OTW balloon remains inflated for duration of EtOH infusion to ensure no reflux into LAD • Balloon cleared with 0.5 cc bolus of normal saline, deflated, and removed • Angiography to confirm 100% occlusion of septal with intact and unchanged LAD

Table 8 (continued)

Step	Description

Post-injection echocardiogram	• Intraprocedural transthoracic echocardiogram is performed
	  – Confirmation of basal septum akinesis
	  – Reassessment of LVOT gradient
	  – Ensure preserved wall motion in the anterior wall and apex
	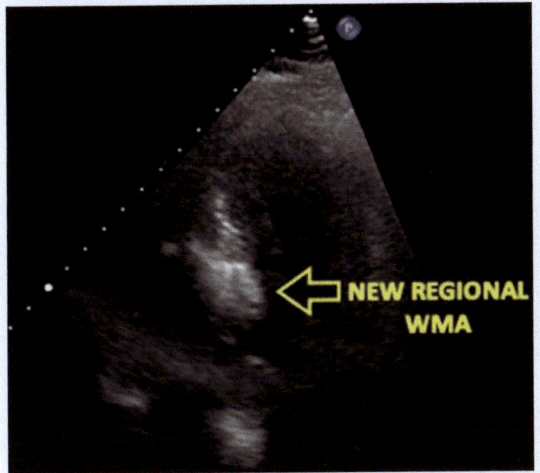

Post-procedural monitoring	• Overnight monitoring in Cardiac Intensive Care Unit • Continuous telemetry to assess for arrhythmia (CHB, VT) • Continuation of transvenous temporary pacemaker backup via IJ • If no pacing, AV block, or pauses, discontinue transvenous pacemaker the next morning and transfer from the CICU to a telemetry unit
Discharge	• Discharge on postprocedural day 3–4 if clinically appropriate

Step-by-step procedural overview of alcohol septal ablation

ACT activated coagulation time, *ASA* alcohol septal ablation, *CHB* complete heart block, *CICU* cardiac intensive care unit, *CVA* cerebrovascular accident, *CXR* chest X-ray, *ICD* implantable cardioverter defibrillator, *IJ* internal jugular, *LAD* left anterior descending artery; *LBBB*, left bundle branch block; *LVOTO*, left ventricular outflow tract obstruction; *MR* mitral regurgitation, *OTW* over-the-wire, *SAM* systolic anterior motion of the mitral valve, *TEE* transesophageal echocardiogram, *TTE* transthoracic echocardiogram, *VT* ventricular tachycardia, *WMA* wall motion abnormality

Table 9 Summary of outcomes and complications for septal reduction therapies

Procedure	Overview of complications	Advantages	Disadvantages
Alcohol septal ablation	• Any procedural complication: 23.2% [72] • Convert to open surgical procedure: 2% [72] • RBBB (60%) [3] • Intraprocedural CHB: 39.6% [71] • Post-op PPM: 8–17% [72, 73] • PPM placed beyond 30 days post-discharge (1.7%) [71] • Hemorrhage requiring transfusion: 1.4% [72] • Pericardial complications: <0.5% [72] • CVA/TIA: <0.5% [72] • DVT/PE: <0.5% [72] • Need for repeat ablation: 17% [71]	• Safety; procedural mortality <1% [74] • Long-term survival = general population [74] • Less invasive • Shorter procedural time • Shorter post-operative LOS [73] • Lower healthcare cost (15–20 k) [72] • Rising prevalence, now greatly outnumbering number of myectomies performed annually [4]	• Should not be performed in patients <21 years old (class III) [2, 57] • Discouraged in patients younger than 40 [2, 57] • Discouraged in patients with septal thickness ≥3 cm or <1.7 cm [2, 57] • Muscle necrosis induced by ASA (16 +/− 7 g) is larger than mass removed by myectomy (6 +/− 4 g) [75] • Variability of treatment effect (up to 25% of ASA cases with necrosis confined to R side of septum, sparing anterior basal septum and LVOTO) [3] • Higher reoperation rate than SM (10%) [76]
Surgical myectomy	• Any procedural complication: 30% [72] • Hemorrhage requiring transfusion: 5.4% [72] • LBBB (50%) [73] • Post-op PPM: 8–10% [65, 72, 73] • PPM placed beyond 30 days post-discharge (4.3%) [71] • Pericardial complications: 0.2% [72] • DVT/PE: 1.5% [72] • Infection: 3.3% [72] • Pressure ulcer: 0.6% [72]	• Safety; procedural mortality <1% [77, 78] • Long-term survival = general population [77] • Direct visualization of outflow tract obstruction by operating surgeon allows more tailored resection to distribution of septal thickening [77] • Permits concomitant correction of other surgical lesions if needed [77] • Survival advantage over symptomatic HCM patients receiving medical management [74] • Lower likelihood of requiring permanent PPM relative to septal ablation [73] • No post-operative intramyocardial scar [77] • Less myocardium affected (6–10 g) [4] • Lower reoperation rate than ASA (1–2%) [76]	• Necessitates median sternotomy, cardiopulmonary bypass • Decreasing familiarity worldwide as percutaneous intervention has become favored approach for majority of patients [65] • Surgical expertise for procedure often necessitates travel to center of excellence [77] • Higher frequency of post-operative bleeding • Longer post-operative LOS [68, 72] • 2–3× Higher mean cost of hospitalization (40–50 k) [72]

Comparison of complications, advantages, and disadvantages of common septal reduction therapies

ASA alcohol septal ablation, *CHB* complete heart block, *CVA* cerebrovascular accident, *DVT* deep vein thrombus, *HCM* hypertrophic cardiomyopathy, *LBBB* left bundle branch block, *LOS* hospital length of stay, *PE* pulmonary embolism, *PPM* permanent pacemaker, *RBBB* right bundle branch block, *SM* surgical myectomy

Chapter Review Questions

1. What patient characteristics would favor surgical myectomy over alcohol septal ablation?
   A. Age <21 years
   B. Baseline RBBB
   C. Septal thickness >3 cm
   D. Prior median sternotomy
   E. SAM
   F. A and C
   G. B and D
   H. All of the above

   Answer: F

   Explanation: Alcohol septal ablation should not be performed in patients less than 21 years of age [57]. Alcohol septal ablation is discouraged in patients younger than 40 years of age, those with extreme septal thickness (≥30 mm), or those with septal thickness <17 mm [2, 73]. The presence of SAM in the absence of intrinsic mitral valve pathology does not favor surgical myectomy. Surgical myectomy is favored over septal ablation when mitral regurgitation is secondary to primary mitral valve disease requiring concomitant MV repair or replacement.

2. A patient with baseline LBBB is undergoing alcohol septal ablation. What is the approximate likelihood that this patient will require permanent pacemaker placement prior to hospital discharge?
   A. <5%
   B. 10%
   C. 25%
   D. 33%
   E. ≥50%

   Answer: E

   Explanation: The prevalence of complete heart block following ASA is 15–20% (Table 7). The prevalence of RBBB following ASA is approximately 60% (Table 9) [3]. For patients with pre-existing LBBB undergoing ASA, the likelihood of requiring a permanent pacemaker post-procedurally is greater than 50%.

3. For the patient with suspected HCM who has inadequate windows on chest wall echocardiogram, the best diagnostic study would be:
   A. Cardiac CT
   B. TEE
   C. CMR
   D. Coronary angiography with right heart catheterization
   E. B or C

   Answer: C

   Explanation: Comprehensive transthoracic echocardiography plays the primary role in establishing the diagnosis of HCM. For patients suspected to have HCM in whom TTE is inconclusive, CMR imaging carries a Class I indication for diagnostic clarification (Fig. 9) [2, 21].

4. For which of the following patients with symptomatic HCM would a stress echocardiogram be indicated?
   A.

   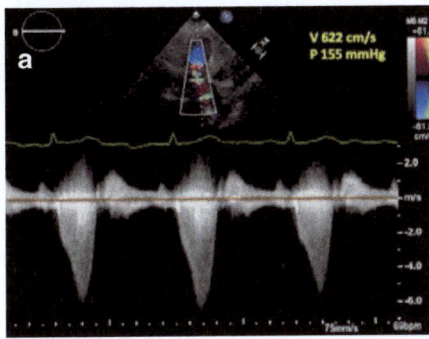

   B.

   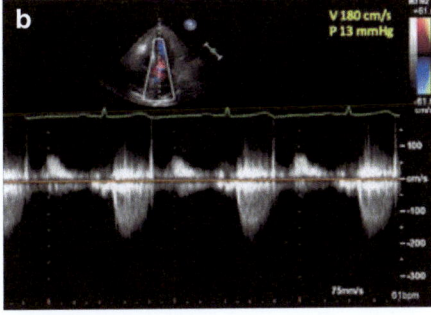

C.

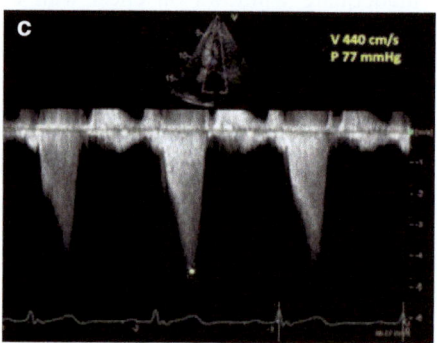

D.

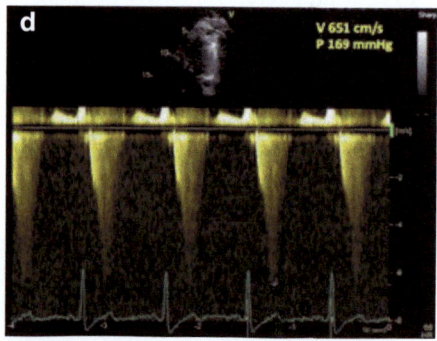

Answer: B

Explanation: LVOT gradients can be dynamic and may be missed on resting echocardiography for up to 50% of patients with obstructive physiology [79]. Stress echocardiography can be most helpful for patients where the presence or severity of LVOTO is uncertain after resting echocardiography. Choice B is the only option above showing a non-diagnostic LVOT gradient; stress echocardiography could be considered for this patient.

5. A 55 year-old woman with past medical history of severe COPD and morbid obesity presents to the Emergency Department after a syncopal event. Her physical examination is notable for a harsh systolic murmur heard along the left sternal border. A transthoracic echocardiogram is ordered and notable for severe left ventricular hypertrophy (septal wall thickness 2.1 cm). Due to limited windows, a gradient across the LVOT could not be measured. Which of the following imaging studies would be the most appropriate diagnostic test for this patient?
   A. Cardiac CT
   B. Transesophageal echocardiogram
   C. Cardiac MRI
   D. Cardiac SPECT
   E. Left and right heart catheterization
   Answer: C

   Explanation: CMR is indicated for diagnostic clarification in cases of suspected obstructive HCM when transthoracic echocardiography is inconclusive (Class I, LOE B-NR) [2].

References

1. Eugene Braunwald DLM, Zipes DP, Libby P, Bonow RO, editors. Braunwald's heart disease: a textbook of cardiovascular medicine, vol. 11. Philadelphia: Elsevier/Saunders; 2015.
2. Ommen SR, et al. 2020 AHA/ACC guideline for the diagnosis and treatment of patients with hypertrophic cardiomyopathy: a report of the American College of Cardiology/American Heart Association joint committee on clinical practice guidelines. J Am Coll Cardiol. 2020;76(25):e159–240.
3. Douglas JS Jr. Current state of the roles of alcohol septal ablation and surgical myectomy in the treatment of hypertrophic obstructive cardiomyopathy. Cardiovasc Diagn Ther. 2020;10(1):36–44.
4. Gimeno JR, Tomé MT, McKenna WJ. Alcohol septal ablation in hypertrophic cardiomyopathy: an opportunity to be taken. Revista Española de Cardiología (English Edition). 2012;65(4):314–8.
5. Matsuda J, et al. Relationship between procedural right bundle branch block and 1-year outcome after alcohol septal ablation for hypertrophic obstructive cardiomyopathy—a retrospective study. Circ J. 2021;85(9):1481–91.
6. Maron MS, Rowin EJ, Maron BJ. How to image hypertrophic cardiomyopathy. Circ Cardiovasc Imaging. 2017;10(7):e005372.
7. Soor GS, et al. Hypertrophic cardiomyopathy: current understanding and treatment objectives. J Clin Pathol. 2009;62(3):226–35.
8. Valente AM, et al. Comparison of echocardiographic and cardiac magnetic resonance imaging in hypertrophic cardiomyopathy sarcomere mutation carriers without left ventricular hypertrophy. Circ Cardiovasc Genet. 2013;6(3):230–7.
9. Germans T, et al. Structural abnormalities of the inferoseptal left ventricular wall detected by cardiac magnetic resonance imaging in carriers of

hypertrophic cardiomyopathy mutations. J Am Coll Cardiol. 2006;48(12):2518–23.
10. Brouwer WP, et al. Multiple myocardial crypts on modified long-axis view are a specific finding in pre-hypertrophic HCM mutation carriers. Eur Heart J Cardiovasc Imaging. 2012;13(4):292–7.
11. Maron MS, et al. Prevalence, clinical significance, and natural history of left ventricular apical aneurysms in hypertrophic cardiomyopathy. Circulation. 2008;118(15):1541–9.
12. Weinsaft JW, et al. LV thrombus detection by routine echocardiography: insights into performance characteristics using delayed enhancement CMR. JACC Cardiovasc Imaging. 2011;4(7):702–12.
13. Authors/Task Force Members, et al. 2014 ESC guidelines on diagnosis and management of hypertrophic cardiomyopathy: the task force for the diagnosis and Management of Hypertrophic Cardiomyopathy of the European Society of Cardiology (ESC). Eur Heart J. 2014;35(39):2733–79.
14. Prinz C, et al. Myocardial fibrosis severity on cardiac magnetic resonance imaging predicts sustained arrhythmic events in hypertrophic cardiomyopathy. Can J Cardiol. 2013;29(3):358–63.
15. Bruder O, et al. Myocardial scar visualized by cardiovascular magnetic resonance imaging predicts major adverse events in patients with hypertrophic cardiomyopathy. J Am Coll Cardiol. 2010;56(11):875–87.
16. O'Hanlon R, et al. Prognostic significance of myocardial fibrosis in hypertrophic cardiomyopathy. J Am Coll Cardiol. 2010;56(11):867–74.
17. Rubinshtein R, et al. Characteristics and clinical significance of late gadolinium enhancement by contrast-enhanced magnetic resonance imaging in patients with hypertrophic cardiomyopathy. Circ Heart Fail. 2010;3(1):51–8.
18. Adabag AS, et al. Occurrence and frequency of arrhythmias in hypertrophic cardiomyopathy in relation to delayed enhancement on cardiovascular magnetic resonance. J Am Coll Cardiol. 2008;51(14):1369–74.
19. Maron MS, et al. Clinical profile and significance of delayed enhancement in hypertrophic cardiomyopathy. Circ Heart Fail. 2008;1(3):184–91.
20. Semsarian C, et al. New perspectives on the prevalence of hypertrophic cardiomyopathy. J Am Coll Cardiol. 2015;65(12):1249–54.
21. Maron BJ, et al. Diagnosis and evaluation of hypertrophic cardiomyopathy: JACC state-of-the-art review. J Am Coll Cardiol. 2022;79(4):372–89.
22. Seidman JG, Seidman C. The genetic basis for cardiomyopathy: from mutation identification to mechanistic paradigms. Cell. 2001;104(4):557–67.
23. Teare D. Asymmetrical hypertrophy of the heart in young adults. Br Heart J. 1958;20(1):1–8.
24. Geisterfer-Lowrance AAT, et al. A molecular basis for familial hypertrophic cardiomyopathy: a β cardiac myosin heavy chain gene missense mutation. Cell. 1990;62(5):999–1006.
25. Coats CJ, Hollman A. Hypertrophic cardiomyopathy: lessons from history. Heart. 2008;94(10):1258–63.
26. Morrow AG, et al. Operative treatment in idiopathic hypertrophic subaortic stenosis. Techniques, and the results of preoperative and postoperative clinical and hemodynamic assessments. Circulation. 1968;37(4):589–96.
27. Sigwart U. Non-surgical myocardial reduction for hypertrophic obstructive cardiomyopathy. Lancet. 1995;346(8969):211–4.
28. Knight C, et al. Nonsurgical septal reduction for hypertrophic obstructive cardiomyopathy: outcome in the first series of patients. Circulation. 1997;95(8):2075–81.
29. Maron BJ, Nishimura RA. Surgical septal myectomy versus alcohol septal ablation: assessing the status of the controversy in 2014. Circulation. 2014;130(18):1617–24.
30. Veselka J, et al. Long-term clinical outcome after alcohol septal ablation for obstructive hypertrophic cardiomyopathy: results from the Euro-ASA registry. Eur Heart J. 2016;37(19):1517–23.
31. Durand E, et al. Non-surgical septal myocardial reduction by coil embolization for hypertrophic obstructive cardiomyopathy: early and 6 months follow-up. Eur Heart J. 2008;29(3):348–55.
32. Greenbaum AB, et al. Transcatheter myotomy to treat hypertrophic cardiomyopathy and enable transcatheter mitral valve replacement: first-in-human report of septal scoring along the midline endocardium. Circ Cardiovasc Interv. 2022;15(6):e012106.
33. Hardarson T, et al. Prognosis and mortality of hypertrophic obstructive cardiomyopathy. Lancet. 1973;302(7844):1462–7.
34. Mandes L, et al. The role of echocardiography for diagnosis and prognostic stratification in hypertrophic cardiomyopathy. J Echocardiogr. 2020;18(3):137–48.
35. Marian AJ, Braunwald E. Hypertrophic cardiomyopathy: genetics, pathogenesis, clinical manifestations, diagnosis, and therapy. Circ Res. 2017;121(7):749–70.
36. Maron MS, et al. Hypertrophic cardiomyopathy is predominantly a disease of left ventricular outflow tract obstruction. Circulation. 2006;114(21):2232–9.
37. Adawi S, et al. Echocardiographic Brockenbrough–Braunwald–Morrow sign. Eur J Echocardiogr. 2011;12(3):E12.
38. Brockenbrough EC, Braunwald E, Morrow AG. A hemodynamic technic for the detection of hypertrophic subaortic stenosis. Circulation. 1961;23(2):189–94.
39. Dybro AM, et al. Randomized trial of metoprolol in patients with obstructive hypertrophic cardiomyopathy. J Am Coll Cardiol. 2021;78(25):2505–17.
40. Bonow RO, et al. Effects of verapamil on left ventricular systolic function and diastolic filling in patients with hypertrophic cardiomyopathy. Circulation. 1981;64(4):787–96.
41. Delatycki MB, Corben LA. Clinical features of Friedreich ataxia. J Child Neurol. 2012;27(9):1133–7.
42. Calore C, et al. Abstract 15703: Hypertrophic cardiomyopathy with normal ECG: clinical

43. O'Hanlon R, Assomull RG, Prasad SK. Use of cardiovascular magnetic resonance for diagnosis and management in hypertrophic cardiomyopathy. Curr Cardiol Rep. 2007;9(1):51–6.
44. Olivotto I, et al. Assessment and significance of left ventricular mass by cardiovascular magnetic resonance in hypertrophic cardiomyopathy. J Am Coll Cardiol. 2008;52(7):559–66.
45. Spiewak M, et al. Comparison between maximal left ventricular wall thickness and left ventricular mass in patients with hypertrophic cardiomyopathy. Kardiol Pol. 2010;68(7):6.
46. Schulz-Menger J, et al. Left ventricular outflow tract planimetry by cardiovascular magnetic resonance differentiates obstructive from non-obstructive hypertrophic cardiomyopathy. J Cardiovasc Magn Reson. 2006;8(5):741–6.
47. Vogel-Claussen J, et al. Cardiac MRI evaluation of hypertrophic cardiomyopathy: left ventricular outflow tract/aortic valve diameter ratio predicts severity of LVOT obstruction. J Magn Reson Imaging. 2012;36(3):598–603.
48. Huang L, et al. MRI native T1 and T2 mapping of myocardial segments in hypertrophic cardiomyopathy: tissue remodeling manifested prior to structure changes. Br J Radiol. 2019;92(1104):20190634.
49. van Dockum WG, et al. Myocardial infarction after percutaneous transluminal septal myocardial ablation in hypertrophic obstructive cardiomyopathy: evaluation by contrast-enhanced magnetic resonance imaging. J Am Coll Cardiol. 2004;43(1):27–34.
50. Henry WL, et al. Mechanism of left ventricular outflow obstruction in patients with obstructive asymmetric septal hypertrophy (idiopathic hypertrophic subaortic stenosis). Am J Cardiol. 1975;35(3):337–45.
51. Levine RA, et al. Papillary muscle displacement causes systolic anterior motion of the mitral valve. Experimental validation and insights into the mechanism of subaortic obstruction. Circulation. 1995;91(4):1189–95.
52. Shah PM, Taylor RD, Wong M. Abnormal mitral valve coaptation in hypertrophic obstructive cardiomyopathy: proposed role in systolic anterior motion of mitral valve. Am J Cardiol. 1981;48(2):258–62.
53. Maron MS, et al. Mitral valve abnormalities identified by cardiovascular magnetic resonance represent a primary phenotypic expression of hypertrophic cardiomyopathy. Circulation. 2011;124(1):40–7.
54. Balaram SK, et al. Role of mitral valve plication in the surgical management of hypertrophic cardiomyopathy. Ann Thorac Surg. 2012;94(6):1990–7.
55. Shah AA, Glower DD, Gaca JG. Trans-aortic Alfieri stitch at the time of septal myectomy for hypertrophic obstructive cardiomyopathy. J Card Surg. 2016;31(8):503–6.
56. Sherrid MV, et al. The mitral valve in obstructive hypertrophic cardiomyopathy: a test in context. J Am Coll Cardiol. 2016;67(15):1846–58.
57. Gersh BJ, et al. 2011 ACCF/AHA guideline for the diagnosis and treatment of hypertrophic cardiomyopathy: a report of the American College of Cardiology Foundation/American Heart Association task force on practice guidelines. Circulation. 2011;124(24):e783–831.
58. Hong JH, et al. Mitral regurgitation in patients with hypertrophic obstructive cardiomyopathy: implications for concomitant valve procedures. J Am Coll Cardiol. 2016;68(14):1497–504.
59. Butzner M, et al. Stable rates of obstructive hypertrophic cardiomyopathy in a contemporary era. Front Cardiovasc Med. 2021;8:765876.
60. Fifer MA. Controversies in cardiovascular medicine. Most fully informed patients choose septal ablation over septal myectomy. Circulation. 2007;116(2):207–16.
61. Spoladore R, et al. Pharmacological treatment options for hypertrophic cardiomyopathy: high time for evidence. Eur Heart J. 2012;33(14):1724–33.
62. Braunwald E, Ebert PA. Hemodynamic alterations in idiopathic hypertrophic subaortic stenosis induced by sympathomimetic drugs*. Am J Cardiol. 1962;10(4):489–95.
63. Desai MY, et al. Myosin inhibition in patients with obstructive hypertrophic cardiomyopathy referred for septal reduction therapy. J Am Coll Cardiol. 2022;80(2):95–108.
64. Spirito P, Rossi J, Maron BJ. Alcohol septal ablation: in which patients and why? Ann Cardiothorac Surg. 2017;6(4):369–75.
65. Kim LK, et al. Hospital volume outcomes after septal myectomy and alcohol septal ablation for treatment of obstructive hypertrophic cardiomyopathy: US Nationwide inpatient database, 2003–2011. JAMA Cardiol. 2016;1(3):324–32.
66. Sorajja P, et al. Outcome of alcohol septal ablation for obstructive hypertrophic cardiomyopathy. Circulation. 2008;118(2):131–9.
67. El Masry H, Breall JA. Alcohol septal ablation for hypertrophic obstructive cardiomyopathy. Curr Cardiol Rev. 2008;4(3):193–7.
68. Geske JB, Gersh BJ. Myectomy versus alcohol septal ablation: experience remains key. JACC Cardiovasc Interv. 2014;7(11):1235–6.
69. Veselka J, Tomasov P, Zemanek D. Long-term effects of varying alcohol dosing in percutaneous septal ablation for obstructive hypertrophic cardiomyopathy: a randomized study with a follow-up up to 11 years. Can J Cardiol. 2011;27(6):763–7.
70. Wells S, et al. Clinical profile of nonresponders to surgical myectomy with obstructive hypertrophic cardiomyopathy. Am J Med. 2018;131(6):e235–9.
71. Batzner A, et al. Survival after alcohol septal ablation in patients with hypertrophic obstructive cardiomyopathy. J Am Coll Cardiol. 2018;72(24):3087–94.
72. Panaich SS, et al. Results of ventricular septal myectomy and hypertrophic cardiomyopathy (from Nationwide inpatient sample [1998–2010]). Am J Cardiol. 2014;114(9):1390–5.

73. Nguyen A, et al. Surgical myectomy versus alcohol septal ablation for obstructive hypertrophic cardiomyopathy: a propensity score-matched cohort. J Thorac Cardiovasc Surg. 2019;157(1):306–315 e3.
74. Ommen SR, et al. Long-term effects of surgical septal myectomy on survival in patients with obstructive hypertrophic cardiomyopathy. J Am Coll Cardiol. 2005;46(3):470–6.
75. Valeti US, et al. Comparison of surgical septal myectomy and alcohol septal ablation with cardiac magnetic resonance imaging in patients with hypertrophic obstructive cardiomyopathy. J Am Coll Cardiol. 2007;49(3):350–7.
76. Cho YH, et al. Residual and recurrent gradients after septal myectomy for hypertrophic cardiomyopathy-mechanisms of obstruction and outcomes of reoperation. J Thorac Cardiovasc Surg. 2014;148(3):909–15.
77. Maron BJ. Controversies in cardiovascular medicine. Surgical myectomy remains the primary treatment option for severely symptomatic patients with obstructive hypertrophic cardiomyopathy. Circulation. 2007;116(2):196–206.
78. Rastegar H, et al. Results of surgical septal myectomy for obstructive hypertrophic cardiomyopathy: the tufts experience. Ann Cardiothorac Surg. 2017;6(4):353–63.
79. Woo A, et al. Clinical and echocardiographic determinants of long-term survival after surgical myectomy in obstructive hypertrophic cardiomyopathy. Circulation. 2005;111(16):2033–41.

Percutaneous Closure of Post-myocardial Infarction Ventricular Septal Rupture

Jessica Raviv and Barry Love

Abstract

Ventricular septal rupture is a rare sequala of myocardial infarction typically appearing in the first week after the initial ischemic insult. Early revascularization strategies have reduced the incidence of post-myocardial infarction ventricular septal defect (PMI-VSD) to less than 1% of all myocardial infarctions however if they occur, the mortality remains high. Surgical closure of PMI-VSD carries a significant mortality risk and high chance of incomplete closure as the friable margins of the defect do not hold sutures well. Transcatheter closure of PMI-VSD was first reported in 1998. Results for primary transcatheter closure of PMI-VSD for large defects associated with shock remain poor. Better outcomes for later close of smaller defects or those who have residual VSD after attempted surgical closure fare better. In this section, we will describe a case of PMI-VSD and the strategies of transcatheter PMI-VSD closure.

Keywords

Myocardial infarction · Post-myocardial infarction ventricular septal defect · Complications of myocardial infarction · Acquired ventricular septal defect · Device closure

Abbreviations

CO	Cardiac output
ECMO	Extracorporeal membrane oxygenation
ELSO	Extracorporeal life support
LV	Left ventricle
MI	Myocardial infarction
PMI-VSD	Post-myocardial infarction ventricular septal defect
RCA	Right coronary artery
RV	Right ventricle
SVR	Systemic vascular resistance
TEE	Transesophageal echocardiography
TTE	Transthoracic echocardiography
VSD	Ventricular septal defect

Test your learning and check your understanding of this book's contents: use the "Springer Nature Flashcards" app to access questions using ▶ https://sn.pub/ambACS.

To use the app, please follow the instructions in the chapter "Transcatheter Aortic Valve Replacement."

J. Raviv · B. Love (✉)
Icahn School of Medicine at Mount Sinai, Mount Sinai Medical Center, NY, New York, USA
e-mail: Jessica.raviv@mssm.edu;
Barry.love@mssm.edu

Learning Objectives

1. Be able to suspect post-myocardial infarction ventricular septal defect by symptoms and clinical signs.
2. Diagnose PMI-VSD by transthoracic and/or transesophageal echocardiography.
3. Understand the high mortality of PMI-VSD when accompanied by shock.
4. Be able to calculate a pulmonary to systemic flow ratio (Qp/Qs) by oximetry measurements.
5. Appreciate bridging strategies including medical therapy, intraaortic balloon pump, impella, ECMO.
6. Appreciate the advantages and disadvantages of surgical and transcatheter treatment options for closure of PMI-VSD.

Case Study

A 55 year old woman with poorly controlled diabetes, active smoker, history of prior strokes with residual aphasia, and paroxysmal atrial fibrillation presented with inferior ST elevation MI after 3 days of chest pain. She was found to have a subtotal occlusion of a dominant right coronary artery and had successful percutaneous coronary intervention (Fig. 1). Despite successful PCI, her clinical condition worsened with progressive shortness of breath and orthopnea. Physical examination revealed a 2/6 holosystolic murmur at the left sternal border. An echocardiogram was obtained showing a basal ventricular septal rupture. She was transferred for management.

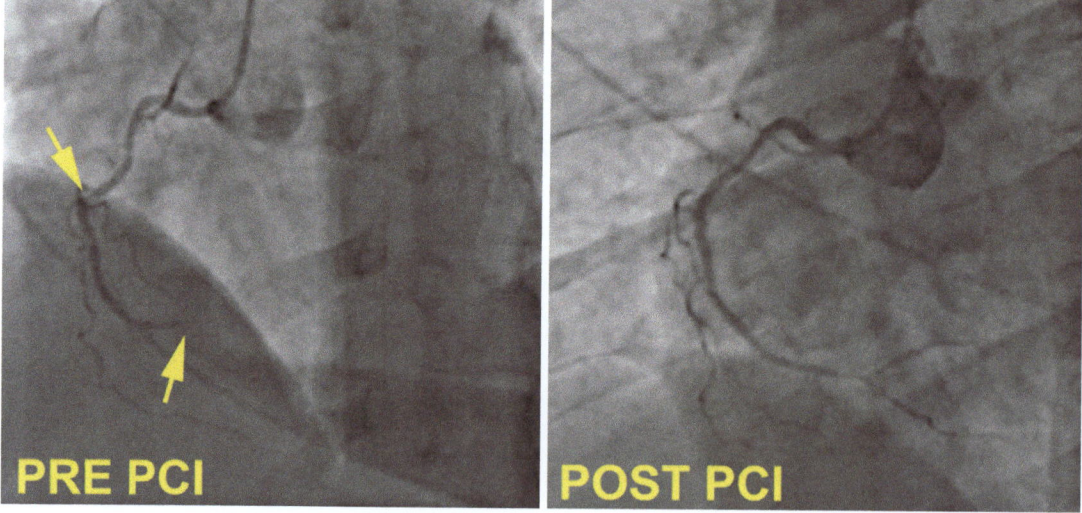

Fig. 1 Selective right coronary angiography showing subtotal mid and total distal RCA occlusion (arrows). Post-PCI flow has been reestablished with perfusion of the posterior descending coronary artery

Background and Definitions

Post-myocardial infarction septal rupture (PMI-VSD) occurs days to weeks after myocardial infarction of a coronary territory supplying the ventricular septum. With better reperfusion strategies for acute myocardial infarction, the incidence of PMI-VSD has decreased and now is encountered in less than 1% of all myocardial infarctions [1]. When PMI-VSD occurs, it typically leads to symptoms of heart failure and low cardiac output as the left ventricular blood is shunted through the VSD to the pulmonary artery and back to the left ventricle. Physical examination will reveal a holosystolic murmur that may be mistaken for mitral regurgitation. Septal infarction at the margins of the heart may also lead to cardiac pseudoaneurysm. Infarction of the LAD territory usually leads to PMI-VSD in the mid-septum to apex whereas infarctions in the posterior descending territory tend to lead to more basal-mid VSDs.

Diagnosis of the VSD is usually made by transthoracic echocardiogram with color Doppler interrogation of the septum in multiple views. Transesophageal echocardiogram can be additionally helpful in obtaining additional views and is used for guiding transcatheter closure. The VSD itself is often serpiginous through the infarcted septum. The extent of the VSD is often underestimated as the margins of the hole itself are surrounded by necrotic tissue that is not stable enough to hold sutures or devices. The extent of LV damage may be underestimated as the LV free-wall function will usually appear hyperdynamic and the overall EF may appear quite good in the face of low afterload with much of the cardiac output being diverted though the VSD to the low-resistance pulmonary system. As the pulmonary to systemic flow ratio (Qp/Qs) increases, the systemic output falls and signs and symptoms of shock emerge. Stabilization of these patients prior to intervention is key as "rushing" to do an intervention (surgical or transcatheter) in the face of this deteriorating clinical situation is invariably fatal. Placement of an intraaortic balloon pump (IABP) and initiation of systemic afterload reduction as the blood pressure allows will decrease the Qp/Qs and increase systemic output. If more support is needed, impella [2] ECMO [3] or other mechanical support can be contemplated but the chances of salvage if that is required become increasingly slim.

In a patient with a large PMI-VSD, the ratio of pulmonary:systemic flow (Qp/Qs) can be calculated with the aid of a pulmonary artery catheter. The formula is as follows:

Qp/Qs = Aortic sat (%) − Mixed venous sat (%)/Pulmonary vein sat (%) − Pulmonary artery sat (%).

The superior vena cava, SVC, saturation obtained from the side port of an internal jugular vein sheath is the best proxy for a mixed venous saturation. The aortic saturation is the arterial saturation obtained from an arterial line or pulse oximeter. The pulmonary vein saturation is the same as the aortic saturation as there is no significant right to left shunt in this lesion, and the pulmonary artery saturation is obtained from the pulmonary artery catheter. It is important to use a co-oximeter to measure the saturation and not use a blood gas machine that calculates an oxygen saturation as this may introduce considerable error. Equally important is to do the Qp/Qs measurements on the lowest amount of oxygen that produces an arterial saturation of 90–95%. Higher inspired O_2 leads to significant dissolved oxygen which may make the calculation less accurate.

The method to estimate Qp/Qs by echocardiography is notoriously inaccurate and should not be used.

In patients with significant PMI-VSD and shock, the Qp/Qs is usually >2:1.

Diagnosis and Pre-procedural Assessment

Transthoracic echocardiogram demonstrated a basal PMI-VSD measuring about 1 cm × 1.4 cm with left to right flow (Figs. 2 and 3). The LV systolic function was normal (EF 55%) and the RV function was moderately depressed. She was initially warm with good urine output and a loud

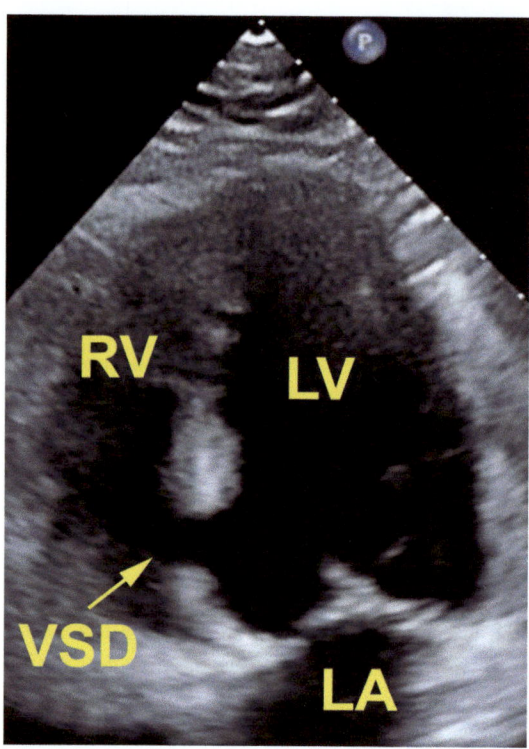 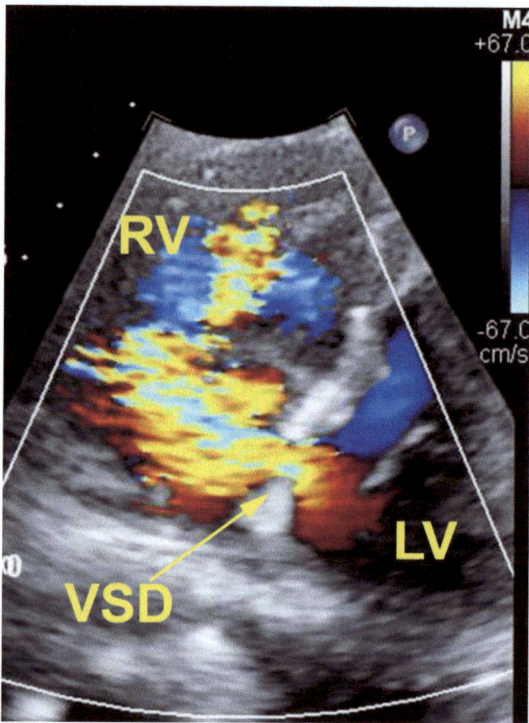

Fig. 2 Transthoracic echo (apical 4 chamber view) showing basal PMI-VSD and proximity to AV valves

Fig. 3 Transthoracic echo with color Doppler (modified apical/parasternal) showing VSD with L to R flow

holosystolic murmur was present. Her mentation was normal. The lactate initially was 0.6 mmol/L with a creatinine of 2.5 mg/dL however over the course of the next 3 days, her creatinine rose to 3.2 mg/dL and the lactate rose to 5.6 mmol/L with corresponding decrease in urine output.

She was taken to the catheterization laboratory where a pulmonary artery catheter was placed. The Qp/Qs was 2.8:1 (PA sat 83% SVC 61% Ao 95%) with a PA pressure of 42/15 (26) and a wedge pressure of 16 mmHg with a simultaneous blood pressure of 92/35 (70). An intraaortic balloon pump (IABP) was placed. In the first few hours, the lactate improved to 0.6 mmol/L and the Qp/Qs came down to 1.8:1. Over the next 3 days with the addition of milrinone, her urine output improved, and the creatinine normalized to 1.3 mg/dL.

Heart Team Approach and Discussion

The patient had been stabilized with medical management and IABP, but there continued to be a significant shunt. It had now been ~12 days since the onset of chest pain.

Left unrepaired, PMI-VSD carried a mortality of 90% within 2 months [4]. Surgical repair of PMI-VSD itself however is not low risk. Mortality has been reported between 19–60% [5]. A retrospective review of the STS database showed a higher operative risk (54%) for those operated on within 7 days of the MI and a lower risk of mortality (18%) for those operated 8 days or more after MI. However, this was a retrospective study and it is likely that those who could wait were also those who were less ill with a less extensive

VSD [5]. Despite the high mortality with surgery, the current American College of Cardiology of American Heart Association Guidelines recommend surgical repair regardless of hemodynamic status [6].

Transcatheter device closure of PMI-VSD has been attempted in lieu of surgery in the acute, subacute and chronic phase as an alternative to surgery and has been reported in case reports and small case series. A larger case series of 29 patients undergoing attempted transcatheter PMI-VSD closure showed 25/29 acute successes but with a mortality of 72% overall. Most of these procedures however were done in patients in the acute phase with 16 patients in shock and all on IABP support [7]. Another study of 17 patient had 12 acute successes with a survival of 65%. Only 5 of the 17 however were on IABP and most of the survivors were those >3 weeks out from MI [8].

Overall, the data is inconclusive favoring surgical or transcatheter closure in the acute phase but it is clear that there is a high risk of mortality for those patients in shock needing mechanical support and that waiting for some time after the acute insult is preferable if the patient's condition can tolerate this.

There are several choices for devices for PMI-VSD closure. Initial experience with the Cardioseal device described by Landzberg and Lock in 1998 was unsatisfactory except for the smallest defects [9]. Development of braided nitinol devices of the Amplatzer family (now a part of Abbott Laboratories) was met with better success. The Amplatzer muscular VSD occluder designed for congenital VSDs comes in a range of sizes from 6 through 18 mm in 2 mm increments. The central waist is 7 mm long and the disks are equal in size and 8 mm larger than the central waist. Abbott also makes a specific device for PMI-VSD [10]. The PMI-VSD occluder is available in sizes from 16 through 24 mm with the disks 10 mm larger than the central waist and a central waist length of 10 mm. The PMI-VSD occluder was available for several years only on an emergency use basis however the device has now received an HDE approval making access to the device somewhat less cumbersome in the United States. One of the problems with the PMI-VSD occluder is that even the largest size may not be sufficiently large for many of the hemodynamically significant lesions. For larger PMI-VSD defects, the Amplatzer Septal Occluder provides a much larger range of sizes with waist diameters up to 38 mm with a left-sided disk 12–14 mm larger than the central waist and a central waist that is 4 mm long. Occlutech and Ceraflex make similarly designed devices available outside the US. For small defects, the Amplatzer Duct Occluder II and the Amplatzer Vascular plugs can also be considered.

Location of the defect and proximity to the AV valves is important in determining the feasibility of transcatheter closure. The device disks cannot be in contact with the AV valves or it will cause regurgitation or perforate the leaflet. Patients who have other lesions that require surgical intervention such as pseudoaneurysm or mitral chordal rupture with flail, or those who require surgical coronary revascularization are also not good candidates for transcatheter PMI-VSD closure. The defect always appears smaller by echocardiography than the needed occluder size because the edges of the defect are necrotic and soft and so anticipating needing to oversize the device by at least 1.5 × compared to the defect size by echocardiography is expected. Larger defects more than 10–15 mm are also much more challenging and prone to failure or complications.

The surgical team felt this patient was a surgical candidate for closure. Her young age and premorbid status (she was living on her own independently) favored a surgical approach but her comorbidities (smoking, diabetes, prior stroke, recent myocardial infarction) made the surgical team cautious. A primary transcatheter closure was discussed. Given the relatively small apparent size of the VSD it was felt that primary transcatheter closure was feasible. However, the basal location of the defect and the proximity to the mitral valve made us cautious that we would not be able to significantly oversize the defect without risk of interference with the mitral valve.

Heart Team Decision

The decision was made to proceed for primary transcatheter closure.

Intraprocedural Imaging Modalities and Measurements

Cath Procedure #1

The access for PMI-VSD closure will depend on the VSD location and the planned device selection. For most larger VSDs, it is preferable to cross the VSD from the LV side as crossing from the RV side is more difficult and the catheter and device can become ensnared in the tricuspid apparatus and RV trabeculations. Additionally, it is preferable to open the LV disk of the device and pull it flush with the septum to create the best seal. After crossing the VSD from the LV side, the wire and catheter are typically easily advanced to the pulmonary artery. The wire can then be snared in the pulmonary artery from a venous approach and exteriorized. The delivery sheath is then advanced over the exteriorized wire from the venous approach through the RA, RV and VSD to the LV where the LV disk is opened, pulled flush with the septum and the RV disk is then formed. For apical VSDs, an internal jugular vein approach is the least tortuous whereas for basal VSDs, a femoral approach is easier.

Access was obtained in the right femoral vein (9 Fr) and right femoral artery (6 Fr). The VSD was first imaged by TEE and the defect appeared to be in the basal septum close to the mitral and tricuspid valves and ~1.3 cm in diameter (Figs. 4 and 5). An LV angiogram was performed showing the basal defect and the size measured ~10 mm by angiography (Fig. 6). The VSD was crossed retrograde with a 6 Fr JR4 catheter (Fig. 7). A 260 cm 0.035 wire was then passed through the catheter and advanced to the pulmonary artery. The wire was then snared in the right pulmonary artery with a 30 mm Gooseneck snare (Fig. 8) and exteriorized out the right femoral vein (Fig. 9). Care needs to be taken when pulling the wire through the heart to also advance the wire and keep the catheter in place on the wire until it is pulled through the heart to avoid the wire acting like a saw and damaging the heart.

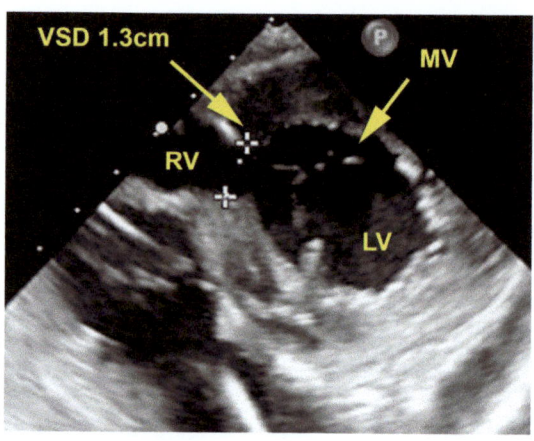

Fig. 4 Transesophageal echo showing basal VSD measuring 1.3 cm. *RV* right ventricle, *LV* left ventricle, *MV* mitral valve. Note VSD proximity to mitral valve

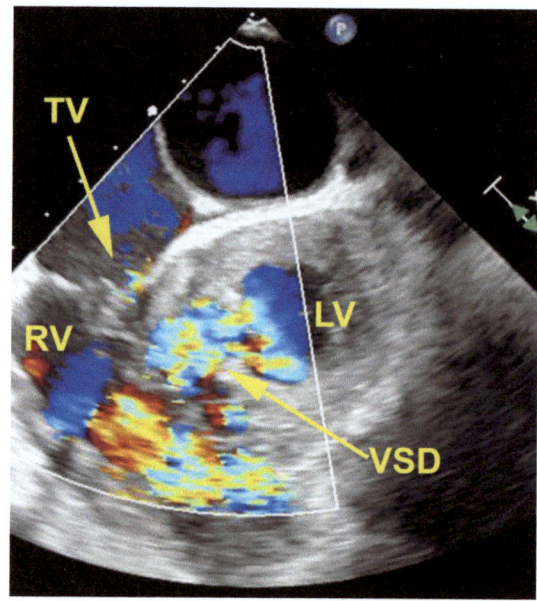

Fig. 5 TEE of PMI-VSD showing color flow from L to R. Note proximity to TV (tricuspid valve)

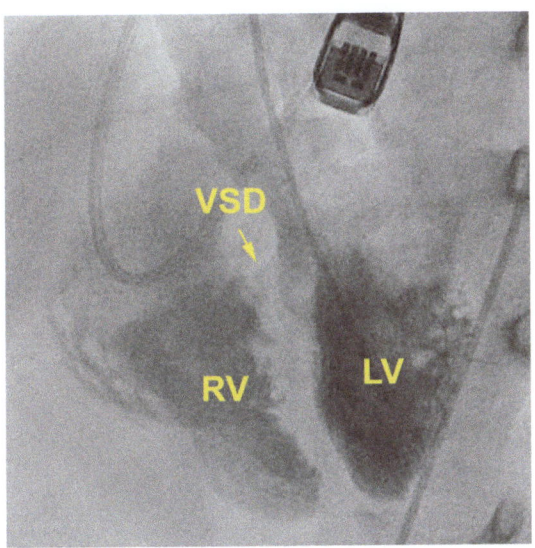

Fig. 6 LV angiogram showing basal VSD with flow to RV

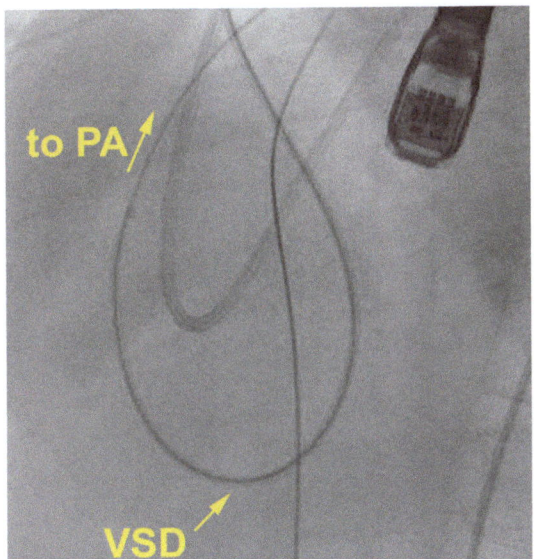

Fig. 7 Angiogram of catheter crossing VSD from LV to RV and wire out to pulmonary artery (to PA)

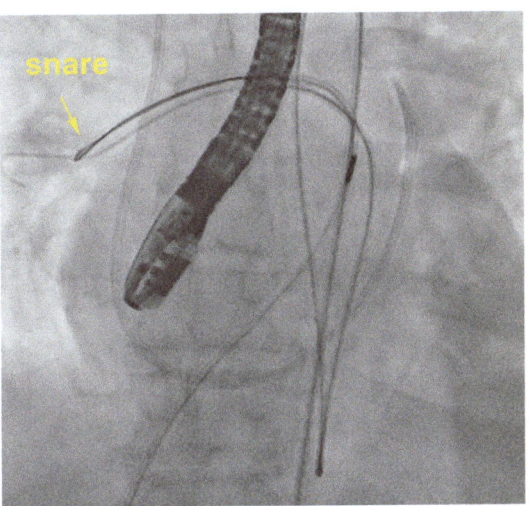

Fig. 8 The wire has passed from the LV through the VSD to the RV and out to the right pulmonary artery (RPA). A 30 mm Gooseneck snare has been advanced form the femoral artery and the wire is snared in the RPA. Other shadows on the image include the TEE probe, the intraaortic balloon pump and the Swan-Ganz catheter in the main pulmonary artery

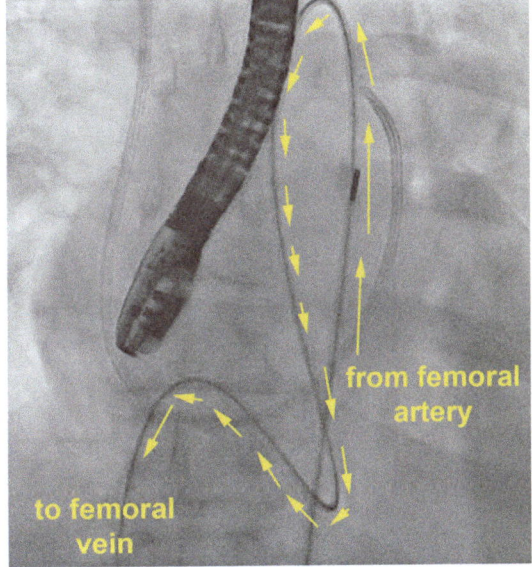

Fig. 9 The snare catheter has pulled the wire out the femoral vein. Arrows denote the complete wire loop from femoral artery, aorta, LV, VSD, RV, RA, IVC, femoral vein

In this patient, we did not have easy availability of the PMI-VSD occluder. Given the anticipated size of the defect however, we thought the largest mVSD occluder would provide a good fit.

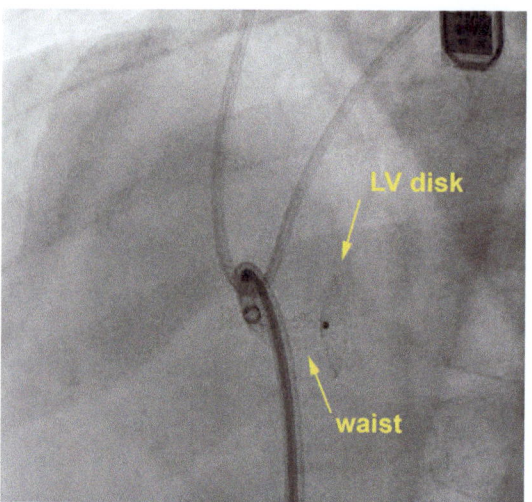

Fig. 10 Deployment of 18 mm Amplatzer mVSD occluder. The LV disk (26 mm in diameter) is gently pulled flush against the septum and the waist is in the VSD

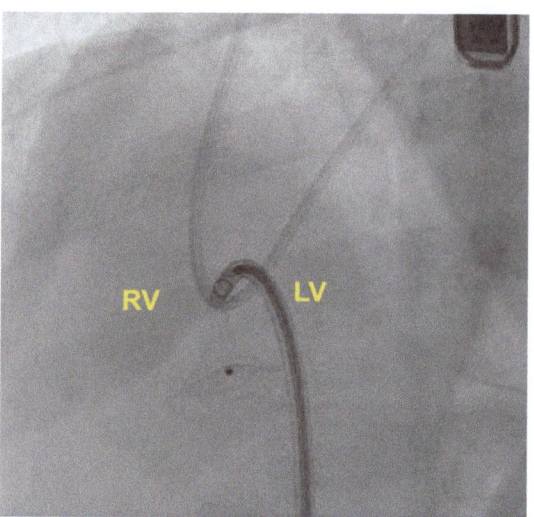

Fig. 11 The defect margins were too friable to hold the device and the 18 mm mVSD occluder prolapsed through the VSD to the RV where it was recaptured and removed

A 9 Fr Amplatzer delivery sheath was advanced over the wire from the femoral vein through the RA, RV, VSD, LV to the ascending aorta. The dilator and wire were removed. An 18 mm mVSD occluder was then advanced and the LV disk and connecting waist opened in the LV and pulled gently against the septum (Fig. 10). However, the defect was obviously larger and not as rigid as we had anticipated and the VSD flow was able to easily push the LV disk (26 mm) through the VSD to the RV (Fig. 11). The device was recaptured in the RV.

We considered recrossing and placing a larger device but the proximity to the mitral valve gave us pause. Given that the 26 mm disk of the device could easily pass through the defect, we anticipated that we would need a device with at least a 30 mm waist. That meant choosing an Amplatzer Septal Occluder that has a larger disk:central waist ratio and we were concerned that would risk interference with the mitral valve. An ad-hoc heart team meeting with the patient on the table was convened and we decided the patient would be better-off with a surgical approach. The sheaths were removed and patient taken back to the ICU with the balloon-pump still in-place, intubated in stable condition.

Surgical Procedure

The following day the patient was taken for surgical VSD closure. On bypass, a longitudinal incision was made in the LV lateral to the posterior descending coronary artery. The VSD was identified and 2–0 pledgeted Ethibond sutures were used to secure a bovine pericardial patch. Given the extent of RV dysfunction, a surgical tricuspid ring was also placed, and the left atrial appendage was clipped. A small residual VSD was seen by TEE post-operatively.

Post-surgical Course

The patient had a difficult post-operative course. She initially weaned from inotropic support but when the balloon pumped was removed, her lactate increased, and she required reinsertion of the IABP and reinitiation of inotropes. She developed renal failure and required hemodialysis. By post-op day 15 it was clear that she was not progressing with medical management. A TEE showed a significant residual VSD with maintained LV function (Fig. 12).

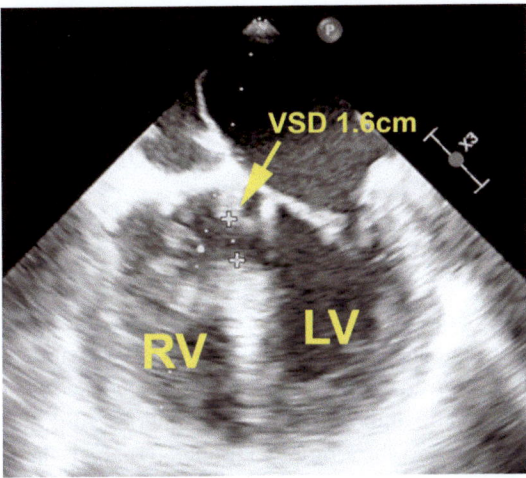

Fig. 12 2 weeks after attempted surgical closure, TEE shows a residual VSD 1.6 cm

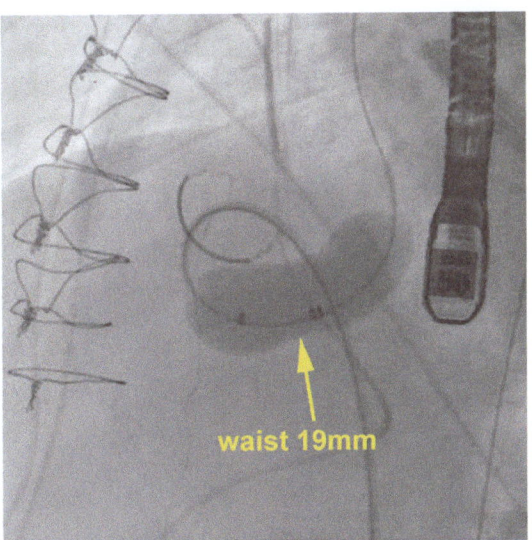

Fig. 14 The VSD was crossed as outlined for attempt #1 and a complete wire loop created. A 24 mm Amplatzer sizing balloon was advanced from the femoral vein and the VSD was balloon-sized with a compliant balloon with a waist of 19 mm

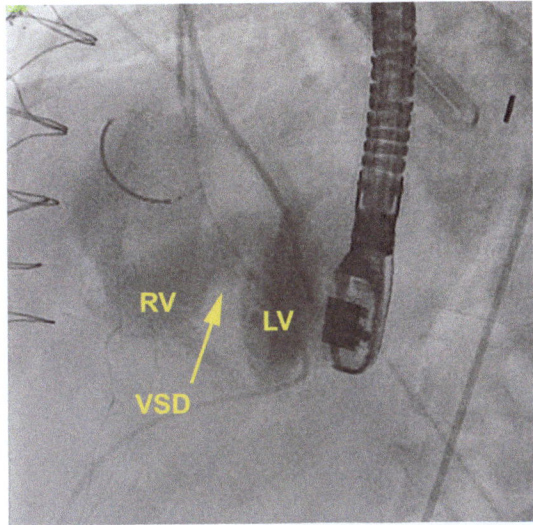

Fig. 13 LV angiogram shows the LV, VSD and RV. Note the tricuspid ring placed at the time of surgery

The heart team reconvened, and we decided that another more aggressive attempt at transcatheter PMI-VSD closure was warranted.

Cath Procedure #2

On post-op day 17 the patient was brought back to the cath lab. Access was obtained in the RFV (12 Fr) and RFA (6 Fr). Angiography from the LV showed a large VSD (Fig. 13). The VSD was crossed retrograde in a similar fashion to attempt #1 and the wire snared in the pulmonary artery and exteriorized. This time, balloon sizing with a 24 mm Amplatzer sizing balloon was performed. The balloon waist measured 19 mm (Fig. 14). Given the prior difficulty with the device pulling through the defect, we decided we needed a device with a waist ~1.5 × the size of the defect. A 30 mm Amplatzer Septal Occluder was chosen. This device has a central waist measuring 30 mm and a left disk that is 44 mm and a right atrial disk that is 42 mm. The femoral sheath was upsized to a 16 Fr short sheath and a 12 Fr Amplatzer delivery sheath passed from the femoral vein through the defect and out the aorta. The left disk was opened in the LV and pulsed flush against the septum (Fig. 15). TEE showed the left disk to be close to, but not touching the mitral valve (Fig. 16). The right disk was then uncovered. Initially the RV disk had a "cobra-head" shape that can occur when there is insufficient room for the disk to form or when there is torque on the device, however the device was stable and was unscrewed from the delivery cable and released (Fig. 17). Over the course of the next 5 min, the right disk slowly reoriented to a more nominal shape.

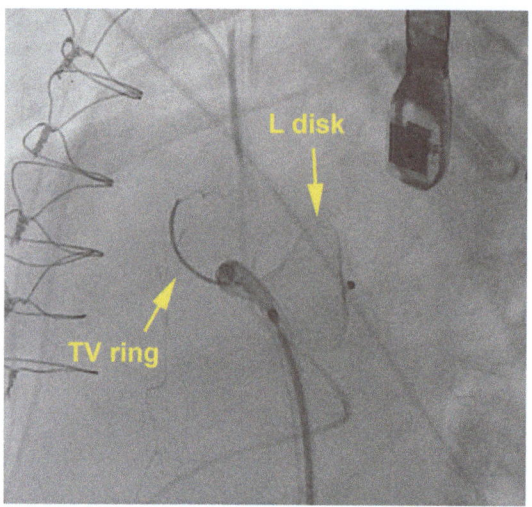

Fig. 15 A 30 mm Amplatzer Septal Occluder was advanced through a 12 Fr delivery sheath. The Left disk was opened in the LV and pulsed flush against the septum

Repeat hemodynamics were much improved with a Qp/Qs of 1.2:1 with a small residual VSD through the device fabric by angiography (Fig. 18) and TEE. TEE also confirmed no increase in tricuspid regurgitation (Fig. 19).

Post Procedural Assessment

The patient improved considerably after the transcatheter VSD closure. The IABP was able to be removed 2 days later and she weaned off all inotropic support. He renal function did not recover and she required a tunneled dialysis catheter. At the time of tunneled dialysis catheter placement 2 weeks after device placement, her hemodynamics were repeated showing a Qp/Qs of 1.14:1 and a wedge pressure of 11 mmHg. Fluoroscopy showed the disks to have reformed

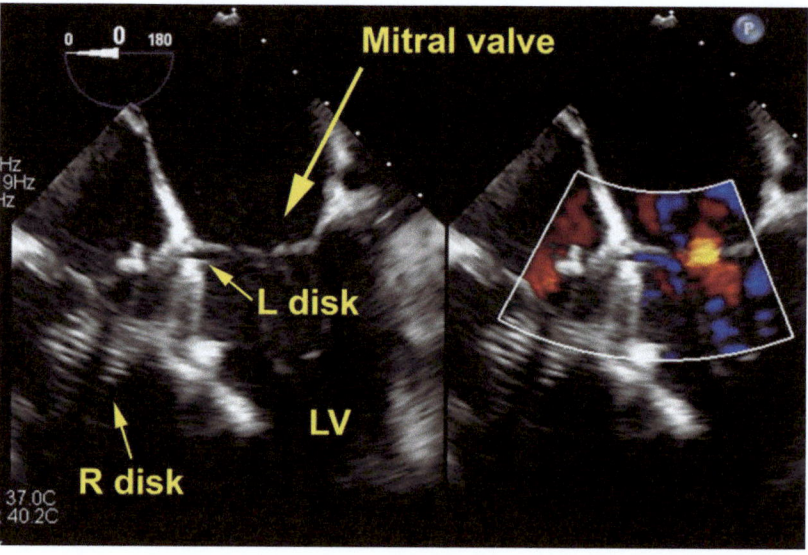

Fig. 16 TEE during deployment of the 30 mm Amplatzer Septal Occluder shows the L disk flush against the septum. The superior aspect of the left disk is close to but doesn't touch the mitral valve annulus

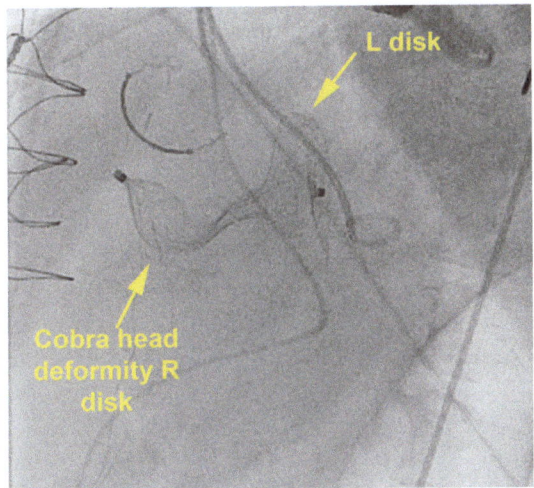

Fig. 17 The right-risk of the 30 mm Amplatzer occluder took a "cobra-head" deformity but we chose to release the device as it was stable

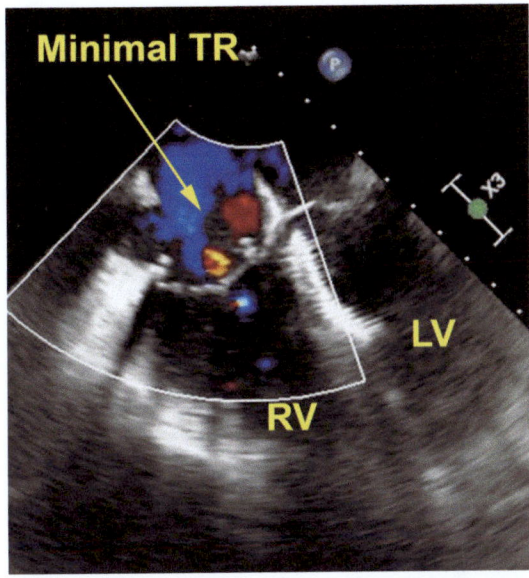

Fig. 19 TEE post-deployment showing the LV disk flush against the septum. Minimal tricuspid regurgitation

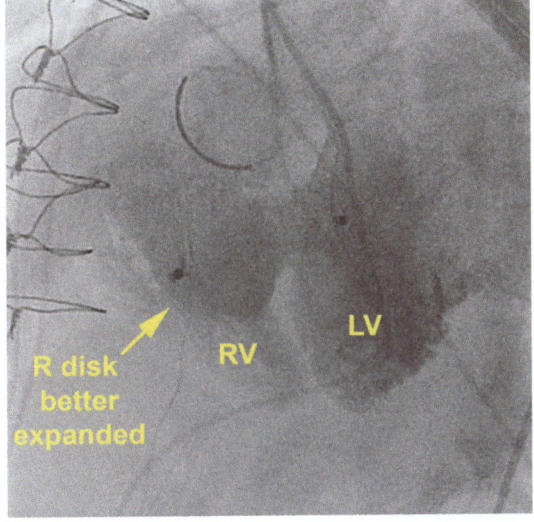

Fig. 18 After 5 min, the device reconfigured and the R sided disk was better expanded. LV angiogram shows some residual flow through the fabric of the device. Note the central waist appears to be completely flush against the VSD margins so we expect the residual flow to diminish/disappear

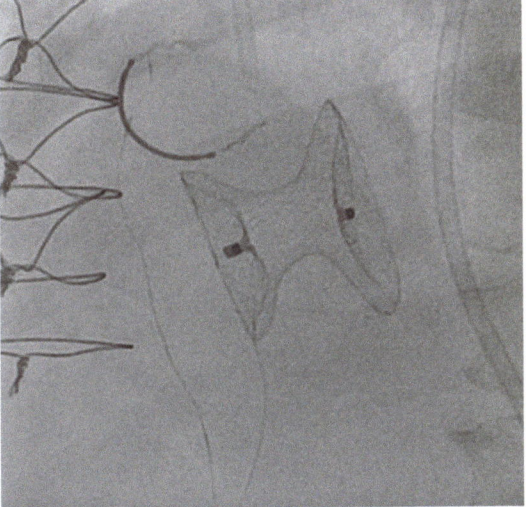

Fig. 20 Fluoroscopy 2 weeks later showing the device has further conformed to its nominal shape

to nominal shape (Fig. 20). Transthoracic echocardiogram showed the device in stable position across the septum with no significant residual shunt and no interference with the mitral or tricuspid valves both with trace-mild regurgitation only (Fig. 21).

The patient was discharged to a rehabilitation facility 3 weeks post-device closure and successfully weaned off the ventilator and discharged home 2 months later.

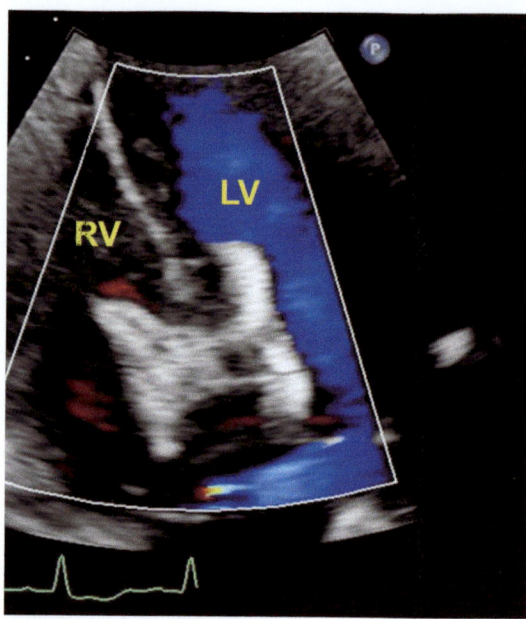

Fig. 21 Transthoracic echocardiogram 2 weeks after placement of the 30 mm Amplatzer Septal Occluder to close the large residual PMI-VSD. No significant residual shunt and no interference with AV valves

Clinical Controversies and Clinical Pearls

- Echo derived Qp:Qs are not accurate and shunt calculations from oxygen saturations is necessary to confirm shunt severity in post MI VSD's.
- Hemodynamic stabilization by dropping SVR and increasing CO is key to decreasing left to right shunt, supporting patient to the time of PMI-VSD closure.
- PMI-VSD's always appear smaller on echocardiography and sizing should be 1.5 times larger than imaging predicts.

Key Points
- PMI-VSD remains a difficult problem. Surgical and transcatheter approaches for hemodynamically significant VSDs with shock are difficult and continue to have a high mortality.
- The best outcomes for transcatheter PMI-VSD closure occur after attempted surgical closure or if the patient can be managed medically for several weeks to allow for the margins of the VSD to become better defined. This may not be possible with large PMI-VSDs.
- Specific devices for transcatheter PMI-VSD closure are often too small for the largest, hemodynamically significant defects but other off-label devices such as ASD Occluders can be used.

Multimodality imaging comparison (table format)

Modality	Advantages	Disadvantages
Transthoracic echo	Can be easily performed bedside	Often underestimates extent of VSD
Transesophageal echo	Better imaging of VSD	More invasive Tends to foreshorten apex also underestimating extent of VSD
Angiography	Better visualization of VSD size	Invasive Doesn't visualize adjacent structures will e.g.: valves Many patients have renal dysfunction increasing risk of contrast nephropathy
CT angiography	Excellent definition of VSD	Usually not able to be performed in patients in critical care

Disclosures Dr. Love is a proctor and consultant for Abbott Laboratories.

Chapter Review Questions

An 84 year old woman presents with shortness of breath after 1 week of chest pain. She is found to have an evolving myocardial infarction. She has a holosystolic murmur at the apex and an echocardiogram shows an LVEF of ~60% and an apical post-MI VSD. The patient has cool extremities and minimal urine output. A Swan-Ganz catheter is placed and a pulmonary artery saturation is 82% with the patient breathing room air. Thermodilution cardiac output is performed and shows a CO of 7 LPM. PA pressure 50/22 (38).

1. Which of the statements is true:
   A. We should be worried—the patient is in shock
   B. We should be reassured—the patient has good cardiac output
   C. We should be reassured—the patient has a small VSD
   D. We should be reassured—the patient has a normal LVEF

   Answer: A

   Explanation: Cool extremities and low urine output indicate shock. The high pulmonary artery saturation of 82% reflects left to right shunt secondary to what must be a significant VSD. The mixed venous saturation is best estimated by the SVC saturation would be low in this patient. Thermodilution will reflect the PULMONARY flow—not the systemic flow. The LVEF is often higher than expected in these patients owing to the low afterload because the majority of the blood is being offloaded to the low resistance pulmonary circuit.

2. To calculate the pulmonary to systemic flow ratio (Qp/Qs) we need the following additional data:
   A. Right atrial and aortic saturation
   B. SVC and aortic saturation
   C. Pulmonary capillary wedge and aortic saturations
   D. Cannot calculate Qp/Qs in this scenario

   Answer: B

   Explanation: In a patient with a large post-MI VSD, the ratio of pulmonary:systemic flow (Qp/Qs) can be calculated with the aid of a pulmonary artery catheter. The formula is as follows:

   Qp/Qs = Aortic sat (%) − Mixed venous sat (%)/Pulmonary vein sat (%) − Pulmonary artery sat (%). The SVC saturation obtained from the side port of an internal jugular vein sheath is the best proxy for a mixed venous saturation. Noteworthy to add that RA sampling can miss small left-to-right shunt due to incomplete mixing of blood entering from SVC, IVC and coronary sinus. The aortic saturation is the arterial saturation obtained from an arterial line or pulse oximeter. The pulmonary vein saturation is the same as the aortic saturation as there is no significant right to left shunt in this lesion, and the pulmonary artery saturation is obtained from the pulmonary artery catheter.

3. Medical optimization of this patient would be best achieved with
   A. Norepinephrine
   B. Intraaortic balloon pump
   C. Epinephrine
   D. Inhaled nitric oxide

   Answer: B

   Explanation: Epinephrine and norepinephrine would increase the systemic vascular resistance and worsen the shunting and worsen systemic output. IABP lowers the systemic resistance favoring systemic flow. The pulmonary artery pressure is high due to high left to right flow. Nitric oxide would further lower the pulmonary vascular resistance and worsen left to right shunt at the VSD.

4. Contraindication for transcatheter post-MI VSD closure in this patient would be
   A. Renal failure
   B. Defect size >10 mm
   C. Apical location
   D. Mitral valve chordal rupture with severe MR

   Answer: D

   Explanation: Additional defects that require surgical repair are contraindications to transcatheter PMI-VSD closure.

5. After successful VSD closure, the patient's LVEF compared to pre-closure would be expected to
   A. Remain the same
   B. Increase
   C. Decrease

   Answer: C

   Explanation: With VSD closure, the lower afterload of the pulmonary system is eliminated and the volume load on the left ventricle decreases. Both the increase in afterload and the decrease in preload will make the LVEF decrease even though the cardiac muscle ability is unchanged.

References

1. Crenshaw BS, Granger CB, Birnbaum Y, Pieper KS, Morris DC, Kleiman NS, et al. Risk factors, angiographic patterns, and outcomes in patients with ventricular septal defect complicating acute myocardial infarction. GUSTO-I (global utilization of streptokinase and TPA for occluded coronary arteries) trial investigators. Circulation. 2000;101:27–32.
2. La Torre MW, Centofanti P, Attisani M, Patane F, Rinaldi M. Posterior ventricular septal defect in presence of cardiogenic shock: early implantation of the impella recover LP 5.0 as a bridge to surgery. Tex Heart Inst J. 2011;38:42–9.
3. Hobbs R, Korutla V, Suzuki Y, et al. Mechanical circulatory support as a bridge to definitive surgical repair after post-myocardial infarct ventricular septal defect. J Card Surg. 2015;30:535–40.
4. Lee WY, Cardon L, Slodki SJ. Perforation of infarcted interventricular septum. Report of a case with prolonged survival, diagnosed ante mortem by cardiac catheterization, and review of the literature. Arch Intern Med. 1962;109:731–41.
5. Arnaoutakis GJ, Zhao Y, George TJ, Sciortino CM, McCarthy PM, Conte JV. Surgical repair of ventricular septal defect after myocardial infarction: outcomes from the Society of Thoracic Surgeons National Database. Ann Thorac Surg. 2012;94:436–43.
6. O'Gara PT, Kushner FG, Ascheim DD, et al. 2013 ACCF/AHA guideline for the management of ST-elevation myocardial infarction: a report of the American College of Cardiology Foundation/American Heart Association task force on practice guidelines. J Am Coll Cardiol. 2013;61:e78–e140.
7. Thiele H, Kaulfersch C, Daehnert I, Schoenauer M, Eitel I, Borger M, et al. Immediate primary transcatheter closure of postinfarction ventricular septal defects. Eur Heart J. 2009;30:81–8.
8. Bialkowski J, Szkutnik M, Kusa J, Kalarus Z, Gasior M, Przybylski R, et al. Transcatheter closure of postinfarction ventricular septal defects using Amplatzer devices. Rev Esp Cardiol. 2007;60:548–51.
9. Landzberg M, Lock JE. Transcatheter management of ventricular septal Pupture after myocardial infarction. Semin Thorac Cardiovasc Surg. 1998;10(2):128–32.
10. Holzer R, Balzer D, Amin Z, Ruiz CE, Feinstein J, Bass J, Vance M, Cao QL, Hijazi ZM. Transcatheter closure of postinfarction ventricular septal defects using the new Amplatzer muscular VSD occluder: results of a U.S. Registry. Catheter Cardiovasc Interv. 2004;61:196–201.

Part III

Interventions in Heart Failure

Interatrial Shunt Devices

Taimur Safder, Sanjiv Shah, and Akhil Narang

Abstract

Heart failure with preserved ejection fraction (HFpEF) remains difficult to manage while contributing to high morbidity and mortality. It is a complex disease state with a pathophysiology based in a multitude of contributing factors. One common aspect of HFpEF is the presence of increased LV end diastolic pressure (LVEDP) resulting in elevated left atrial (LA) pressure. Increased LA pressure may also be the best guide in assessing if dyspnea is the result of elevated LA pressures leading to pulmonary congestion. In this chapter, we will discuss the evolving field of interatrial shunt devices (IASD) which target elevated LA pressures as a possible therapeutic option in patients with HFpEF. This chapter will discuss prevalence, morbidity and mortality of HFpEF, along with the pathophysiology of elevated left atrial pressures in HFpEF, and treatment options using interatrial shunt devices. Lastly, an example case of a patient undergoing an IASD placement with pre, intra and post procedural imaging guidance will be reviewed.

Keywords

Heart failure with preserved ejection fraction treatment · Heart failure with mild range ejection fraction treatment · Interatrial shunt device · Left atrial hypertension · Diastolic dysfunction

Abbreviations

ACEi	Angiotensin-converting enzyme inhibitors
ARB	Angiotensin II receptor blockers
ARNI	Angiotensin receptor-neprilysin inhibitor
CABG	Coronary artery bypass graft
CAD	Coronary artery disease
EF	Ejection fraction
HF	Heart failure
HFimrEF	Heart failure with improved EF
HFmrEF	Heart failure with mildly reduced ejection fraction
HFrEF	Heart failure with reduced ejection fraction

Supplementary Information The online version contains supplementary material available at https://doi.org/10.1007/978-3-031-50740-3_9.

T. Safder · S. Shah (✉) · A. Narang
Bluhm Cardiovascular Institute, Northwestern Memorial Hospital, Chicago, IL, USA
e-mail: Taimur.Safder@nm.org; Sanjiv.Shah@northwestern.edu; Akhil.Narang@nm.org

IAS	Interatrial septum
IASD	Interatrial shunt device
KCCQ	Kansas City Cardiomyopathy Questionnaire
LA	Left atrium
LV	Left ventricle
LVEDP	Left ventricle end diastolic pressure
MRA	Mineralocorticoid receptor antagonists
PA	Pulmonary artery
PCWP	Pulmonary capillary wedge pressure
PVD	Pulmonary vascular disease
PVR	Pulmonary vascular resistance
RA	Right atrium
RV	Right ventricle
WU	Wood units

Test your learning and check your understanding of this book's contents: use the "Springer Nature Flashcards" app to access questions using ▶ https://sn.pub/ambACS. To use the app, please follow the instructions in the chapter "Transcatheter Aortic Valve Replacement."

Learning Objectives

1. Review prevalence, morbidity and mortality and the definitions of HFpEF.
2. Understand the interplay of HFpEF and left atrial hypertension and how left atrial decompression may be a viable and effective treatment option in patients with HFpEF.
3. Review the currently available literature in the field of interatrial shunts for HFpEF.
4. Understand the factors that are important to identify in the pre-procedural stage that could make the imaging and the procedure more challenging.
5. Understand the key steps for a IASD procedure and the optimal imaging needed to support it.
6. Understand post procedural imaging goals and possible complications that can occur.

Case Study

A 70-year-old male presents to clinic for worsening dyspnea. He has a history of CAD status post three vessel coronary artery bypass graft, HFpEF, permanent atrial fibrillation status post left atrial appendage occlusion device, hypertension, hyperlipidemia and obesity. Patient reports he can only walk 1–2 blocks before having significant dyspnea that limits his activity.

Transthoracic echocardiogram was notable for normal LV size and function (LVEF 65%), mildly dilated RV, bi-atrial enlargement, no significant valvular abnormalities. LV global longitudinal strain −15%.

For further evaluation of etiology of the patient's symptoms, a right heart catheterization (RHC) with exercise bike was done with results noted in Table 1.

Table 1 RHC with exercise bike results prior to IASD

	Rest	Peak exercise
RA (mean, mmHg)	6	22
RV (mean, mmHg)	8	
PA (mean, mmHg)	29	51
PCWP (mmHg)	11	32
CI (L/min/m^2)	2.5	3.6
PVR (woods units)	3.5	

Background and Definitions

Despite significant advances in the field of heart failure (HF) management, HF remains a challenging diagnosis for clinicians. The combined prevalence of HFpEF and HFmrEF exceeds HFrEF and possess a significant challenge to clinicians [1–5]. HFpEF, and to a certain extent HFmrEF, represent a distinct entity than HFrEF [6] (Table 2). HFpEF, in particular, is a complex multiorgan syndrome that has layers of different pathophysiological mechanisms that are built upon the traditional diastolic heart failure paradigm. Despite this complex underpinning of

HFpEF, one common thread that binds these patients is elevated LVEDP and LA pressure at rest and/or with exercise [7]. Elevated LVEDP leads to an increased LA pressure and remodeling, which further leads to increased pulmonary pressures and lung gas exchange abnormalities resulting in the characteristic symptom of dyspnea [8]. With modest success of medical therapies, one new focus of treatment in HFpEF and HFmrEF patients has become ways to help reduce the elevated LA pressure.

Left atrial decompression by a way of an iatrogenic interatrial shunt is one strategy currently being investigated. This strategy developed from historical observations of patients with left sided valvular disease and atrial septal defects (ASD), such as Lutembacher syndrome. These patients were found to tolerate their valvular disease better than patients with valvular disease but no ASD. In addition, closure of ASDs has shown to result in abrupt increases of LA pressure and HF exacerbations [1] (Fig. 1). Utilizing this framework, this novel device-based treatment strategy of iatrogenic interatrial shunt is currently being pursued and several shunt devices are in various stages of development for patients with HF (Fig. 2).

Data from clinical trials using the Corvia IASD device has been promising (Fig. 3). Phase I data from the REDUCE LAP-HF trials demonstrated safety and efficacy of the Corvia IASD device in patients with LVEF ≥40% (Table 3). Although the overall phase 3 randomized control trial failed to show an overall difference in the primary end point (CVD death or non-fatal ischemic stroke at 12 months, total HF events up to 24 months, and change in KCCQ overall summary score at 12 months) between sham and treatment arm, the study did note a positive signal of benefit in patients without PVD (PVR <1.8 WU). This may represent a subsegment of patients that may benefit from IASD therapy [9]. At this stage, IASD therapy remains promising and further studies are needed to establish it as an evidence based therapy for HF patients.

Table 2 Definitions of HF by LVEF, adapted from ACC/AHA/HFSA 2022 HF guidelines

HF types	Definition
HF with reduced EF	LVEF ≤40%
HF with improved EF	Previous LVEF ≤40% but now LVEF ≥40%
HF with mildly reduced EF	LVEF 41–49%
HF with preserved EF	LVEF ≥50%

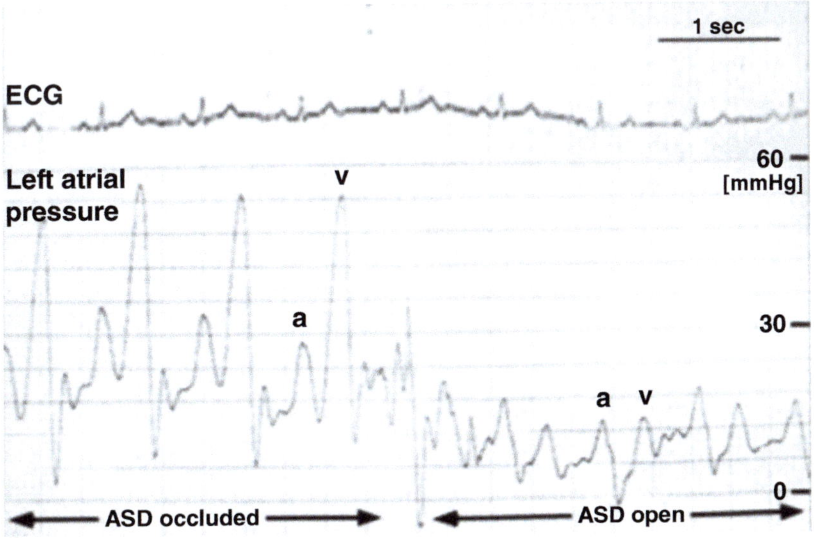

Fig. 1 Left atrial pressure tracing showing increased LA pressures when ASD is occluded and decrease of LA pressures when ASD is opened

Device	Corvia	V-Wave	Occlutech	Edwards	Alleviant	NoYA	InterShunt
Type	Implant	Implant	Implant	Implant	Procedure	Procedure	Procedure
Description	Nitinol stent	Nitinol/PTFE hourglass	Nitinol braid with central orifice	Tubular nitinol device with retention arms	Coring catheter	RF catheter	Cutting catheter
Shunt flow	LA → RA	LA → RA	LA → RA	LA → CS	LA → RA	LA → RA	LA → RA
Shunt size	8 mm	5.1 mm	4, 6, 8, 10 mm	7 mm	6 mm	4-12 mm	4 mm
Development stage	Phase 3 RCT	Phase 3 RCT	Open-label studies	FIH complete	Animal studies	FIH complete	FIH complete

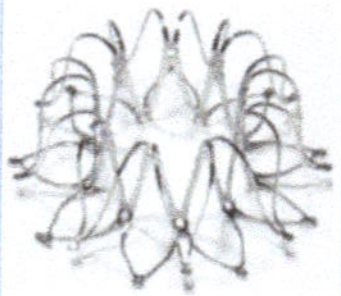

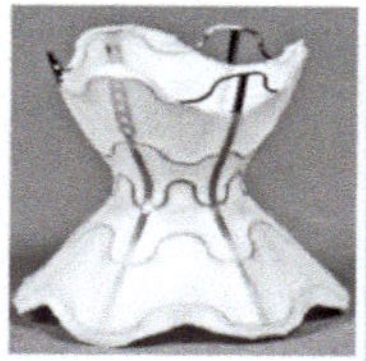

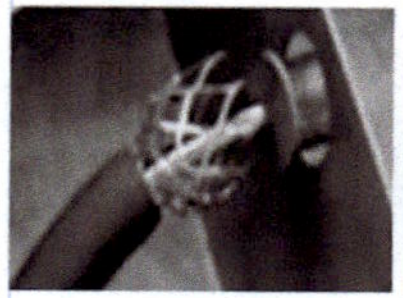

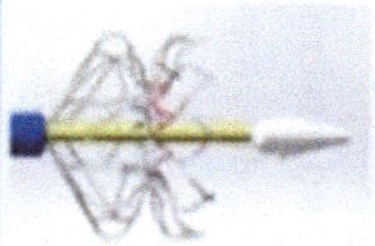

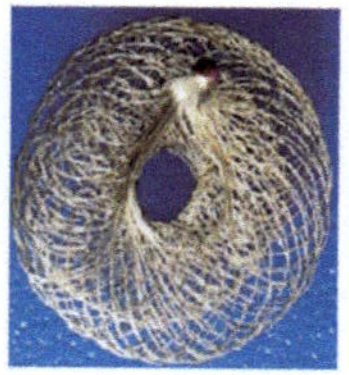

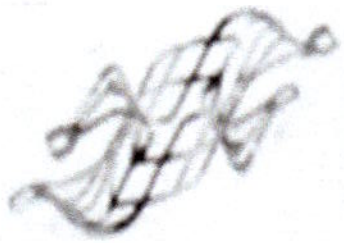

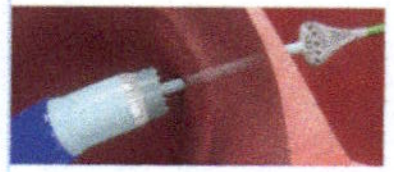

Fig. 2 List of the current interatrial shunt devices/procedures under investigation

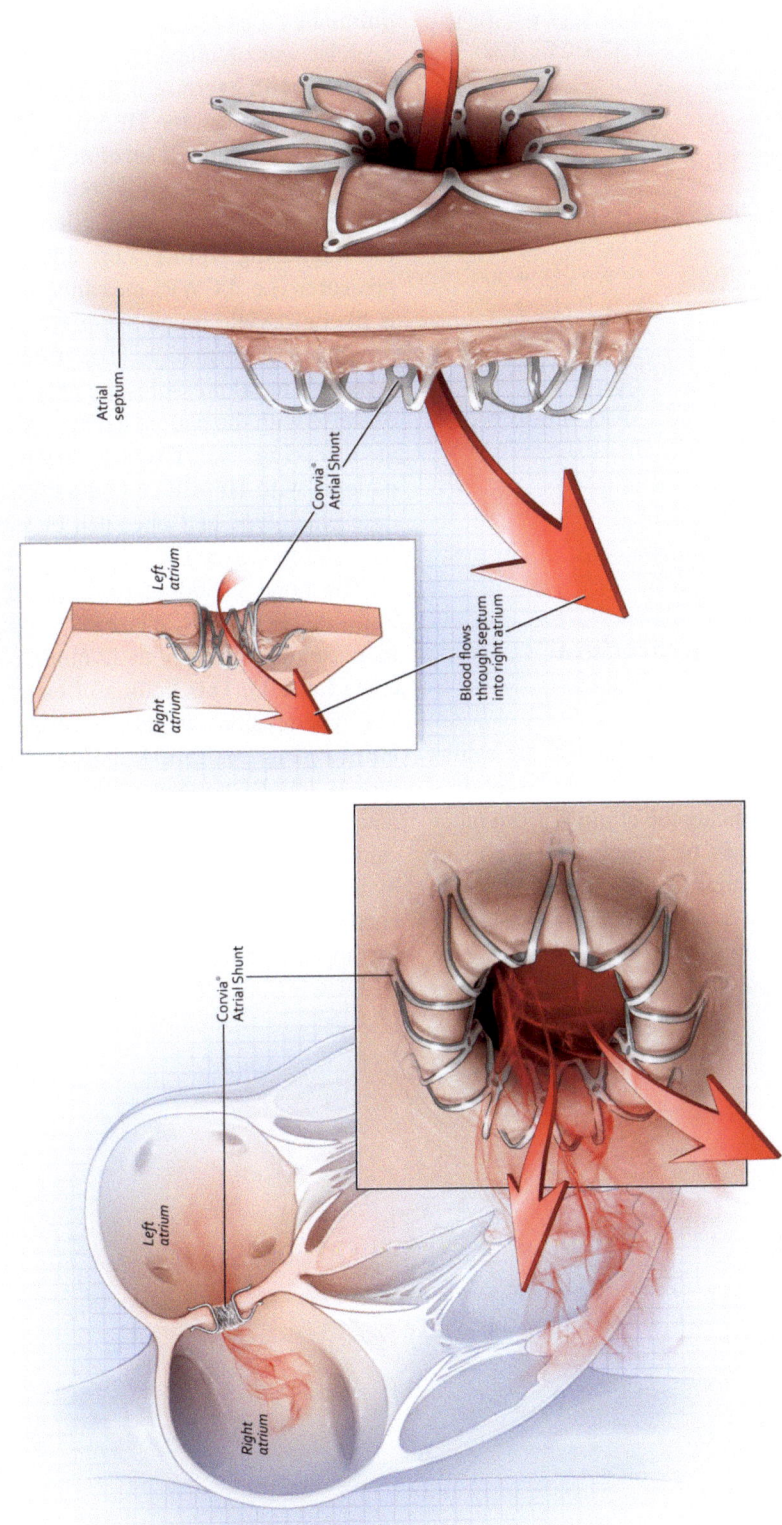

Fig. 3 Proposed mode of action for Corvia device: dynamic decompression of overloaded LA chamber by shunting blood from LA → RA (Qp:Qs 1.2–1.3)

Table 3 Summary of REDUCE LAP-HF trials

	Shah et al. REDUCE LAP-HF II (2022)
Baseline characteristics	
N	314 (treatment arm)
Age (years)	73 (median)
Male (%)	36
LVEF (%)	60 (median)
PCWP at rest (mmHg) Baseline Post-procedure	Percent of patients with: PCWP <15 → 30% PCWP >15 → 70%
Functional status outcomes	
NYHA Baseline Post-procedure	Change in median NYHA −0.5 (−1 to 0)**
Median change in KCCQ (IQR) from baseline to 12 months	10.2 (−1.8 to 26.8)*

*Not statistically significant
**Statistically significant

Diagnosis and Pre-procedural Assessment

When patients with suspected HFpEF are evaluated for IASD, their symptoms must be interrogated fully as to delineate the etiology from other comorbidities that may be present in this patient population (i.e. anemia, COPD). Exercise stress echocardiogram can be a helpful tool in assessing diastolic dysfunction in patients presenting with unexplained dyspnea. After a comprehensive evaluation which excluded ischemia, anemia, or pulmonary disease in our patient, a RHC with exercise was obtained.

RHC with exercise is an important and often underutilized test for HFpEF. When done correctly and interpreted accurately, the information can be revealing. Resting measurements of cardiac filling pressures alone often lack sensitivity for diagnosing HFpEF. Left sided cardiac filling pressures (i.e. PCWP) measured during exercise is likely to yield much better HF diagnostic and prognostic information [10]. Occasionally elevated left atrial pressures are only elicited during exercise with the patient having normal pressures at rest (Fig. 4). Exercise hemodynamics in patients with HFpEF can help classify their disease phenotype and one such classification system is proposed in Fig. 5.

The notable finding from our patients RHC notes a resting PCWP of 13 mmHg, which increases significantly to 32 mmHg at peak exercise (Table 1). This finding of exercised induced LA hypertension categorizes our patient as type I HFpEF (Fig. 5). Type I, and to a smaller extent type II, HFpEF patients represent the ideal candidate for an IASD (Fig. 6). Patients with significant right heart failure and/or pulmonary arterial hypertension are unlikely to benefit from an IASD and are poor candidates for shunt based therapy (these patients were also excluded from REDUCE LAP-HF II trials).

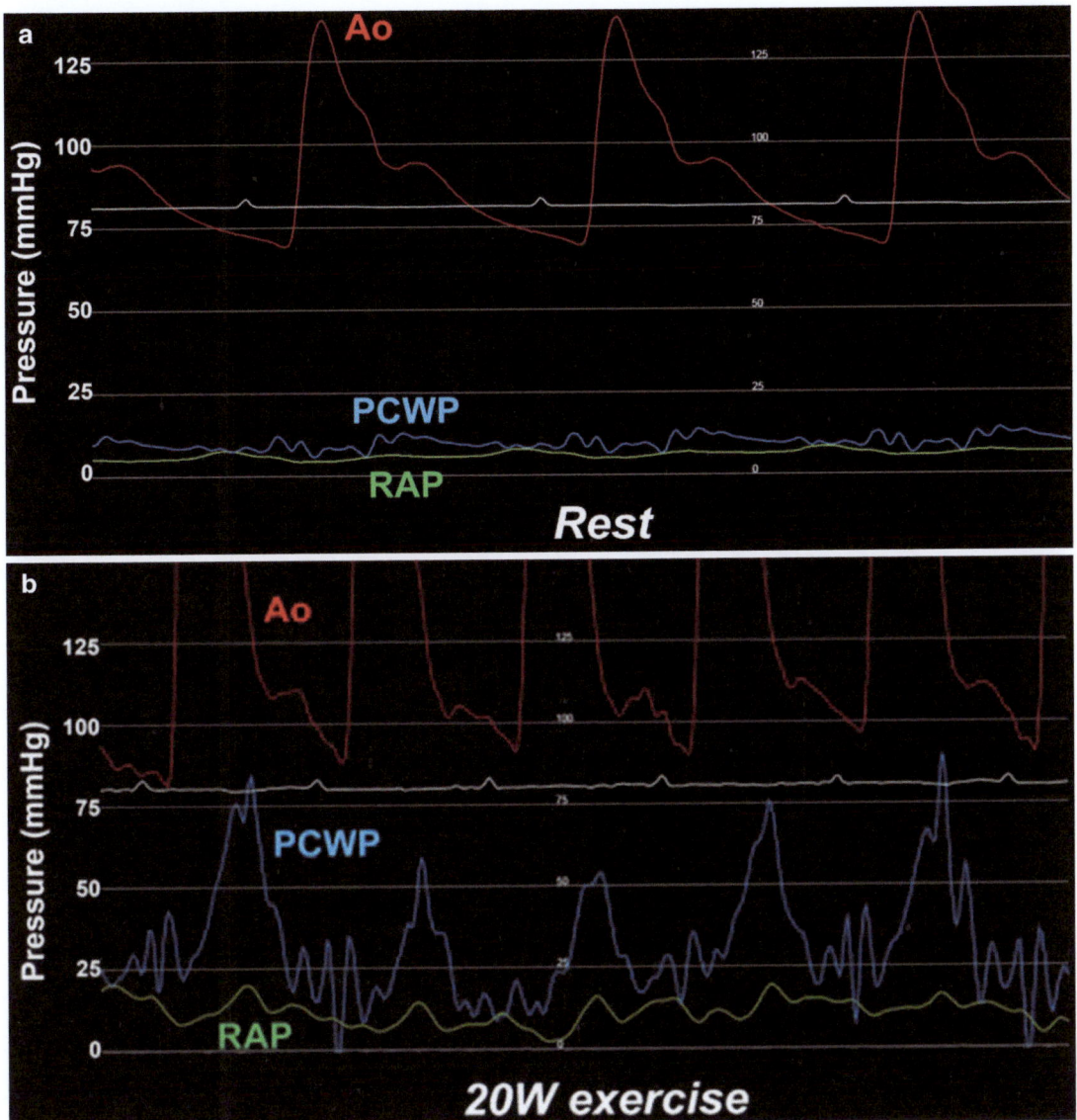

Fig. 4 Hemodynamic measurements at rest (Panel **a**) showing normal values and the same patient undergoing exercise with hemodynamic measurements (Panel **b**), showing significant increase in the PCWP

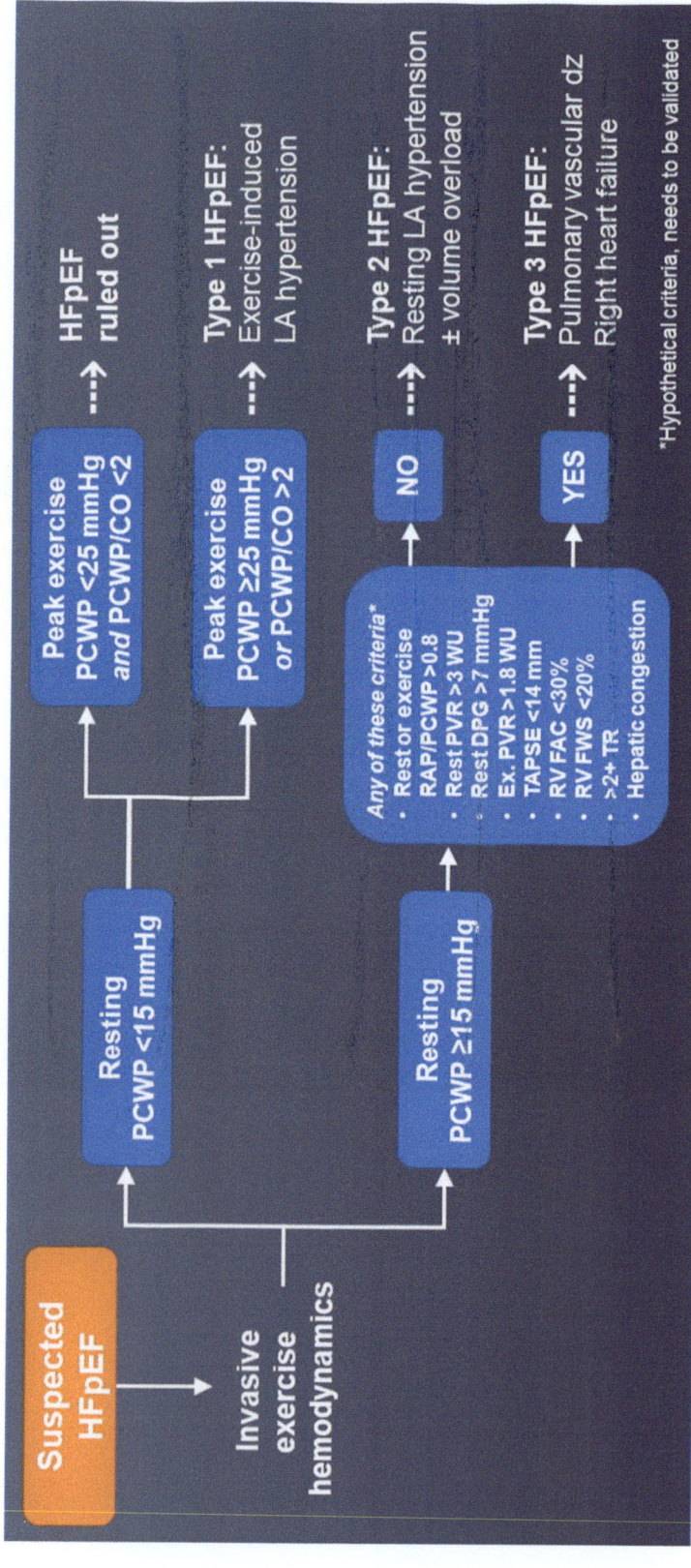

Fig. 5 Phenotype guided approach to HfpEF

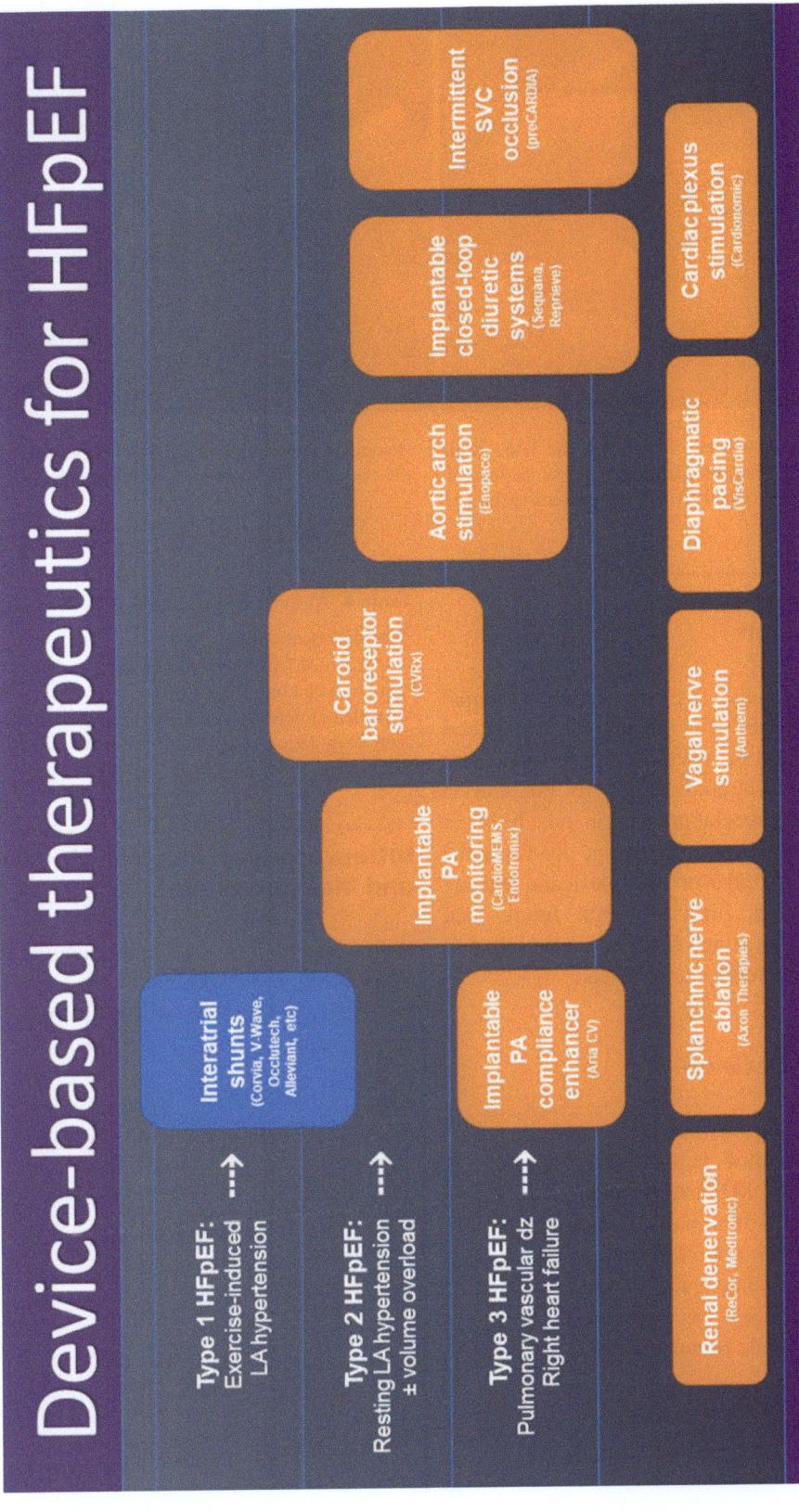

Fig. 6 Device based therapeutics for HFpEF

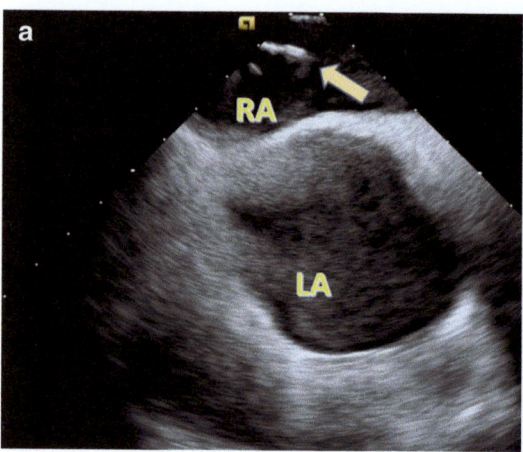 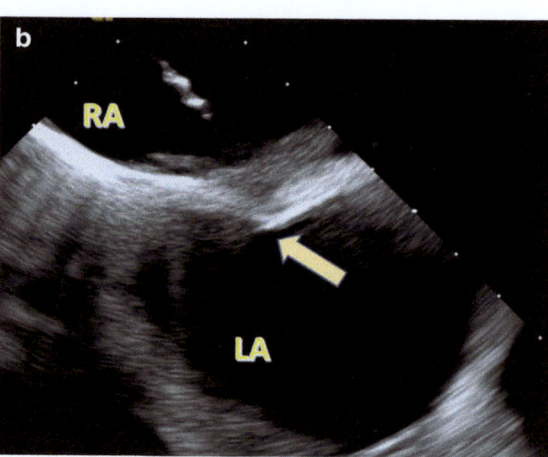

Fig. 7 ICE Bi-caval view visualizing the IAS. Right atrium (RA), Left atrium (LA), Arrow-points towards catheter tip in RA (Panel **a**) and shows tenting of IAS (Panel **b**) into LA at the optimal location of transeptal puncture, near the center of foramen ovale

Heart Team Approach and Discussion

Once a determination is made as to the potential benefit of an IASD for the patient, procedural feasibility should be assessed. While there are a few absolute contraindications to the Corvia IASD (Table 4), special precaution must be taken with the presence of intracardiac leads as the device could impinge or trap the leads causing lead malfunction, difficulty with future lead exchange or worsening of tricuspid regurgitation due to increased tension on the lead.

Heart Team Decision

Since our patient was confirmed to have type I HFpEF with hemodynamic exercise testing, it was likely he would benefit from an IASD based therapy option. Additionally, our patient did not meet any absolute contraindications and did not have any intracardiac leads and so likelihood of procedural success was deemed to be high. Decision was made to move forward with IASD implantation.

Table 4 Absolute contraindication for Corvia IASD

Absolute contraindications
HCM, constrictive pericarditis, infiltrative cardiomyopathies (i.e. amyloid, sarcoid)
Unable to tolerate procedural or post-procedural anti-coagulation/anti-platelet regimen
Significant RV dysfunction

Intraprocedural Imaging Modalities and Measurements

Below are the key steps and imaging highlights of an IASD, more specifically the Corvia device, deployment using ICE. Alternatively, a TEE can also be used for device deployment.

Key procedural steps	Key imaging highlights	Correlated video/figure
Transeptal puncture	– Confirm presence of adequate space for placement of IASD without impinging on other structures (20 mm diameter when fully deployed) – Optimal position of transeptal puncture is center of fossa ovalis	– Figure 7 – Video 1

Interatrial Shunt Devices

Key procedural steps	Key imaging highlights	Correlated video/figure
Delivery system guidance	– Aid in guidewire positioning in to the LA and pulmonary vein followed by advancing of delivery system over the wire and into the left atrium	– Figure 8
Device positioning	– The catheter tip should be positioned in the mid-LA cavity	
Device deployment	– The LA legs and barrel of the device are deployed first – Next, the delivery system is retracted until the LA legs make contact with the interatrial septum. A slight amount of tension is held on the septum with the LA legs while echocardiographic visualization confirms good positioning of the device and good LA legs-septal contact – While maintaining that slight tension on the septum, the RA legs are deployed – Deployment of the RA legs releases the device from the delivery system – It is important to note presence and positioning of any intra-cardiac leads as to avoid entrapment of the leads within the device	– Figures 9, 10, 11 and 12 – Videos 2, 3 and 4
Delivery system withdrawal	– Under fluoroscopic and echocardiographic guidance, confirm slow withdrawal and position of the delivery system into the RA – Once in the RA, the closed delivery system can be fully removed but the guidewire is kept in place until post deployment evaluation can confirm good device deployment and function	
Evaluation post deployment	– Proper positioning and function of the device is confirmed with echocardiographic and fluoroscopic imaging – Direction of shunt flow should be confirmed by echocardiography – After confirmation of proper placement and function of device, guidewire can be carefully removed as not to get it entangled within the device	– Figure 13 – Video 5

Post procedural Assessment

Possible adverse events associated with IASD implantation include the same risks associated with other cardiac catheterization procedure with instrument manipulation within the cardiovascular system. They range from access site complications, arrhythmias, to cardiac perforation,

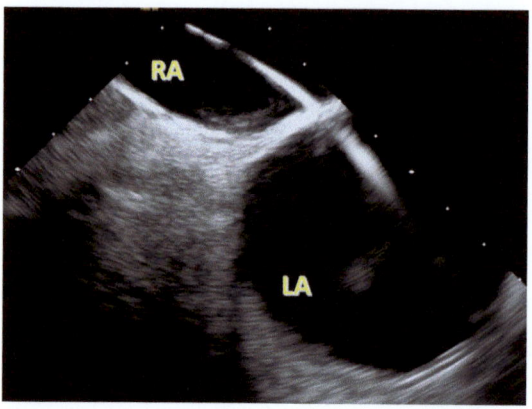

Fig. 8 ICE Bi-caval view confirming successful septal puncture and positing of guidewire in LA. Right atrium (RA), left atrium (LA)

tamponade and cardiac arrest to name a few notable ones. Complications related more specifically to the IASD device include embolization of the device, device thrombus formation, and intracardiac lead malfunction due to entrapment within the device.

Most patients, barring any procedural complications, recover well and are able to go home the next day. Our patient did well post-procedure and was discharged home the next day. Follow up plan can vary depending on institution protocols but follow up in clinic is typically in 1 month with a TTE follow up in 4–6 months. Decision on anti-platelet and anti-coagulation therapy varies with patient characteristics (i.e. atrial fibrilla-

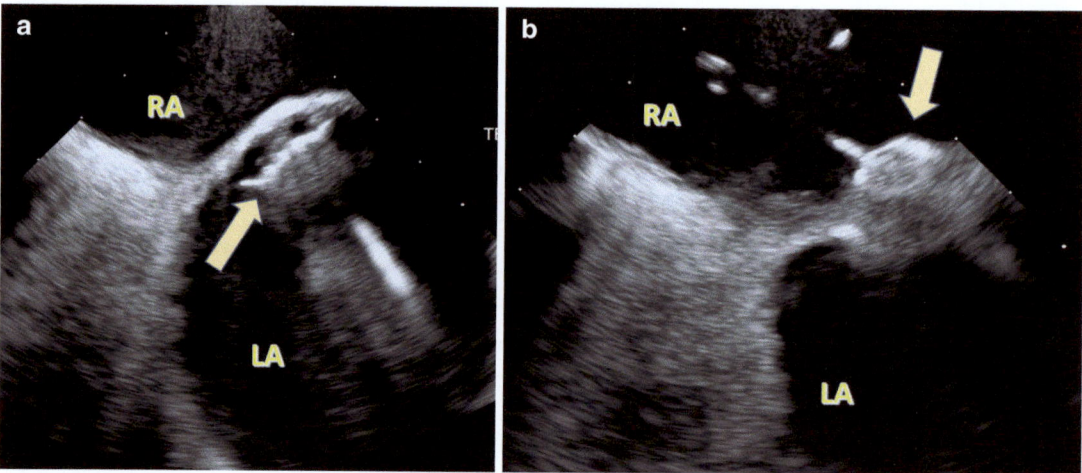

Fig. 9 ICE Bi-caval view. Arrow shows deployment of device legs on the LA side with septal contact (Panel **a**). Arrow (Panel **b**) shows deployment of device legs on the RA side

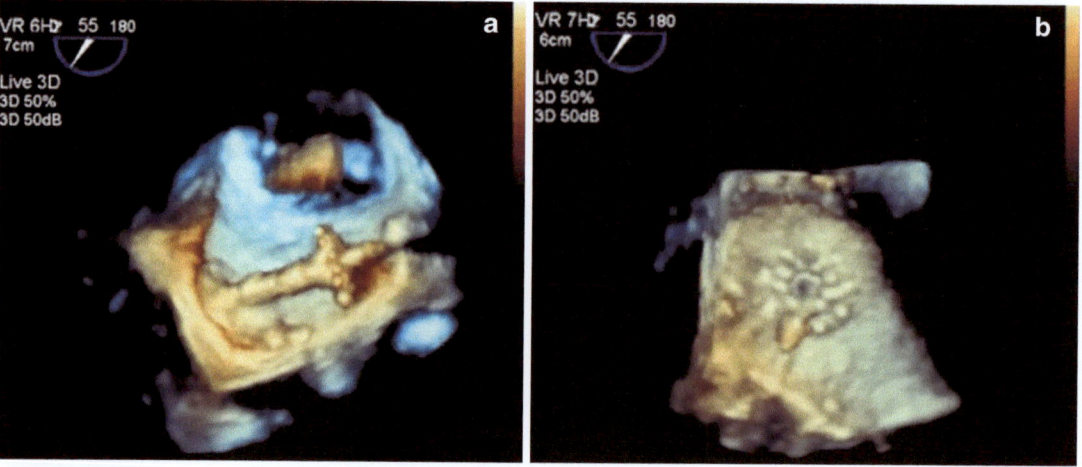

Fig. 10 TEE 3D image showing LA legs deployed in LA but prior to retraction of device towards the septum (Panel **a**), while panel **b** showing a fully deployed IASD device from LA

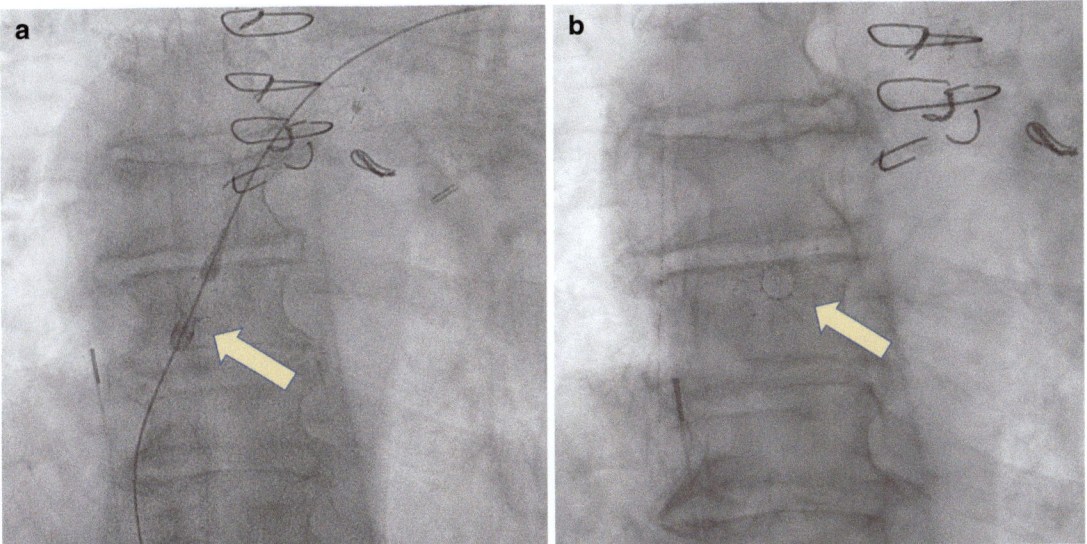

Fig. 11 RAO cranial fluoroscopic view shows (arrow) position of partially deployed device with legs in the LA (Panel **a**). RAO caudal fluoroscopic view showing (arrow) fully deployed device (Panel **b**)

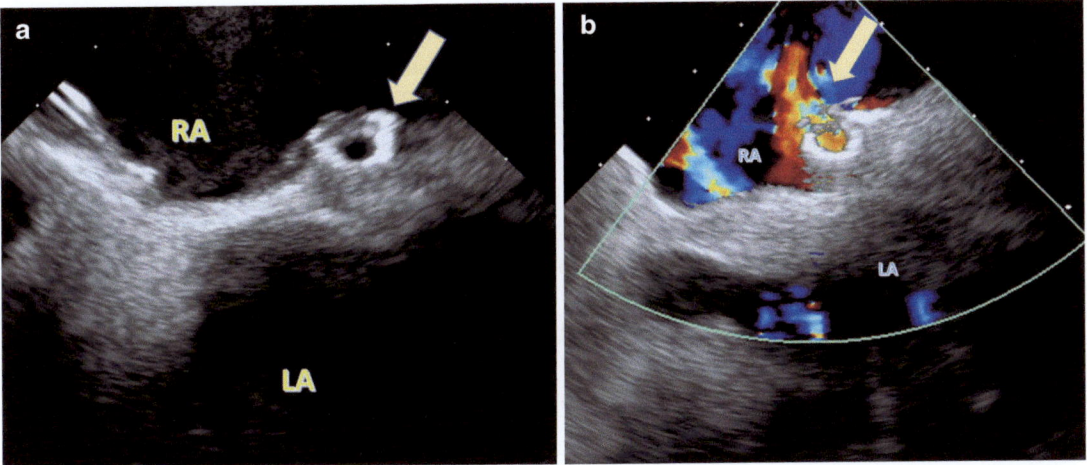

Fig. 12 Stable position of the device (arrow) immediately after deployment (Panel **a**) and color Doppler through the device where Left to right shunt flow (arrow) can be appreciated (Panel **b**). Right atrium (RA), left atrium (LA)

tion). But generally, dual anti-platelet therapy is administered for 6 months and then can typically be discontinued. If a patient is on oral anticoagulant for a different indication prior to device implantation, the OAC can continued post procedure. Our patient was on OAC due to his atrial fibrillation and he was instructed to continue his OAC at discharge.

At subsequent follow ups, our patient reported significant improvement in his dyspneic symptoms. At 4 months, patient reported he was able to walk a mile without significant symptoms. Patient was designated to have NYHA I–II symptoms (improved from NYHA III). His 6 month follow up TTE noted stable position of IASD and continued left to right shunt (Fig. 13).

Patients with HFpEF remain a challenging group of patients to manage but IASD therapy appears to be a promising therapeutic option in appropriately selected patients.

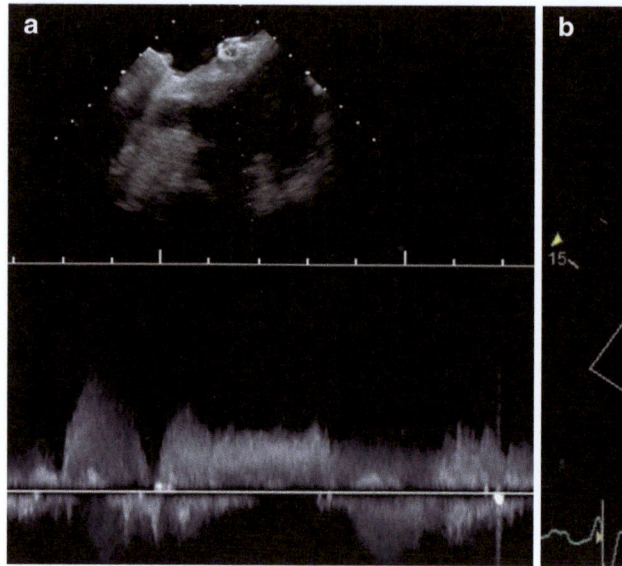

Fig. 13 ICE Bi-caval view with continuous wave Doppler through the device which shows predominantly continuous left to right shunt flow (Panel **a**). Six month follow up TTE (subcostal view) showing patent left to right flow from IASD (Panel **b**)

Key Points
- HFpEF is a complex disease process with a multifactorial etiology and thus treatment options for these patients must be individualized to their specific risk factors.
- Categorizing HFpEF patients by specific phenotypic classes (type I, II or III) may help guide device based therapy.
- Symptomatic HFpEF patients with elevated LA pressures but without significant PH or RV dysfunction, may benefit from LA decompression therapy with an ISAD.

Chapter Review Questions

1. In the context of findings from REDUCE LAP-HF II trial, a patient with which of the following hemodynamic profile might benefit from a IASD therapy?
    A. Peak exercise PCWP 14 mmHg, Exercise PVR 1 WU, TAPSE 20 mm, RV FAC 45%
    B. Peak exercise PCWP 26 mmHg, Exercise PVR 3 WU, TAPSE 20 mm, RV FAC 45%
    C. Peak exercise PCWP 26 mmHg, Exercise PVR 1.4 WU, TAPSE 20 mm, RV FAC 45%
    D. Peak exercise PCWP 26 mmHg, Exercise PVR 1.4 WU, TAPSE 8 mm, RV FAC 20%

Answers
A. Incorrect. These are essentially normal values and would not benefit from a IASD
B. Incorrect. While this patient does have elevated left sided cardiac pressures, as evidenced by an elevated exercise PCWP, the significant PVD (PVR 3 WU) likely makes this patient a poor candidate for IASD therapy
C. Correct answer. This patient might benefit from IASD therapy. In a sub-group analysis of REDUE LAP-HF II, a positive signal was found in patients with elevated left sided pressures but without significant PVD(peak exercise PVR <1.74 WU).
D. Incorrect. The significant RV dysfunction in this patient makes them a poor candidate for IASD therapy as these patients were excluded from IASD trials.

2. Which of the following is not an absolute contraindication for the Corvia IASD?
   A. Intracardiac leads
   B. Severe RV dysfunction
   C. Infiltrative cardiomyopathy
   D. Recent history of life threatening bleeding episode

   Answer

   Correct answer A. Presence of intracardiac leads should be noted pre-procedurally and caution should be taken during procedure as not to entangle device with leads but it does not preclude placement of an IASD as a possible treatment option. The other choices are all absolute contraindications.

3. What is the optimal position for a transeptal puncture for the Corvia IASD?
   A. Center of fossa ovalis
   B. Midpoint of IAS
   C. Anywhere in the top 1/3 of IAS
   D. Anywhere in the bottom 1/3 of IAS

   Answer

   Correct Answer A. Center of fossa ovalis is the most optimal position for transeptal puncture.

4. Which of the following classes of medications have shown mortality benefit in patients with HFpEF?
   A. Beta blockers
   B. ACEi/ARBs
   C. ARNI
   D. SGLT2 inhibitors
   E. None of the above

   Correct answer D. So far, only SGLT2 inhibitors have shown mortality benefit in a robust RCT in patients with HFpEF. EMPEROR-PRESERVED showed that SGLT2 use reduced the combined risk of CVD death or HF hospitalization in HFpEF patients.

References

1. Emani S, Burkhoff D, Lilly SM. Interatrial shunt devices for the treatment of heart failure. Trends Cardiovasc Med. 2021;31(7):427–32. https://doi.org/10.1016/J.TCM.2020.09.004.
2. Maggioni AP, Dahlström U, Filippatos G, et al. EURObservational research Programme: regional differences and 1-year follow-up results of the heart failure pilot survey (ESC-HF pilot). Eur J Heart Fail. 2013;15(7):808–17. https://doi.org/10.1093/EURJHF/HFT050.
3. Tsao CW, Lyass A, Enserro D, et al. Temporal trends in the incidence of and mortality associated with heart failure with preserved and reduced ejection fraction. JACC Hear Fail. 2018;6(8):678–85. https://doi.org/10.1016/J.JCHF.2018.03.006.
4. Roger VL. Epidemiology of heart failure. Circ Res. 2021;128:1421–34. https://doi.org/10.1161/CIRCRESAHA.121.318172.
5. Heidenreich PA, Bozkurt B, Aguilar D, et al. 2022 AHA/ACC/HFSA guideline for the management of heart failure: a report of the American College of Cardiology/American Heart Association joint committee on clinical practice guidelines. Circulation. 2022;145(18):e895–e1032. https://doi.org/10.1161/CIR.0000000000001063.
6. Borlaug BA, Redfield MM. Diastolic and systolic heart failure are distinct phenotypes within the heart failure spectrum. Circulation. 2011;123(18):2006–13. https://doi.org/10.1161/CIRCULATIONAHA.110.954388.
7. Shah SJ, Borlaug BA, Kitzman DW, et al. Research priorities for heart failure with preserved ejection fraction: National Heart, Lung, and Blood Institute working group summary. Circulation. 2020;141:1001–26. https://doi.org/10.1161/CIRCULATIONAHA.119.041886.
8. Griffin JM, Borlaug BA, Komtebedde J, et al. Impact of interatrial shunts on invasive hemodynamics and exercise tolerance in patients with heart failure. J Am Heart Assoc. 2020;9(17):16760. https://doi.org/10.1161/JAHA.120.016760.
9. Shah SJ, Borlaug BA, Chung ES, et al. Atrial shunt device for heart failure with preserved and mildly reduced ejection fraction (REDUCE LAP-HF II): a randomised, multicentre, blinded, sham-controlled trial. Lancet. 2022;399:1130–40. https://doi.org/10.1016/S0140-6736(22)00016-2.
10. Eisman AS, Shah RV, Dhakal BP, et al. Pulmonary capillary wedge pressure patterns during exercise predict exercise capacity and incident heart failure. Circ Heart Fail. 2018;11(5):e004750. https://doi.org/10.1161/CIRCHEARTFAILURE.117.004750.

Part IV

Percutaneous Therapeutic Intervention in Adult Congenital Heart Diseases

Patent Foramen Ovale and Atrial Septal Defect

Aken Desai, Edward Gill, and John Carroll

Abstract

Patent Foramen Ovale (PFO) is the most common congenital cardiac abnormality and found in ~25% of all adults. PFO results from the failed closure of the foramen ovale and is associated with an increased risk of stroke in symptomatic patients and recent trials have demonstrated the utility of PFO closure for the prevention of recurrent stroke in patients with cryptogenic stroke and PFO. Imaging plays an important role in determining both the presence of a PFO as well as its suitability for closure in a patient with cryptogenic stroke. Atrial septal defects are the third most common congenital defect (after PFOs and bicuspid aortic valve) but are often asymptomatic until adulthood. Complications of undetected ASDs include arrythmia, paradoxical embolization, cerebral abscess, right ventricular (RV) volume overload with late RV failure, and potentially irreversible pulmonary hypertension. This chapter explores the indications and important imaging features in diagnosis, preprocedural planning and interventional closure of PFOs and ASDs. The heart team discussion highlights the multifactorial approach regarding surgical vs. percutaneous closure and device choice.

Keywords

Atrial septal defect · Patent foramen ovale · Inter-atrial shunting · Percutaneous closure devices

Supplementary Information The online version contains supplementary material available at https://doi.org/10.1007/978-3-031-50740-3_10.

A. Desai (✉) · E. Gill · J. Carroll
Division of Cardiology, University of Colorado School of Medicine, Aurora, CO, USA
e-mail: aken.desai@cuanschutz.edu; edward.gill@cuanschutz.edu; john.carroll@cuanschutz.edu

> Test your learning and check your understanding of this book's contents: use the "Springer Nature Flashcards" app to access questions using ▶ https://sn.pub/ambACS.
>
> To use the app, please follow the instructions in the chapter "Transcatheter Aortic Valve Replacement."

Learning Objectives
1. Identify the indication for closure of inter-atrial shunts
2. Understand the differences in the evaluation of patent foramen ovale and atrial septal defects
3. Understand the role of multimodality imaging in atrial septal defects
4. Understand sizing of devices for patent foramen ovale and atrial septal defects
5. Understand the intra-procedural imaging needs for patent foramen ovale and atrial septal defects

> **Case Study**
> A 34-year old woman with no major medical history presents with acute left sided weakness and aphasia approximately 90 min prior to arrival. A CT angiogram reveals an acute right middle cerebral artery territory ischemic stroke of the M3 segment. She undergoes acute thrombectomy with retrieval of a small thrombus from the M3 segment. Her symptoms resolve and she is admitted to the neurology service for post-stroke care.

Background and Definitions

PFO: Inter-atrial shunts encompass a broad variety of defects, most of which are discovered in childhood given increased awareness in the pediatric community. Of those which make it into adulthood without treatment, the vast majority are patent foramen ovale with a smaller number of patients presenting with true atrial septal defects, most commonly ostium secundum defects. PFOs are not considered atrial septal defects by many as they are not a true deficiency of tissue but a remnant of fetal circulation [1]. For the purposes of this chapter, we will focus on patent foramen ovale given it is the predominant lesion that seen in adults while addressing issues important to the management of true atrial septal defects. At least in a small series of adults presenting with paradoxical embolism, PFO was seen in 57% of patients vs ASD in 43% of patients [2].

The patent foramen ovale is a remnant of the fetal circulation that is a flap like defect. The PFO begins in the fossa ovalis on the right atrial side and ends with the ostium secundum on the left atrial side. In fetal circulation, this structure is open due to the right atrial pressure being higher than left atrial pressure. With the first breath after birth, the left atrial pressure becomes higher than the right atrial pressure and the septum primum on the left side compresses onto the secundum on the right side. These two layers then fuse and create the largely impermeable inter-atrial septum. However, incomplete fusion results in a the patent foramen ovale [1]. Autopsy studies have shown this incomplete fusion to be present in about 25% of the population but there is a wide spectrum of patency ranging from only probe patent to widely patent and shunting significantly without provocative maneuvers [3].

Other types of atrial septal defects can be found in the evaluation of patients with cryptogenic stroke as all defects are associated with some degree of right to left shunting.

ASD: ASDs represent the third most common congenital defect (after PFO and bicuspid aortic valve). The most common type of atrial septal defect in adults is a septum secundum defect and this represents 60–80% of atrial septal defects. These are typically caused by incomplete formation of the fossa ovalis and surrounded by in-folded atrial wall that forms the rims of the defects. Septum primum defects are likely better referred to as atrio-ventricular septal defects as they are commonly associated with abnormalities of the atrio-ventricular valves, atrio-ventricular conduction and left ventricular outflow tract. These are most seen in patients with Downs' syndrome. Sinus venosus ASDs are due to either vena cava (most commonly the superior vena cava) over-riding the inter-atrial septum and are associated with anomalous pulmonary venous return. Lastly, coronary sinus ASDs are due to deficiency of the coronary sinus—atrial wall with drainage directly into the left atrium and are associated with persistent left SVCs [4].

Diagnosis and Pre-procedural Assessment

Given the patient's MCA stroke, an evaluation for embolic source is warranted. As the initial evaluation for potential cardiac sources of emboli, the patient underwent transthoracic echocardiography with microbubble injection revealing an intermittent right to left shunt at rest (thus no Valsalva was performed) (Fig. 1 and Video 1).

Additionally, further testing for potential causes of stroke was undertaken. A thorough evaluation for hypercoagulable disorders was unrevealing. Guideline directed malignancy screening should be considered in appropriate patients and was negative in this case. She is not found to have atrial fibrillation on telemetry while admitted and a post-discharge 14-day event monitor shows no significant arrhythmias. No deep venous thrombosis is found on venous duplex imaging. She is discharged 3 days after presentation with no residual neurologic deficits on aspirin and clopidogrel.

In patients with cryptogenic stroke, there are five primary goals to pre-procedure imaging: understanding the mechanism of stroke, the presence of intra-cardiac shunts, the anatomy of the shunt, the physiologic significance of the shunt (degree of shunting) and lastly identification of anatomies which may prove challenging for device closure.

PFO: Anatomically, patent foramen ovales are evaluated based on degree of right to left shunting and features that correlate with increased likelihood of paradoxical embolization. Although several different methods of quantifying the degree of shunt exist, for the purposes of determining eligibility for the trials that demonstrated efficacy of PFO closure for reducing recurrent stroke, large shunts are typically defined as greater than 20–25 microbubbles seen within 4 beats after arrival on the right sided chambers. "Massive" shunts are typically called when there

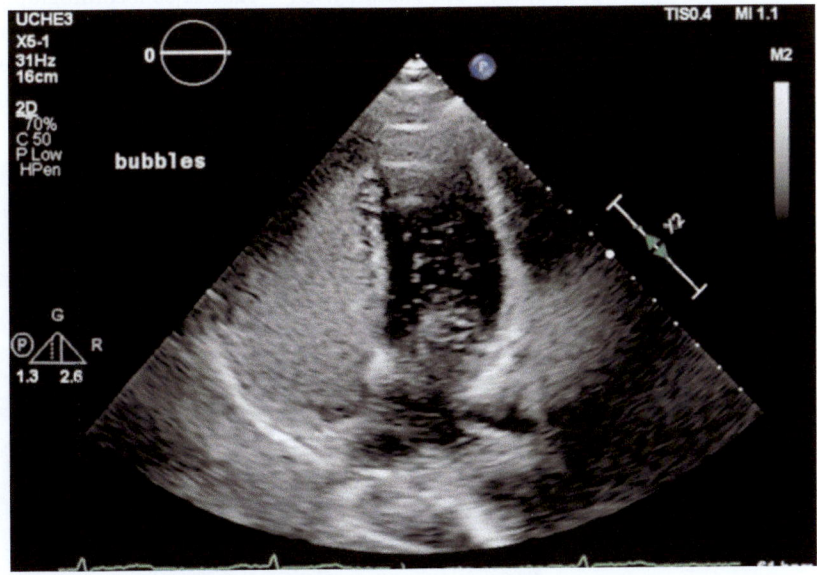

Fig. 1 Transthoracic 4 chamber view of microbubble injection revealing right to left shunt at rest

is rapid and complete whiteout of the left sided chambers. To augment venous return and thus accentuate the opening of the PFO, a Valsalva maneuver or cough can be helpful to reveal PFOs that at rest may not be apparent.

The timing of bubble arrival on the left side can be used to delineate whether the shunt is truly intra-cardiac. It is thought that bubbles arriving later (>6 beats after arrival on the right side) may represent extracardiac shunting. However, there may be exceptions to this such as low cardiac output states, Valsalva (which during the strain phase lowers venous return), deep inspiration or cough [5]. Alternatively, if the source of bubbles seen on the left side can be ascertained (emanating from a pulmonary vein vs. emanating from the interatrial septum), then this can be used in lieu of the number of beats to differentiate intracardiac vs. extracardiac shunting. Then, certain anatomic features can help identify higher risk features such as atrial septal aneurysms (Fig. 2), Chiari networks and prominent Eustachian ridges (Fig. 3) [6, 7].

Given the presence of intracardiac shunting on TTE, a TEE is performed for the purpose of identifying high risk features associated with cryptogenic stroke and whether challenges for device closure may be present. Challenges to percutaneous closure include: redundant tissue, fenestrations, thicker/lipomatous septum secundum, small retroaortic rim, the presence of chiari networks and atypical pulmonary vein anatomy. Of note, PFO size is typically measured by TEE in its maximum diameter with color flow Doppler (Fig. 4), however, this underestimates defect size relative to sizing balloon because PFOs typically remain closed during imaging and gentle inflation with a sizing balloon more closely approximates the PFOs true shape and size [8]. On TEE with color doppler, there is intermittent flow across the PFO (Fig. 5). A small shunt is seen on TEE bubble study (Fig. 6 and Video 2) no Valsalva is performed. TEE will typically underestimate the degree of shunting due to the effect of sedation on degree of shunting and its effect on filling pressures and provocative maneuvers. As a result, we primarily use TTE for the assessment of the degree of shunting while relying on TEE to visualize the PFO and detect atrial septal aneurysm. No other intra-cardiac thrombi are noted on the TEE. No atrial septal aneurysm was identified, the retro-aortic rim was >5 mm and the septum secundum appeared to be of normal thickness. The Eustachian ridge was prominent, but no Chiari networks were seen. Assuming four pulmonary veins, the pulmonary veins were all seen and noted to connect to the left atrium. There were no fenestrations noted in the interatrial septum and there was a clear tunnel that measured about 10 mm (measured as the length of overlap between the flap and the septum secundum). No aortic dilation was noted (Video 3).

Given the high likelihood of PFO (rather than a true atrial septal defect), consideration was given to directly proceeding with PFO closure and intracardiac echocardiography at the time of the procedure and forgoing preprocedural TEE. However, our institutional operator preference is to undertake pre-procedure TEE to not only ensure the cor-

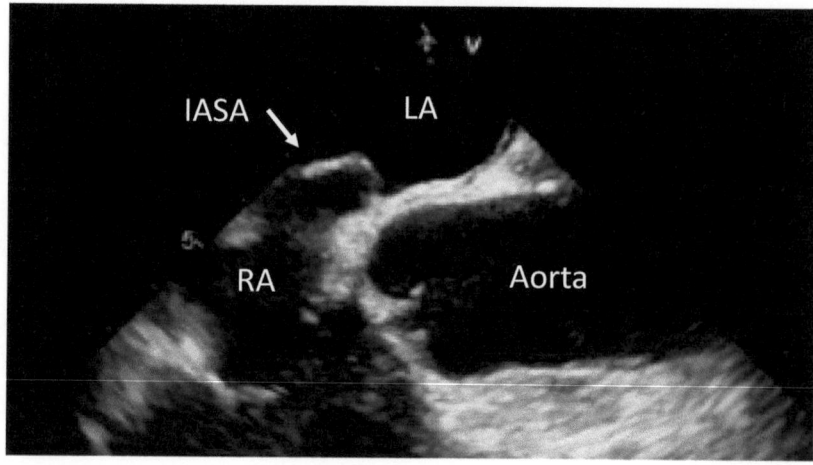

Fig. 2 Transesophageal image of interatrial septum demonstrating interatrial septal aneurysm with bowing of the septum toward the left atrium. *LA* left atrium; *IASA* interatrial septal aneurysm; *RA* right atrium

Fig. 3 Transesophageal image of prominent Eustachian ridge. *LA* left atrium; *RA* right atrium

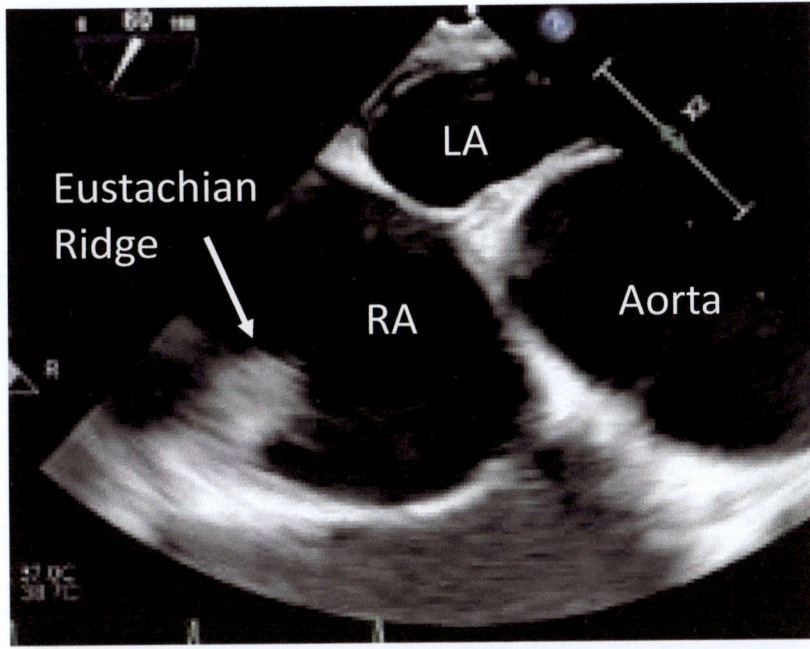

Fig. 4 Intracardiac echo image of interatrial septum with color Doppler over patent foramen ovale, and maximum diameter measured

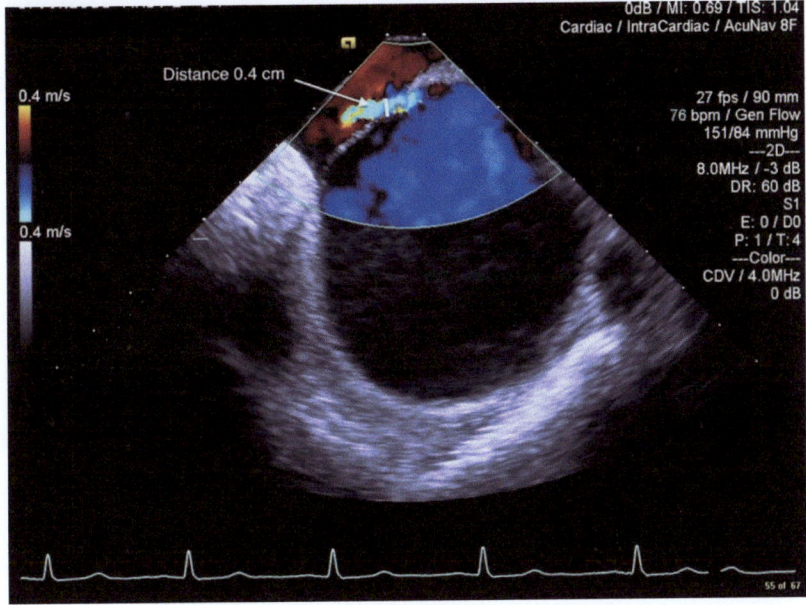

rect defect is identified but also for device selection purposes. There have been cases where a PFO was suspected but during the procedure, a complex fenestrated defect was found or a secundum ASD was found, which can dramatically change the procedural plan and device selection. Additionally, TEE has increased sensitivity for other potential sources of cardiac emboli such as left atrial or ventricular thrombi, myxoma, papillary fibroelastoma, endocarditis and Lamble's excrescence. Lastly, the in-hospital evaluation for mechanism is often incomplete for many reasons. There is rarely sufficient length of telemetry monitoring to rule out paroxysmal atrial fibrillation and thrombophilia workups are delayed in the setting of acute clot as well and are often not back prior to discharge. For these reasons, closure during the index hospitalization is rare.

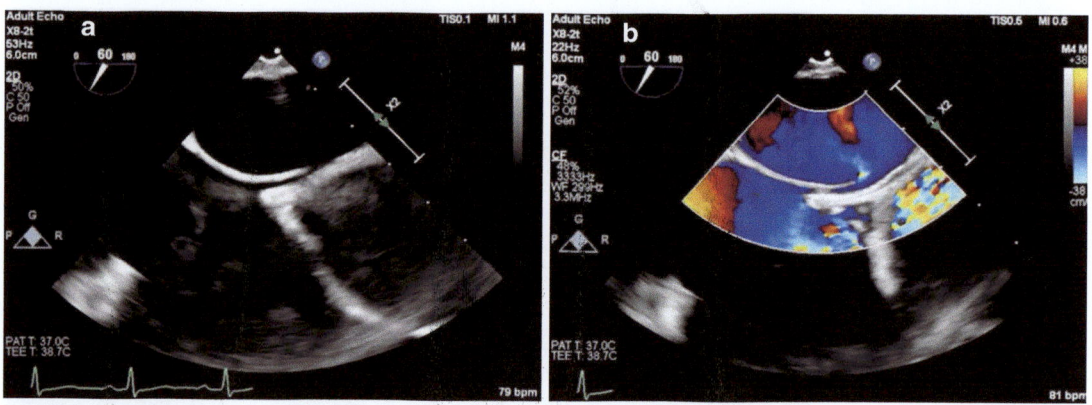

Fig. 5 (a) TEE bicaval view of PFO on the left image and (b) TEE bicaval view of PFO with color Doppler on right image showing resting right to left shunt

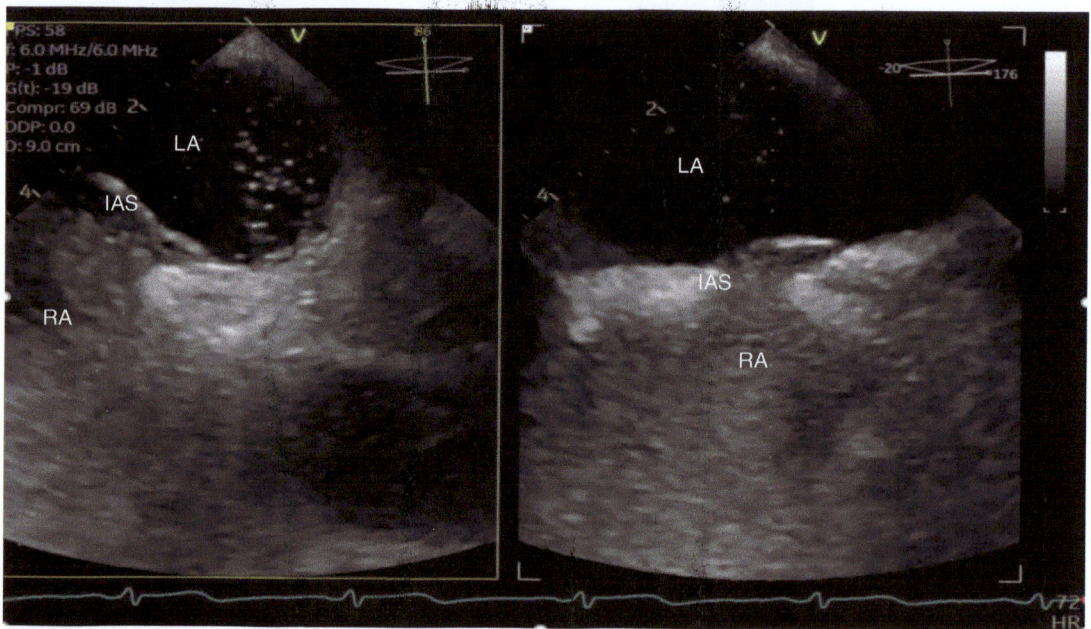

Fig. 6 Transesophageal echocardiogram of interatrial septum obtained in mid esophagus in 2 orthogonal planes

ASD: For secundum atrial septal defects (Video 4) in particular, pre-procedure imaging plays an important role in determining whether a defect is appropriate for trans-catheter closure. Our practice is to obtain 3D TEE measurements of the defect as this has been shown to correlate closely with 2D balloon sizing (Fig. 7). Additionally, even large defects (up to 44 mm) have been closed with transcatheter techniques, particularly if the defect is oval with a shorter minor axis and adequate rims. During pre-procedure assessment of secundum ASDs, important issues to pay attention to are ensuring all four pulmonary veins are visualized as there is an association of partial anomalous pulmonary venous return with secundum ASDs. A sinus venosus defect can be seen in the midesophageal bicaval (120°) view. Ideally, rims should be visualized (as discussed in the intra-procedural guidance section). The degree of mitral regurgitation should be assessed as post-ASD closure, this

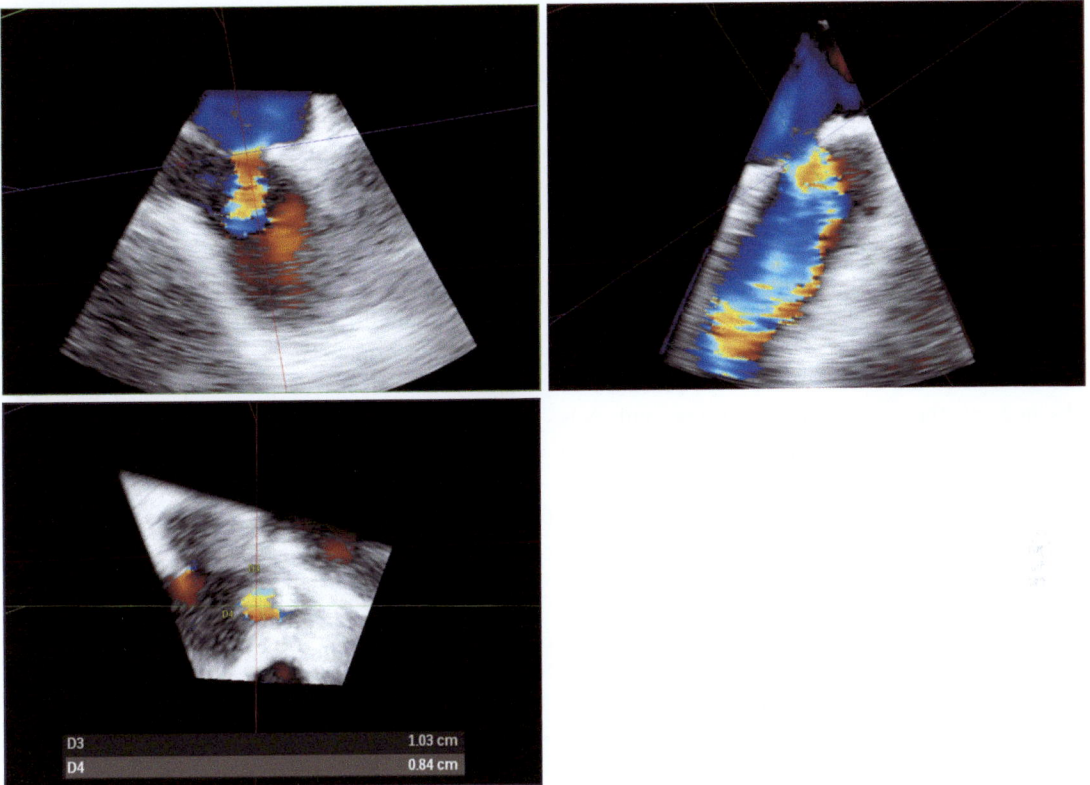

Fig. 7 3D rendering of atrial septal defect with orthogonal B-mode image slices in top 2 panels and short axis of atrial septal defect measured in bottom left panel

can increase due to the increase in left sided volumes and can worsen significant mitral valve disease.

Cross sectional imaging (gated cardiac CT and MRI) is not particularly helpful in evaluation of PFOs but can be helpful in understanding the three-dimensional anatomy of atrial septal defects as well as investigating congenital anomalies associated with them. This can be particularly useful in the identification of complex ASDs that may require multiple devices or lead to significant interaction with surrounding cardiac structures, such that surgical closure might be more effective and safer. While CT has superior spatial resolution and can be used to plan for closure with virtual placement of devices as well as 3D printing of complex defects to assist with case planning, MRI can be used for these purposes as well as hemodynamic evaluation of ASDs through calculation of cardiac output, shunt fractions, and Qp/QS via phase contrast imaging.

Anatomically precise 3D reconstructions of ASD anatomy through pre-procedure cross-sectional imaging have also allowed for increasing use of intraprocedural intra-cardiac echocardiography rather than TEE for guidance of closure. Overall, specifically for the purposes of initial PFO and ASD evaluation, echocardiography in its various forms remains the mainstay of diagnostic evaluation as well as procedural guidance during percutaneous closure procedures.

PFO: Importantly, two main scores assessing the likelihood that a cryptogenic stroke was due to a PFO have been developed. The initial Risk of Paradoxical Embolism (RoPE) score was developed and internally validated from 3023 patients in 12 combined databases of patients with cryptogenic stroke [9]. The resulting parsimonious bedside model incorporates six features of patient history and demographics to determine stroke relatedness to the PFO with a small observational study indicating a cutpoint of 7 (PFO-attributable stroke was 0% [95% CI 0–7.5] for RoPE <7 and 71.1% [95% CI: 35–87.3] for ROPE >7). The model has subsequently been validated for the relative risk reduction of device vs. medical therapy [10]. Importantly, the RoPE score does not take into account known "high risk" features of PFOs, including atrial septal aneurysm (defined as ≥10 mm excursion of the atrial septum from the midline) or hemodynamic consequence (large shunt was defined as >20 bubbles in the left atrium on TEE). The PASCAL classification system combines the ROPE score with presence or absence of these high-risk features and was derived and validated from a cohort of 3740 patients in six randomized clinical trials of PFO closure plus medical therapy versus PFO closure alone in patients aged 18–60. The PFO-Associated Stroke Causal Likelihood (PASCAL) Classification System improved upon the ROPE score's ability to discriminate those that were most likely to benefit from PFO closure, indicating the potential importance of high-risk imaging features in determining the potential benefit that may be derived from percutaneous PFO closure.

Heart Team Approach and Discussion

The patient was seen in the multi-disciplinary PFO/stroke clinic to discuss the etiology of her stroke as well as management options. Vascular neurology reviewed her brain imaging and agreed that the location of the stroke as typical of a cardio-embolic stroke and she had no other compelling data to suggest an alternative cause such as vasculitis, early atherosclerosis, a hypertensive stroke or that there was an arterial hypercoagulable state that may have contributed. Her RoPE [9, 10] score was calculated at eight and her PASCAL classification [11] was probable given RoPE score of 8 and presence of a large shunt. Taken together, these scores suggests that (1) there is an increased likelihood of her stroke being "PFO-related" and (2) she would derive substantial reduction in recurrent stroke rate with PFO closure and a low risk of peri-procedural atrial fibrillation. Given this, it was felt reasonable to proceed with closure of the patent foramen ovale to decrease her risk of recurrent stroke with a lower risk of peri-procedure atrial fibrillation.

The interventional cardiologist then met with the patient to discuss percutaneous closure vs. medical management. At this point, given the variety of percutaneous closure devices available as well as the clinical trial data in support of percutaneous PFO closure over antithrombotic or anticoagulant therapy, surgical closure of PFOs is rarely appropriate. The patient and interventional cardiologist discussed the compelling data supporting that the patient experienced a stroke due to paradoxical embolization via the patent foramen ovale was probable. The options of antiplatelet therapy alone or anticoagulation were discussed as part of a shared decision-making process. Given the patients young age and potential for future pregnancies as well as desire to not be on life-long anticoagulation, percutaneous PFO closure was decided upon.

The role of medical therapy in PFO is minimal in patients otherwise deemed appropriate for PFO closure. Current guidelines recommend against anti-thrombotic or anti-coagulation therapy instead of PFO closure in patients with PFO related stroke [12]. RESPECT [13] and REDUCE [14, 15] led to the approval of the two currently commercially available devices based on their long-term results. Specifically, in longer-term follow up, it was shown that PFO closure reduced the rate of recurrent ischemic strokes. It was a patient-level data meta-analysis [16] that have led to a understanding of the treatment effect with a relative risk of recurrent stroke of 0.42. This and many other similar meta-analyses led to the eventual shift from the term "cryptogenic stroke in the presence of a PFO" to "PFO-related stroke". Additionally, this meta-analysis showed that there was an increased risk of atrial fibrillation with device closure. Though no RCT exists, this data has been extended to cover peripheral paradoxical embolization as well.

The other clear indication for PFO closure is hypoxemia with exertion or upright position that cannot be explained by another etiology, platypnea-orthodeoxia syndrome. The mechanism is with upright or standing position, intrathoracic and intracardiac conditions cause a PFO to be in an open position, and shunting across the PFO increases, leading to systemic hypoxemia and dyspnea. This is typically also caused by abnormalities that cause the PFO to be deformed such that it is opened to a greater degree or "slides" open; for example: aortic aneurysm, atrial enlargement, paralyzed hemi-diaphragm or mediastinal shifting. Other conditions that lead to increase right atrial pressures may also cause increased right to left shunting via the PFO [17, 18]. In our experience, these shunts are often massive on TTE and if only a small shunt is noted, one should question the diagnosis of platypnea-orthodeoxia syndrome.

Decompression sickness (DCS) with scuba diving may be more prevalent in divers with PFOs and that closure may reduce this risk. The pathophysiology of DCS causing neurologic symptoms is the formation of nitrogen gas bubbles in the systemic venous circulatory system during rapid ascent some of which can bypass the lung filtering mechanism when a PFO is present, and subsequent arterial manifestations can include neurologic symptoms, cutaneous changes (Cutis marmorata) and joint "bends". The current recommendation is counseling on the increased risk of DCS with PFO and avoidance of high-risk diving. SCAI guidelines recommend against PFO closure for prevention of DCS given no clear evidence to suggest benefit [12] though allow for closure if the patient and physician participate in a shared decision making process.

Perhaps the most controversial condition associated with PFO is migraine. Migraines are disabling and can be incredibly challenging to treat so this has led to many different procedural solutions, one of which is PFO closure. PFO stroke study sub-group analyses first discovered a reduction of migraine days among PFO closure patients. There are many proposed mechanisms by which PFOs are thought to contribute to migraine including chemicals crossing the PFO instead of being blocked by the blood brain barrier, micro-emboli and cerebral hypoxia. However, three RCTs testing device closure for treating migraine headaches (MIST [19], PREMIUM [20] and PRIMA [21]) were unable to achieve their primary outcomes. Despite this, there remains significant hope that PFO closure might benefit this difficult to treat entity. A new study, RELIEF [22], is currently recruiting patients to test whether the Gore CARDIOFORM PFO occluder in patients that have migraines responsive to P2Y12 therapy may derive benefit from PFO closure.

ASD: True atrial septal defects can have a significant degree of left to right shunting and are associated with right sided volume overload; therefore, right sided chamber dilation, pulmonary hypertension and atrial arrhythmias can be seen. The indication for ASD closure include the presence of RVE, suggesting significant left to right shunting, even in the asymptomatic child. Some patients with long-standing untreated ASDs will develop pulmonary vascular disease, that when severe can reverse shunting leading to cyanosis. Decision-making regarding closure is more complex and if pulmonary vascular resistance is greater than 8 Woods' units or two-thirds systemic vascular resistance or mean PA pressure greater than two-thirds of systemic blood pressure, closure is not pursued in favor of treating underlying pulmonary hypertension first [23–25]. Iatrogenic ASD's following different procedures involving transeptal catheterization may spontaneously close but if it causes substantial shunting, including systemic hypoxemia, closure is indicated.

There are some findings during initial evaluation that are contraindications to PFO and ASD closure until there is resolution. Percutaneous closure should not be pursued in patients who have active thrombi in the ileo-femoral venous system, inferior vena cava or atria as there is risk of embolization. Additionally, active infection is a contraindication due to the risk of device endocarditis.

PFO: There are two commercially available devices in the United States specifically for PFO closure. The Abbott Amplatzer PFO Occluder and Gore Cardioform PFO Occluder. PFOs with concomitant septum primum fenestrations can also be treated with the Abbott Amplatzer Cribiform Occluder. Very large PFOs may be amenable to closure with the Abbott Amplatzer

Septal Occluder used for ASDs. Gore also has developed an ASD occluder which can treat large PFOs as well.

Device selection for PFO and ASD closure is determined by multiple factors including the size and characteristics of the septal defect, the devices that are approved by the regulatory system of the country, operator experience and preferences, and some patient-specific features related to potential complications such as device erosion, nickel allergy, and potential need for future transseptal access to the left atrium. Atrial septal defect sizing often involves balloon sizing, i.e. inflating a sizing balloon across the defect until shunting ceases and the "waist" on the balloon is measured by ultrasound or X-ray. PFO sizing to select the size of device to be used can utilize balloon sizing but often a stiff wire across the defect holds the septum primum in an open position and allows echocardiographic measurement of the PFO size. Atrial septal aneurysms of the septum primum and lipomatous septum secundum are further modifiers of PFO device selection. Long tunnels can often be closed by both devices unless the tissue is non-compliant, preventing tunnel collapse and deforming the devices. Under-sizing of the device needed for both ASD and PFO closure can lead to incomplete closure and even device embolization.

Device sizing recommendations are included in the instructions for use for the Amplatzer device. PFOs that are "simple" with a non-prominent atrial septal aneurysm (<20 mm excursion), tunnel length <10 mm, and normal thickness septum secundum (<10 mm) can be closed with a 25 mm device. Those that do not meet those criteria, will likely require a larger device. All these measurements are easily found on a thorough TEE.

Device selection for PFO closure is based on experience and availability. There are no randomized data comparing the two PFO closure devices available in the US and they performed well in their respective clinical trials. Some finer points of device selection have been identified. In the presence of a small aortic rim, the Cardioform device may be safer given it is more flexible and without rigid edges. Device erosion, often associated with deficient rims, by the Amplatzer PFO Occluder is very rare, more so than with the Amplatzer ASD Occluder. To date, there have been no case reports of erosion with the Cardioform PFO device though there are reports of wire fracture causing tamponade [26]. However, the Cardioform may come with a slightly greater increased risk of atrial fibrillation in the early post-procedure period after PFO closure [15]. Given the lack of a randomized comparison involving patients with a diversity of PFO anatomy, it is not possible to say whether the two devices differ in terms of the completeness of PFO closure.

The last consideration may be a nickel allergy. Our practice is to counsel the patient regarding the unsettled nature of whether a cutaneous nick allergy is even relevant to the risk of an allergic reaction to an intravascular device. The suspicion of nickel allergy is often uncovered with a through history. Skin patch testing for nickel allergy is standard but does not accurately predict if a systemic reaction may occur from an implanted device containing nitinol, an alloy of nickel and titanium. Therefore, a nickel allergy is not an absolute contraindication to percutaneous device closure but given case reports of systemic reactions after PFO or ASD closure, careful counseling is recommended prior to proceeding with percutaneous PFO closure in patients with significant nickel allergies. Surgical closure can be entertained in this patient population if there is enough concern and the patient desires PFO closure without nickel containing materials [27]. New techniques of PFO closure using a transcatheter suture deployment system may be considered, although complete data are not yet available on other outcomes versus device-mediated closure techniques.

The role of PFO closure in patients with hypercoagulable states is less clear. The newest SCAI guidelines do suggest PFO closure in patients with a PFO related stroke, even with thrombophilia requiring anticoagulation [12]. However, the determination of whether a stroke is PFO related versus not in patients with a significant thrombophilia, such as anti-phospholipid antibody may be quite challenging. Given this, it would be reasonable to involve vascular neurology as well as hematology experts to provide individualized recommendations to patients. PFO closure may be reasonable as an "additive" therapy given there may be instances during which patients who would otherwise be on long-term anticoagulation cannot be on it, but this would need to be weighed against the risk of device related thrombosis.

Heart Team Decision: Percutaneous PFO Closure

In patients who do not have other indications for cardiac surgery, percutaneous closure of patent foramen ovale is recommended as it was in this patient's case. Surgical closure of a PFO requires surgical access to the heart (sternotomy), cardiopulmonary bypass, and a prolonged recovery versus device-closure often being performed with conscious sedation on an outpatient basis with minimal recovery.

Intraprocedural Imaging Modalities and Measurements, (Discussion Between Members of the Heart Team)

Intraprocedural imaging for closure is usually done with intra-cardiac echocardiography or transesophageal echocardiography. Less frequently, the procedure is performed with TTE and angiographic guidance. Though limited in use, fluoroscopy only guided closure of PFOs has been shown in small studies to be safe and effective [28, 29].

Trans-esophageal echo cardiography offers the ability to both perform the screening TEE and therapeutic procedure in a single setting but typically this requires deep sedation or general anesthesia. Intracardiac echocardiography (ICE) allows the performance of the closure procedure to be done with conscious sedation, which may allow for same-day discharge due to faster recovery. Studies have shown the two methods to be equivalent [30–32].

Typically, if the procedure is performed with ICE guidance, the interventionalist manipulates the catheter and has catheterization laboratory staff operate the imaging console with capture of key images. However, with the advent of 3D ICE, the presence of an echocardiographer experienced in acquiring 3D datasets and interpretation can be quite helpful. Regardless of modality, the procedural imaging follows the same general cadence. The use of fluoroscopy is also useful to the interventionalist who can see the position of the device relative to cardiac borders and ensure the discs are deployed fully.

First, a repeat assessment of key cardiac structures is performed to ensure no other possible sources of emboli (in the case of stroke patients) are found. TEE offers the advantage of once again assessing for the presence of LA and LV thrombi, which may not be as easily visualized with ICE. On TEE, the inter-atrial septum is imaged in a bicaval and short axis view. On ICE, a septal view is obtained by retroflexion and clockwise rotation from the "home" view with the catheter in the right atrium (Video 5) The catheter is then advanced slightly cranial, which shows the SVC rim. Then, a short axis view which is like the TEE short axis view (other than in ICE the right atrium is at the apex of the imaging cone whereas in TEE the left atrium is at the apex of the imaging cone) is obtained by rotating clockwise and then retroflexing further with slight leftward deflection or using newer catheters, with bi-plane of the septal view. This shows the aortic rim in detail [33].

The PFO is then assessed at rest, paying attention to key features: the aortic rim, the presence and excursion of an atrial septal aneurysm, tunnel length, thickness of the septum secundum and degree of shunting by bubble. Not infrequently, if lower extremity injection was not performed as part of the screening TTE or TEE, with a bubble injection into the femoral vein, the degree of shunting becomes far more impressive.

After this, the defect is crossed, often without much effort with a standard J-tipped guidewire and multi-purpose diagnostic catheter. Imaging guidance can assist if there is difficulty in ensuring the guidewire is positioned in the tunnel to cross the PFO (Video 6). If despite visualization of the J-wire in the tunnel, the wire is unable to cross, this may lead one to consider that the PFO may be too small to be the cause of a cryptogenic stroke or certainly, hypoxemia. One can try with hydrophilic guidewires or different shaped catheters if there is a strong indication for closure.

After crossing, echo guidance can help position the wire and catheter in the left upper pulmonary vein, which provides the best trajectory for insertion of the delivery sheath. Once positioned in the vein, the wire is exchanged for a stiff guidewire. Echo is used to ensure the wire is indeed in the pulmonary vein as fluoroscopically, the left atrial appendage is in a similar position. Should the wire be in the LAA, this can be a cause of perforation given the thin-walled nature of the LAA. At this point, the PFO is maximally "propped" open (Video 7). Measurements of the PFO width are performed by measuring the width of the color jet on the right atrial side (Fig. 8). The tunnel length often also becomes more apparent as one can measure the length of the septum primum from the right atrial entrance to the tip of the primum on the left atrial side. A general rule is the right atrial disc width should be at least two times the width of the PFO or tunnel length. This is because the PFO devices are not self-centering since the central portion is connecting pin rather than a true disc and therefore, when sizing, one must assume that the device may be pushed entirely into one corner of the defect and therefore, the radius of the device must be large enough to close the defect.

Once a device is chosen, echo guidance is used to ensure the delivery sheath tip is free in the left atrium (Video 8). Then, the left atrial disc is unsheathed and then pulled back such that it is pulled against the inter-atrial septum without prolapsing into the tunnel (Videos 9 and 10). Echo guidance is key for this step as if the LA disc falls into the tunnel, the device can be easily recaptured and torqued to allow the LA disc to sit against the septum. Then, while maintaining some tension, the right atrial disc is deployed and pushed against the septum. Again, echo guidance allows for visualization to ensure the entirety of the right atrial disc is on the right atrial side (Videos 11 and 12). At this point, the device is evaluated to ensure that there is no interaction with the aorta or SVC (Video 13), which if seen, is a marker for erosion. Fluoroscopically, in the LAO cranial view, the discs of the device should be separate and there may even be motion of the discs, reflecting the motion of the tissue in between the two discs. A push-pull test is performed to demonstrate stability. If a disc is seen within the tunnel, then the device should be

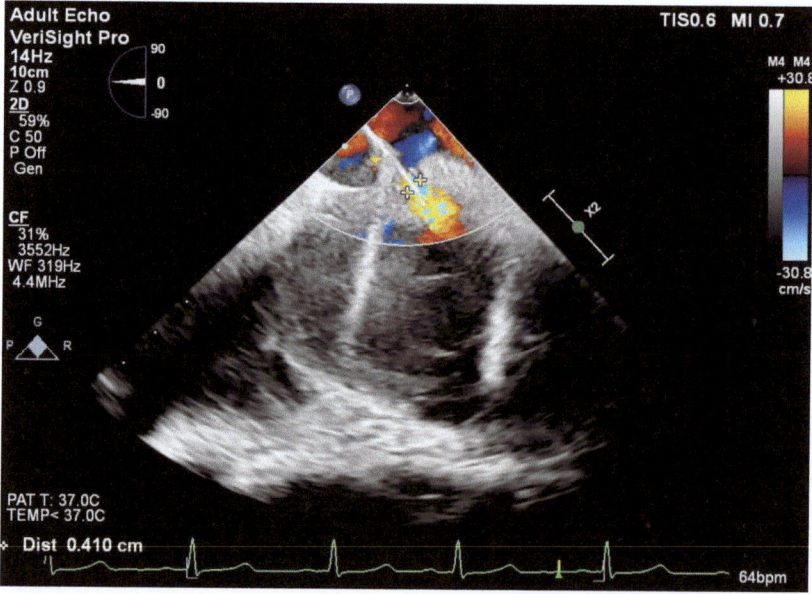

Fig. 8 ICE image with color Doppler, wire over interatrial septum with measurements of the PFO width performed by measuring the width of the color jet on the right atrial side

upsized. If the device is felt to be well positioned and sized, the device is released. Often, with release, there is dramatic shifting in the device as it orients to the natural lie of the inter-atrial septum. The device is re-inspected to ensure both discs remain well positioned. A repeat bubble study can be performed to verify closure. Repeat color doppler should also be performed of the inter-atrial septum to document that there were no "missed" small atrial septal defects.

ASD: In contrast, atrial septal defect closure guidance at our center remains largely guided by TEE except in the cases of well defined, small ASDs with large rims on pre-procedure imaging; most often iatrogenic ASDs. Rims are best assessed with 2D views. For each ASD, we recommend measuring rims in the following views: SVC and IVC rims in the mid-esophageal 90° view (Fig. 9), aortic and posterior rims in the 45° mid-esophageal view (Fig. 10), mitral and atrial rims in the 0° mid-esophageal view (Fig. 11). Most commonly, as in the case demonstrated here, aortic rims are deficient and this is not a contraindication to percutaneous closure. Often, particularly with external referrals, these measurements are done on the table at the time of the closure procedure.

During the procedure, the defect size is confirmed using 3D TEE. Then after crossing, balloon sizing is performed (Fig. 12). The 34 mm balloon can be used for all ASDs since it is longer and will shift less with inflation so many tend to only use this size but care must be taken to not over-inflate the balloon and rupture the inter-atrial septum.

After sizing, the delivery catheter is advanced into the LA and TEE can be used to ensure the catheter is in the left upper pulmonary vein (Fig. 13). The LA disc is deployed and pulled against the septum (Fig. 14), then the RA disc is deployed (Fig. 15). Before release, views are obtained to ensure no significant leaks (Fig. 16) and that there has been no impact on the surrounding structures: SVC and IVC flow, mitral valve function and the aortic root. A gentle tug test is performed to ensure stability and if so, the device is released and further evaluation for leaks is performed (Fig. 17) as with shifting of the device, new leaks may be identified as tension from the delivery cable is released.

Both available devices in the United States have been reported to close defects up to 40-44 mm in diameter though strictly labeled, the Amplatzer can treat defects up to 38 mm and the Gore up to 35 mm by stop flow balloon sizing. Typically, with the Amplatzer device, a 5 mm rim of tissue is needed for device stability and to decrease the risk of erosion. The major risk fac-

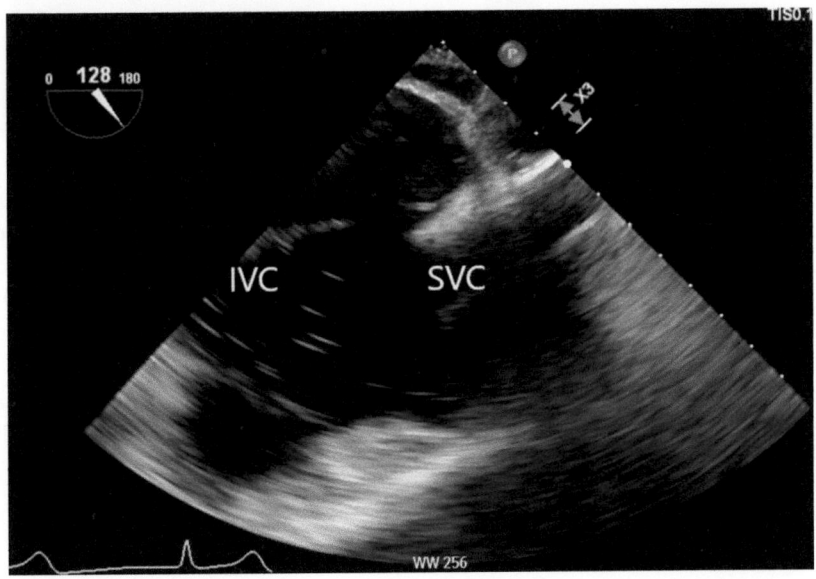

Fig. 9 ICE image of measurements of SVC and IVC rims of ASD in the mid-esophageal 90° view

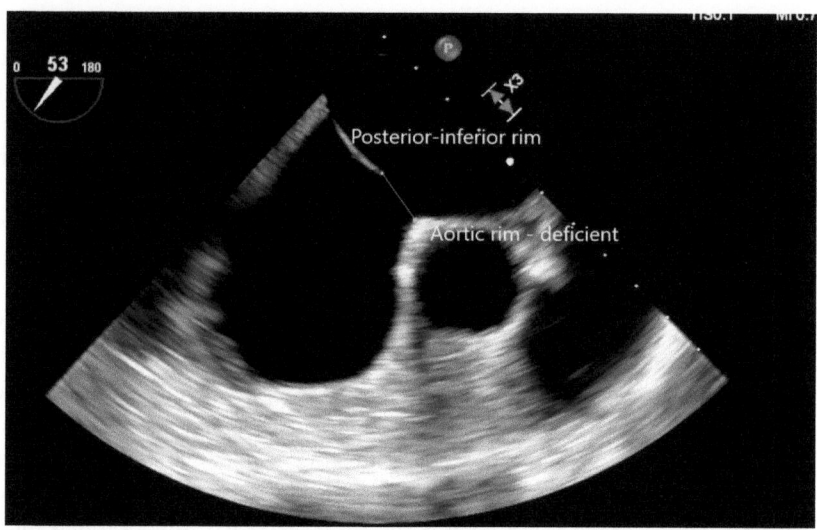

Fig. 10 ICE image of measurement of aortic and posterior rims of ASD in the 45° mid-esophageal view

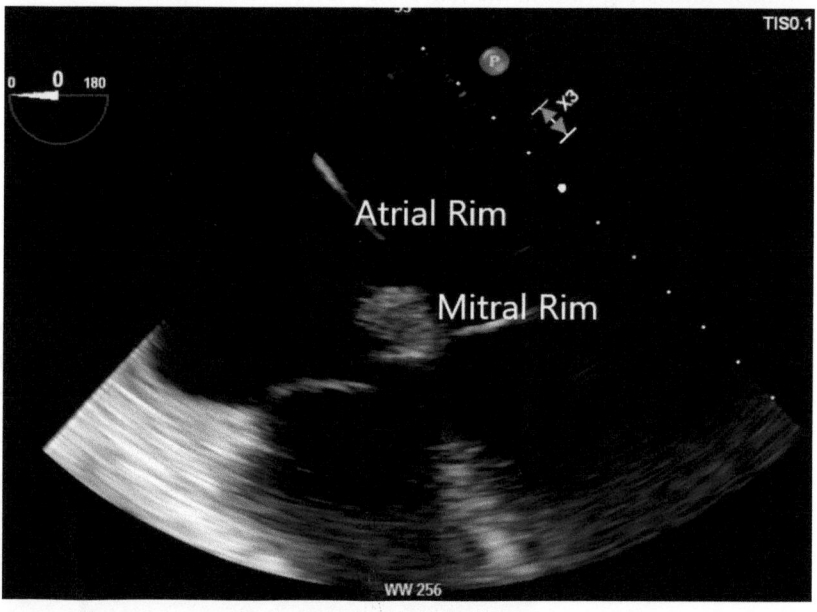

Fig. 11 ICE image of measurement of mitral and atrial rims of ASD in the 0° mid-esophageal view

tors for erosion with the Amplatzer device are: deficient rims (particularly inferior), a balloon sized stop flow diameter 5 mm greater than the static diameter or a low weight to device size ratio [34]. Given the design of the Gore device, these rims may not be as necessary for erosion risk but tissue rim is needed for device stability. A deficient rim from the defect to the AV valves can lead to AV valve dysfunction. There are many different techniques and tricks described to optimally place these devices in complex anatomy that are not covered in this chapter given its focus on imaging. In fact, there have been cases in which multiple devices can be used to close large defects (Fig. 18) where the first device is left in place and a second device from a second access site is deployed, essentially using the first as the "rim" for the second.

Fig. 12 Biplane TEE image of balloon crossing interatrial defect while balloon sizing is performed

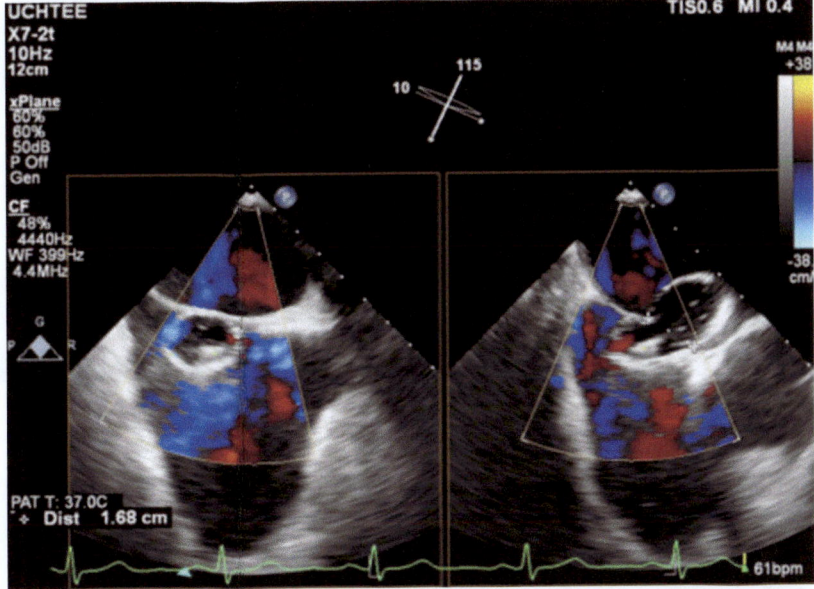

Fig. 13 3D TEE image of the delivery catheter advanced into the LA to ensure the catheter is in the left upper pulmonary vein

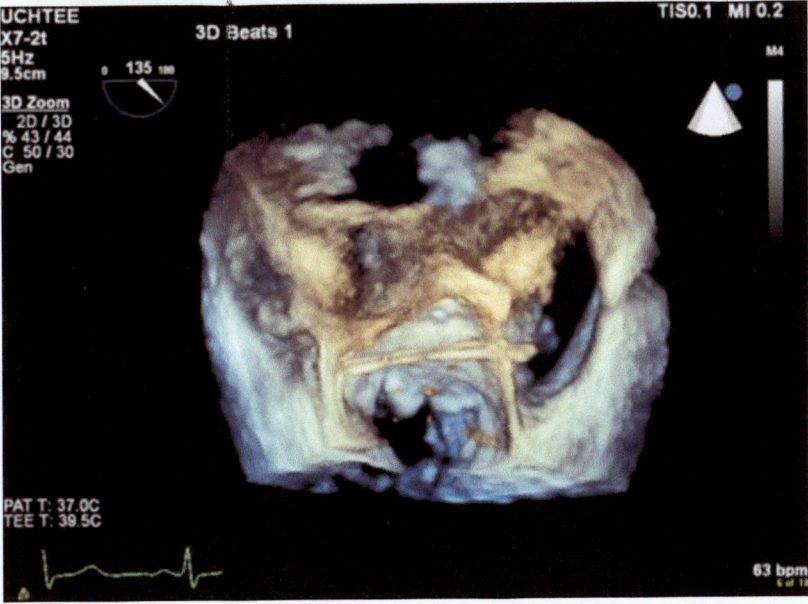

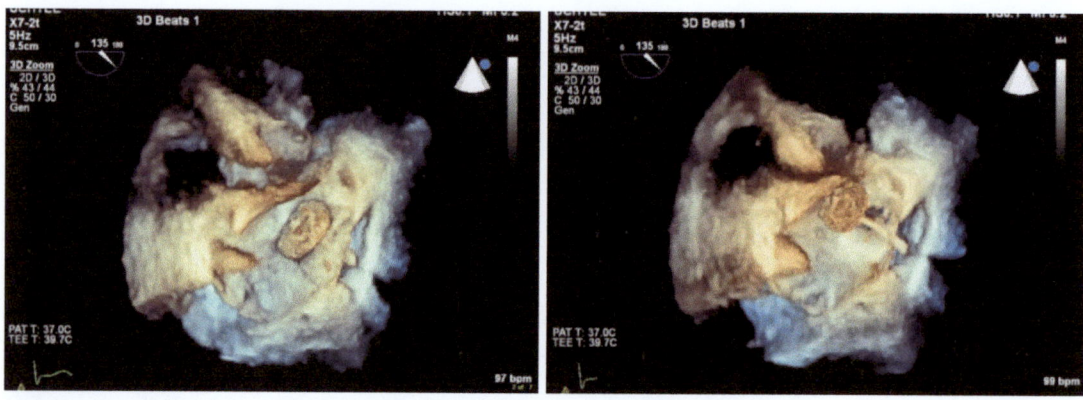

Fig. 14 3D TEE image of LA disc deployed and pulled against the septum

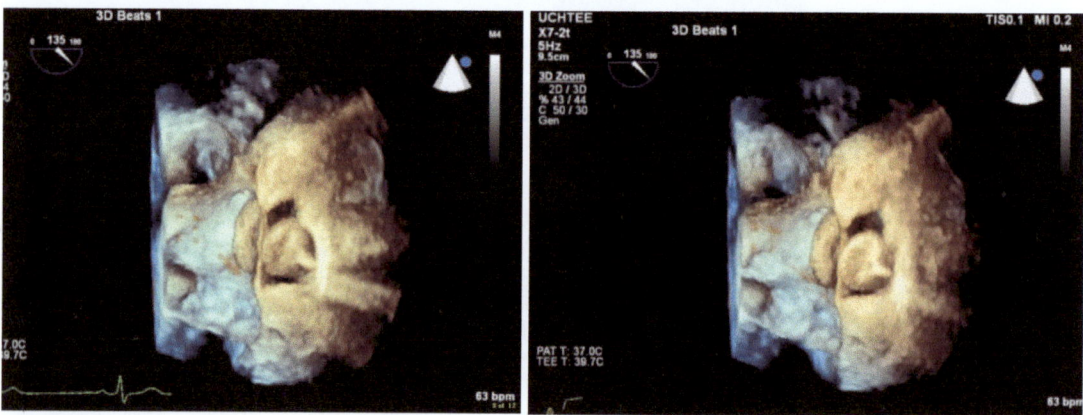

Fig. 15 3D TEE image of the RA disc is deployed

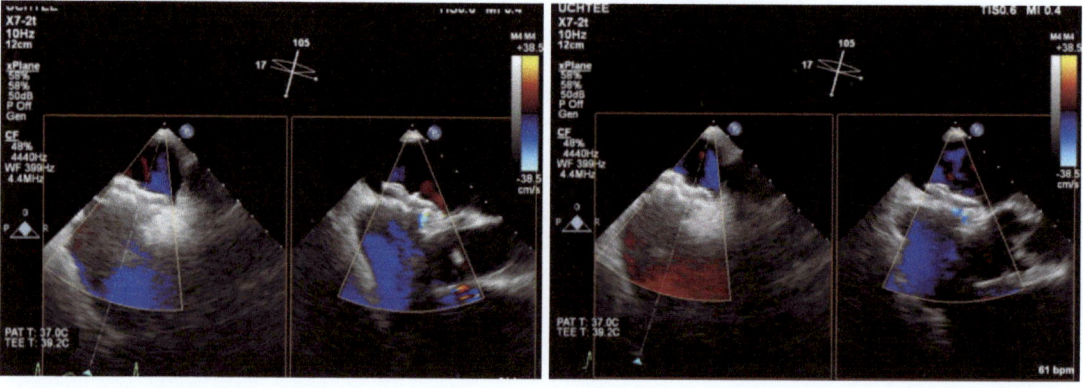

Fig. 16 Biplane ICE images with color Doppler are obtained during tug test to ensure no significant leaks or impingement on the surrounding structures: SVC and IVC flow, mitral valve function and the aortic root before release

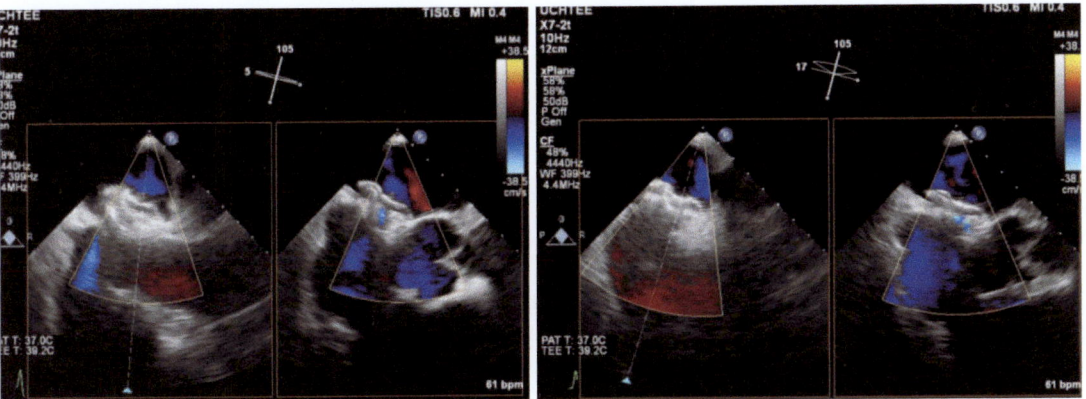

Fig. 17 Biplane ICE images with color Doppler after device is released and further evaluation for leaks is performed

Fig. 18 ICE image of large ASD with first device is left in place and a second device from a second access site is deployed, essentially using the first as the "rim" for the second

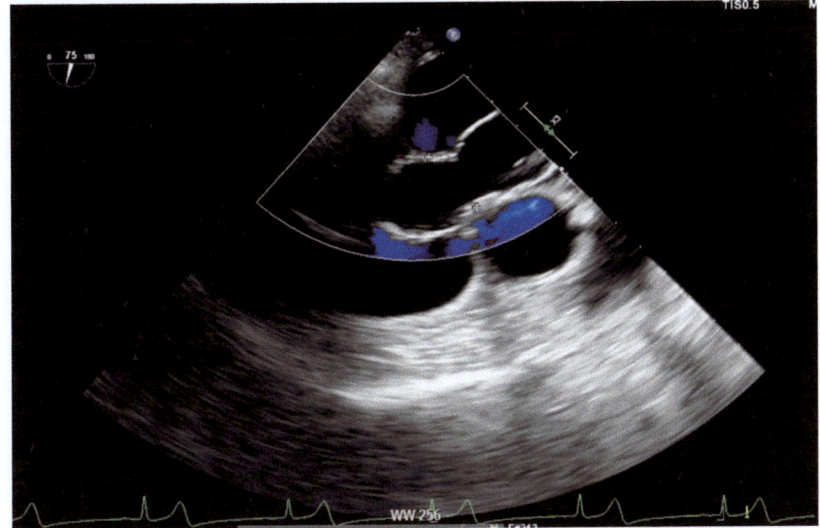

Post Procedural Assessment

ASD and PFO: After the procedure, a transthoracic echocardiography is performed to document the position of the device and a bubble study to document any residual shunting (Video 14). Though not in this case, in many cases, a tiny shunt remains, especially with provocative maneuvers. This should not by itself be a cause for alarm as most times, with endothelialization, the follow up TTE shows no residual shunting. It often takes a full year to be able to assess the final degree of closure because endothelialazation is a slow process. Additionally, the echo should be reviewed for any sign of pericardial fluid as this may be an early sign of erosion or intra-procedural injury of cardiac chambers. If new pericardial fluid is noted, it may be worth keeping the patient overnight for a repeat echo in the morning instead of discharging them after recovery. Post-PFO closure, recommendations are usually for at least 1 month of dual anti-platelet therapy following by indefinite low dose aspirin therapy in patients with prior stroke [12]. SBE prophylaxis is recommended for a minimum of 6 months. In patients closed for non-stroke indications such as right sided chamber dilation or platypnea-orthodeoxia, our practice is to stop aspirin after 6 months.

Repeat imaging usually consists of another TTE and bubble study sometime between 3 and

6 months post procedure. After that, routine imaging is not recommended unless there are new clinical events that would suggest device related complications such as new strokes, infection, or new arrhythmias.

Multimodality imaging comparison

Modality	Degree of shunting	Anatomic characterization	Procedural guidance	Post procedure
TTE	+++	+	++	++
TEE	+++	+++	+++	+++
ICE	+++	+++	+++	–
MRI	++ (ASD)	+ (PFO), ++ (ASD)	–	++
CT	–	– (PFO), ++ (ASD)	–	++
Angiography	+	+	+	–

Clinical Controversies and Pearls

- The presence of anatomic "high risk" features, such as atrial septal aneurysm and "large" shunt (defined as greater than 20 bubbles seen in the left atrium on TEE imaging) increase the likelihood of recurrent stroke and are predictive of benefit from closure in patients with PFO and cryptogenic stroke
- Device selection for PFO closure is based on operator experience and device availability as randomized head to head data are lacking. The cardioform device may be preferred in the setting of deficient atrial rims due to a perceived lower risk of device erosion
- For ASDs, cardiac MRI may be considered as part of the primary evaluation due to the ability to assess chamber size, pulmonary vein and great vessel anatomy, as well as cardiac hemodynamics (Qp/Qs, shunt fraction, cardiac output) ion a single exam, and provide 3D reconstructions for 3D printing or other applications in a single exam.

Key Points
- TTE with bubble study is the first step in evaluation of right to left shunting, however, the use of lower extremity injection and Valsalva may be needed to increase the sensitivity of the bubble study
- TEE is the preferred modality for the anatomic characterization of inter-atrial shunts
- Procedural guidance can be achieved successfully with intra-cardiac echocardiography or TEE
- ASD guidance may be better with TEE given the higher degree of complexity of the closure procedure as well as need for accurate characterization of tissue rims which may not always be seen with 2D ICE
- CT and MRI are helpful to evaluate true atrial septal defects but are limited in the evaluation of patent foramen ovale due to the dynamic nature of shunting

Chapter Review Questions

1. A 25-year-old woman presents with cryptogenic stroke. Which of the following findings is not typical for patent foramen ovale?
   A. Positive bubble study at rest that increases with Valsalva
   B. Right ventricular dilation
   C. Bubble study only positive with Valsalva
   D. Inter-atrial septal aneurysm

   Answer: B

   Explanation: As patent foramen ovales are flap-like, they typically are only associated with right to left shunting though a small amount of bidirectional shunting can be seen when "stretched" open. If right ventricular dilation, pulmonary hypertension, or right atrial dilation are seen, suspicion for an atrial septal defect or congenital abnormalities

should increase. Of note, inter-atrial septal aneurysms are commonly seen in PFOs and are an imaging marker of high risk of stroke recurrence. Bubble studies may be positive either at rest, or with Valsalva, or both, depending on the relative RA and LA pressures.

2. A 40-year-old woman presents with symptoms of dyspnea without hypoxemia and right ventricular enlargement is seen on TTE as well as color flow Doppler of the inter-atrial septum showing left to right shunting. Which defect is statistically most likely?
   A. Patent foramen ovale
   B. Septum primum
   C. Septum secundum
   D. Sinus venosus
   E. Unroofed coronary sinus

   Answer: C

   Explanation: Septum secundum defects are the most common type of atrial septal defect. Patent foramen ovale would not typically be associated with dyspnea unless hypoxemia is seen.

3. A 78-year-old man presents with severe hypoxemia upon standing and with exertion. He has no history of lung disease and PFTs are normal. A TTE performed with agitated saline in an antecubital vein shows complete white out of the left sided chambers within two heart beats of the bubbles arriving in the right atrium. Which concomitant abnormality should be ruled out?
   A. Aortic aneurysm
   B. Cirrhosis
   C. Arterio-venous fistula
   D. Lung cancer

   Answer: A

   Explanation: Aortic aneurysms can cause shifting of the inter-atrial septum leading to opening of a previously closed patent foramen ovale. B and C would be suggested by the late arrival of bubbles in the left atrium.

4. A 25-year-old man presents with cryptogenic stroke. TTE bubble study is negative at rest. Due to a high index of suspicion, a TEE is performed and a PFO with inter-atrial septal aneurysm is found. Additionally, a prominent eustachian valve is noted. Which maneuvers could have discovered the PFO on the initial TTE?
   A. Injection of a higher volume of agitated saline
   B. Lower extremity injection
   C. Valsalva
   D. Use of echo microbubble contrast

   Answer: B and C

   Explanation: Both Valsalva maneuvers and lower extremity injection can increase the sensitivity of agitated saline microbubble studies. Generally, the initial TTE should always include provocative maneuvers. Lower extremity injections are rarely needed.

5. A 38-year-old woman underwent closure of an inter-atrial shunt of unknown type 2 years prior with an unknown device in the setting of an embolic stroke. She presents with cardiac tamponade and bloody fluid is removed. A TEE reveals hematoma surrounding the aortic root. A device is seen but poorly visualized. Which of the following factors is least likely to be involved?
   A. Deficient aortic rim
   B. Gore Cardioform PFO Occluder 30 mm
   C. Amplatzer PFO Occluder 35 mm
   D. Amplatzer ASO Occluder

   Answer: B

   Explanation: Deficient aortic rims are associated with increased risk of erosion with Amplatzer type devices. The frequency of erosion is one case per several thousand implants of the Amplatzer ASO device and is even more rare with larger Amplatzer PFO occluders.

References

1. Gill EA. Definitions and pathophysiology of the patent foramen ovale: broad overview. Cardiol Clin. 2005;23(1):1–6.
2. Bannan A, et al. Characteristics of adult patients with atrial septal defects presenting with paradoxical embolism. Catheter Cardiovasc Interv. 2009;74(7):1066–9.
3. Hagen PT, Scholz DG, Edwards WD. Incidence and size of patent foramen ovale during the first 10 decades of life: an autopsy study of 965 Normal hearts. Mayo Clin Proc. 1984;59(1):17–20.

4. Surkova E, et al. International journal of cardiology congenital heart disease the ACHD multi-modality imaging series: imaging of atrial septal defects in adulthood. Int J Cardiol Congenital Heart Disease. 2021;4:100188.
5. Gill EA, Quaife RA. The echocardiographer and the diagnosis of patent foramen ovale. Cardiol Clin. 2005;23(1):47–52.
6. Radico F, et al. The 'dreaded PFO': anatomical and functional features of high risk for stroke. Eur Heart J Suppl. 2021;23(Supplement_E):E189–93.
7. Nakayama R, et al. Identification of high-risk patent foramen ovale associated with cryptogenic stroke: development of a scoring system. J Am Soc Echocardiogr. 2019;32(7):811–6.
8. Kumar P, Rusheen J, Tobis JM. A comparison of methods to determine patent foramen ovale size. Catheter Cardiovasc Interv. 2020;96(6):E621–9.
9. Kent DM, et al. An index to identify stroke-related vs incidental patent foramen ovale in cryptogenic stroke. Neurology. 2013;81(7):619–25.
10. Kent DM, et al. Risk of paradoxical embolism (RoPE)-estimated attributable fraction correlates with the benefit of patent foramen ovale closure: an analysis of 3 trials. Stroke. 2020;51(10):3119–23.
11. Kent DM, et al. Heterogeneity of treatment effects in an analysis of pooled individual patient data from randomized trials of device closure of patent foramen ovale after stroke. JAMA. 2021;326(22):2277–86.
12. Kavinsky CJ, et al. SCAI guidelines for the management of patent foramen ovale. J Soc Cardiov Angiogr Interv. 2022;1:100039.
13. Saver JL, et al. Long-term outcomes of patent foramen ovale closure or medical therapy after stroke. N Engl J Med. 2017;377(11):1022–32.
14. Kasner SE, et al. Patent foramen ovale closure with GORE HELEX or CARDIOFORM septal Occluder vs. antiplatelet therapy for reduction of recurrent stroke or new brain infarct in patients with prior cryptogenic stroke: design of the randomized Gore REDUCE clinical study. Int J Stroke. 2017;12(9):998–1004.
15. Søndergaard L, et al. Patent foramen ovale closure or antiplatelet therapy for cryptogenic stroke. N Engl J Med. 2017;377(11):1033–42.
16. Mojadidi MK, et al. Transcatheter patent foramen ovale closure after cryptogenic stroke. JACC Cardiov Interv. 2017;10(21):2228–30.
17. Chen GP-W, Goldberg SL, Gill EA Jr. Patent foramen ovale and the platypnea-orthodeoxia syndrome. Cardiol Clin. 2005;23(1):85–9.
18. Mojadidi MK, et al. The effect of patent foramen ovale closure in patients with platypnea-orthodeoxia syndrome. Catheter Cardiovasc Interv. 2015;86(4):701–7.
19. Dowson A, et al. Migraine intervention with STARFlex technology (MIST) trial. Circulation. 2008;117(11):1397–404.
20. Mojadidi MK, et al. Pooled analysis of PFO Occluder device trials in patients with PFO and migraine. J Am Coll Cardiol. 2021;77(6):667–76.
21. Mattle HP, et al. Percutaneous closure of patent foramen ovale in migraine with aura, a randomized controlled trial. Eur Heart J. 2016;37(26):2029–36.
22. Ahmed Z, Sommer RJ. Reassessing the PFO-migraine trials: are we closer to closure? J Am Coll Cardiol. 2021;77(6):677–9.
23. Faccini A, Butera G. Atrial septal defect (ASD) device trans-catheter closure: limitations. J Thorac Dis. 2018;10(S24):S2923–30.
24. Poommipanit P, Amin Z. Considerations for ASD closure. Understanding the devices and proper anatomic evaluation to prevent and manage possible complications. Cardiac Interv Today. 2014:30–9.
25. Wiktor DM, Carroll JD. ASD closure in structural heart disease. Curr Cardiol Rep. 2018;20(6):37.
26. Thomson JDR, Qureshi SA. Device closure of secundum atrial septal defect's and the risk of cardiac erosion. Echo Res Pract. 2015;2(4):R73–8.
27. Spina R, et al. Nickel hypersensitivity reaction following Amplatzer atrial septal defect occluder device deployment successfully treated by explantation of the device. Int J Cardiol. 2016;223:242–3.
28. Wahl A, et al. Safety and feasibility of percutaneous closure of patent foramen ovale without intraprocedural echocardiography in 825 patients. Swiss Med Wkly. 2008;138(39):567.
29. Siddiqui IF, Michaels AD. Percutaneous patent foramen ovale closure using Helex and Amplatzer devices without Intraprocedural echocardiographic guidance. J Interv Cardiol. 2011;24(3):271–7.
30. Alqahtani F, et al. Intracardiac versus transesophageal echocardiography to guide transcatheter closure of interatrial communications: nationwide trend and comparative analysis. J Interv Cardiol. 2017;30(3):234–41.
31. Vigna C, et al. Echocardiographic guidance of percutaneous patent foramen ovale closure: head-to-head comparison of transesophageal versus rotational intracardiac echocardiography. Echocardiography. 2012;29(9):1103–10.
32. Moon J, et al. Comparison of intracardiac echocardiography and transesophageal echocardiography for image guidance in percutaneous patent foramen ovale closure. Medicina. 2020;56(8):401.
33. Kim SS, et al. The use of intracardiac echocardiography and other intracardiac imaging tools to guide noncoronary cardiac interventions. J Am Coll Cardiol. 2009;53(23):2117–28.
34. Mcelhinney DB, et al. Relative risk factors for cardiac erosion following transcatheter closure of atrial septal defects. Circulation. 2016;133(18):1738–46.

Percutaneous Ventricular Septal Defect Closure

Kamel Shibbani, Karim A. Diab, Damien Kenny, and Ziyad M. Hijazi

Abstract

Percutaneous Ventricular Septal Defect (VSD) closure has become a viable alternative to surgery for certain perimembranous and most muscular ventricular septal defects. Various devices exist that cater to the unique anatomical variations in each patient. Given the variability in size and location of such defects, a detailed anatomical assessment is vital to allow the care team to make the most appropriate decision regarding surgical vs percutaneous VSD closure. Transthoracic echocardiography is essential in preprocedural planning, with transesophageal echocardiography playing an equally important intraprocedural role. Rarely, advanced cross-sectional imaging with a CT/MRI might be helpful in complex VSDs. In this chapter, we look at the standard transthoracic and transesophageal imaging assessment for percutaneous closure of perimembranous and muscular VSDs using a case-based illustrated approach.

Keywords

Percutaneous · Ventricular septal defect · Perimembranous · Muscular · Transesophageal · Transthoracic · Echocardiography

Supplementary Information The online version contains supplementary material available at https://doi.org/10.1007/978-3-031-50740-3_11.

K. Shibbani
Division of Cardiology, Department of Pediatrics, Rady Children's Hospital, San Diego, CA, USA

K. A. Diab (✉)
Division of Cardiology, Department of Pediatrics, Lurie Children's Hospital, Northwestern Feinberg School of Medicine, Chicago, IL, USA

Division of Cardiology, Department of Pediatrics, Inova Children's Hospital, Fairfax, VA, USA

D. Kenny
Department of Pediatric and Congenital Cardiology, Children's Health Ireland at Crumlin, Dublin, Ireland

Z. M. Hijazi
Sidra Heart Center, Sidra Medicine, Weill Cornell Medicine, Doha, Qatar

Abbreviations

CT	Computed tomography
ECG	Electrocardiography
LAX	Long axis
MPA	Main pulmonary artery
MRI	Magnetic resonance imaging
mVSD	Muscular ventricular septal defect
pmVSD	Perimembrenous ventricular septal defect
RA	Right atrium
RV	Right ventricle
RVOT	Right ventricular outflow tract
SAX	Short axis
TEE	Transesophageal echocardiography
TTE	Transthoracic echocardiography
VSD	Ventricular septal defect

> Test your learning and check your understanding of this book's contents: use the "Springer Nature Flashcards" app to access questions using ▶ https://sn.pub/ambACS.
>
> To use the app, please follow the instructions in the chapter "Transcatheter Aortic Valve Replacement."

Learning Objectives

1. Identify the best transthoracic echocardiographic imaging planes to assess perimembranous and muscular ventricular septal defects
2. Identify the best transesophageal echocardiographic imaging planes to assess perimembranous and muscular ventricular septal defects
3. Identify essential intra-operative and post-procedural echocardiographic checklists
4. Understand the inclusion and exclusion criteria for percutaneous VSD device closure, especially those identified by echocardiography

Muscular VSD

> **Case Study**
>
> A 31-year-old male involved in a motorcycle accident was admitted in severe hypovolemic shock. Workup included an ECG that revealed a right bundle branch block and a transthoracic echo that revealed a large apical muscular VSD that measured about 18 mm in diameter. Echocardiography also revealed an avulsed tricuspid valve with severe regurgitation. The defect had a gradient of 55 mmHg with left to right shunting (Qp:Qs was 2:1 on hemodynamic assessment).

Background and Definitions

A muscular VSD is a defect in the interventricular septum that has exclusive muscular borders. Muscular VSDs represent the second most common type of VSDs in children, accounting for approximately 10–15% of such defects [1]. They are less common in adults but can be seen after blunt chest trauma [2], as described herein. These defects are categorized according to their location as being mid muscular vs apical (in relation to the moderator band), and anterior vs posterior. They can exist as a single defect, or as multiple simultaneous defects (Swiss-cheese type of VSD, when consisting of 4 or more defects) [3].

Diagnosis and Pre-procedural Assessment

Preprocedural evaluation is of paramount importance to determine not just eligibility for percutaneous closure of a mVSD, but also to define the characteristics of the VSD and to plan for the best percutaneous approach, as well as to anticipate any potential post-procedural complications. Evaluation begins with a transthoracic echocardiogram (TTE) to identify the location, number, and size of mVSDs, and to determine the presence or absence of any associated cardiac defects. Pre-procedural TTE also plays an important role in evaluating the hemodynamic significance of mVSD through assessing the size of the left heart chambers and helps in estimating the amount of shunt (Qp:Qs). It is worth noting that most small mVSDs are often not hemodynamically significant. These small mVSDs are sometimes difficult to visualize on TTE by 2D and may necessitate color Doppler evaluation. Important views to obtain by TTE for the assessment of mVSD include the parasternal short and long axis views and the 4-chamber view. The parasternal short axis view with a sweep beginning at the base of the heart and progressing to the apex is of particular importance in evaluating mVSDs. In this view, posterior mVSDs will appear between 7 and 10 o'clock, mid-muscular VSDs will appear between 10 and 12 o'clock, and anterior mVSDs will appear between 12 and 2 o'clock [4]. The parasternal long axis view is also helpful to assess the location and size of mVSD with particular sweeps across the septum using color Doppler. Additional views to assess mVSD location and number include the apical 4-chamber sweep. In the apical view, visualization of the defect at the level of the atrioventricular valves indicates a posterior mVSD, whereas visualization at the level of the outflow tracts indicates an anterior mVSD. In addition, the location along the long axis plane (apical vs mid vs basal) can be interrogated in this view. These various views are also essential to assess for left sided chamber dilatation and estimating the gradient across the VSD shunt. In younger patients and children, the subcostal sagittal view is also helpful to assess the mVSD shunt and location.

Transesophageal echocardiography (TEE) plays an important intraprocedural role during mVSD closure. TEE can help with accurate sizing, localization of the defect (s), and identification of total number of defects prior to closure. It can also be used to monitor closure through assessing the stability of the device, impingement on surrounding structures, and residual shunts post device deployment. TEE views during percutaneous VSD closure include a trans-gastric short axis view of the left ventricle, mid-esophageal four chamber view, and the transgastric basal short axis view [5, 6]. These views are essential to evaluate the shunt location and size during the intra-operative procedure and for selecting which VSD to approach first especially in the setting of multiple or Swiss Cheese mVSDs. TEE also provides accurate measurement of the size of the mVSD which is usually done by 2D and color in order to decide on the size of the device needed. After other associated abnormalities are studied and after chamber sizes and function are assessed, more imaging is performed concentrating on the VSD and nearby structures, namely, the papillary muscles, moderator band, and the chordae tendinae. The atrioventricular valves are interrogated at baseline for any regurgitation.

The VSD is measured in multiple views including the frontal 4-chamber and basal short-axis views. Tissue rims and distances from aortic and tricuspid valves are also measured in the above views to determine adequacy for device closure. The appropriate device size is usually chosen to be 1–2 mm larger than the VSD size as assessed by TEE with color Doppler and angiographic evaluation (maximal size at end-diastole). During the closure procedure, the TEE mid-esophageal 4-chamber view is a helpful home view to help guide passage of the guidewire and the delivery system across the defect into the LV cavity and to monitor the subsequent deployment of the LV disk followed by aligning the device in the appropriate position against the ventricular septum. This real-time monitoring of the device by TEE is essential to help the operator maneuver or reposition the device when needed and for avoiding any damage to close-by structures such as the mitral, tricuspid and aortic valves. It is also essential to check for any residual shunting and if significant then to allow the operator to redeploy a larger device if needed.

Heart Team Approach and Discussion

Multiple surgical approaches for mVSD closure have been reported including staged repair with pulmonary artery banding as a first step in young patients, or single stage repair via a right atriotomy, right ventriculotomy, or left ventriculotomy [7]. A left ventriculotomy offers ideal visualization of these defects but leaves the patient susceptible to myocardial dysfunction and aneurysm formation [7, 8]. A right ventriculotomy, while associated with less ventricular dysfunction, is hindered by the fact that visualization of muscular septal defects can be challenging in the setting of dense trabeculations that are intrinsic to the right ventricle [7, 9]. A right atriotomy makes visualization of apical VSDs difficult [10]. Staged repair, now rarely used and done mostly with complicated congenital defects, is associated with up to 50% early reoperation for pulmonary artery band revision [11].

Alternatively, as more devices made their way into the market, percutaneous mVSD closure has become a viable alternative to surgical repair. For a mVSD to be considered suitable for percutaneous closure, it must be of significant size to be considered hemodynamically significant and the patient should be at least 5 kg although more contemporary device design may facilitate closure in smaller infants. On the other hand, exclusion criteria for percutaneous mVSD closure include evidence of irreversible pulmonary vascular disease, proximity to the semilunar or AV valves (defined as <4 mm) [12] and patients with contraindications to anti-platelet therapy. Though a variety of devices exist for percutaneous, VSD closure, the catheter-based approach is generally similar and involves crossing the mVSD retrograde from the LV using a soft wire. Device delivery can be antero-grade when the operator snares the wire from the right side (pulmonary artery or superior vena cava) and exteriorizes it either from the femoral vein or right internal jugular vein based on the location of the mVSD, and then advancing the delivery sheath over this wire to mid LV cavity. Alternatively, the delivery sheath can be positioned retrogradely over this wire into the mid RV cavity and deployment of the device first in RV, then defect and finally the LV desk into the LV.

Heart Team Decision

The ideal approach for closure of the mVSD in our patient was discussed among the surgical and interventional teams. The apical nature of the mVSD would make surgical closure via a right atriotomy challenging, and the team wished to avoid a ventriculotomy unless necessary. The patient was scheduled for surgical repair of his tricuspid valve, and decision was made to perform a hybrid procedure by closing the VSD through direct perventricular access to the right ventricle.

Intra and Post-procedural Assessment

Intra-procedural and immediate post-procedural evaluation is typically done by fluoroscopy and TEE while the patient is in the catheterization laboratory to assess the position of the device, any residual shunting through the device, any affected structures close to the device as well as any change in cardiac function and pericardial effusion. In addition, the presence of additional mVSDs should be identified as small mVSD that are difficult to identify during pre-procedural assessment can have significantly more flow across them immediately after closure of a larger mVSD.

Initial angiography in our case confirmed the presence of a large apical mVSD. The defect was also visualized by TEE, which revealed a defect that measured approximately 18 mm in diameter (Fig. 1).

As this case was performed in the operating room due to the need for tricuspid valve repair, fluoroscopy was not used during the device closure. Under TEE guidance, a wire was used to cross the defect from the right into the left ventricle. A delivery sheath was then advanced over the wire and positioned in the mid LV (Fig. 2). An 18 mm Amplatzer muscular VSD occluder was advanced through the sheath. Deployment of the device was done under TEE guidance to ensure adequate positioning across the apical mVSD (Fig. 3). Prior to release, TEE showed

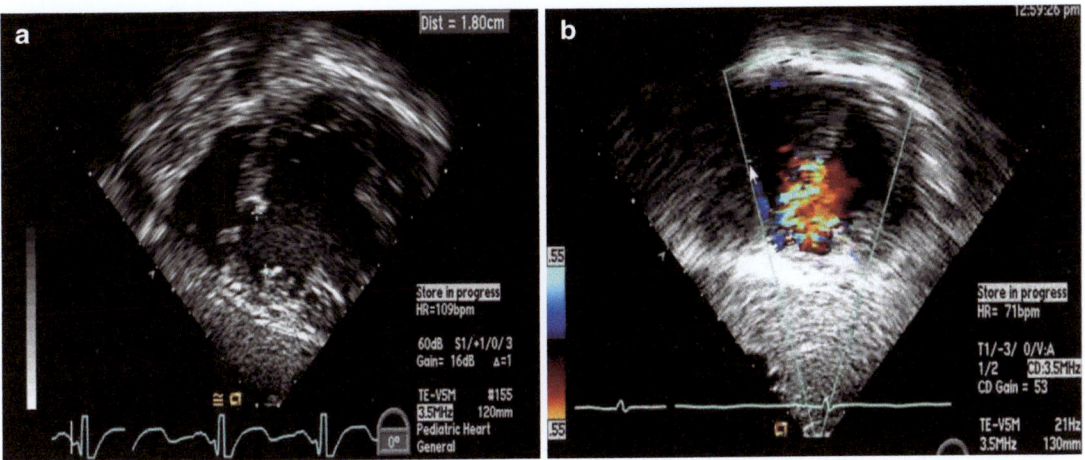

Fig. 1 (**a**) Trans-gastric basal SAX showing the VSD in 2D. (**b**) Trans-gastric basal SAX showing the VSD with color

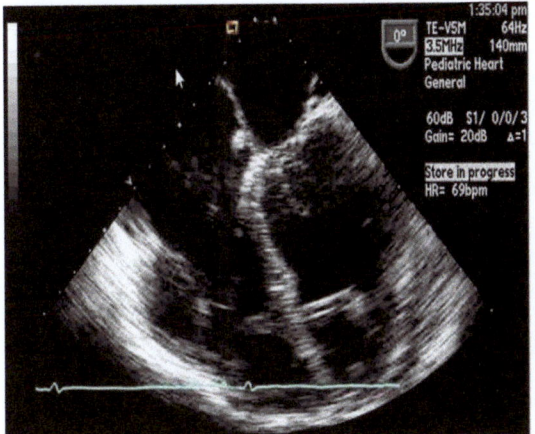

Fig. 2 TEE mid-esophageal 4 chamber view showing the sheath crossing through mVSD

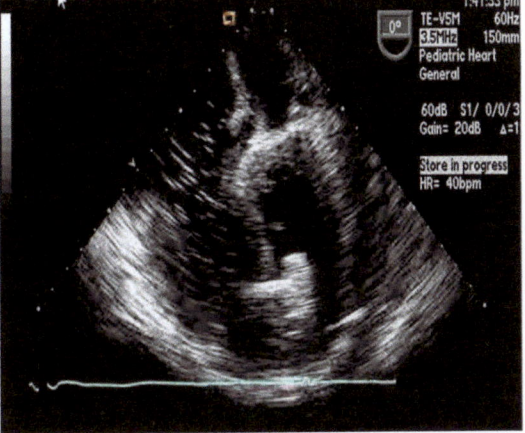

Fig. 3 TEE mid-esophageal 4 chamber view showing the device across the mVSD with the LV disc on the left side

minimal flow across the device. Immediate postprocedural assessment by TEE revealed a well seated device with minimal residual flow through it (Fig. 4).

Subsequent assessment is typically done by TTE on the first day post procedure and at subsequent follow up at 4–6 weeks. This assessment should focus on the presence or absence of residual flow through and around the device, any presence of pericardial effusion, and assessment of cardiac function. In rare instances, when a mVSD is large and not pressure restrictive, closure could result in a significant increase in LV afterload leading to systolic dysfunction.

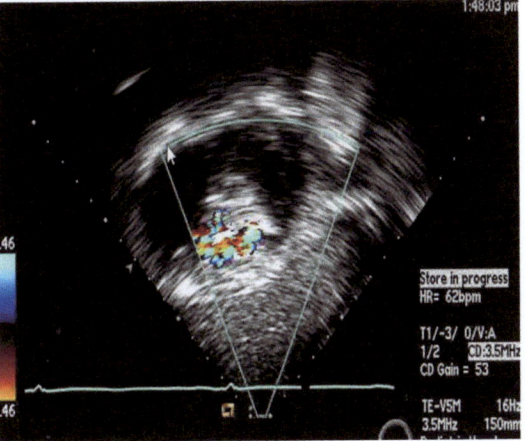

Fig. 4 TEE trans-gastric SAX view showing the device in place with minimal flow across it

Clinical Controversies and Clinical Pearls

- Visualization of mVSD is sometimes difficult by 2D TTE and may necessitate color Doppler evaluation. Important views are parasternal short and long axis views and the 4-chamber view.
- In adults with poor image quality, TTE has limited value for precise anatomical and hemodynamic assessment.
- Percutaneous closure of mVSD is becoming a viable alternative option to surgical closure.
- Surgical closure via left ventriculotomy is ideal for defect visualization with the risk of left myocardial dysfunction and aneurysm formation. A right ventriculotomy, while associated with less ventricular dysfunction, is hindered by the fact of difficult visualization of mVSD due to RV dense trabeculations

Key Points

- The mVSD is an interventricular septum defect exclusively surrounded by muscular borders and are categorized according to their location as being mid muscular vs apical (in relation to the moderator band), and anterior vs posterior.
- Pre-procedural imagining is done mainly via TTE and focuses on identifying location, number, and size of the defects, as well as helping to identify hemodynamically significant defects that require closure and the presence or absence of any associated cardiac defects
- The appropriate device size is usually chosen to be 1–2 mm larger than the VSD size as assessed by TEE with color Doppler and angiographic evaluation (maximal size at end-diastole).
- Percutaneous closure relies heavily on intraprocedural use of TEE and fluoroscopy to ensure appropriately positioned device with minimal residual flow and no damage to adjacent structures.
- Post procedural assessment is typically done by TTE on the first day post procedure and at subsequent follow up at 4–6 weeks
- Exclusion criteria for percutaneous mVSD closure include evidence of irreversible pulmonary vascular disease, proximity to the semilunar or AV valves (defined as <4 mm) [12] and patients with contraindications to antiplatelet therapy.

Perimembrenous VSD

Case Study

Our patient is a 63-year-old male with a history of bicuspid aortic valve with mild-moderate aortic regurgitation, recurrent streptococcus sanguis septecemia leading to infective endocarditis, and a perimembranous VSD (pmVSD) with communication to the right atrium. He also had coronary artery disease with percutaneous coronary intervention on the right coronary artery, left anterior descending coronary artery, and the left circumflex coronary artery. He presented for percutaneous closure of his pmVSD in the setting of significant left to right shunt across the pmVSD and a high-pressure gradient of 105 mmHg across it.

Background and Definitions

A pmVSD, sometimes called central, subaortic, membranous, and paramembranous VSD, is a defect that exists within the membranous septum of the heart. Such defects are located behind the septal leaflet of the tricuspid valve and below the right or non-coronary leaflet of the aortic valve [3]. They are the most common type of VSDs and represent about 80% of all ventricular septal defects [1].

Diagnosis and Pre-procedural Assessment

As in the case of mVSD, pre-procedural assessment of pmVSD provides critical information about the feasibility of percutaneous closure. Here again, the TTE plays a pivotal role in assessing the size of the defect and proximity to surrounding structures including the tricuspid valve and the aortic valve. This is of paramount importance, since the pmVSD exists in fibrous continuity with the tricuspid valve in the right ventricle and the aortic valve in the left ventricle [4]. As such, care must be taken to identify the presence or absence of tricuspid valve attachment to the margins of the VSD and the presence or absence of aortic valve prolapse through the VSD. TTE is also used to estimate the amount of shunting and to assess left chamber sizes to help determine the hemodynamic significance of the pmVSD. Pulmonary artery pressure and right ventricular pressure should also be assessed. Identifying the presence of an aneurysm, also known as a windsock deformity, in the perimembranous area is also an important part of pre-procedural TTE evaluation as it could affect the type of device used for percutaneous closure.

Characterization of the pmVSD through TTE is best done in the parasternal short and parasternal long axis views, as well as the apical view. Typically, in the parasternal short axis view, the pmVSD is visualized at the level of the base between the tricuspid valve annulus and the 12'o clock position. In the parasternal long axis view, the defect is seen just beneath the aortic valve. This view is particularly helpful in identifying any prolapse of the aortic valve cusps. Here, too, the distance between the superior rim of the defect and the aortic valve can be measured to determine adequacy of the rims for percutaneous device closure (at least a 2 mm rim between the aortic valve and the defect is required for percutaneous closure). Those views are also helpful to determine the size of the defect by 2D and color Doppler and to determine the pressure gradient across the defect and the degree of aortic insufficiency, if any. The apical 4-chamber and 5-chamber views help assess the VSD and determine any enlargement of the left-sided chambers.

Intraprocedural TEE also plays an important role to ensure safe closure of a pmVSD, perhaps more so than a mVSD. Here, the operator must deploy the device without affecting the tricuspid or aortic valve leaflets. Important TEE windows to visualize a pmVSD include the four-chamber and five-chamber mid-esophageal view, the mid-esophageal long axis view, and the mid-esophageal short axis view. As is the case with mVSDs, full assessment is performed including assessing chamber sizes and function as well as the atrioventricular valves before focusing on the pmVSD. The above views are often used to assess the VSD size and rims. The TEE mid-esophageal 4-chamber view is then used to help guide the passage of the delivery system and device, as well as its deployment. Transesophageal echocardiography ensures adequate size and absence of significant impingement on the atrioventricular valves and their structures and allows the operator to check on any significant residual shunting before release of the device.

In addition to TEE, Intracardiac Echocardiography (ICE) can also be utilized during pmVSD device closure and can potentially avoid the use of general anesthesia in adult cases [6]. After introduction of the ICE catheter through the femoral vein, it is advanced from the inferior vena cava and placed in the right atrium in a neutral position. The ultrasound plane is oriented such that it passes through the tricuspid valve. This provides the operator with the "home view", which allows visualization of the right atrium (RA), right ventricle (RV), right ventricular outflow tract (RVOT), and the membranous septum where the pmVSD is located. Next, the operator can flex the catheter slightly such that the transducer remains in the RA but assumes a slight anterior angulation towards the atrial septum to provide a 4-chamber view. From there, the operator can flex the catheter posteriorly and rotate the entire system clockwise such that the transducer will sit within the tricuspid valve annulus. This will provide the subaortic short axis view. Using these three views, pmVSD characterization can be done and appropriate device deployment and release can be monitored [6]. It is worth noting that current ICE systems require at least an 8 Fr sheath, which limits their use to older children and adults.

Heart Team Approach and Discussion

Percutaneous pmVSD closure has been gaining traction as a safe and effective alternative to surgical repair over the past 20 years. Indeed, a recent meta-analysis that looked at 6762 such procedures noted a success rate of 97.8%. Complete heart block, which had been an early stumbling block for percutaneous pmVSD closure, occurred in 1.1% of cases. In an RCT comparing percutaneous vs surgical pmVSD closure, there were no cases of complete heart block in either arm. As a matter of fact, minor adverse events were noted to be significantly higher in the surgical arm as compared to the percutaneous arm [13]. In addition, newer devices for pmVSD percutaneous closure have been reported as potentially having lower risk of complete heart block. For example, several studies assessing the risk of heart block with Konar-MF, vascular plug II, Nit-Occlud Le VSD-Coil, and the ADO II have shown rates ranging from 0 to 1.4% [14].

When considering such an approach, inclusion criteria consist of a 2 mm rim between the VSD defect and the aortic valve, and a defect <12 to 14 mm [15]. Patients are excluded from consideration, however, if the VSD is associated with other cardiac malformations that require surgical repair, if there is irreversible pulmonary vascular disease, severe aortic valve prolapse, or if there is malalignment of the ventricular septum [15, 16]. Here too, patients with contraindications to antiplatelet therapy may be considered for surgical closure.

Heart Team Decision

In our patient, the history of significant coronary artery disease in the setting of mild to moderate aortic valve regurgitation and infective endocarditis led to a discussion about the possibility of avoiding cardiopulmonary bypass. The surgical and catheterization teams discussed the feasibility of percutaneous closure. Given that there was no evidence of aortic prolapse and no significant septal malalignment, the team felt comfortable proceeding with percutaneous pmVSD closure.

Intra and Post-procedural Assessment

Intra-procedural and immediate post-procedural assessment is done by TEE while the patient is still in the catheterization laboratory. In percutaneous pmVSD device closure, immediate post-procedural TEE assessment should focus on the presence or absence of tricuspid valve regurgitation and aortic regurgitation. Flow across the device should also be assessed, as well as stability of the device. In addition, any change in cardiac function and presence of pericardial effusion is assessed, as in any intervention.

In our patient, initial angiography showed a pmVSD with left ventricle to right atrial communication. This was confirmed by Intraprocedural TEE, which showed a moderate pmVSD seen best in the mid-esophageal aortic valve short-axis views (Fig. 5). There was evidence of mild aortic regurgitation by TEE at baseline, however there was no evidence of ventricular septal malalignment.

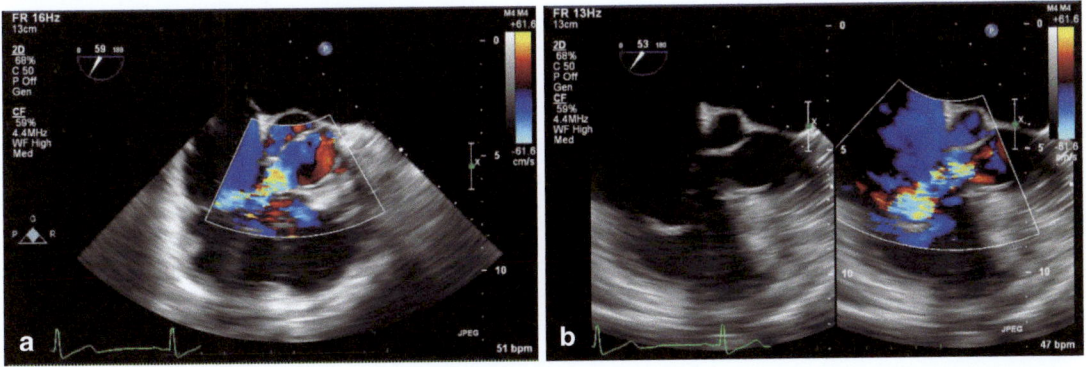

Fig. 5 (**a**) TEE mid-esophageal SAX showing the pmVSD shunt with a LV-RA jet. (**b**) TEE mid-esophageal SAX view with 2D and color showing the defect

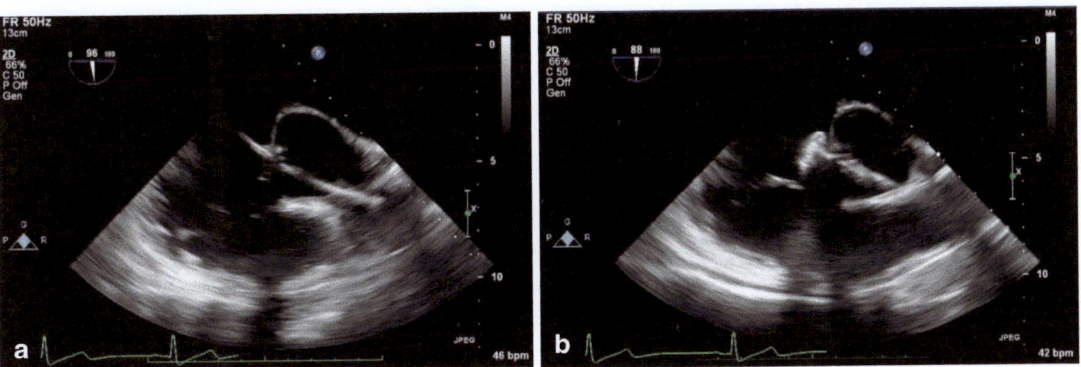

Fig. 6 (**a**) TEE mid-esophageal view with angulation showing the wire crossing the LV into the RA across the pmVSD. (**b**) Same TEE view showing one disk of the device deployed into the RA side

After crossing the pmVSD from the left ventricle under fluoroscopic and TEE guidance, the wire was advanced into the superior vena cava. An 8 Fr sheath was advanced over the stiff wire and positioned across the VSD. Under both fluoroscopic and echocardiographic guidance, a Lifetech Symmetric membranous VSD occluder was deployed. The device sat across the defect on the right atrial aspect rather than the right ventricular aspect (Fig. 6). Here, TEE images ensured not only adequate positioning, but also verified the normal function of the aortic and tricuspid valves and ensured the absence of any regurgitation secondary to impingement of the device (Fig. 7). Further imaging showed the device in good position with no residual shunting (Fig. 8).

Subsequent assessment is done exclusively by TTE, with the first echo typically on the first day post-procedure and a follow up echo done at 4–6 weeks thereafter. Aside from valvular regurgitation, subsequent assessment should focus on pericardial effusion, myocardial dysfunction, presence of residual flow through and around the pmVSD device, and the presence of additional ventricular septal defects not seen prior to pmVSD closure. Additionally, stability and position of the device can be assessed by TTE.

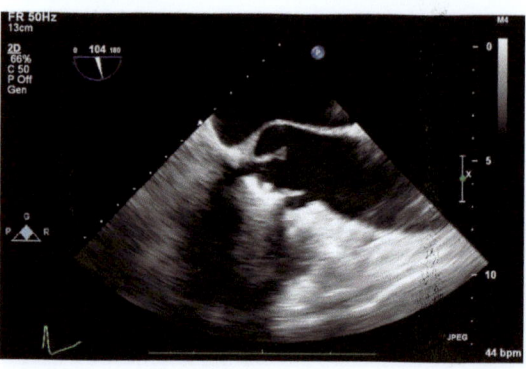

Fig. 7 TEE mid-esophageal LAX showing no impingement of the device on the aortic valve

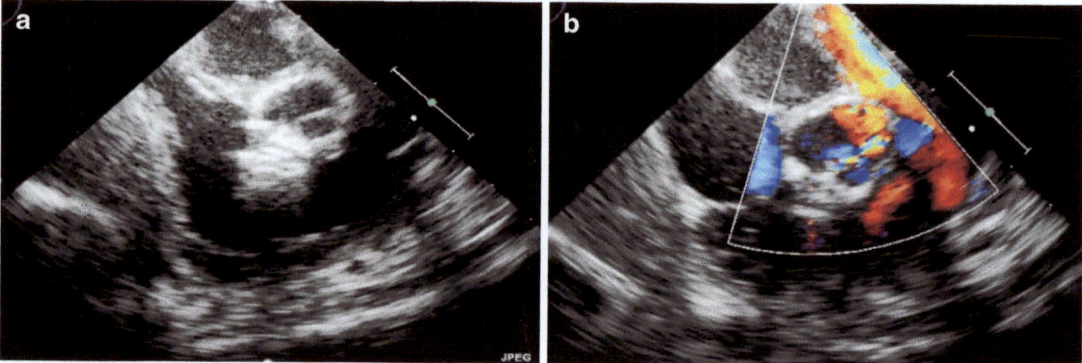

Fig. 8 TEE mid-esophageal view with 2D (**a**) and color (**b**) after device deployment showing the VSD device in good position with no residual shunting by color

Clinical Controversies and Clinical Pearls

- Surgical vs. transcatheter closure of pmVSD: A randomized control trial comparing surgical vs transcatheter approach for closure of pmVSD showed fewer side effects in the percutaneous group
- TEE is a common method for intra-procedural and immediate post-procedural assessment focusing on the presence or absence of tricuspid valve regurgitation and aortic regurgitation, residual shunting across the device as well as proper position and stability of the device. Some centers use ICE during pmVSD device closure and avoid general anesthesia.

Key Points
- Perimembranous VSDs are the most common type of VSDs exist is in the membranous septum located behind the septal leaflet of the tricuspid valve and below the right or non-coronary leaflet of the aortic valve.
- Transthoracic echocardiography has a pivotal role in pmVSD by assessing the size of the defect and proximity to surrounding structures including the tricuspid valve and the aortic valve, while TEE, ICE and angiography are the mainstay of intraprocedural evaluation.
- At least a 2 mm rim between the aortic valve and the defect and a defect size <12-14 mm is suggested for percutaneous closure.

- Usually patients are excluded from VSD percutaneous closure. if the VSD is associated with other cardiac malformations that require surgical repair, if there is irreversible pulmonary vascular disease, severe aortic valve prolapse, or if there is malalignment of the ventricular septum.

Imaging study	Benefits	Disadvantages
Echocardiogram	– TTE has the key role in diagnosis mVSD and providing anatomical, and physiological data such as shunt direction and (Qp:Qs) volume overload, RV and PA pressures, LV function. – Real time imaging TEE is ideal imaging modality for intra procedural evaluation – Rules out other anatomical lesions. ICE can be utilized for intraprocedural assessment. – No radiation	– In adults with poor image quality TTE has limited value for precise anatomical and hemodynamic assessment
CT	– Detailed anatomic evaluation. – Can help evaluate the ventricular function	– No hemodynamic information. – Radiation exposure
MRI	– Provides detailed anatomical evaluation, shunt flow assessment, (Qp:Qs), associated anomalies as well as accurate ventricular function. – No radiation	-Some form of sedation is commonly needed in children with <6 years age and older patients with cognitive impairment

Chapter Review Questions

1. What is the most common type of ventricular septal defect?
   A. Inlet VSD
   B. Muscular VSD
   C. Perimembrenous VSD
   D. Outlet VSD
   Answer: C
   Explanation: Of all VSDs, perimembrenous VSD constitute about 80% with muscular VSD being a distant second at 10–15%.

2. Which of the following constitutes an exclusion criterion for percutaneous perimembranous VSD closure?
   A. Decreased left ventricular systolic function
   B. Severe aortic valve prolapse
   C. Presence of a patent foramen ovale
   D. A defect measuring 10 mm in diameter-
   Answer: B
   Explanation: Severe aortic valve prolapse is a contraindication for perimembranous VSD device closure. Other contraindications include presence of other congenital cardiac defects that require surgical closure, malalignment of the ventricular septum, and the presence of irreversible pulmonary hypertension.

3. Which of the following TEE views is most useful in the evaluation a perimembranous VSD?
   A. Trans-gastric mid-papillary short axis view
   B. Mid-esophageal bicaval view
   C. Trans-gastric basal short axis view
   D. Mid-esophageal 2 chamber
   E. Mid-esophageal long axis view
   Answer: E
   Explanation: The following TEE views are most helpful in evaluation of a perimembranous VSD: Mid-esophageal long axis view, mid-esophageal aortic valve short axis view, and mid-esophageal 4 chamber view.

4. Which of the following statements about surgical VSD closure is INCORRECT?
   A. Left ventriculotomy is associated with aneurysm formation
   B. Right atriotomy provides an ideal view for the correction of an apical muscular VSD
   C. Right ventricular trabeculations can make the visualization of muscular VSD difficult via a right ventriculotomy

   Answer: B

   Explanation: By virtue of its location, an apical muscular VSD is difficult to visualize via a right atriotomy and might require a ventriculotomy for surgical closure. A left ventriculotomy might offer the best views of ventricular septal defects but is associated with ventricular dysfunction and aneurysm formation. A right ventriculotomy is associated with less dysfunction, though muscular septal defects can be difficult to visualize given the extensive trabeculations of the right ventricular septum.

5. Which of the following is not part of the immediate post-procedural TEE assessment of perimembranous VSD percutaneous device closure?
   A. Impingement on the aortic valve
   B. Left ventricular outflow tract obstruction
   C. Impingement on tricuspid valve
   D. Evidence of endocarditis

   Answer: D

   Explanation: All the choices provided, except for endocarditis, are possible complications of percutaneous perimembranous VSD closure that can be evaluated for by immediate post-procedure TEE assessment.

References

1. Diab KA, Cao QL, Hijazi ZM. Device closure of congenital ventricular septal defects. Congenit Heart Dis. 2007;2:92–103.
2. Diab K, Shibbani K, Nigro J, Pophal S, Alboliras ET. Perventricular and percutaneous closure of traumatic ventricular septal defects following blunt chest trauma. J Struct Heart Disease. 2016;2:3–101.
3. Moss and Adams' heart disease in infants, children, and adolescents. Wolters Kluwer; 2016.
4. Echocardiography in pediatric and congenital heart disease. Wiley Blackwell 2016.
5. Hijazi ZM, Shivkumar K, Sahn DJ. Intracardiac echocardiography during interventional and electrophysiological cardiac catheterization. Circulation. 2009;119:587–96.
6. Cao QL, Zabal C, Koenig P, Sandhu S, Hijazi ZM. Initial clinical experience with intracardiac echocardiography in guiding transcatheter closure of perimembranous ventricular septal defects: feasibility and comparison with transesophageal echocardiography. Catheter Cardiovasc Interv. 2005;66:258–67.
7. Kitagawa T, Durham LA 3rd, Mosca RS, Bove EL. Techniques and results in the management of multiple ventricular septal defects. J Thorac Cardiovasc Surg. 1998;115:848–56.
8. Wollenek G, Wyse R, Sullivan I, Elliott M, de Leval M, Stark J. Closure of muscular ventricular septal defects through a left ventriculotomy. Eur J Cardiothorac Surg. 1996;10:595–8.
9. Shetty V, Shetty D, Punnen J, Chattuparambil B, Whitlock R, Bohra D. Single-stage repair for multiple muscular septal defects: a single-Centre experience across 16 years. Interact Cardiovasc Thorac Surg. 2017;25:422–6.
10. Myhre U, Duncan BW, Mee RB, Joshi R, Seshadri SG, Herrera-Verdugo O, et al. Apical right ventriculotomy for closure of apical ventricular septal defects. Ann Thorac Surg. 2004;78:204–8.
11. Seddio F, Reddy VM, McElhinney DB, Tworetzky W, Silverman NH, Hanley FL. Multiple ventricular septal defects: how and when should they be repaired? J Thorac Cardiovasc Surg. 1999;117:134–9; discussion 139–140.
12. Holzer R, Balzer D, Cao QL, Lock K, Hijazi ZM. Device closure of muscular ventricular septal defects using the amplatzer muscular ventricular septal defect occluder: immediate and mid-term results of a U.S. Registry. J Am Coll Cardiol. 2004;43:1257–63.
13. Yang J, Yang L, Yu S, Liu J, Zuo J, Chen W, et al. Transcatheter versus surgical closure of perimembranous ventricular septal defects in children: a randomized controlled trial. J Am Coll Cardiol. 2014;63:1159–68.
14. Leong MC, Alwi M. Complete atrio-ventricular heart block, a not to be forgotten complication in transcatheter closure of perimembranous ventricular septal defect—a case report and review of literature. Cardiol Young. 2021;31:2031–4.
15. Yang J, Yang L, Wan Y, Zuo J, Zhang J, Chen W, et al. Transcatheter device closure of perimembranous ventricular septal defects: mid-term outcomes. Eur Heart J. 2010;31:2238–45.
16. Butera G, Carminati M, Chessa M, Piazza L, Micheletti A, Negura DG, et al. Transcatheter closure of perimembranous ventricular septal defects: early and long-term results. J Am Coll Cardiol. 2007;50:1189–95.

Coronary Cameral Fistula Closure

Anita Sadeghpour, Ata Firouzi, and Zahra Hosseini

Abstract

Coronary-cameral fistulas (CCFs) are abnormal communications between coronary arteries and cardiac chambers. Predominant symptoms are angina and heart failure, although the majority are asymptomatic, particularly small CCFs. The therapeutic approach consists of a medical, surgical, or transcatheter approach. However, the optimal strategy is controversial and percutaneous transcatheter closure (TCC) is increasingly applied with promising results as an effective and safe alternative to surgery. In evaluating a patient with CCFs, the following parameters should be considered: Location (proximal vs distal), size (small vs large) and number of the CCFs (single vs multiples). Symptomatic patients with moderate or large size CCF should be discussed in the multidisciplinary team and carefully selected for TCC considering that myocardial infarction (MI) is a major complication of this procedure. In this section, we will discuss the role of cardiac imaging in diagnosis of CCFs and pre and post-procedural assessment of the patients who are candidate for TCC.

Keywords

Coronary-cameral fistulas · Coronary artery fistula · Congenital heart disease · Continuous murmur · Transcatheter closure · Echocardiography · Cardiac imaging

Supplementary Information The online version contains supplementary material available at https://doi.org/10.1007/978-3-031-50740-3_12.

A. Sadeghpour (✉)
MedStar Cardiovascular Corelabs, MedStar Health Research Institute and Georgetown University, Washington, DC, USA
e-mail: anita.sadeghpour@medstar.net

A. Firouzi · Z. Hosseini
Cardiovascular Intervention Research Center, Rajaie Cardiovascular Medical and Research Center, Tehran, Iran

Abbreviations

CAFs	Coronary artery fistulas
CCF	Color flow imaging
CT	Computed tomography
LA	Left atrium
LMCA	Left main coronary artery
LV	Left ventricle
MI	Myocardial infarction
NYHA	New York Heart Association
RA	Right atrium
RV	Right ventricle
TEE	Transesophageal echocardiography
TTE	Transthoracic echocardiography

> Test your learning and check your understanding of this book's contents: use the "Springer Nature Flashcards" app to access questions using ▶ https://sn.pub/ambACS.
> To use the app, please follow the instructions in the chapter "Transcatheter Aortic Valve Replacement."

Learning Objectives

1. Identify CCFs and choose the appropriate imaging modality for the optimal management.
2. Know the indications for CCFs closure and preprocedural considerations of TCC vs surgical repair.
3. Know the early and late outcomes and complications of transcatheter CCFs closure.
4. Learn appropriate imaging modality for the follow up and investigation interval.

> **Case 1**
> A 34-year-old woman was referred to the outpatient clinic for evaluation of recent onset atypical chest pain, and dyspnea on exertion (NYHA functional class II). Physical examination was unremarkable except for a continuous murmur (grade II) heard at the mid-chest wall. Electrocardiogram (ECG) showed a normal sinus rhythm with a normal axis, without any abnormal ST-T segment changes.

Background and Definitions

Coronary artery fistulas (CAFs) are congenital or acquired abnormal vascular communications between the coronary arteries and the cardiac chambers or any segment of the systemic or pulmonary circulation, without an intervening capillary network. The prevalence of CAFs visualized by computed tomographic (CT) angiography is reported to be as high as 0.9%, which is higher than the previously reported prevalence of 0.002% to 0.3% in invasive angiography [1, 2]. More than 90% of CAFs are congenital, while acquired CAFs result from iatrogenic events such as myocardial infarction, myectomy, coronary stent placement, coronary bypass surgery, trauma, chest irradiation, intracardiac device implantation, endomyocardial biopsies, and coronary vasculitis. CAFs can be detected in any age group with no predilection for either sex. Although most patients with CAFs are asymptomatic, clinical symptoms have been reported in 19% of patients aged younger than 20 years and in 63% of older patients [3]. Patients with medium or large CAFs are usually referred for the evaluation of loud continuous murmurs, electrocardiographic (ECG) changes, or clinical symptoms such as exertional dyspnea, chest pain, myocardial infarction, infective arteritis, arrhythmia, syncope, and congestive heart failure. The severity of the symptoms depends on the amount of the coronary steal syndrome, presence of concomitant congenital anomalies, and the degree of the left-to-right shunting which is determined by the origin, the site of the drainage, the size of the fistula, and the number of involved coronary vessels. Accordingly, a precise evaluation of the anatomy of CAFs defining the origin, course, and termination site of the fistula is vital.

Coronary-cameral fistulas (CCFs) are a subset of coronary artery fistulas (CAFs) defined as an abnormal communication between coronary arteries and cardiac chambers. Patients with CCFs have left-to-right shunt, determined by the size of the fistula, the pressure of the drainage site, and the degree of the fistula flow. Those with a modest left-to-right shunt flow present with right heart volume overload, and high cardiac output state, whereas those with a significant left-to-left shunt tend to present with left ventricular volume overload and arterial runoff similar to aortic insufficiency. Spontaneous closure of CAFs could occur in 1–2% of patients. The natural course is the progressive dilation of the fistulous tract, which may progress to aneurysm formation, intimal ulceration, medial degeneration, intimal rupture, atherosclerotic deposition, calcification, side-branch obstruction, mural thrombosis, and rarely, rupture [4]. Complications secondary to CAFs are present in 11% of patients younger than 20 years of age and in 35% of patients aged above 20 years [5].

Diagnostic Workup

Physical Exam: In the physical examination of patients with significant CAFs, the most typical finding is a loud, soft, crescendo-decrescendo continuous murmur on the chest wall depending on the entry site. It is often lower than the murmur of a patent ductus arteriosus (PDA) and *peaks in mid-to-late diastole at the drainage site*. In the differential diagnosis of this murmur, PDAs, ruptured sinuses of Valsalva, anomalous origin of the left coronary artery (LCA) or the right coronary artery (RCA) from the pulmonary artery, aortopulmonary windows, and pulmonary arteriovenous fistulas should be considered.

ECG: ST-T changes is dependent on the magnitude of ischemia and left or right ventricular volume overload, although ECG is normal in about 50% of patients.

Echocardiogram: In 2D transthoracic echocardiography (TTE), the hemodynamic effect of CAFs (the size and function of the left and right chambers), regional wall motion abnormality, valvular insufficiency secondary to papillary muscle dysfunction, pulmonary artery pressure, and the dilated fistulous course should be assessed carefully. *Color flow imaging (CFI) is helpful in showing high velocity continuous turbulent flow at the site of termination of the CCFs*. However, detailed anatomy and course of coronary arteries are more difficult to evaluate by echocardiography. Additionally, echocardiography could demonstrate any concomitant anomalies such as atrial septal defects, ventricular septal defects, PDAs, pulmonary atresia with an intact ventricular septum, and the tetralogy of Fallot [6].

Coronary Angiography: Invasive coronary angiography is the gold-standard modality for the detection of CAFs, their origins, courses, and terminal sites. Not only can this modality determine the size and location of fistulous tracts and the number of involved vessels but also it can facilitate the hemodynamic assessment by right heart catheterization. Nevertheless, the efficacy of invasive coronary angiography is undermined by its inability to accurately determine some CAFs with complex courses.

Cardiac CT: ECG-gated CT angiography and 3D volume-rendered imaging are the imaging alternatives and preferred method by some authorities as they can render a precise delineation of the origin, course, and drainage site of CAFs by better temporal and spatial resolution even in complex cases. Furthermore, it assists in selecting the appropriate treatment approach (surgical or transcatheter closure [TCC]) in the preprocedural planning and appropriate device selection before invasive angiography, and finding the optimal fluoroscopic angles. So, Cardiac CT angiography is suggested as a pre-procedural planning imaging modality by defining the fistula's origin, size, anatomic course, and termination site. The evaluation of the presence of other intrathoracic vascular communications requires a wide field of view, including the chest wall.

Cardiac magnetic resonance (CMR): CMR is another modality for the anatomic assessment of CAFs, and myocardial perfusion imaging is a functional test for the evaluation of the severity of myocardial ischemia related to CAFs.

CAF Classification

According to the Sakakibara CAF classification, a CAF can be classified as a proximal or distal segment on the basis of its origin. When the fistula originates within the proximal one-third of the coronary arteries, the proximal feeding arteries tend to be dilated, and the diameter of the coronary arteries distal to the CAF origin remains normal (type A). In the distal type, which usually terminates on the right side of the heart, the feeding arteries originating from the distal coronary arteries tend to be of the end-artery type with dilatation of the entire vessel. (type B) [7]. CAFs can be [8] classified as small fistulas, which are smaller than the largest diameter of the coronary artery not feeding the coronary fistula and absence of coronary artery dilatation; medium-sized fistulas, which are one or two times larger than the largest diameter of the non feeding coronary artery; and large fistulas, which are larger than twice of the largest diameter of the non feeding coronary artery. In another classification, small fistulas are defined as those with a vessel diameter of less than 2 mm, medium-sized fistulas as those with a vessel diameter of between 2 and 8 mm, and large fistulas as those with a vessel diameter of over 8 mm [9].

Concerning the origin sites of CAFs, the RCA is the most frequent (55%), followed by the left anterior descending artery (35%) and the left circumflex artery (LCX) (5–20%) [10]. The most common drainage site is right sided chambers with the following order: right ventricle, pulmonary artery, right atrium, the left ventricle, the coronary sinus, the superior vena cava, and the left atrium [11]. Interestingly, 90% of all CAFs terminate to the right cardiac chambers [12]. However, the site of the origine and drainage of CAF varies between studies. The left main coronary has also been suggested as a common locations where CAF originates. Coronary artery-to-coronary sinus fistulas constitute the most frequent underlying cause of huge aneurysmal formation, congestive heart failure, myocardial infarction, and even sudden cardiac death and are associated with several postprocedural complications (either surgical or TCC) such as myocardial infarction [13].

Management of CAFs

The 2009 American College of Cardiology/American Heart Association (ACC/AHA) guideline for the Management of Adults with Congenital Heart Disease, suggested that percutaneous or surgical closure is a Class I recommendation with the level of evidence C for: 1. Large fistulas regardless of symptoms and 2. For moderate to small-sized fistulas with evidence of myocardial ischemia, arrhythmia, systolic or diastolic dysfunction, ventricular enlargement, or endarteritis. The patients with small, asymptomatic coronary arteriovenous fistulas should not undergo defect closure [14]. The updated 2018 guidelines of the ACC/AHA emphasized the importance of a heart team approach to evaluate the appropriateness and feasibility of CAF closure at centers with expertise in both percutaneous and surgical closure techniques [15].

TCC Techniques

TCC is an invasive strategy associated with fewer complications than the surgical approach. The aim of TCC is to occlude the CAF as distally as possible and close to its termination point to avoid coronary branch occlusion that feeds the normal myocardium. TCC is a suitable strategy with a high success rate in patients with proximal CAFs, single drainage sites, non-tortuous vessels, distal narrowing with accessible routes for the closure device and in the absence of important branches or other cardiac disorders [16]. The most appropriate approach in those with CAFs is trans-arterial technique and in those with CCFs is trans-venous approach.

Diagnosis and Pre-procedural Evaluation in Case 1

As the initial evaluation for a patient with symptoms and signs suggestive for structural heart disease, patient underwent TTE which demonstrated: mild left and right atrium and left ventricular (LV) enlargement with suboptimal contractility (ejection fraction ~50%). Right ventricular (RV) size and function was normal without any valvular heart disease. CFI showed an abnormal continuous turbulent flow originating from left coronary artery with a tortuous course and terminating in the right atrium (RA), near the interatrial septum.

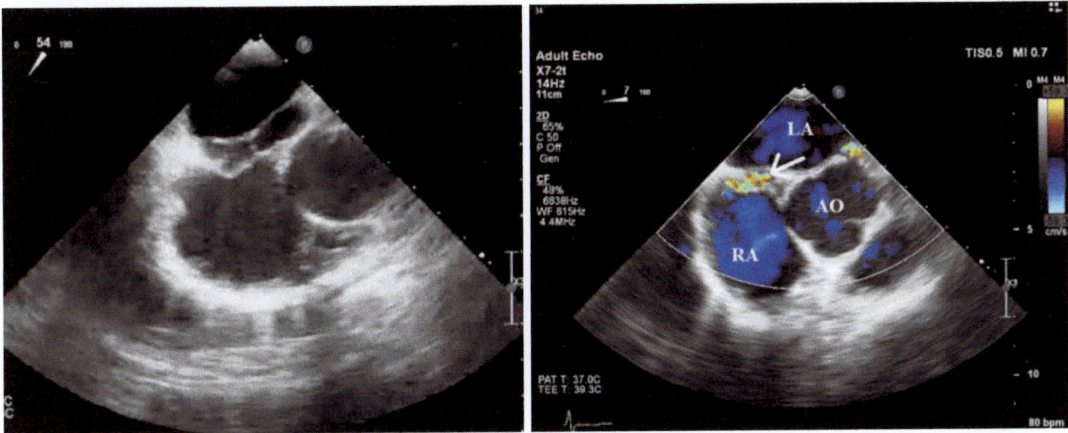

Fig. 1 Transesophageal echocardiography, short-axis view showing fistulus tract by 2D study (Left panel), and dilated left main coronary artery (LMCA) with an anomalous course of the left coronary artery to the interatrial septum (white arrows) and drainage into the right atrium (RA), left atrium (LA), Aorta (AO)

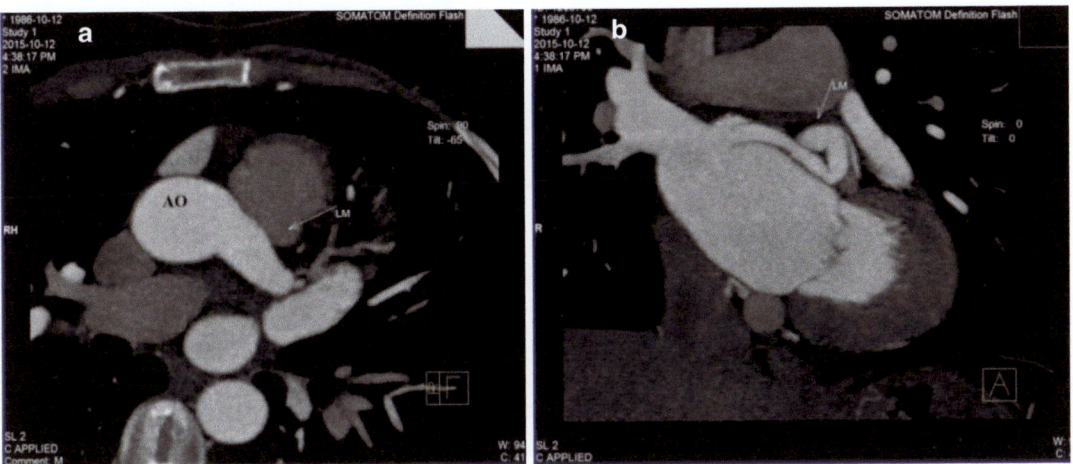

Fig. 2 (**a** and **b**) Coronary computed tomography angiography showed a dilated left main coronary artery (LMCA) (**a**) with an anomalous course of the left coronary artery to the interatrial septum (**b**). Aorta (AO)

Transesophageal echocardiography (TEE) performed for better evaluation of abnormal turbulent flow origin and termination. TEE revealed a dilated left main coronary artery (1.2 cm) (Fig. 1, Videos 1–3) with an abnormal continuous turbulent flow, tortuous course drained into the RA, adjacent to the interatrial septum. The finding was suggestive for CCF originated from the left main with extension and draining to the RA.

Computed tomography (CT) angiography reported a dilated left main, which trifurcated to three branches: the left circumflex artery, left anterior descending artery, and another tortuous and elongated fistulous tract. This finding confirmed the diagnosis of a large single tortuous CCF (Fig. 2a and b).

Heart Team Approach and Decision

Given the patient's history of chest pain, exercise stress echocardiography was requested to find the latent ischemia due to steal phenomenon.

However, the test was terminated in stage I due to symptoms and new wall-motion abnormality.

Based on the symptoms related to the sizable CCFs and chamber dilatation suggestive for significant left to right shunt, patient was candidate for CCFs closure (either TCC or surgically).

In properly selected patients with symptomatic medium or large-size CAFs, TCC is an effective and relatively safe alternative procedure to surgery with reported complete occlusion of 90–95% [17]. The heart team approach is highly recommended [15].

The main parameters to be considered are:

1. Location of CAFs: As proximal or distally located. In other words, the CAFs originating from proximal or distal of the main coronary artery.
2. Size of coronary artery proximal to the CAFs particularly if it is enlarged with diameter ≥10 mm.
3. If the CAFs are simple or complex regarding the number of origins, clarity of the pathway, and termination site (Simple has a single origin, pathway, and termination vs. complex CAFs that are large with multiple origins, tortuous pathway, and plexiform appearance).

In an enlarged proximal coronary artery with diameter ≥10 mm or CAFs with significant myocardium at risk, surgery with bypass graft is suggested since there is a risk of thrombosis and myocardial infarction [18].

In this case, based on the heart team decision making and patient's preference, she was deemed a candidate for TCC of the fistulae.

Procedural Technique

Under conscious sedation and hemodynamic monitoring, after insertion of right common femoral artery and vein sheaths (6-F), IV Heparin was completed to achieve activating clotting time (ACT) more than 200 s. Selective left main (LM) injection confirmed a large fistulous tract which originated from LM trunk and drained to the right atrium (RA-A). After wiring of the LM with a 0.014″ inch coronary guidewire (BMW), the wire was advanced to the right atrium, right ventricle, and the pulmonary artery (B). The wire was snared and exteriorized from the right femoral vein. Through the femoral vein, a long delivery sheath (an 8-F Occlutech) was advanced toward the LM (C). An 8/10 Occlutech patent ductus arteriosus occluder (Occlutech International AB, Sweden) was passed through the sheath. After multiple injections, the occluder was deployed as distally as possible to the LM (D). The final selective LM injection denoted the appropriate position of the device with no residual shunting (E) (Fig. 3).

Case 2

A case of left main coronary artery (LMCA) fistula drainage to the LA: Transesophageal echocardiography (TEE) with CFI showing an abnormal continuous turbulent flow originating from left coronary sinus of Valsalva with a tortuous course and terminating in the LA in a 33-year-old lady with complaint of exertional dyspnea (NYHA functional class III) (Fig. 4a–c).

Computed tomography (CT) angiography reported a dilated left main (13 mm) terminated to the LA via a very tortuous and elongated fistulous tract. So, the diagnosis of a large single tortuous CCF between LM and LA was verified (Fig. 5a–c).

Based on the fistula size (5 mm) estimated by CTA, a Vascular plug III occluder device (10 mm) was chosen for implanting as distally as possible. The final LM injection demonstrated complete obliteration of the fistula flow without complications (Figs. 6 and 7).

Case 3

A 31 year old woman with chief complaint of atypical chest pain shows CCF from LAD to PA. Fig. 8 and Videos 4 and 5.

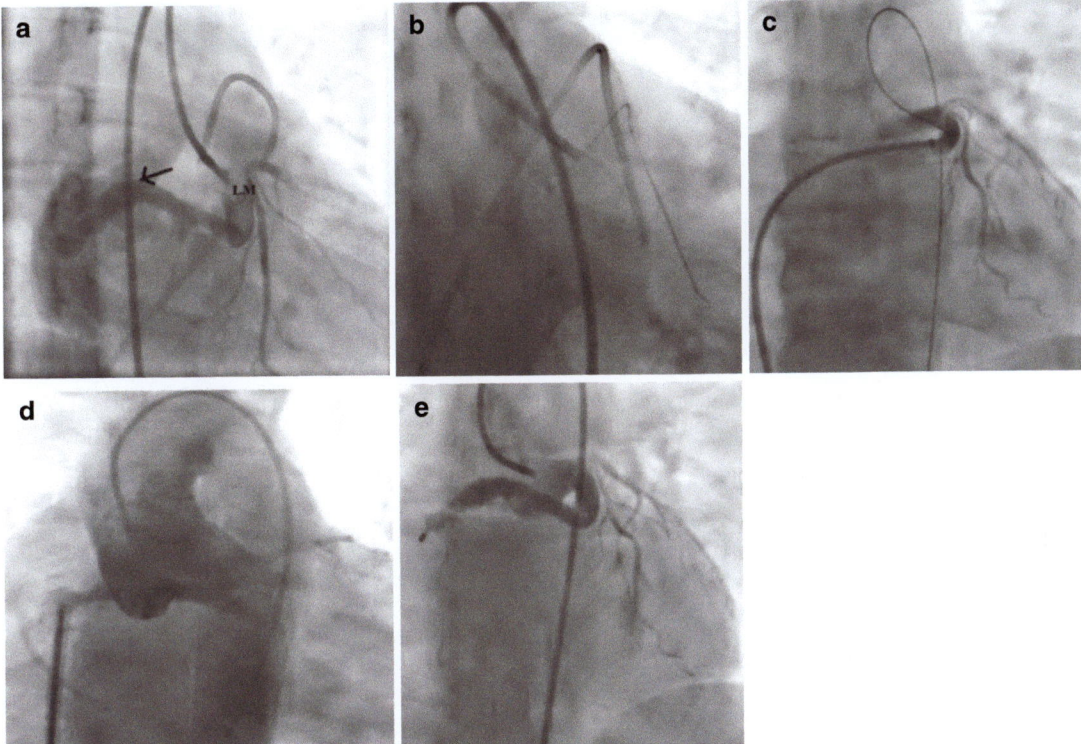

Fig. 3 (a–e) Selective left main coronary artery (LM) injection shows an aneurysmal and elongated LM, draining into the right atrium (a coronary-cameral fistula) (**a**). After wiring of the LM with coronary guidewire (BMW), the wire was advanced to the right atrium, the right ventricle, and the pulmonary artery (**b**). The wire was snared and exteriorized from the right femoral vein. Through the femoral vein, a long delivery sheath (an 8-F Occlutech) was advanced toward the LM (**c**). An 8/10 Occlutech patent ductus arteriosus occluder (Occlutech International AB, Sweden) was passed through the sheath. After multiple injections, the occluder was deployed as distally as possible to the LM (**d**). The final selective LM injection illustrated the appropriate position of the device with no residual shunting (**e**)

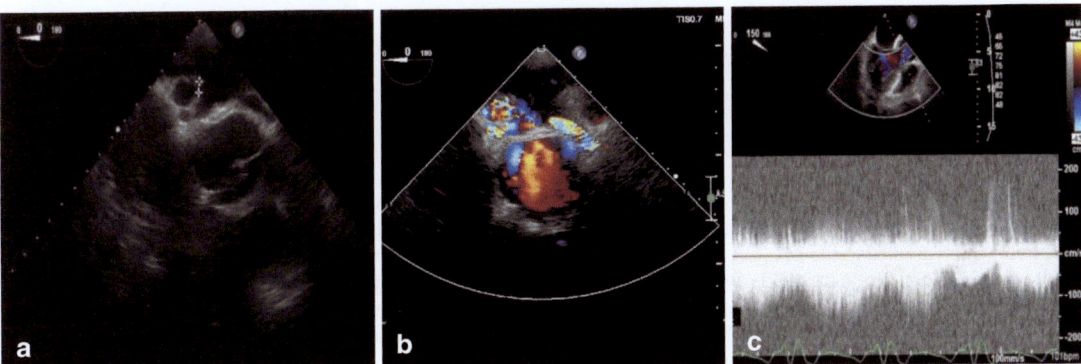

Fig. 4 (a–c) In TEE, dilated LM is denoted and the diameter of the fistula origine is 5 mm (**a**). A turbulent flow originating from the left main coronary artery (LMCA) which is drained to the LA is shown in (**b**). An abnormal continuous flow is demonstrated in Doppler mode (**c**). No evidence of PDA, ruptured sinuses of Valsalva, anomalous origins of the left coronary artery (LCA) or the right coronary artery (RCA) from the pulmonary artery was detected

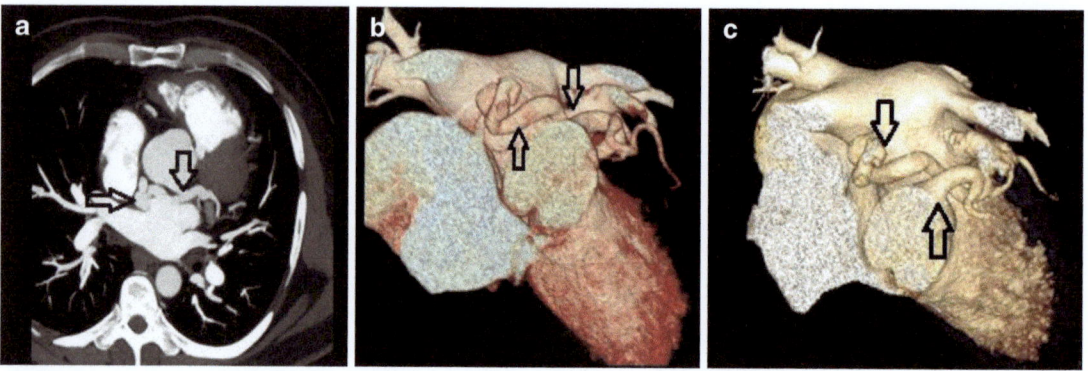

Fig. 5 (**a–c**) Coronary computed tomography angiography shows a dilated left main coronary artery (LMCA) (**a**) with a very tortuous and elongated single fistulous tract (**b**) which is terminated to the LA (**c**) demonstrated by arrows

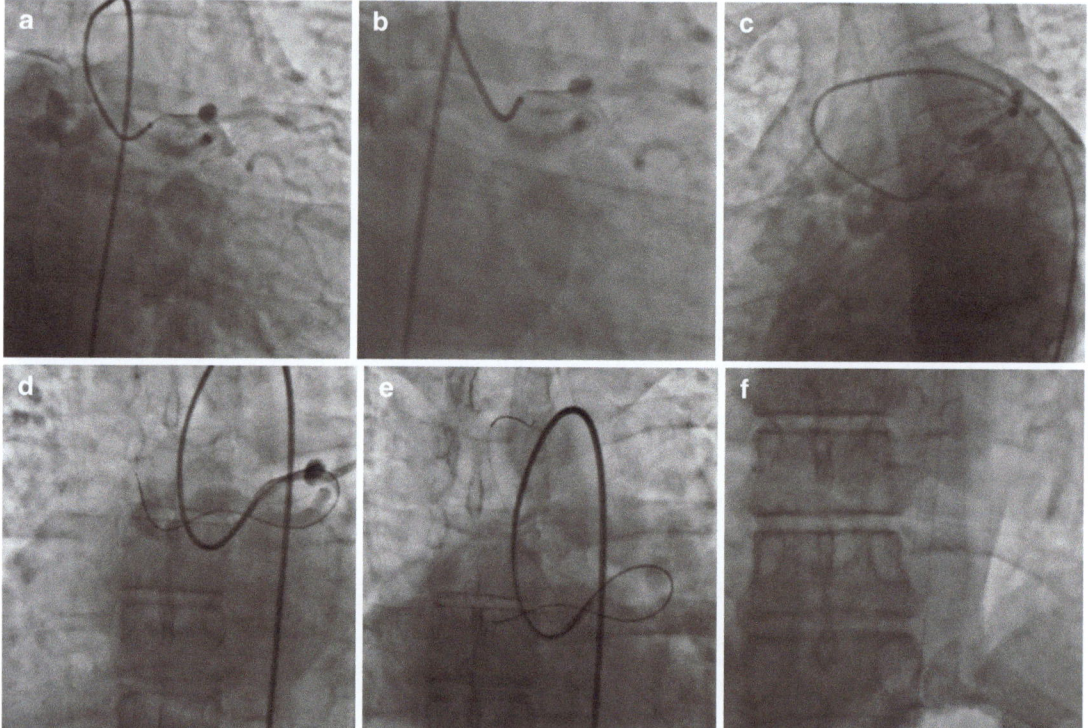

Fig. 6 (**a–l**) Selective LM injection illustrated dilated LM trunk with a very tortous and elongated single fistulous tract which drained to the LA [LA border is denoted] (**a–c**). A 0.014-inch coronary guide wire (Whisper-MS) under support of the microcatheter (Caravel 150 cm) was directed from the LM toward the fistulous tract, LA, LV, and ascending aorta (**d, e**). Then, the wire was snared in ascending aorta from the contralateral CFA (**f**) and the microcatheter was advanced over the wire toward the left CFA and the wire was exchanged with a 0.014-inch Gladius (300 cm) guide wire (**g**). There after, A kink resistant long delivery sheath (5F) was passed over the microcatheter toward the LM (**h**). By repetitive contrast injection through the sheath and LM, the appropriate position of the closure site (as distally as possible) was confirmed (**i**). By retracting the delivery sheath, first, the distal disk of the selected occluder device (Vascular plug-III 10 mm) was deployed and it's correct position was confirmed by contras injection and finally, the proximal disk was deployed (**j**). By several injections through the LM and the sheath and confirming the proper position of the device, the device was released. Final LM injection demonstrated complete obliteration of the fistulae flow without any complications (**l**)

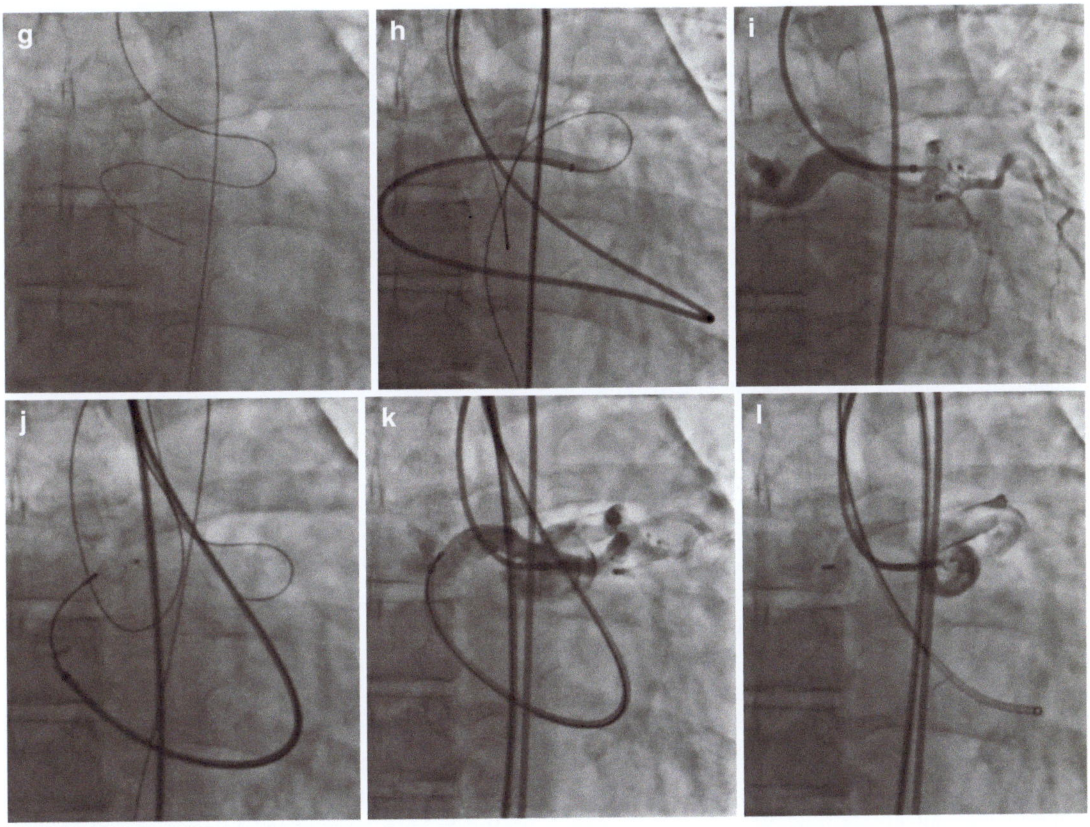

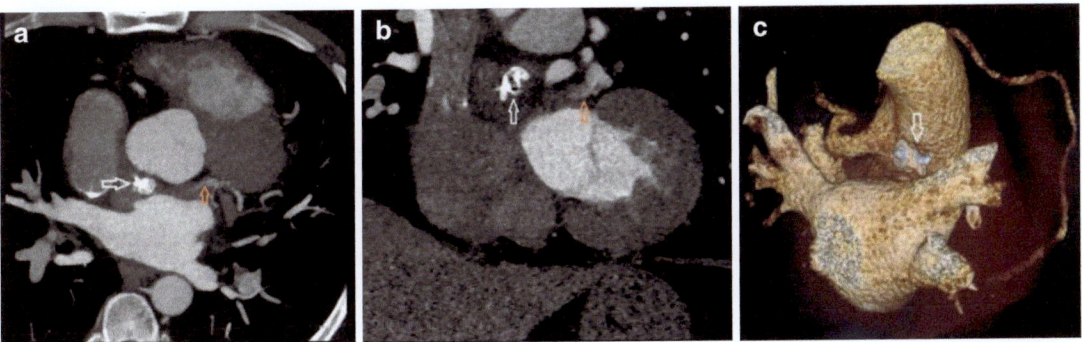

Fig. 6 (continued)

Fig. 7 (**a–c**) Follow-up coronary CT angiography (3 weeks later) illustrated almost complete obliteration of the CCF (white arrow: occluder device, orange arrow: the residual origin of the fistula which opacified and after that the fistulae is thrombosed) (**a, b**). The device position and configuration (white arrow) is appropriate without any compromising effect on the other vessels (**c**)

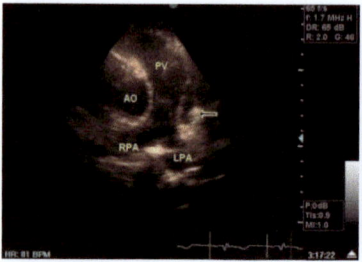 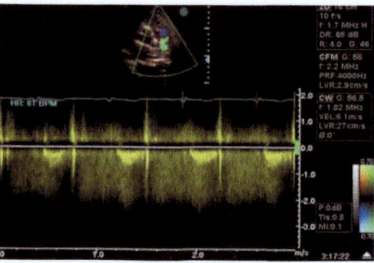 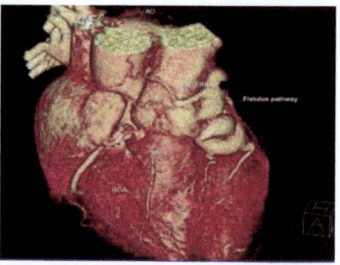

Fig. 8 Left: Transthoracic echocardiography, short-axis view showing echo free space adjacent to the main pulmonary artery Middle: Continuous flow by Continuous wave Doppler study. Right: Fistulous tract from LAD to main PA confirmed by Coronary CT angiography, Aorta (AO), Pulmonary valve (PV), Left pulmonary Artery (LPA), and Right Pulmonary Artery (RPA)

Challenges and Controversies

Although the natural history of CAFs is variable and many fistulas are incidental findings on angiography, *small fistulas in asymptomatic children should be monitored clinically for the signs of growth and increased flow. The CAFs tend to grow with age in children*, hence many authors recommend treating symptomatic CAFs. Be that as it may, the topic is still the subject of debate in patients without symptoms. Some investigators have recommended the closure of CAFs even in asymptomatic patients to prevent fistula-related complications such as the aneurysmal dilatation of the feeder artery, thrombus formation and distal embolization, aneurysmal rupture, heart failure, endocarditis, and myocardial ischemia [19]. TEE, selective coronary artery angiography, CMR and 3D CT angiography can accurately demarcate not only the anatomical characteristics of CAFs such as the origin of the fistula (whether proximal or distal), the presence of multiple feeders, the tract of the fistulae, the tortuosity of the vessel, any aneurysmal fistulous tract, the terminal site, and any adjacent side branch at the drainage site but also the physiologic effects of the fistula such as the size of the feeder vessel, the Qp/Qs ratio, the size of the left and right chambers, and the pressure of the pulmonary artery.

Surgical CAF closure via epicardial or endocardial ligations with or without distal bypass grafting is the standard treatment of CAFs, especially in patients with distally located fistulas and proximal artery aneurysm formation (≥10 mm), with a high success rate [3, 20, 21]. Cheung et al [22] found that 96.9% of the patients in their series remained asymptomatic at a mean follow-up of 9.1 years. In addition, approximately 10% of their study population had a demonstrable recurrence of fistulas without hemodynamic disturbances.

A previously published surgical series consisting of 71 patients (81 fistulas) showed a 1.4% mortality rate (secondary to myocardial infarction), a 6.17% arrhythmia incidence rate, a 1.4% incidence rate of transient ischemic changes on ECG, and a 1.4% incidence rate of stroke. No late postoperative deaths were reported [23, 24].

On the strength of recent advances in equipment and devices, in combination with innovations in percutaneous closure techniques, TCC is now considered the preferred strategy for CAFs and CCFs closure except in some high-risk cases such as multiple drainage sites, extreme vessel tortuosity, aneurysm formation, acute angulation, the proximity of a side branch to a drainage site, and the distal location of the lesion precluding the delivery of a catheter.

In patients with coronary-cameral fistulas (especially the LCX to the coronary sinus) or extremely tortuous and large distal fistulas requiring extra support for advancing the equipment, an arteriovenous loop is highly suggested. In these cases, the fistula is wired with a 0.014″ coronary guidewire or a 0.035″ hydrophilic wire from the arterial side. Subsequently, the wire is advanced to the terminal chamber or circulation (Over 90% of CAFs drain into the low-pressure venous system or the right heart chambers). The wire is then snared in the superior and inferior venae cavae, the right atrium, or the pulmonary arteries before it is exteriorized from the venous access. Through the venous access, a kink-resistant long delivery sheath is advanced forward to pass the terminal site and the fistula, and it is stabilized in the distal part of the origin artery. We usually wire the arterial side with a 0.014″ coronary guidewire under the support of a 150 cm microcatheter; and when the microcatheter is positioned in the terminal chamber or circulation, we exchange the previous wire with an RG3 guidewire (0.01″, 330 cm, 3 g, ASAHI). After snaring the RG3 wire from the venous side, we advance the long delivery sheath over it. During the whole procedure, we keep this wire to further stabilize the delivery sheath and lest we lose the arteriovenous rail in the case of inappropriate device selection [25].

In this chapter, we introduced some selected high risk patients who despite of high risk features (aneurysmal feeder arteries [more than 10 mm], tourtous and aneurysmal fistulae tract, and distal drainage site) underwent successful TCC approach closure.

The success rate of TCC ranges between 80 and 100% in small case series in minimum 1-year follow-ups with appropriate case selection [26, 27]. One of the most considering issues in these patients is the chance of recanalization, so, follow-up coronary CT angiography is highly suggested. Our default treatment is single antiplatelet therapy for at least 1 year in patients without aneurysmal dilatation in the feeder artery and lifelong anticoagulant therapy in patients with aneurysm formation, particularly in those with fistulas to the systemic circulation [25].

Conclusion

One of the most common coronary artery anomalies is CAF, which is detected incidentally in most cases. The natural course of CAFs is progressive dilatation by aging; therefore, even in small fistulas, follow-up helps to prevent subsequent complications. In the patients with medium to large-sized, CAFs the management (either surgical ligation or TCC) should be discussed in the multidisciplinary team. In the current era of advances in equipment and devices, innovations in percutaneous closure techniques and preprocedural imaging, TCC is now regarded as the preferred strategy for CAF and CCF closure except in some very high-risk cases. A comprehensive heart team, comprising an interventional cardiologist, a cardiac imager, and a cardiac surgeon, in a tertiary heart center is the integral component of planning. As the previous studies are all small single-center case series with limited long-term follow-ups, it seems that more multicenter trials with long-term clinical follow-ups are needed to accurately define the best treatment options and the long-term complications after closure.

Clinical Pearls and Follow up Consideration:

- An enlarged proximal coronary artery with a diameter ≥10 mm has a higher risk of thrombosis and myocardial infarction after closure due to low flow state in the proximal part of closed dilated coronary artery. Simple CAFs has a single origin, pathway, and termination vs. complex CAFs that are large with multiple origins, tortuous pathway, and plexiform appearance.
- In CAFs originate more proximally from the main coronary arteries, more dilatation is anticipated and for those originates more distally more tortuousity is anticipated and are difficult for transcatheter closure.
- Even in the complex CAF and CCF, TCC can be done successfully in the hands of the expert interventionis and an equipped cath-lab.
- In transcatheter occlusion: coil or device embolization, transient T-wave abnormality or bundle branch block, and myocardial infarction have been reported as rare complications and in the patients with surgically repaired CCFs, postoperative myocardial infarction

might happen because of the dilated coronary artery at proximal to fistula and low flow state.

> **Key Points**
> - *Coronary-cameral fistulas (CCFs) as a subset of coronary artery fistulas (CAFs) are abnormal communication between coronary arteries and cardiac chambers.*
> - *The most common CAFs originate from the right coronary system and drain the right ventricle or right atrium.*
> - *2D and color Doppler study by transthoracic echocardiography is valuable by demonstrating the dilated coronary artery at origin and high velocity continuous turbulent flow at the site of termination of the CCFs.*
> - *Cardiac CT angiography is the pre-procedural planning imaging modality that defining the fistula's origin, size, anatomic course, and termination site.*
> - *In properly selected patients with symptomatic medium or large-size CAFs, transcatheter closure is an effective and safe alternative procedure to surgery with reported complete occlusion of 80–95% considering that heart team approach is highly recommended.*

Imaging study	Benefits	Disadvantages
Echocardiogram	- Screening tool providing the hemodynamic effect of CAFs (the size and function of the cardiac chambers), regional wall motion abnormality, valvular insufficiency secondary to papillary muscle dysfunction, and visualizing the dilated fistulous course. Color flow imaging (CFI) showing high velocity continuous turbulent flow at the site of termination of the CCFs. - Echocardiogram could demonstrate concomitant congenital anomalies - No radiation	- Limited value for providing detail anatomy and course of coronary arteries [28]
CT	- *ECG-gated CT angiography and 3D volume-rendered imaging are preferred pre-procedural planning imaging modality by providing a precise delineation of the origin, course, and drainage site of CAFs.* - *CT is helpful in choosing appropriate treatment approach (surgical or transcatheter closure [TCC]) and device selection and finding the optimal fluoroscopic angles.* - *Additionally it is helpful in the evaluation of the presence of other intrathoracic vascular communications or associated congenital anomalies*	- Radiation exposure - Risk of iodinated contrast nephropathy
CMR	- Provides with the cardiac chambers, accurate ventricular function, shunt flow assessment (Qp:Qs), and associated anomalies - No radiation. - valuable for the anatomic and hemodynamic assessment of CAFs, and myocardial perfusion imaging can be added for evaluating the CCFs related ischemia	- Needs patient's cooperation and sometimes deep sedation - Sub optimal imaging in the setting of arrhythmias or irregular heart rate

Disclosures *There are no conflicts of interest to disclose.*

Chapter Review Questions

1. A 43-year-old man with a continuous murmur underwent transthoracic echocardiography. He had a possible diagnosis of LAD to the right ventricle coronary cameral fistula (CCF). Which of the following findings are NOT consistent with the diagnosis of CCF:
   A. Ischemic chest pain
   B. Cardiac chamber enlargement
   C. Left ventricular systolic dysfunction
   D. Cyanosis

   Answer: D

   Explanation: Sizable fistulas may result in significant left to right shunt and causing cardiac chamber dilatation or myocardial ischemia distal to coronary fistula due to steal phenomenon and consequently left ventricular dysfunction.

2. A 55-year-old woman with typical ischemic chest pain and past medical history of MVR was diagnosed with sizable coronary cameral fistulas (CCF). The proximal diameter of the feeding coronary artery was 10 mm. She underwent transcatheter closure of the CCFs based on the heart team's decision. The patient complained of chest pain before discharge. Which of the following is the most possible diagnosis in this patient:
   A. Coil embolization
   B. Myocardial infarction due to thrombus formation
   C. Mitral prostheses malfunction due to interference of prostheses with the CCF's occluder
   D. It is a normal finding after CCFs closure with no clinical significance

   Answer: B

   Explanation: Although complications are rare in properly selected patients for CCF transcatheter closure, we should be aware that coil embolization, transient T-wave abnormality or bundle branch block, and myocardial infarction might happen. An enlarged proximal coronary artery with a diameter ≥10 mm has a higher risk of thromboses and myocardial infarction after closure.

3. The most common type of coronary artery fistulas (CAFs) are:
   A. RCA origin draining into the RA or RV
   B. LCX origin draining into the LA or LV
   C. LAD origin draining in to the RV
   D. LCX draining into the RV

   Answer: A

   Explanation: The most common type of CAF's originates from the right coronary system and drains the right ventricle or right atrium.

4. Which cardiac imaging is recommended for the preprocedural evaluation of a patient with a suspected coronary cameral fistula (CCF)?
   A. 2D transthoracic echocardiography (TTE) is adequate for preprocedural planning.
   B. Cardiac MRI is more valuable than cardiac CT in identifying the whole course of the coronary anatomy and is preferred for preprocedural planning, with the added benefit of lack of radiation exposure for the patient.
   C. Transesophageal echocardiogram with 3D imaging of the CCF origin is preferred for pre-procedural planning.
   D. Cardiac CT is the preferred imaging modality for pre-procedural planning.

   Answer: D

   Explanation: Cardiac CT is the preferred imaging modality for pre-procedural planning.

   Initial identification of CCF's is best made by TTE to evaluate the etiology and site of termination of high-velocity continuous flow of CCF's. Preprocedural planning however requires a more comprehensive evaluation of the course of the CCF as can be obtained from the CT.

   Answer B is not correct. Cardiac MRI provides excellent visualization of the proximal course of the CCF but is not adequate for comprehensive pre-procedural planning. TEE imaging may identify the proximal blood flow into CCF with the opportunity to visualize the termination on color flow imaging, but is inadequate for pre-procedural planning.

References

1. Lim JJ, Jung JI, Lee BY, Lee HG. Prevalence and types of coronary artery fistulas detected with coronary CT angiography. AJR Am J Roentgenol. 2014;203(3):W237–43.
2. Kim MS, Jung JI, Chun HJ. Coronary to pulmonary artery fistula: morphologic features at multidetector CT. Int J Cardiovasc Imaging. 2010;26(suppl 2):273–80.
3. Mavroudis C, Backer CL, Rocchini AP, Muster AJ, Gevitz M. Coronary artery fistulas in infants and children: a surgical review and discussion of coil embolization. Ann Thorac Surg. 1997;63:1235–42.
4. Challoumas D, Pericleous A, Dimitrakaki IA, Danelatos C, Dimitrakakis G. Coronary arteriovenous fistulae: a review. Int J Angiol. 2014;23(1):1–10. https://doi.org/10.1055/s-0033-1349162.
5. Gillebert C, Van Hoof R, Van De Werf F, Piessens J, De Geest H. Coronary artery fistulas in an adult population. Eur Heart J. 1986;7(5):437–43.
6. Fernandes ED, Kadivar H, Hallman GL, Reul GJ, Ott DA, Cooley DA. Congenital malformations of the coronary arteries: the Texas Heart Institute experience. Ann Thorac Surg. 1992;54:732–40.
7. Sakakibara S, Yokoyama M, Takao A, Nogi M, Gomi H. Coronary arteriovenous fistula: nine operated cases. Am Heart J. 1966;72:307–14.
8. Latson LA. Coronary artery fistulas: how to manage them. Cathet Cardiov Interv. 2007;70(1):110–6.
9. Said SA, Van Der Werf T. Dutch survey of coronary artery fistulas in adults: congenital solitary fistulas. Int J Cardiol. 2006;106(3):323–32.
10. Ata Y, Turk T, Bicer M, Yalcin M, Ata F, Yavuz S. Coronary arteriovenous fistulas in the adults: natural history and management strategies. J Cardiothorac Surg. 2009;4(1):62.
11. Dodge-Khatami A, Mavroudis C, Backer CL. Congenital heart surgery nomenclature and database project: anomalies of the coronary arteries. Ann Thorac Surg. 2000;69(3 Suppl 1):270–7.
12. Moe TG. The multidisciplinary heart team approach to management of coronary artery fistula with the assistance of 3D image reconstruction*. JACC Case Rep. 2020;2(11):1739–41.
13. Valente AM, Lock JE, Gauvreau K, et al. Predictors of long-term adverse outcomes in patients with congenital coronary artery fistulae. Circ Cardiovasc Interv. 2010;3(2):134–9.
14. Warnes CA, Williams RG, Bashore TM, et al. ACC/AHA 2008 guidelines for the management of adults with congenital heart disease: executive summary—a report of the American College of Cardiology/American Heart Association Task Force on practice guidelines (Writing committee to develop guidelines for the management of adults with congenital heart disease). Circulation. 2008;118(23):2395–451. 67.
15. Stout KK, Daniels CJ, Aboulhosn JA, et al. 2018 AHA/ACC guideline for the management of adults with congenital heart disease: executive summary: a report of the American College of Cardiology/American Heart Association Task Force on clinical practice guidelines. J Am Coll Cardiol. 2019;73:1494–563.
16. Buccheri D, Chirco PR, Geraci S, Caramanno G, Cortese B. Coronary artery fistulae: anatomy, diagnosis and management strategies. Heart Lung Circ. 2018;27(8):940–51. https://doi.org/10.1016/j.hlc.2017.07.014.
17. Al-Hijji M, El Sabbagh A, El Hajj S, AlKhouli M, El Sabawi B, Cabalka A, et al. Coronary artery fistulas: indications, techniques, outcomes, and complications of transcatheter fistula closure. J Am Coll Cardiol Intv. 2021;14(13):1393–406.
18. Boyle S, Jesuthasan LSB, Jenkins C, Challa P, Ranjan S, Dahiya A. Coronary-cameral fistula. Circ Cardiov Imaging. 2019;12(5):e008691.
19. Kamiya H, Yasuda T, Nagamine H, et al. Surgical treatment of congenital coronary artery fistulas: 27 years' experience and a review of the literature. J Card Surg. 2002;17:173–7.
20. Dimitrakakis G, Otto von Oppell U. eComment: surgical treatment of coronary arteriovenous fistulas. Interact Cardiovasc Thorac Surg. 2011;13:674–5.
21. Wang S, Wu Q, Hu S, et al. Surgical treatment of 52 patients with congenital coronary artery fistulas. Chin Med J. 2001;114(7):752–5.
22. Cheung DL, Au WK, Cheung HH, Chiu CS, Lee WT. Coronary artery fistulas: long-term results of surgical correction. Ann Thorac Surg. 2001;71(1):190–5.
23. Carrel T, Tkebuchava T, Jenni R, Arbenz U, Turina M. Congenital coronary fistulas in children and adults: diagnosis, surgical technique and results. Cardiology. 1996;87:325–30.
24. Goto Y, Abe T, Sekine S, Iijimaa K, Kondoha K, Sakurada T. Surgical treatment of the coronary artery to pulmonary artery fistulas in adults. Cardiology. 1998;89:252–6.
25. Firouzi A, Alemzadeh-Ansari MJ, Mohebbi B, Khajali Z, Khalilipur E, Baay M, Bayatian A, Taherian M, Khosropour A, Hosseini Z. Diverse transcatheter closure strategies in coronary artery fistulas a state-of-the-art approach. Curr Probl Cardiol. 2021;47:101010.
26. Qureshi SA. Coronary arterial fistulas. Orphanet J Rare Dis. 2006;1(1):51. https://doi.org/10.1186/1750-1172-1-51.
27. Ilkay E, Celebi OO, Kacmaz F, et al. Percutaneous closure of coronary artery fistula: long-term follow-up results. Postepy Kardiol Interwencyjnej. 2015;11:318–22.
28. Frommelt P, Lopez L, Dimas VV, Eidem B, Han BK, Ko HH, Lorber R, Nii M, Printz B, Srivastava S, Valente AM, Cohen MS. Recommendations for multimodality assessment of congenital coronary anomalies: a guide from the American Society of Echocardiography: developed in collaboration with the Society for Cardiovascular Angiography and Interventions, Japanese Society of Echocardiography, and Society for Cardiovascular Magnetic Resonance. J Am Soc Echocardiogr. 2020;33(3):259–94. https://doi.org/10.1016/j.echo.2019.10.011.

Transcatheter Closure of Ruptured Sinus of Valsalva

Y. Hejazi, Z. M. Hijazi, and A. Sadeghpour

Abstract

Sinus of Valsalva Aneurysm (SOVA) typically is caused by congenital weakness in the aortic wall of one of three aortic sinuses (most commonly right) and resulting in outpouching protrusion into nearby cardiac chambers. Men are more affected (4:1), and there is a higher reported incidence in Asian groups. SOVA is either congenital or acquired. Congenital ones are seen in connective tissue disorders and in some forms of congenital heart diseases, like ventricular septal defects (VSDs) and bicuspid aortic valve. Most of these defects are asymptomatic. Acquired SOVAs are seen in patients who suffered abrupt deceleration trauma; infections such as bacterial endocarditis, syphilis, and even tuberculosis and degenerative diseases. Though rare, rupture and fistulous connections with one of the adjacent cardiac chambers will give signs and symptoms of heart failure. If left untreated, the disease has poor prognosis. Multi-modality imaging plays crucial role in detecting this rare disease and in guiding management. Surgery has been traditionally the treatment of choice. However, several studies reported safety and efficacy of transcatheter treatment. In this chapter, we will discuss multiple imaging modalities implemented in diagnosis and transcatheter treatment of ruptured SOVAs, and briefly compare surgical and transcatheter treatments approach.

Keywords

Structural heart · Sinus of Valsalva · Ruptured · Multimodality imaging · Transcatheter closure

---

Y. Hejazi
Department of Cardiovascular Diseases, Sidra Medicine & Weill Cornell Medicine, Doha, Qatar

Z. M. Hijazi (✉)
Weill Cornell Medicine, Sidra Medicine, Doha, Qatar
e-mail: zhijazi@sidra.org

A. Sadeghpour
Advanced Cardiovascular Imaging, MedStar Health Research Institute, Georgetown University, Washington, DC, USA
e-mail: anita.sadeghpour@medstar.net

Test your learning and check your understanding of this book's contents: use the "Springer Nature Flashcards" app to access questions using ▶ https://sn.pub/ambACS.

To use the app, please follow the instructions in the chapter "Transcatheter Aortic Valve Replacement."

© The Author(s), under exclusive license to Springer Nature Switzerland AG 2024
A. M. Kelsey et al. (eds.), *Cardiac Imaging in Structural Heart Disease Interventions*,
https://doi.org/10.1007/978-3-031-50740-3_13

Learning Objectives

1. To draw cardiologists' attention to sinus of Valsalva aneurysm, an uncommon disease, which can present with nonspecific signs and symptoms, and can be easily misdiagnosed
2. To review pre-procedural multi-modality imaging modalities in the evaluation of ruptured sinus of Valsalva
3. Review intra procedural imaging which plays an important role in successful transcatheter closure of ruptured SOVA
4. Briefly compare surgical vs transcatheter approach for ruptured SOVA

> **Case Study**
>
> 36-year-old female patient was referred to cardiology clinic for evaluation of signs and symptoms of heart failure. She was complaining of exertional dyspnea, easy fatigability, palpitations and atypical chest pain for around 6 months. Physical exam was remarkable for hyperdynamic precordium, grade III continuous murmur over the left lower sternal border. ECG: sinus rhythm, non-specific intraventricular conduction delay, LVH, and no ischemic changes.

Background and Definitions

The sinuses of Valsalva can be identified as small dilatations in the aortic wall just above each cusp of the aortic valve, precisely between the annulus and Sino tubular (ST) junction. They allow aortic valve opening during systole without occlusion of coronary artery ostia [1]. Defect in aortic wall resulting in outpouching protrusion into nearby cardiac chambers is known as Sinus of Valsalva Aneurysm (SOVA). SOVA was first described by Hope in 1839. Edward and Burchell's reported that SOVAs are secondary to failure of the aortic media to fuse with the heart during prenatal development. The estimated incidence varies between 0.09 up to 0.96% [2–5]. Ethnicity plays an important role in this variable incidence. Chue et al. [6] reported five times higher incidence of ruptured SOVA (RSOVA) in Far Eastern patients than in Westerns.

SOVAs comprise 0.1–3.5% of all congenital cardiac defects [1]. Typically, men are more affected (4:1), and there is a higher reported incidence in Asian groups. Most of these defects are asymptomatic. However, rupture and fistulous connections with one of the adjacent cardiac chambers will give signs and symptoms of heart failure. If ruptured SOVAs remain untreated, the prognosis is poor, with a life expectancy of 1-year [1].

Causes and Pathophysiology

Embryologically, SOVA forms first as a blind diverticulum secondary to pressure forces on the aortic root [7]. Thus, congenital defects potentiating these pressure forces can lead to development of a SOVA [1]. SOVA is either congenital or acquired. Whether congenital or acquired, SOVA is a consequence of weakness of the elastic lamina at the junction of the aortic media and the annulus fibrosis [8]. Congenital ones are seen in connective tissue disorders such as Marfan syndrome [9] or Ehlers-Danlos syndrome [10–14]. Also, there are several congenital defects commonly associated with SOVA. For example, ventricular septal defects (VSDs), with or without aortic regurgitation have been reported in 12% and up to 78% of SOVA patients [15, 16], most commonly with aneurysm of right coronary sinus. Aortic valve abnormalities such as bicuspid aortic valve has been reported in at least 10% of SOVA patients [9, 15].

On the other hand, acquired SOVAs are seen in patients who suffered abrupt deceleration trauma; infections such as bacterial endocarditis, syphilis, and even tuberculosis and degenerative diseases, such as cystic medial necrosis and atherosclerosis. Additionally, intense physical activity can cause rupture of an existing SOVA [17].

SOVA arises from the right sinus of Valsalva in 80–85% cases, from the non-coronary sinus in 5–15%, and rarely from the left sinus [4]. This notable difference in distribution is thought to be related to the role of outlet septum defects in the genesis of SOVAs. The right coronary cusp of aortic valve adjoins a big part of the outlet septum, while left coronary cusp does not originate from the outlet septum [17].

Diagnosis and Pre-procedural Assessment

A transthoracic Echocardiogram (TTE) was performed, and showed severe aortic regurgitation along with dilated left ventricle with preserved ventricular function. However, when the case was discussed at cardiac-cardiothoracic surgical meeting, possibility of ruptured sinus of Valsalva aneurysm (SOVA) was raised considering history and hyperdynamic precordium associated with continuous murmur over the left lower sternal border.

Heart Team Approach, Discussion and Decision

As no definite diagnosis was agreed on, and after reviewing TTE images thoroughly, cardiac CT was done and confirmed the diagnosis of ruptured right sinus of Valsalva to right atrium. Surgical closure was suggested. However, we conducted extensive discussion with the patient, she was not in favor for a major open-heart surgery and she preferred transcatheter approach if feasible. The team decision was to proceed with diagnostic cardiac catheterization to obtain detailed imaging, with intraprocedural Transesophageal Echocardiogram (TEE) and close percutaneously if feasible.

Clinical Presentation

Unruptured SOVA

Usually asymptomatic, but occasionally, continuous murmur can be heard due to the flow in and out of the intact aneurysmal pouch [18]. Unruptured lesions can result in significant arrhythmias including ventricular tachycardia, atrial fibrillation, and complete heart block through extension into the interventricular septum and compression of the atrioventricular (AV) node and His bundle [18]. Cases of coronary artery compression secondary to compression of coronary flow by unruptured SOVA have been reported [19]. SOVA can uncommonly cause RVOT obstruction. Rarely (Fig. 1), thrombus formation within the SOVA can lead to thromboembolic cerebrovascular accidents Fig. 2 [20].

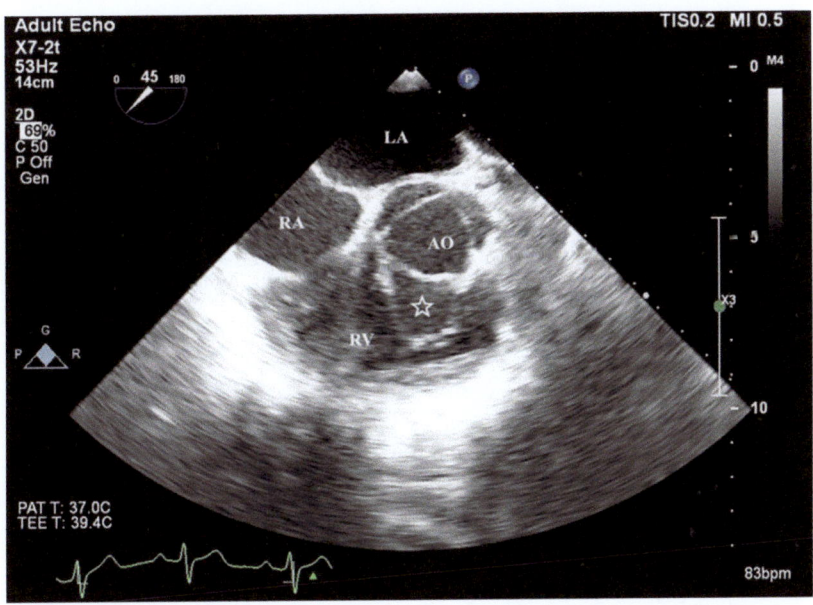

Fig. 1 Transesophageal echocardiogram in short axis view showing right sinus of Valsalva aneurysm (asterixis) protruding to the right ventricular outflow tract. Aorta (AO), RA, right atrium; left atrium (LA); right ventricle (RV)

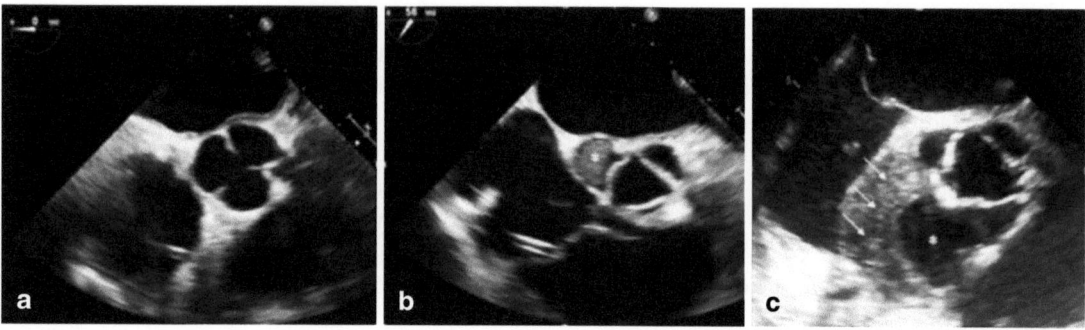

Fig. 2 A 72-year-old female patient admitted with decompensated heart failure secondary to severe mitral regurgitation from an anterior leaflet flail. Two years prior, she required pacemaker placement for complete heart block. The patient underwent surgical repair of the mitral valve. Intraoperative TEE did not reveal any apparent pathology on the mid-esophageal short-axis view of the aortic valve (**a**). However, further assessment of the sinus of Valsalva at the level of the annular plane (**b**) revealed a non-coronary SOVA with adherent mural thrombus (asterisk) (**c**). A 52-year-old male patient admitted with an inferior ST elevation myocardial infarction. Mid-esophageal short-axis view on TEE demonstrated a large right SOVA (asterisk) with severe adherent mural thrombus (arrows in panel **c**). With permission from Xu B, Kocyigit D, Betancor J, Tan C, Rodriguez ER, Schoenhagen P, Flamm SD, Rodriguez LL, Svensson LG, Griffin BP. Sinus of Valsalva Aneurysms: A State-of-the-Art Imaging Review. J Am Soc Echocardiogr. 2020, Elsevier

Ruptured SOVA

The anatomical location of a SOVA will determine the clinical significance and manifestations of aneurysm rupture. Right and noncoronary sinuses rupture leads to connection between the aorta and right ventricle outflow tract or the aorta and the right atrium (RA). Left SOVA is more benign and results in connection between the left atrium and left ventricular outflow tract [1].

SOVA can rupture at any age, but typically between 20 and 40 years of age. Clinical outcome is largely dependent on how fast the rupture occurs, in addition to the size of ruptured orifice, and to which chamber the rupture occurs (receiving chamber) [9]. The most common location for rupture is the right ventricle followed by the right atrium [21].

There are two distinct clinical scenarios for ruptured SOVA: acute rupture of large SOVA which manifests with severe substernal chest pain, upper abdominal pain or severe dyspnea with abrupt hemodynamic compromise [18]. Physical stress, blunt chest trauma, or iatrogenic trauma during percutaneous procedures are often preceding events. On the other hand, small and/or very gradual rupture presents insidiously. Patients will usually remain asymptomatic, and they may have mild dyspnea prior to progression to heart failure. Sudden cardiac death can result from tamponade, ischemia, arrhythmia and/or conduction issues [22].

The right ventricle receives around 75% of ruptured right SOVAs (Fig. 3). Unruptured right coronary SOVAs often protrude into right ventricular outflow tract resulting in obstruction. These lesions may distort pulmonary valve and cause pulmonic and tricuspid regurgitation [18]. Most noncoronary SOVAs rupture into right atrium.

Diagnostic Evaluation

Both ruptured and unruptured SOVAs have non-specific clinical presentation. As shown in our case, clinical presentation and even initial diagnostic evaluation may not easily lead to proper diagnosis. Therefore, multi-modality imaging is of crucial role in establishing precise diagnosis and guiding management.

CXR

On frontal film, SOVA may manifest as bulging of the aorta to the right of caval shadow. Ruptured

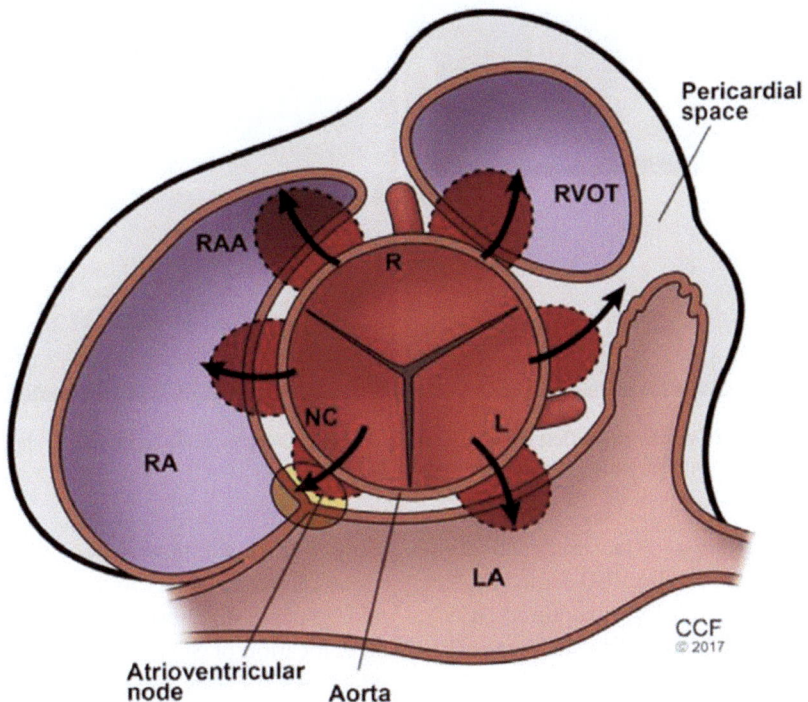

Fig. 3 Schematic figure demonstrating the different aortic sinuses that could be affected by SOVA and anatomical relation to the cardiac chambers in projected SOVA or rupture. Note to the noncoronary sinus which is related to both LA and RA although mostly ruptures to the RA and the right sinus of Valsalva which is related to the RA and RV although mostly ruptures to the RV. *L* left coronary; *LA* left atrium; *LAA* left atrial appendage; *NC* noncoronary cusp; *R* right coronary; *RA* right atrium; *RAA* right atrial appendage; *RVOT* right ventricular outflow tract; *SOVA* sinus of Valsalva aneurysm. With permission from Xu B, et al. Sinus of Valsalva Aneurysms: A State-of-the-Art Imaging Review. J Am Soc Echocardiogr. 2020, Elsevier

SOVA can result in enlarged cardiac silhouette, pulmonary plethora and pulmonary venous hypertension.

Transthoracic Echocardiogram (TTE)

Aortic root can be adequately imaged and evaluated by TTE. Parasternal long-axis, modified apical five chamber and three chamber views provide accurate assessment and measurements of aortic root [23]. As per American Society of Echocardiography (ASE) guidelines, it is recommended to measure SOVA diameter perpendicular to the long axis of the ascending aorta in the parasternal long axis view at end diastole using the leading edge–to–leading-edge method [23]. A single-center study comparing TTE and surgical findings in 212 patients with SOVAs undergoing surgery has shown that the sensitivity, specificity, and accuracy of TTE for diagnosing SOVAs were 93.9%, 99.9%, and 99.8%, respectively [23]. In ruptured SOVAs, color Doppler images would show a continuous turbulent flow between the ruptured sinus and the receiving chamber (Fig. 4). A significant diastolic flow reversal is usually seen in the aorta. If the rupture involves a large part of the SOVA, a "windsock" deformity may be noted, which indicates a large, ruptured sinus expanding and contracting through the cardiac cycle. Differentiating isolated SOVA rupture from SOVA rupture with VSD is a diagnostic challenge. If the aneurysm or the prolapsing cusp of the aortic valve occludes it, VSD may be missed [24]. Cheng et al. have suggested that the short-axis view should be checked to differentiate the relatively thin-walled and fibrous SOVA or prolapsed cusp from the thicker myocardial wall to avoid a misdiagnosis [24]. Another common diagnostic challenge when there is coexist-

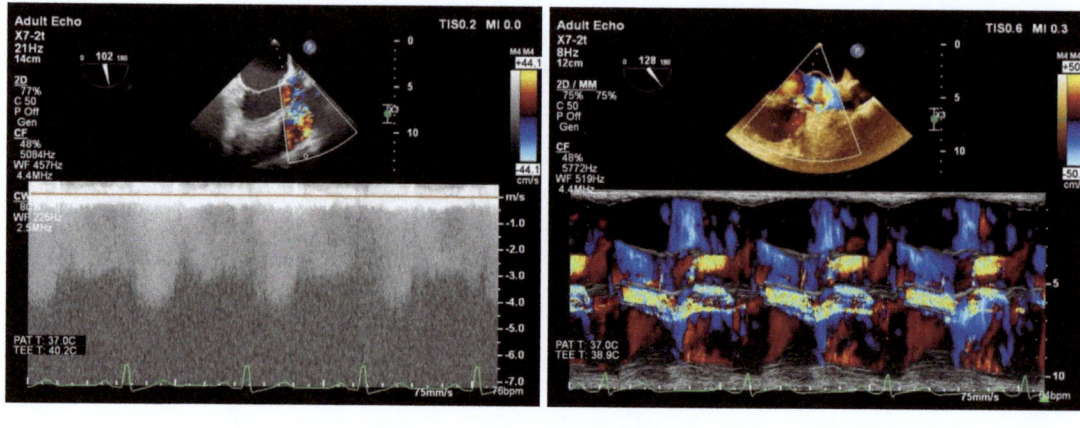

Fig. 4 Continuous wave Doppler study (left panel) and color M-mode Doppler study (right panel) showing continuous flow from ruptured right sinus of Valsalva to the right ventricle

ing aortic regurgitation. The diastolic aortic regurgitant flow and systolic VSD jet may create a Doppler flow jet similar to a ruptured SOVA, even in the absence of rupture. In such scenarios, the Doppler waveform patterns would be helpful in differentiating the two anomalies. SOVA shunt rupture begins in mid diastole and gradually increases toward end diastole. Aortic regurgitation, if present, usually begins in early diastole and continues throughout the diastole in a decrescendo fashion [25] (Fig. 3).

Transesophageal Echocardiography (TEE)

Aortic valve, aortic root and ascending aorta can be evaluated with high resolution images through mid-esophageal long axis (120–150) and short axis (at 30–60) views (Figs. 5 and 6). Relationship between the aneurysm and right ventricle, aortic valve cusps and coronary arteries can be precisely assessed by long and short axis imaging [23]. It may be necessary to use off axis views and to advance the probe away from the aortic root toward the annular plane. Doppler studies in both TTE and TEE are helpful in diagnosis of associated cardiac abnormalities and/or potential complications of SOVAs such as rupture, aortic regurgitation, compressive effects on cardiac structures, and thrombus or vegetations. TEE is the diagnostic modality of choice during interventional procedures for SOVAs. One should keep in mind; TEE is semi-invasive procedure.

However, for adults with poor images, TEE provides improved image quality. 3D imaging can add valuable diagnostic information in regard to size, location of SOVAs and their relationship to adjacent structures. Real time 3D TEE is increasingly being used to guide the percutaneous closure of SOVAs. It helps in selecting appropriate devices and also avoiding procedure related complications, such as device embolization, significant residual shunting, and obstruction of an adjacent cardiac chamber [26].

Multi Detector Computed Tomography (MDCT)

MDCT is becoming an essential diagnostic modality in cardiovascular imaging especially because of continuous improvement in spatial and temporal resolution. It can provide valuable additional information, such as evaluation of coronary arteries, entire thoracic aorta, SOV diameter, SOVA or rupture and related chambers, dynamic assessment of aortic valve motion, quantification of left ventricle (LV) ejection fraction, and post processing (e.g., volume rendering) [27]. Typically, the wall of the aortic root or ascending aorta aneurysms is not thickened and measures around 1 mm [23].

Evaluation of SOV diameters can be done by two methods: sinus-to-sinus and sinus-to-commissure on MDCT/CMR.

In both methods SOV diameters measurement is based on the inner to inner edges in double-

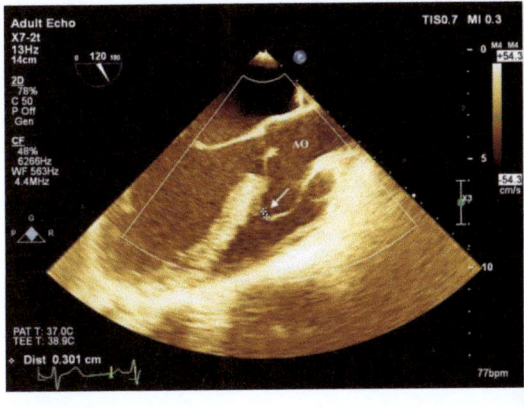 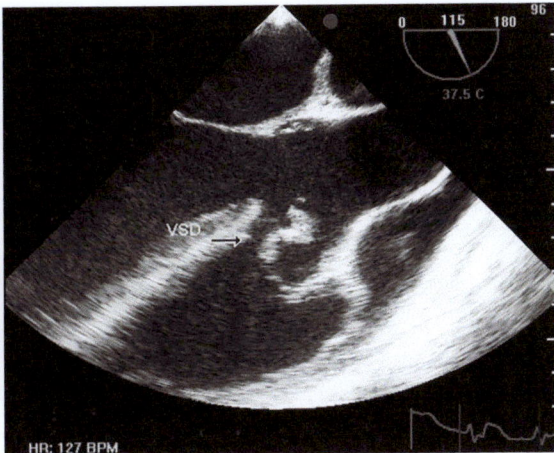

Fig. 5 TEE mid esophageal long axis views showing rupture of right SOVA without associated ventricular septal defect (VSD) (left panel) and rupture of right SOVA associated with VSD (right panel). Note that VSD is below the aortic valve and rupture of SOVA is above aortic annulus

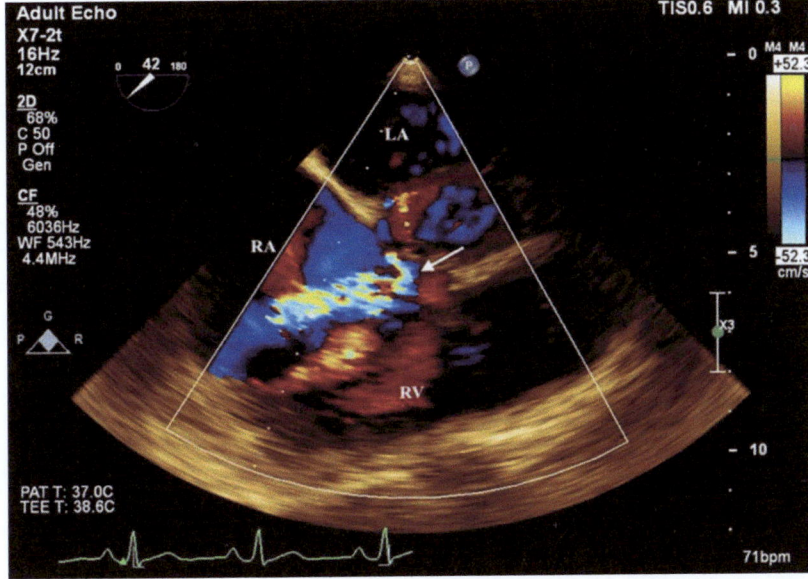

Fig. 6 Rupture of right sinus of Valsalva to right atrium just above tricuspid valve illustrated by continuous turbulent flow (white arrow)

oblique technique with the planes parallel to the aortic annular and perpendicular to the long axis of the proximal ascending Ao (Fig. 7).

Based on 2015 Guidelines for Multimodality Imaging of Diseases of the Thoracic Aorta in Adults, sinus to sinus measurement in end diastole is the recommended method to measure aortic sinuses [28]. These measurements are averaged if sinuses are symmetric, and reported individually if sinuses are not symmetric. Recent recommendations by The Society of Cardiovascular Computed Tomography in Transcatheter Aortic Valve implantation/replacement (TAVI/TAVR) suggested sinus-to-commissure method which means measuring from the commissure to the opposite sinus. This method generally results in 2 mm smaller SOV mean diameter compared to the sinus-to-sinus method [29]. The typical SOVA can be seen on CT as thin walled-out pouching in proximity to the wall of aorta. If disconnected from the aortic wall, once should suspect ruptured SOVA [27]. The main disadvantages of MDCT are radiation exposure, low temporal resolution, and lack of

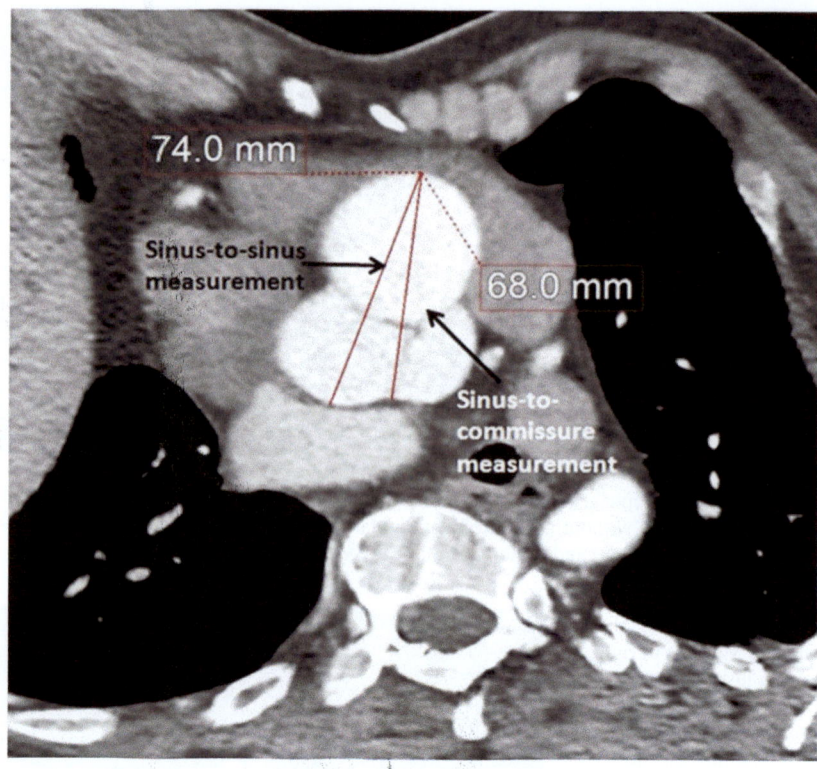

Fig. 7 Cardiac computed tomography angiography showing two methods of measurement sinus of Valsalva diameter. (Sinus-to-sinus versus sinus-to-commissure with permission from Xu B, et al. Sinus of Valsalva Aneurysms: A State-of-the-Art Imaging Review. J Am Soc Echocardiogr. 2020, Elsevier

flow information, for which it can miss small rupture, VSD and aortic regurgitation.

Cardiac MRI

CMR provides comprehensive assessment of the aorta, including aortic measurements and relationship of the SOVAs with the cardiac chambers. Beside accurate delineation of cardiac and aortic anatomy, CMR assesses cardiac function and flow, and has higher sensitivity than MDCT in detection of thrombi through delayed enhancement imaging [30]. Dynamic assessment of SOVA morphology and its impact on the adjacent structures can be nicely reviewed by cine loops of bright blood images. CMR has important advantages over MDCT in the evaluation of SOVAs. It has better temporal resolution (20–50 ms in CMR vs. 83–135 ms in MDCR), lacks radiation, and its capacity of functional evaluation. For example, in case of suspected SOVAs rupture, Qp:Qs ratio can be calculated by velocity-encoded cine phase-contrast sequences acquired through both outflow tracts [30]. Despite CMR being an attractive imaging modality, it has a few significant drawbacks such as: lower spatial resolution, its limited accessibility, longer acquisition time which may result in claustrophobia for some patients, and being not safe in hemodynamically compromised patients.

Angiography

Based on the shape of left to right shunt jet on aortic root angiography, Liu S et al. [31] divided SOVA angiographically into four types (Fig. 8): Type I: window-like, in which the jet scattered immediately right after the rupture site; type II, aneurysmal; type III, tubular with long waist; type IV, other rare types. Type I was the most common in their series of 30 patients. In types I and II, they used small-waist double-disk occluders, while muscular occluders were used in type III. Success rate was 93.3% at discharge and during a median follow up of 18.5 months.

Also, SOVAs, have been classified based on their site of origin and rupture by Sakakibara and Konno in 1962. The original classification system defined only four types of SOVA,

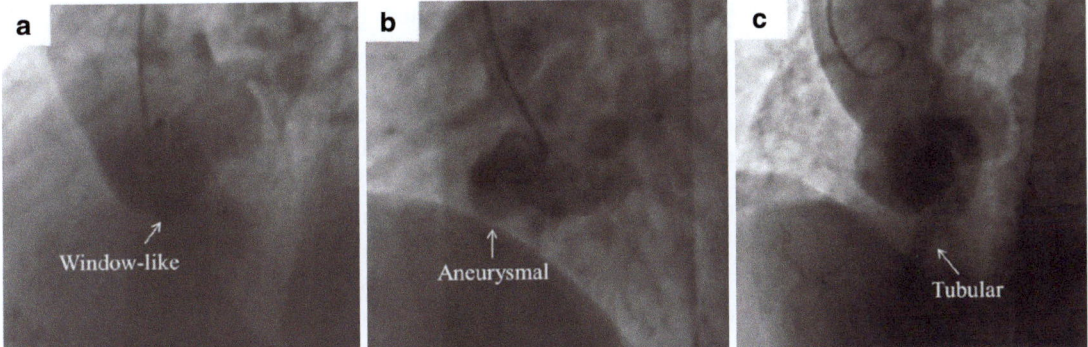

Fig. 8 Types I, II, and III in the angiographic classification system for ruptured sinus of Valsalva aneurysm. (**a**) In the type I, window-like, the shunt jet is scattered immediately after crossing the ruptured site; (**b**) In the type II, aneurysmal, the shunt jet is aneurysmal shape after crossing the ruptured site; (**c**) In the type III, tubular, the shunt jet is long and the diameter in the left and right sides of the ruptured site is the same. With permission from Liu S, Xu X, Chen F, Zhao Z, Zhang Y, Wang C, Xiang J, Wu G, Chen X, Zhao X, Qin Y. Angiographic features of ruptured sinus of Valsalva aneurysm: New classification. Journal of Cardiology. 2014. Elsevier

including those arising from the right coronary sinus or the noncoronary sinus.

Consequently, modified classification system proposed as a simple and more practical classification for clinical use (Table 1) [32, 33].

Management

Although, surgical closure (SC) is the mainstay therapy for ruptured SOVA with excellent results, many studies showed favorable outcomes for transcatheter closure of ruptured SAV in selected patients [8]. In general, approach to the unruptured SOV aneurysm is similar to the aortic root aneurysm since there is no specific guidelines in this regard [28].

Noteworthy to consider that patients with congenital ruptured SOVA have more congenital associated lesions such as the VSD as the most common coexisting finding followed by aortic regurgitation (AR) and BAV, making aortic valve surgery for AR necessary in addition to repairing the RSOVA [34].

Surgical Repair

Surgery is the standard traditional method for RSOVA repair. It can be done either by direct suture closure or patch integration. The procedure has low mortality rate and 90% survival rate at 10 years [35, 36]. In one study reported freedom from postoperative grade 3 or worse AR at 10 years was found to be 93% [37]. Kuriakose et al., reported reintervention for aneurysm recurrence up to 3.2%, with 4.2% re operation for aortic regurgitation (AR). On follow up, 6.8% developed new or progressive AR [8]. Indeed, residual or progressive AR was the main influencing factor in prognosis.

Transcatheter Closure of Ruptured SOVA

In 1992 Hourihan et al. [5], reported the first successful transcatheter closure (TC). This was followed by several case reports and small series using different types of devices and approaches [7, 38–45]. Currently, there is no recommendation in terms of SC vs TC of ruptured SOVA but obviously decision should be made based on the precise evaluating of the site, size and number of the ruptured sinus of valsalva aneurysm (RSVA) redundancy of the SOVA, proximity to the coronary arteries and associated VSD, AR and BAV. Surgery remains the treatment of choice in patients with complex anatomy of RSVA, cases with significant AR and any other associated lesion that needs surgical repair. Undoubtedly, the *heart team approach helps to assess the feasibility and appropriateness of each procedure.*

Device Selection and Procedure Details

Pre-procedure evaluation involves determining the sinus involved, site of rupture, number of rupture if more than one site, defect size at the aortic end and exit site, redundancy of the aneurysmal

Table 1 Sakikabara original and modified classification that are based on the ruptured sinus of Valsalva aneurysm (RSVA) anatomic location and protrusion site

Type	Sakakibara classification	Modified Sakakibara classification
I	Originating from left part of right coronary sinus, protruding into conus of right ventricle, just beneath commissure of right and left pulmonary valves	Protrusion and rupture into right ventricle just beneath pulmonary valve
II	Originating from central part of right coronary sinus, protruding into right ventricle, penetrating crista supraventricularis	Penetration and rupture into or just beneath crista supraventricularis of right ventricle
IIIa	Originating from posterior part of right coronary sinus, protruding into right ventricle, just beneath septal leaflet of tricuspid valve, penetrating membranous septum	Penetration and rupture into right ventricle adjacent to or at tricuspid annulus
IIIb	Originating from posterior part of right coronary sinus, protruding into right atrium, near commissure of septal and anterior leaflets of tricuspid valve	Penetration and rupture into right atrium adjacent to or at tricuspid annulus
IV	Originating from right part of noncoronary sinus, protruding into right atrium, near septal leaflets of tricuspid valve	Protrusion and rupture into right atrium
V		Other rare conditions (e.g., rupture into left atrium, pulmonary artery, left ventricle, or other structures)

tissue, right ventricular outflow tract obstruction, aortic cusp prolapse, aortic regurgitation, and if any additional shunt lesions exist. More importantly, distance between SOVA aortic opening to coronary ostium should be measured. Procedure is usually performed under fluoroscopic and TEE guidance [43–46]. Device selection has crucial role in procedure success. Galeczka et al. reported 23 patients in which 26 devices were used (22 Duct Occluders, 3 muscular VSD and 1 atrial septal occluder) [47]. The size of Duct Occluder was selected based on SOVA shape. Precise delineation of ruptured SOVA anatomy plays major role in selecting type of occluders to achieve better sealing effect and minimize complication as well as residual defect. Notably, they had one patient with left coronary artery to RSVA distance of less than 5 mm who experienced ST segment depression suggestive for coronary artery compression [47]. Balloon sizing of SOVA can be helpful in device selection, but it can cause further damage to a fragile tissue around the defect. Generally speaking, it is recommended to oversize the Occluder by at least 2 mm larger than the entrance diameter of SOVA on angiographic imaging. In a study by Tong et al. there was no device related complication when they selected duct occluder up to 1–3 mm larger than the maximal size of the RSVA opening site [48].

Window-like or aneurysmal type defects with surrounding soft tissue have been preferably treated with small-waist double disk VSD Occluders. The small-waist matches the entrance diameter of window-like and aneurysmal SOVA. The shape usually recovers well after release and does not obstruct enough to affect aortic valve function. Tubular shaped SOVA or those close to the tricuspid valve, are best managed with PDA Occluder with long connecting waist. This device preserves tricuspid valve function and has less chance of residual shunt and/or Occluder dislodgment which may occur when aortic end is pulled into the side of aneurysm.

Several techniques have been reported for transcatheter closure of the ruptured SOVA. (a) **Antegrade closure using conventional duct occluders**: This is by far the most commonly adapted technique due to its safety and high success rate (and this is the technique we followed in our case). Arteriovenous wire loop needs to be formed as follows [50]: advance a multipurpose coronary catheter from a femoral artery sheath until the mouth of sinus of Valsalva aneurysm. Then advance a Balance 0.014″/300 cm coronary Guidewire (ACS, Temecula, CA) retrograde through the aneurysm into the right atrium through rupture. This can be facilitated with the help of a 3 Fr transit catheter (Cordis). Using a 10 mm Goose Neck Snare (Microvena, White

Bear Lake, MN), advanced through an 8 Fr right femoral (or internal jugular) venous sheath, snare the coronary guidewire in the right atrium and exteriorize it out through the venous access (Figs. 9 and 10). Over the exteriorized wire, AGA delivery sheath (AGA Medical, Golden Valley, MN) is advanced antegrade into the aneurysm. Finally, an appropriate size ADO (AGA Medical) is advanced and placed to close the defect (Fig. 11). **(b) Retrograde approach using muscular ventricular septal occluders:** Aortogram is first done using a pigtail catheter. A right Judkins or Multipurpose catheter is used to cross the defect. Then Mullins sheath is introduced over 0.035″ or 0.038″ Amplatz exchange guidewire. Using a muscular ventricular septal occlude with waist diameter exceeding the defect size by 2 mm, the defect was closed retrogradely. Finally, device is released after confirming correct position with echocardiography and Aortogram. **(c) Retrograde approach using ADO-II devices:** same technique as described in B (Table 2).

Procedure Challenges and Pitfall

1. The windsock of the SOVA and adjacent areas are thin, which provide little support for the device deployment. Interventionists can reduce risk of embolization by oversizing the device by 2–4 mm or using additional disc on either side of the defect [46].
2. When the aneurysm has excessive large windsock, this may prevent proper opening of the Occluder resulting in device malalignment.

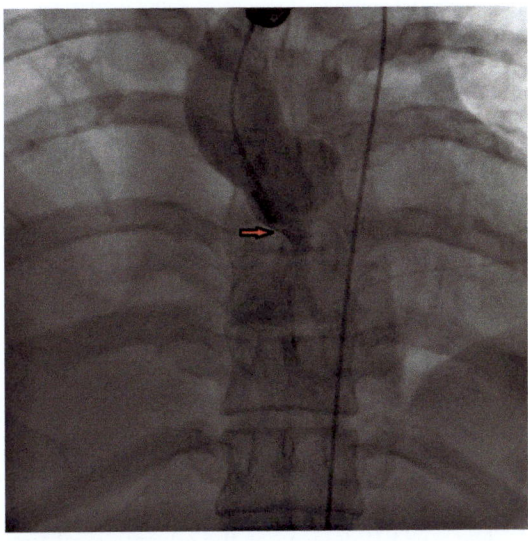

Fig. 10 Zoomed still image, aortic root angiography through a pigtail catheter showing ruptured SOVA of the right sinus, red arrow, angiographic type III (tubular)

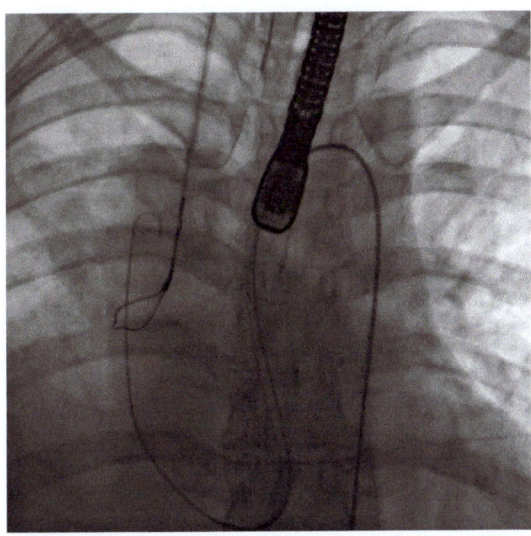

Fig. 9 Fluoroscopic image, RAO view, showing a Guidewire advanced retrograde from a femoral artery sheath through a multipurpose coronary catheter. The wire was then snared using a Goose Neck Snare advanced from a right internal jugular venous sheath

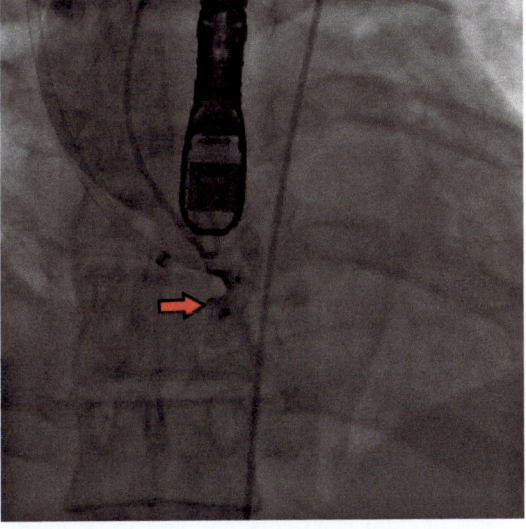

Fig. 11 Still image, aortic root angiography, RAO view, zoomed, after release of ADO I, red arrow, showing no residual shunt across the ruptured SOVA. Amplatzer Duct Occluder I, 10/8 mm was advanced anterograde from the right internal jugular sheath, red arrow. SOVA: sinus of Valsalva aneurysm

Table 2 Comparison of the two appoaches to device closure of SOVA

Antegrade approach	Retrograde approach
Better profile of duct Occluders, less bulky	Bulky design with discs on both sides
Can be deployed only through venous end	No need for AV loop formation, less hardware
Longer fluoroscopic time	Less fluoroscopic time
Single arterial puncture	Bilateral femoral arterial access
Better to oversize slightly (flimsy rims)	Retention discs on both sides, better support
Two devices may be deployed if needed	B/L retention skirts may prevent multiple devices
More experience, cost effective	Lesser experience

Moreover, the excessive tissue may cause RVOT obstruction which may get worse by device oversizing.

3. TEE is recommended and is superior to TTE for procedural guidance. Use of TTE may underestimate worsening aortic regurgitation as reported by Mahimarangaiah J and colleagues [46].
4. The ADO-II device has the advantage of low profile and can be delivered through Judkin's right coronary guide catheter. It is considered good option to close small size defects, or residual leaks. However, risk of embolization and/or residual defect are considerable concerns.
5. Moderate size defects can be closed by the retrograde approach using muscular VSD Occlude. Attention needs to be taken to avoid entrapment of the atrioventricular valves or causing inflow obstruction.
6. Large defect can still be closed percutaneously. Largest device used by Mahimarangaiah J and colleagues was 18/20 mm ADO-I device.
7. Operator will need two orthogonal projections for complete assessment and visualization of the rupture site and receiving chamber. Right or non-coronary sinus rupture into the RA or right ventricular inflow can be nicely evaluated in anteroposterior (AP) or right anterior oblique (RAO) views with minimal cranial angulations [46]. Right sinus ruptures into the RVOT or pulmonary artery (PA) are examined in left anterior oblique (LAO) views with cranial angulations.
8. It is important to recognize that even the surrounding structures are diseased. So, it is crucial to evaluate the patients on regular basis and look for residual leaks, new sites of rupture, and or aortic regurgitation. Interventionist should be mindful for rare, but high-risk defects, such as left coronary sinus to pulmonary artery SOVA. Galeczka et al. reported an abandoned case due to ischemic changes on ECG immediately after deployment of Amplazter duct Occluder, presumably secondary to coronary artery compression [47].

Comparison of Clinical Results Between Percutaneous Closure and Surgical Repair

Both, percutaneous and surgical treatment are relatively effective and safe. Recent review by Yang et al. compared surgical vs percutaneous closure [51]. Percutaneous approach was used in 26 patients while surgical closure done in 108 patients. Propensity matched scoring was done for three variables (age, sex and rupture size), so that 32 patients matching percutaneous closure group were selected. No immediate procedure related mortality, myocardial infarction or embolization was reported. On the other hand, surgical closure was performed in 108 patients. In Surgical Repair group and Matched group, there was no in hospital death, ventricular arrhythmia, or third-degree AV block [51].

Post Procedural Assessment

Follow Up and Long-Term Outcome

Generally, the procedure carries high success rate ranging from 83 to 97% in other reports [47, 49]. Follow up protocol would vary between centers. Outpatient clinic visits at 1, 3, 6 and 12 months post procedure would be reasonable. This includes physical exam, ECG and Echocardiography. In the previously mentioned report by Yang et al., the Percutaneous Group patients were followed for 1–84 months. Postoperative mild-moderate AR did not worsen on follow up. A tiny residual shunt was noticed in two patients, one of them disappeared after 25 months of follow up. Recurrence of SOVA did happen in one patient 6 years after procedure. More severe complications such as infective endocarditis, device embolization or hemolysis were not observed during follow up. No late death was reported. Xioa et al., in their series of 29 patients, reported no residual shunt, thrombosis or device related aortic valve disease on follow up period of (89.4 ± 34.9) months [49]. Three patients required re intervention for a second SOVA in a series of 23 patients reported by Galeczka et al. [47]. Same in this report, no serious complications were reported.

In our case, the patient was followed in cardiology clinic at 1, 6, and then 12 months post procedure. She did very well. ECG showed sinus rhythm, and TTE revealed significant reduction in LV size 12 months after the procedure with no residual shunt.

Multimodality Imaging Comparison

Table 3 summarizes goals of imaging in evaluation of sinus of Valsalva aneurysm.

> **Key Points**
> - SOVA is a rare structural heart disease, which can be treated with high success rate and low morbidity and mortality. However, can lead to devastating outcome if left untreated.
> - Multi-modality imaging approach is highly needed in this rare disease, to

Table 3 Summarizes the goals of imaging in evaluating the sinus of Valsalva aneurysm

Goals of imaging	Details
1. Aortic root anatomy	
2. Confirmation of diagnosis	
3. Distinguish from prolapsed aortic cusp, VSD, and aortic root aneurysm	
4. Aneurysm anatomy	(a) Sinus of origin (RCS: 72–85%, NCS: 5–22%, LCS: 5–6%) (b) Chamber of penetration (RV > RA > RVOT > LV > IVS > LA > pericardial space) (c) Signs of rupture (d) Shunt quantification (MRI)
5. Origin and relationship of coronary artery with aneurysm	
6. Other structural cardiac defects and complications such as aortic valve regurgitation, VSD, infective endocarditis and compression of adjacent structures	
7. Standard reporting format	(a) Aortic root anatomy with SOVA identification (b) Number, origin and drainage site (if ruptured) SOVA (c) Presence of compression due to SOVA and look for any thrombus within it (d) Assessment of coronaries (distance between SOVA neck and coronary origin from the same sinus is calculated) (e) Assessment of both atrioventricular and semilunar valves with special focus on the aortic valve to rule out aortic regurgitation (f) Assessment of cardiac chambers (especially right sided chambers) for dilation/failure (g) Presence of pulmonary arterial and venous hypertension and any lung parenchymal changes

IVS interventricular septum; *LA* left atrium; *LCS* left coronary sinus; *LV* left ventricle; *NCS* non-coronary sinus; *RA* right atrium; *RCS* right coronary sinus; *RVOT* right ventricle outflow tract; *RV* right ventricle; *VSD* ventricular septal defect

properly delineate anatomy and effects on adjacent structures, to help provide the best treatment strategy.
- Transcatheter approach is considered safe and efficient method of treatment, with good long-term outcome, but should be done in center with good experience and after thorough pre-procedural evaluation.

Acknowledgements The authors wish to thank Dr. Younes Boudjemline for providing the clinical case scenario and Figs. 9, 10, and 11.

Disclosures ZMH is a consultant for NuMED Inc. Other authors have no conflict of interest.

Chapter Review Questions

1. 40 y/o male construction worker was brought to emergency department with sudden onset severe chest pain and dyspnea. On examination, HR is regular at a rate of 120 bpm/min, BP 145/60 mmHg and a loud continuous murmur is heard. ECG showed sinus tachycardia and no ischemic changes. What is the most likely diagnosis?
   A. Patent ductus arteriosus
   B. Post Myocardial infarction VSD
   C. Ruptured sinus of Valsalva aneurysm (SOVA)

Answer: C

   Explanation: PDA would not give such an acute presentation. Post MI VSD can manifest as above but the murmur is systolic. However, there should be some evidence of ischemia on ECG.

2. Ruptured sinus of Valsalva aneurysm (SOVA) has been confirmed by TTE and patient was stabilized and admitted to CICU. What would be the best next step in management?
   A. Transesophageal Echocardiogram
   B. Obtain cardiac CT/MR
   C. Urgent cardiac catheterization

Answer: C

   Explanation: as the patient has hemodynamically significant ruptured SOVA, he will obviously require urgent intervention. Traditionally, surgery has been the modality of choice. However, percutaneous closure is considered an option as discussed in the chapter above. As diagnosis is confirmed, TEE can be done during cardiac Cath and would not be of much value in such symptomatic patient. Cardiac CT/MR would be very reasonable in asymptomatic or mildly symptomatic patients to delineate anatomy and effect on adjacent structures.

3. Transesophageal echocardiography reveals an unruptured sinus of Valsalva aneurysm (SOVA) in a patient evaluated for widened mediastinum on chest X-ray and chest discomfort. What is the next best step in management?
   A. Cardiac MR/Cardiac CT for confirmation of the aneurysm, and, if confirmed, immediate surgical consultation
   B. Follow up echocardiogram in 6 weeks
   C. Holter monitor
   D. Referral for outpatient cardiothoracic surgery consultation

Answer: A

   Explanation: Sinus of Valsalva aneurysm can cause compression of the adjacent coronary arteries resulting in myocardial ischemia and infarction. This can be best evaluated with cardiac CT/MR. If patient found to have coronary artery disease, this can be addressed during percutaneous or surgical closure of SOVA.

References

1. Weinreich M, Yu PJ, Trost B. Sinus of Valsalva aneurysms: review of the literature and an update on management. Clin Cardiol. 2015;38(3):185–9. https://doi.org/10.1002/clc.22359. Epub 2015 Mar 10.
2. Taguchi K, Sasaki N, Matsuura Y, Uemura R. Surgical correction of aneurysm of the sinus of Valsalva. A report of forty-five consecutive patients including eight with total replacement of the aortic valve. Am J Cardiol. 1969;23(2):180–91. https://doi.org/10.1016/0002-9149(69)90065-4.

3. Edwards JE, Burchell HB. The pathological anatomy of deficiencies between the aortic root and the heart, including aortic sinus aneurysms. Thorax. 1957;12(2):125–39. https://doi.org/10.1136/thx.12.2.125.
4. van Son JA, Danielson GK, Schaff HV, Orszulak TA, Edwards WD, Seward JB. Long-term outcome of surgical repair of ruptured sinus of Valsalva aneurysm. Circulation. 1994;90(5 Pt 2):II20–9.
5. Hourihan M, Perry SB, Mandell VS, Keane JF, Rome JJ, Bittl JA, et al. Transcatheter umbrella closure of valvular and paravalvular leaks. J Am Coll Cardiol. 1992;20:1371–7.
6. Chu SH, Hung CR, How SS, et al. Ruptured aneurysms of the sinus of Valsalva in oriental patients. J Thorac Cardiovasc Surg. 1990;99:288–98.
7. Arora R, Trehan V, Rangasetty UMC, Mukhopadhyay S, Thakur AK, Kalra GS. Transcatheter closure of ruptured sinus of Valsalva aneurysm. J Interv Cardiol. 2004;17:53–8.
8. Kuriakose EM, Bhatla P, McElhinney DB. Comparison of reported outcomes with percutaneous versus surgical closure of ruptured sinus of Valsalva aneurysm. Am J Cardiol. 2015;115(3):392–8. https://doi.org/10.1016/j.amjcard.2014.11.013. Epub 2014 Nov 13.
9. Takach TJ, Reul GJ, Duncan JM, et al. Sinus of Valsalva aneurysm or fistula: management and outcome. Ann Thorac Surg. 1999;68:1573–7.
10. Oka N, Aomi S, Tomioka H, Endo M, Koyanagi H. Surgical treatment of multiple aneurysms in a patient with Ehlers-Danlos syndrome. J Thorac Cardiovasc Surg. 2001;121(6):1210–1. https://doi.org/10.1067/mtc.2001.111644.
11. Thomas P, Bossan A, Lacour JP, Chanalet S, Ortonne JP, Chatel M. Ehlers-Danlos syndrome with subependymal periventricular heterotopias. Neurology. 1996;46(4):1165–7. https://doi.org/10.1212/wnl.46.4.1165.
12. Takahashi T, Koide T, Yamaguchi H, Nakamura N, Ohshima Y, Suzuki J, Murao S, Hino H. Ehlers-Danlos syndrome with aortic regurgitation, dilation of the sinuses of Valsalva, and abnormal dermal collagen fibrils. Am Heart J. 1992;123(6):1709–12. https://doi.org/10.1016/0002-8703(92)90833-h.
13. Cupo LN, Pyeritz RE, Olson JL, McPhee SJ, Hutchins GM, McKusick VA. Ehlers-Danlos syndrome with abnormal collagen fibrils, sinus of Valsalva aneurysms, myocardial infarction, panacinar emphysema and cerebral heterotopias. Am J Med. 1981;71(6):1051–8. https://doi.org/10.1016/0002-9343(81)90341-7.
14. Leier CV, Call TD, Fulkerson PK, Wooley CF. The spectrum of cardiac defects in the Ehlers-Danlos syndrome, types I and III. Ann Intern Med. 1980;92(2 Pt 1):171–8. https://doi.org/10.7326/0003-4819-92-2-171.
15. Dong C, Wu Q-Y, Tang Y. Ruptured sinus of Valsalva aneurysm: a Beijing experience. Ann Thorac Surg. 2002;74:1621–4.
16. Mayer ED, Ruffmann K, Saggau W, et al. Ruptured aneurysms of the sinus of Valsalva. Ann Thorac Surg. 1986;42:81–5.
17. Ott DA. Aneurysm of the sinus of valsalva. Semin Thorac Cardiovasc Surg Pediatr Card Surg Annu. 2006;9:165–76. https://doi.org/10.1053/j.pcsu.2006.02.014.
18. Feldman DN, Roman MJ. Aneurysms of the sinuses of Valsalva. Cardiology. 2006;106(2):73–81. https://doi.org/10.1159/000092635. Epub 2006 Apr 12.
19. Jiang Z, Tang M, Liu H, Mei J. Surgical management of giant left Sinus of Valsalva aneurysm causing left anterior descending coronary artery occlusion. Ann Thorac Surg. 2017;104(1):e27–9. https://doi.org/10.1016/j.athoracsur.2017.01.099.
20. Stöllberger C, Seitelberger R, Fenninger C, Prainer C, Slany J. Aneurysm of the left sinus of Valsalva. An unusual source of cerebral embolism. Stroke. 1996;27(8):1424–6. https://doi.org/10.1161/01.str.27.8.1424.
21. Nakamura Y, Aoki M, Hagino I, Koshiyama H, Fujiwara T, Nakajima H. Case of congenital aneurysm of sinus of Valsalva with common arterial trunk. Ann Thorac Surg. 2014;97(2):710–2. https://doi.org/10.1016/j.athoracsur.2013.06.107.
22. Munk MD, Gatzoulis MA, King DE, Webb GD. Cardiac tamponade and death from intrapericardial rupture [corrected] of sinus of Valsalva aneurysm. Eur J Cardiothorac Surg. 1999;15(1):100–2. https://doi.org/10.1016/s1010-7940(98)00269-3. Erratum in: Eur J Cardiothorac Surg 1999 Mar;15(3):379.
23. Xu B, Kocyigit D, Betancor J, Tan C, Rodriguez ER, Schoenhagen P, Flamm SD, Rodriguez LL, Svensson LG, Griffin BP. Sinus of Valsalva aneurysms: a state-of-the-art imaging review. J Am Soc Echocardiogr. 2020;33(3):295–312. https://doi.org/10.1016/j.echo.2019.11.008.
24. Cheng TO, Yang YL, Xie MX, Wang XF, Dong NG, Su W, Lü Q, He L, Lu XF, Wang J, Li L, Yuan L. Echocardiographic diagnosis of sinus of Valsalva aneurysm: a 17-year (1995-2012) experience of 212 surgically treated patients from one single medical center in China. Int J Cardiol. 2014;173(1):33–9. https://doi.org/10.1016/j.ijcard.2014.02.003. Epub 2014 Feb 15.
25. Guo DW, Cheng TO, Lin ML, Gu ZQ. Aneurysm of the sinus of Valsalva: a roentgenologic study of 105 Chinese patients. Am Heart J. 1987;114(5):1169–77. https://doi.org/10.1016/0002-8703(87)90193-1.
26. Vatankulu MA, Tasal A, Erdogan E, Sonmez O, Goktekin O. The role of three-dimensional echocardiography in diagnosis and management of ruptured sinus of valsalva aneurysm. Echocardiography. 2013;30(8):E260–2. https://doi.org/10.1111/echo.12248. Epub 2013 May 11.
27. Hoey ET, Gulati GS, Singh S, Watkin RW, Nazir S, Ganeshan A, Rafique A, Sivananthan MU. The role of multi-modality imaging for sinus of Valsalva aneurysms. Int J Cardiovasc Imaging. 2012;28(7):1725–

38. https://doi.org/10.1007/s10554-011-0001-5. Epub 2012 Jan 12.
28. Goldstein SA, Evangelista A, Abbara S, Arai A, Asch FM, Badano LP, Bolen MA, Connolly HM, Cuéllar-Calàbria H, Czerny M, Devereux RB, Erbel RA, Fattori R, Isselbacher EM, Lindsay JM, McCulloch M, Michelena HI, Nienaber CA, Oh JK, Pepi M, Taylor AJ, Weinsaft JW, Zamorano JL, Dietz H, Eagle K, Elefteriades J, Jondeau G, Rousseau H, Schepens M. Multimodality imaging of diseases of the thoracic aorta in adults: from the American Society of Echocardiography and the European Association of Cardiovascular Imaging: endorsed by the Society of Cardiovascular Computed Tomography and Society for Cardiovascular Magnetic Resonance. J Am Soc Echocardiogr. 2015;28(2):119–82. https://doi.org/10.1016/j.echo.2014.11.015.
29. Blanke P, Weir-McCall JR, Achenbach S, Delgado V, Hausleiter J, Jilaihawi H, Marwan M, Nørgaard BL, Piazza N, Schoenhagen P, Leipsic JA. Computed tomography imaging in the context of transcatheter aortic valve implantation (TAVI)/transcatheter aortic valve replacement (TAVR): an expert consensus document of the Society of Cardiovascular Computed Tomography. JACC Cardiovasc Imaging. 2019;12(1):1–24. https://doi.org/10.1016/j.jcmg.2018.12.003.
30. O'Donnell DH, Abbara S, Chaithiraphan V, Yared K, Killeen RP, Cury RC, Dodd JD. Cardiac tumors: optimal cardiac MR sequences and spectrum of imaging appearances. AJR Am J Roentgenol. 2009;193(2):377–87. https://doi.org/10.2214/AJR.08.1895.
31. Liu S, Xu X, Chen F, Zhao Z, Zhang Y, Wang C, Xiang J, Wu G, Chen X, Zhao X, Qin Y. Angiographic features of ruptured sinus of Valsalva aneurysm: new classification. J Cardiol. 2014;64(2):139–44. https://doi.org/10.1016/j.jjcc.2013.12.004. Epub 2014 Feb 1.
32. Xin-jin L, Li X, Peng B, Guo H, Wang W, Li S, et al. Modified Sakakibara classification system for ruptured sinus of Valsalva aneurysm. J Thorac Cardiovasc Surg. 2013;146(4):874–8.
33. Sakakibara S, Konno S. Congenital aneurysm of the sinus of Valsalva: anatomy and classification. Am Heart J. 1962;63:405–24.
34. Wang Z-J, Zou C-W, Li D-C, Li H-X, Wang A-B, Yuan G-D, Fan Q-X. Surgical repair of sinus of Valsalva aneurysm in Asian patients. Ann Thorac Surg. 2007;84:156–60.
35. Breatnach CR, Walsh KP. Ruptured sinus of Valsalva aneurysm and Gerbode defects: patient and procedural selection: the key to Optimising outcomes. Curr Cardiol Rep. 2018;20(10):90. https://doi.org/10.1007/s11886-018-1038-z.
36. Vural KM, Sener E, Taşdemir O, Bayazit K. Approach to sinus of Valsalva aneurysms: a review of 53 cases. Eur J Cardiothorac Surg. 2001;20(1):71–6. https://doi.org/10.1016/s1010-7940(01)00758-8.
37. Murashita T, Kubota T, Kamikubo Y, Shiiya N, Yasuda K. Long-term results of aortic valve regurgitation after repair of ruptured sinus of Valsalva aneurysm. Ann Thorac Surg. 2002;73(5):1466–71. https://doi.org/10.1016/s0003-4975(02)03493-8.
38. Chang C-W, Chiu S-N, Wu E-T, Tsai S-K, Wu M-H, Wang J-K. Transcatheter closure of a ruptured sinus of Valsalva aneurysm. Circ J. 2006;70:1043–7.
39. Szkutnik M, Kusa J, Glowacki J, Fiszer R, Bialkowski J. Transcatheter closure of ruptured sinus of Valsalva aneurysms with an Amplatzer occluder. Rev Esp Cardiol. 2009;62:1317–21.
40. Kerkar PG, Lanjewar CP, Mishra N, Nyayadhish P, Mammen I. Transcatheter closure of ruptured sinus of Valsalva aneurysm using the Amplatzer duct occluder: immediate results and mid-term follow-up. Eur Heart J. 2010;31:2881–7.
41. Sivadasanpillai H, Valaparambil A, Sivasubramonian S, Mahadevan KK, Sasidharan B, Namboodiri N, et al. Percutaneous closure of ruptured sinus of Valsalva aneurysms: intermediate term follow-up results. EuroIntervention. 2010;6:214–9.
42. Liu S, Xu X, Ding X, Liu G, Zhao Z, Zhao X, et al. Comparison of immediate results and mid-term follow-up of surgical and percutaneous closure of ruptured sinus of Valsalva aneurysm. J Cardiol. 2014;63:239–43.
43. Fang Z-F, Huang Y-Y, Tang L, Hu X-Q, Shen X-Q, Tang J-J, et al. Long-term outcomes of transcatheter closure of ruptured sinus Valsalva aneurysms using patent ductus arteriosus occluders. Circ J. 2014;78:2197–202.
44. Liu S, Xu X, Zhao X, Chen F, Bai Y, Li W, et al. Percutaneous closure of ruptured sinus of Valsalva aneurysm: results from a multicentre experience. EuroIntervention. 2014;10:505–12.
45. Xiao J-W, Wang Q-G, Zhang D-Z, Cui C-S, Han X, Zhang P, et al. Clinical outcomes of percutaneous or surgical closure of ruptured sinus of Valsalva aneurysm. Congenit Heart Dis. 2018;13:305–10.
46. Mahimarangaiah J, Chandra S, Subramanian A, Srinivasa KH, Usha MK, Manjunath CN. Transcatheter closure of ruptured sinus of Valsalva: different techniques and mid-term follow-up. Catheter Cardiovasc Interv. 2016;87(3):516–22. https://doi.org/10.1002/ccd.26107. Epub 2015 Aug 10.
47. Galeczka M, Glowacki J, Yashchuk N, Ditkivskyy I, Rojczyk D, Knop M, Smerdzinski S, Cherpak B, Szkutnik M, Bialkowski J, Fiszer R, Lazoryshynets V. Medium- and long-term follow-up of transcatheter closure of ruptured sinus of Valsalva aneurysm in Central Europe population. J Cardiol. 2019;74(4):381–7. https://doi.org/10.1016/j.jjcc.2019.03.012. Epub 2019 Apr 23.
48. Tong S, Zhong L, Liu J, Yao Q, Guo Y, Shu M, Song Z. The immediate and follow-up results of transcatheter occlusion of the ruptured sinus of Valsalva aneurysm with duct occluder. J Invasive Cardiol. 2014;26(2):55–9.
49. Xiao JW, Wang QG, Zhang DZ, Cui CS, Han X, Zhang P, Hou C, Zhu XY. Clinical outcomes of percutaneous or surgical closure of ruptured sinus of Valsalva aneurysm. Congenit Heart Dis. 2018;13(2):305–10. https://doi.org/10.1111/chd.12572. Epub 2018 Feb 5.

50. Fedson S, Jolly N, Lang RM, Hijazi ZM. Percutaneous closure of a ruptured sinus of Valsalva aneurysm using the Amplatzer Duct Occluder. Catheter Cardiovasc Interv. 2003;58(3):406–11. https://doi.org/10.1002/ccd.10401.

51. Yang K, Luo X, Tang Y, Hu H, Sun H. Comparison of clinical results between percutaneous closure and surgical repair of ruptured sinus of Valsalva aneurysm. Catheter Cardiovasc Interv. 2021;97(3):E354–61. https://doi.org/10.1002/ccd.29216. Epub 2020 Aug 31.

Transcatheter Approach to Coarctation of Aorta and Isolated Interrupted Aortic Arch in Adults

Ata Firouzi, Anita Sadeghpour, and Zahra Hosseini

Abstract

Isolated coarctation of the aorta (COA) is a localized aortic narrowing (usually post-ductal, near subclavian artery) that mainly remains undiagnosed in adulthood and is detected incidentally in a hypertensive patient with Radial-Femoral pulse delay. Untreated patients have poor prognoses. Previously, the gold standard of treatment was the surgical repair. However, during the last two decades, balloon angioplasty with stenting has perceived their roles and long-term outcome trials confirmed the safety and effectiveness of transcatheter (TC) coarctoplasty in adulthood. Interrupted aortic arch (IAA) is aortic luminal disruption between ascending and descending aorta, a complex congenital heart disease commonly associated with other congenital anomalies. Although, the surgical approach was the first option for those with associated other anomalies, in selected cases, percutaneous reconstruction of IAA before surgical repair of other defects, facilitates the surgeon's point of view. In this section, we will discuss the role of cardiac imaging in diagnosing COA and IAA and their roles in characterizing the appropriate cases for the TC approach, the interventional tackle, and post-procedure follow-up.

Keywords

Coarctation of aorta · Hypertension · Transcatheter coarctoplasty · Interrupted aortic arch · Luminal disruption · Surgical repair · Cardiac imaging

Abbreviations

BAV   Bicuspid aortic valve
BES   Balloon-expandable stent
CMRI Cardiac magnetic resonance imaging
COA   Coarctation of aorta
CTA   Computed tomography angiography
HTN   Hypertension
IAA   Interrupted aortic arch
PDA   Patent ductus arteriosus
SES   Self-expandable stent
TC   Trans-catheter
TEVAR Thoracic endovascular aortic repair
TS   Turner syndrome

Supplementary Information The online version contains supplementary material available at https://doi.org/10.1007/978-3-031-50740-3_14.

A. Firouzi · Z. Hosseini (✉)
Cardiovascular Intervention Research Center, Rajaie Cardiovascular Medical and Research Center, Tehran, Iran

A. Sadeghpour
MedStar Cardiovascular Corelabs, MedStar Health Research Institute, Georgetown University, Washington, DC, USA
e-mail: anita.sadeghpour@medstar.net

© The Author(s), under exclusive license to Springer Nature Switzerland AG 2024
A. M. Kelsey et al. (eds.), *Cardiac Imaging in Structural Heart Disease Interventions*,
https://doi.org/10.1007/978-3-031-50740-3_14

| TTE | Transthoracic echocardiography |
| VSD | Ventricular septal defects |

Test your learning and check your understanding of this book's contents: use the "Springer Nature Flashcards" app to access questions using ▶ https://sn.pub/ambACS.
To use the app, please follow the instructions in the chapter "Transcatheter Aortic Valve Replacement."

Learning Objectives

1. *Emphasis on the timely diagnosis of COA.*
2. *Know the indications for coarctoplasty and appropriate therapeutic approach*
3. *Know the role of imaging in diagnosis and interventional therapeutic approach and surveillance.*

Case 1
A 29 year-old-man was referred to the outpatient clinic for more evaluation of refractory systemic hypertension despite full guideline directed medications. In physical examination, Radial-Femoral pulse delay was evident; upper extremities BP: 160/90 mmHg, right lower popliteal artery BP: 100/60 mmHg. There was an interscapular systolic murmur (Grade II) in his heart auscultation. The Electrography (ECG) demonstrated LVH pattern with a strain pattern in pericardial leads.

Background and Definitions

Coarctation of aorta (COA) is a congenital juxta ductal localized aortic narrowing (usually post-ductal in adults) with a ridge consisting of localized medial thickening and infolding with superimposed neo-intimal tissue. Most commonly, it is located at the junction of the ductus arteriosus with the aortic arch, just distal to the left subclavian artery. COA accounts for 5–8% of children born with congenital heart disease, which is often associated with other congenital cardiac anomalies including: VSD, PDA, Hypoplastic aortic arch, Shone complex, and Bicuspid aortic valve (BAV) [1].

BAV is commonly associated with COA and is present in more than half of COA patients which can lead to AI, AS or aortic dilatation and dissection. Intracranial aneurysms may also occur (2–10%). Timely diagnosis of COA is mandatory for a good prognosis since early treatment is associated with lower risk of long-term morbidity and mortality. The natural history of this condition is miserable, with death ensuring on average in the fourth decade of life and three-quarters of patients dying before their 50th birthday [2].

The most common causes of death are congestive heart failure, aortic dissection, rupture of the aorta, infective endocarditis, premature coronary artery disease, and intra-cranial hemorrhage [3]. In adults, the most common presentation is systemic hypertension, accounts for 0.2% of all hypertension cases in adults.

The transverse aortic arch (TAA) is a segment of the arch between the innominate artery and the left subclavian artery (LSA). Isthmus is a portion of aorta distal to LSA. If TAA diameter is <60% of ascending aortic diameter, it is called hypoplastic. Isthmus is hypoplastic if its diameter is <40% of ascending aortic diameter. Normally, aortic isthmus is 80–90% of TAA diameter and almost equal to that of aorta at the diaphragmatic level [4].

An Interrupted aortic arch (IAA), is an anomaly that can be considered the most severe form of coarctation of the aorta. In an IAA, there is an anatomical and luminal disruption between the ascending and descending aorta. The incidence is about 1.5% in patients with congenital cardiac anomaly [5]. If untreated, 90% of the affected infants may die in the first year of life, with the majority in the first few days. In the few cases reported in adults, the presentation varies from being asymptomatic to differential blood pressure recordings in the extremities, refractory systemic arterial hypertension, headache, claudication, and congestive heart failure [6]. Survival into adulthood is dependent upon the development of collateral circulation. Although in neonates the most common type of the IAA is type B (The disruption is located between the left carotid artery and the left subclavian artery), in adults, type A is the most frequent type (The disruption is located distal to the left subclavian artery) [7].

Diagnostic Workup

Physical Examination: Radial-Femoral pulse delay is evident unless significant AI coexists. The systolic blood pressure gradient ≥20 mmHg between the upper (right arm) and lower extremities suggests significant CoA that requires therapeutic intervention. The differential systolic blood pressure of at least 10 mmHg can be indicative for CoA. CoA patients might have interscapular early to mid-systolic or continuous murmurs (due to collateral vessels) in auscultation.

ECG: various degrees of LVH are seen. **CXR**; So called "figure-3" configuration and rib notching (in about 50% of cases) are diagnostic [8, 9].

Transthoracic Echocardiogram (TTE):

- Suprasternal window provides the best view for visualizing the narrowing of the aorta and accelerated flow proximal to the narrowing.
- Continuous wave Doppler study of the coarctation site has a characteristic pattern called "Sawtooth" appearance which is turbulent antegrade systolic flow extending to the diastole. However, it might be difficult to find the narrowing and typical Doppler findings in adult patients.
- In significant CoA, pulse wave Doppler study of the abdominal Aorta shows delayed and low velocity systolic flow that extends to the diastole with absent early diastolic flow reversal.
- The width and length of the stenotic segment, gradients and collateral vessels should be searched by TTE. Even in the absence of a significant gradient through the stenotic segment, a slow systolic upstroke and an antegrade diastolic flow on spectral Doppler suggest significant COA or IAA with collateral vessels.
- Additionally, TTE should provide data about the biventricular function, aortic valve (eg, bicuspid aortic valves, aortic stenosis, and aortic insufficiency), left ventricular outflow tract obstructions associated with ventricular septal defects, patent ductus arteriosus.

In CoA and IAA, cardiac magnetic resonance (CMR) imaging and computed tomography (CT) angiography are recommended as class I indications for initial and follow-up evaluation. The exact location, width and length, site of the stenosis, collateral vessels, and the size of the aorta at the level of the sinus of Valsalva, ascending, proximal arch, transverse arch, descending aorta at the level of the diaphragm, and any other anomalies should be evaluated. Also they assist in selecting the appropriate treatment approach (surgical or transcatheter approach [TC]) in the preprocedural planning and appropriate device selection before invasive angiography and finding the optimal fluoroscopic angles especially in those with IAAs.

The standard management of native coarctation in infants and young children is surgical repair, with preferred therapy in older children, adolescents, and adults being percutaneous intervention [10].

Significant aortic coarctation (native or recurrent) based on the AHA/ACC 2018 guideline is defined as [10]:

- Resting upper extremity to lower extremity peak-to-peak gradient >20 mmHg or mean systolic Doppler pressure gradient >20 mmHg
- Upper extremity to lower extremity pressure gradient >10 mmHg or mean systolic Doppler gradient >10 mmHg in the presence of

decreased LV systolic function or aortic regurgitation
- Upper extremity to lower extremity gradient >10 mmHg or mean Doppler pressure gradient >10 mmHg in the presence of collateral flow

Therapeutic intervention recommendations based on the ESC 2020 Guideline [9]:

Class I: In a hypertensive patient with peak-to-peak gradient ≥20 mmHg, stenting is preferred over surgery when technically feasible.

Class IIa: In a hypertensive patient with a peak-to-peak gradient is <20 mmHg, but aortic narrowing ≥50% relative to the diameter of the aorta at the diaphragm, catheter treatment (stenting) should be considered when technically feasible. In a normotensive patient with peak to peak gradient ≥20 mmHg, stenting should be considered when technically feasible.

Class IIb: In a normotensive patient with peak-to-peak gradient <20 mmHg, but aortic narrowing ≥50% compared to the diameter of the aorta at the diaphragm, stenting may be considered when technically feasible

Diagnosis and Pre-procedural Evaluation in Case 1

As the patient was highly suspicious of the COA, 2-D TTE was done and showed: Normal size and function left ventricle with moderate concentric LVH. There was BAV without AS and mild to moderate eccentric AI. Aortic root and ascending aorta evaluation revealed annulus-aortic ectasia with ST junction effacement and aneurysmal ascending aorta: 5.3 cm (Fig. 1a). There was significant narrowing with systolic turbulency in proximal part of the thoracic descending aorta with systolic PG: 64 mmHg and diastolic antegrade flow (diastolic tail—Fig. 1b), limited abdominal aorta pulsatility with early systolic upstroke consistent with COA (Fig. 1c). There was no other associated cardiac abnormality (Fig. 2).

CTA confirmed the echocardiography diagnosis of bicuspid aortic valve, aneurysmal dilatation of aortic root and ascending aorta with juxtaductal discrete COA and associated multiple large collaterals.

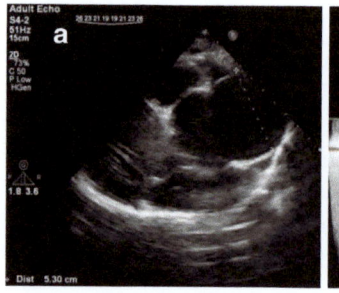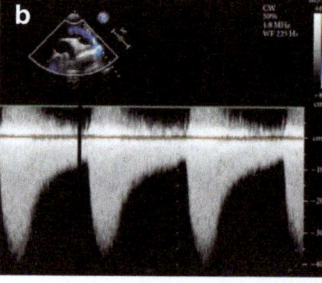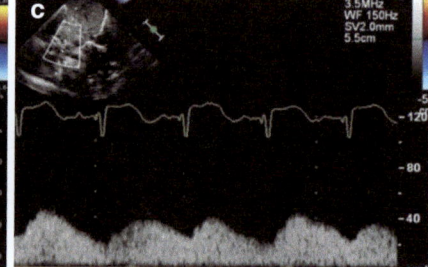

Fig. 1 (**a–c**) In TTE, Annulus-aortic ectasia with ST junction effacement is denoted (**a**). A significant narrowing with systolic turbulency in the proximal part of the thoracic descending aorta with the diastolic antegrade flow (diastolic tail) resulting typical Sawtooth pattern (**b**). Abdominal aorta pulse wave Doppler study shows slow and low-velocity systolic flow extending to the diastole with absent early diastolic flow reverse consistent with severe COA (**c**)

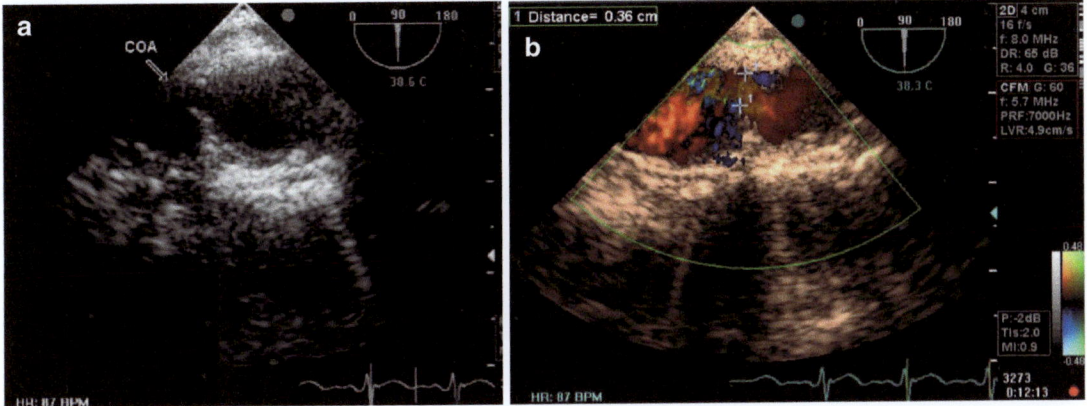

Fig. 2 (**a, b**) Transesophageal echocardiogram in long axis view of thoracic Aorta showing CoA narrowing by 2D and color Doppler study

Heart Team Approach and Decision

In neonates and adolescents with coarctation, surgical approach has been the gold standard treatment.

However, in recent decades, coarctoplasty and primary stenting techniques have been suggested for young adults and adults as the best therapeutic approach considering the technical improvement in this field. There are several surgical methods; while end-to-end anastomosis and subclavian flap repair have a high risk of re-coarctation (10%), patch aortoplasty has a high risk of aneurysm formation (10%).

Our patient was a candidate for the transcatheter approach regarding refractory hypertension and significant focal CoA to facilitate the surgical aortoplasty as the next step.

Procedural Technique

Under conscious sedation, after right CFA sheath (6F) insertion, 5000 units IV Heparin was injected. A Multipurpose catheter wiring of the narrowed segment was done with 0.035-inch hydrophilic wire (260 cm), then the wire was exchanged with a supper-stiff long wire. Aortic root injection in LAO projection showed: BAV with no AS and mild AR and aneurysmal dilatation of the aortic root. After that, aortic arch injection was done to characterize the residual segment, length, the distance to the left subclavian artery and the size of the aorta before and after the coarctatrion (Fig. 3a and b). After advancing a long delivery sheath (Cook-10F) toward the aortic arch, the dilator was removed and the sheath was de-aired. According to the size of the aortic arch (22 mm) and distal aortic size (26 mm), a self-expandable stent (Sinus-XL 22*60) was chosen. The delivery stent was passed through the sheath to reach the tip of the sheath. In LAO view by aortography through the sheath, the correct position of the stent was confirmed. For optimal stent positioning, we covered the proximal stent with the delivery sheath and slowly expanded the distal part of the stent to its full size, then by pulling the sheath off of the stent catheter, the remainder of the stent was deployed across the coarctation segment. Following stent deployment, postdilatation was performed by ATLAS GOLD 18*40 balloon (Fig. 3c). A Pigtail catheter was passed to obtain simultaneous pressure measurements across the stent and to rule out any complications after multiple angiograms in LAO and RAO projections. The procedure was terminated with good final result without any residual gradient (Fig. 3d).

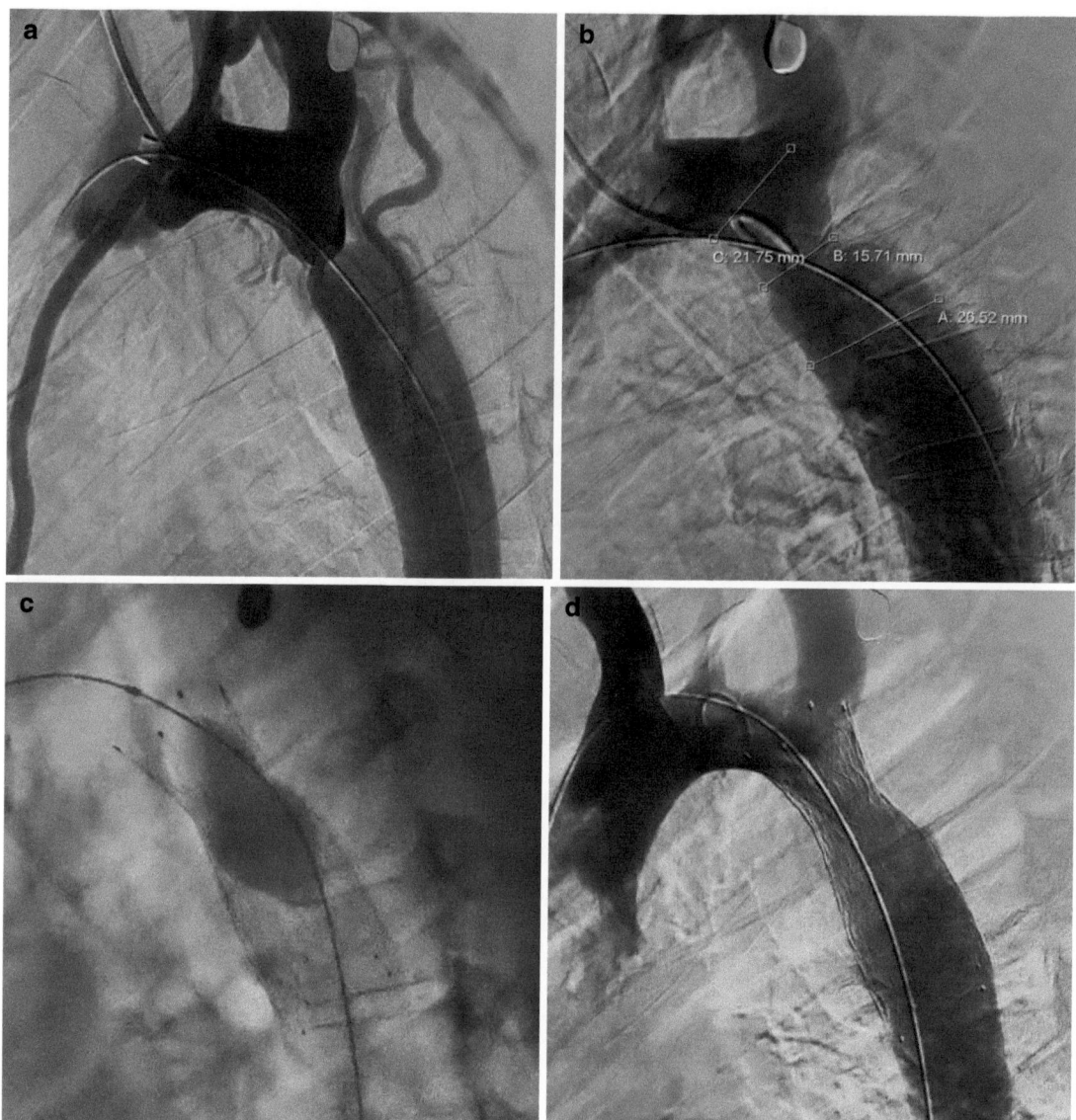

Fig. 3 (**a–d**) Aortic arch injection in deep LAO projection demonstrated a discrete juxtaductal coarctation (COA) with multiple well developed collateral vessels (**a**). Sizing of the proximal and distal to the COA was done and a self-expandable stent (Sinus-XL 22*60) was selected based on the size of the aorta at the level of the transverse arch (**b**). The delivery stent was passed through the sheath to reach the tip of the sheath. In LAO view and angiography through the sheath, the correct position of the stent was confirmed. For optimal stent positioning, we covered the proximal stent with the delivery sheath and slowly expanded the distal stent to its full size, then by pulling the sheath off of the stent catheter, the remainder of the stent was deployed across the coarctation segment. As the waist of the stent was not dilated appropriately, postdilatation was done by ATLAS GOLD balloon (18*40) (**c**). Final aortography in multiple projections confirmed well expanded stent without any complications and the final residual gradient was zero (**d**)

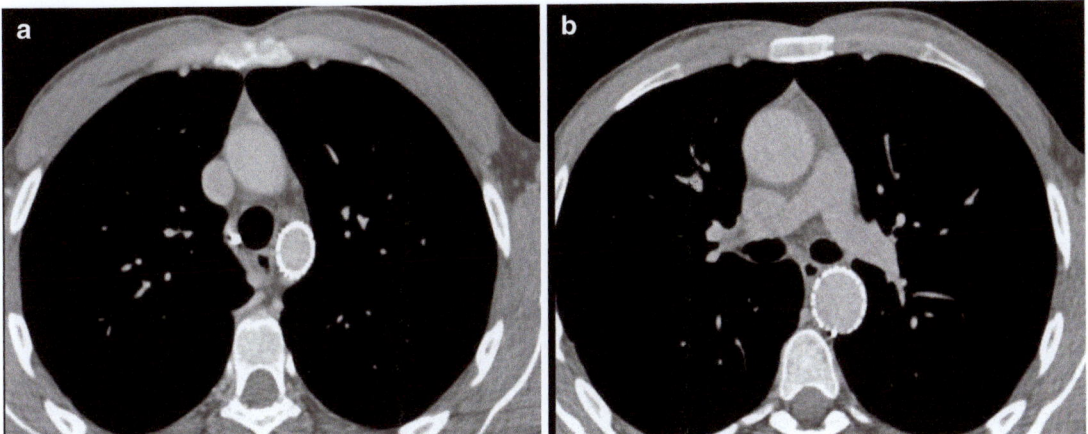

Fig. 4 (**a** and **b**) Follow-up aortic CTA 1 month later demonstrated patent stent at proximal and distal portions of descending aorta, no evidence of recoarctation, and no sign of complication at the site of stenting (**a** and **b**)

Post-procedural Follow Up

In our case, aortic CTA, 1 month later, denoted: Patent stent at the proximal portion of descending aorta, no evidence of recoarctation, no sign of complication at the site of stenting (Fig. 4a and b).

All CoA patients require regular annual follow up. 2-D TTE is the first imaging modality to estimate the immediate and late residual gradient and also to evaluate the degree of the AI and aortic size in patients with concomitant BAV.

However, CTA or preferably MRA are suggested imaging modalities to assess the postinterventional anatomy (Fig. 5) and possible complications every 3–5 years, although it might be different based on the aortic pathology [9, 10].

> **Case 2**
>
> A 25-year-old lady (G1P0), was referred to the outpatient clinic with a history of abortion 2 months ago (at 22 weeks of gestation). She was a known case of uncontrolled hypertension 5 years ago and was under guideline-directed medical therapy. In physical examination, the general appearance was normal. Bilateral upper extremities BP was 150/90 mmHg and right lower popliteal artery BP was 70/30 mmHg. Undetectable femoral pulses bilaterally.

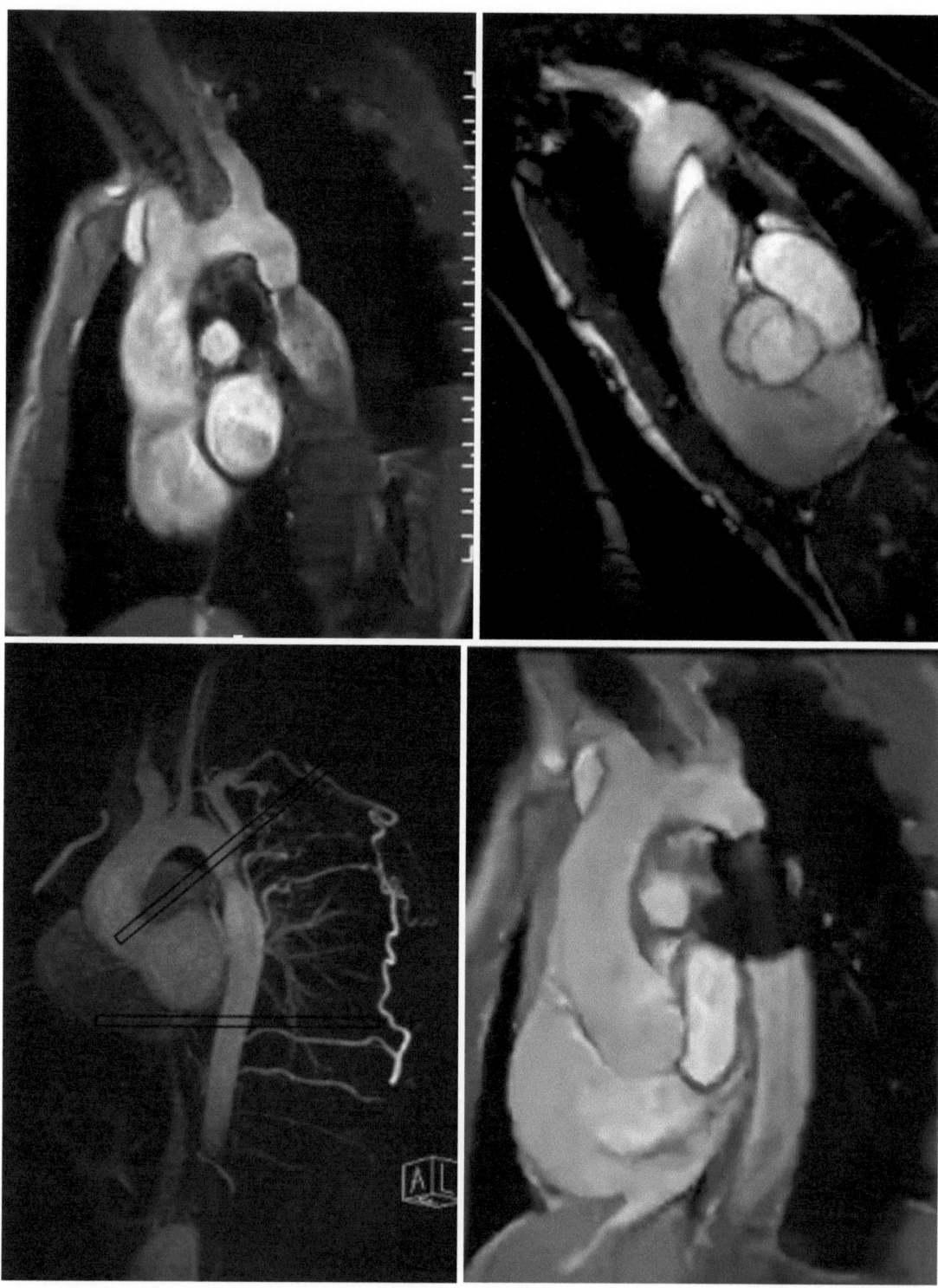

Fig. 5 CMR of a patient with severe CoA and flow acceleration at the site of stenosis (Left upper image, Movie 1). Associated bicuspid aortic valve in steady-state free precession CMR (right upper image, Movies 2 and 3), significant collaterals with reversal of intercostal flow, in 3D contrast-enhanced magnetic resonance angiography (MRA), note that collateral flow can be assessed via flow differential between proximal and distal aorta (Left lower panel) Status post aortic stent placement with reduced aortic gradient from 46 to 6 mmHg and reduced collateral (Right lower, Movie 4)

Diagnosis and Pre-procedural Evaluation

2-D TTE illustrated: Tricuspid AV, with normal size ascending aorta. In the supra sternal view, the descending thoracic aorta after left subclavian artery was not visible (Fig. 6 left panel) There was significant turbulent flow at the site of the interruption with multiple collateral vessels and *no significant gradient* (Fig. 6 right panel). Abdominal aorta Doppler study showed continuous low systolic and antegrade diastolic flow in favor of sever COA or interrupted aorta (IAA).

Interestingly, CT angiography of the aorta revealed interrupted aortic arch just before left subclavian artery origin with no residual lumen, the length of the interruption: 6 mm, tapered proximal and distal ends—Fig. 7a–c). Numerous well developed collateral vessels were visible (Fig. 7d). The best working view to characterize the alignment of the end parts: RAO 10 and caudal 22.

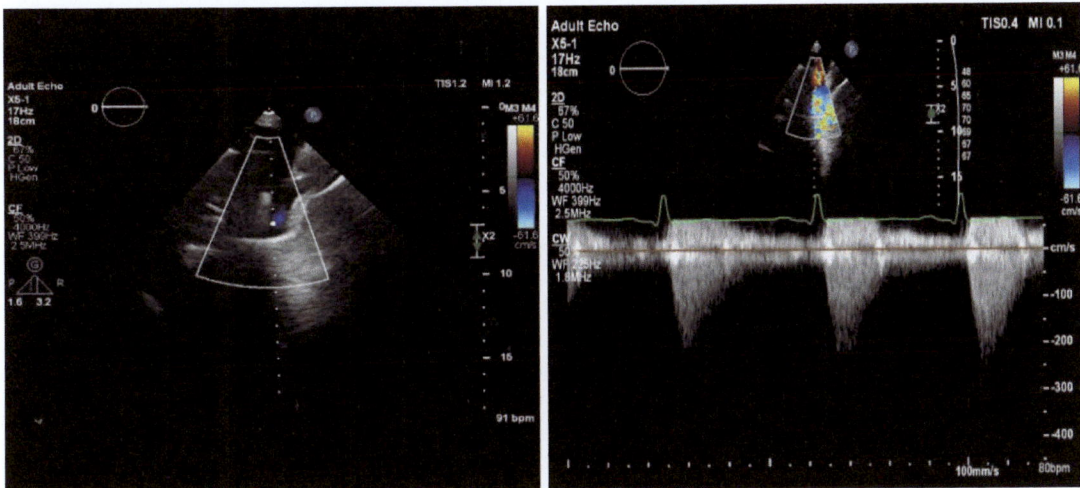

Fig. 6 In TTE, descending aorta was not evaluable after left subclavian artery with significant turbulent flow at the site of the interruption (left panel) and nonsignificant gradient at the site of the obstruction (right panel)

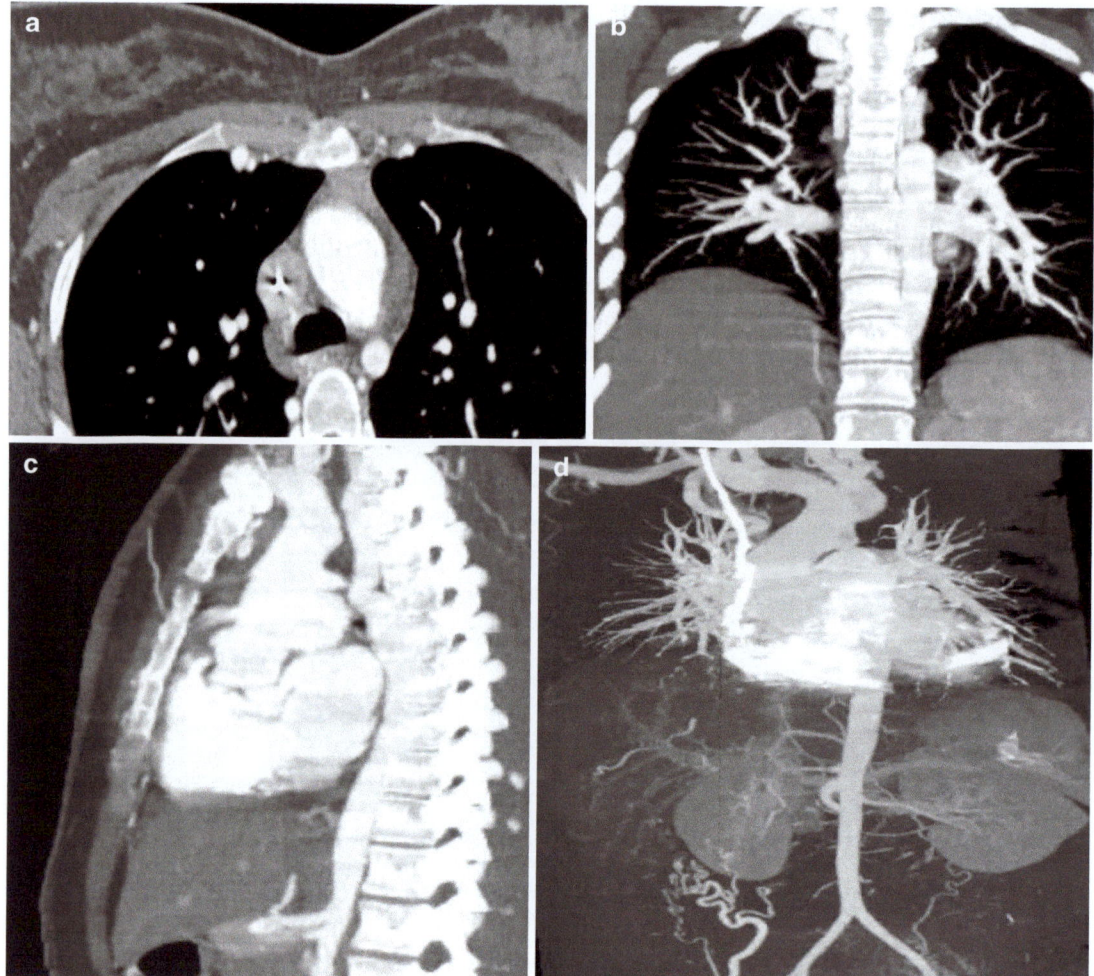

Fig. 7 (**a–d**) In axial, coronal and sagittal views, short interrupted aorta just before the origin of left subclavian artery is demonstrated (**a–c**). Numerous collateral vessels and the size of the descending aorta at the level of the diaphragm and lower extremities are shown (**d**)

Procedural Technique

Under conscious sedation, after ultra-sonography guided right CFA puncture and sheath (6F) insertion, and right radial artery access, 5000 units IV Heparin was injected (the base-line gradient was 70 mmHg). Right CFA angiography showed an acceptable diameter of the SFA, CFA, EIA, and CIA (Fig. 8a). So, 2 Perclose Proglide™ [Abbott Medical, Santa Clara, CA, USA] was inserted in the right CFA. Simultaneous antegrade and retrograde aortography at the level of the aortic isthmus and descending aorta with Pigtail catheter and Multipurpose catheter at deep LAO and AP projections depicted interrupted aorta just at the level of left subclavian artery (Fig. 8b). The interrupted segment length was discrete and both proximal and distal ends were tapered and their alignment in the suggested working view by CTA was not complex. Under meticulous hemodynamic monitoring, antegrade wiring was performed by CTO guidewire (Gaia 2nd) and after confirming the position of the wire to be in the true lumen by aortography in several projections

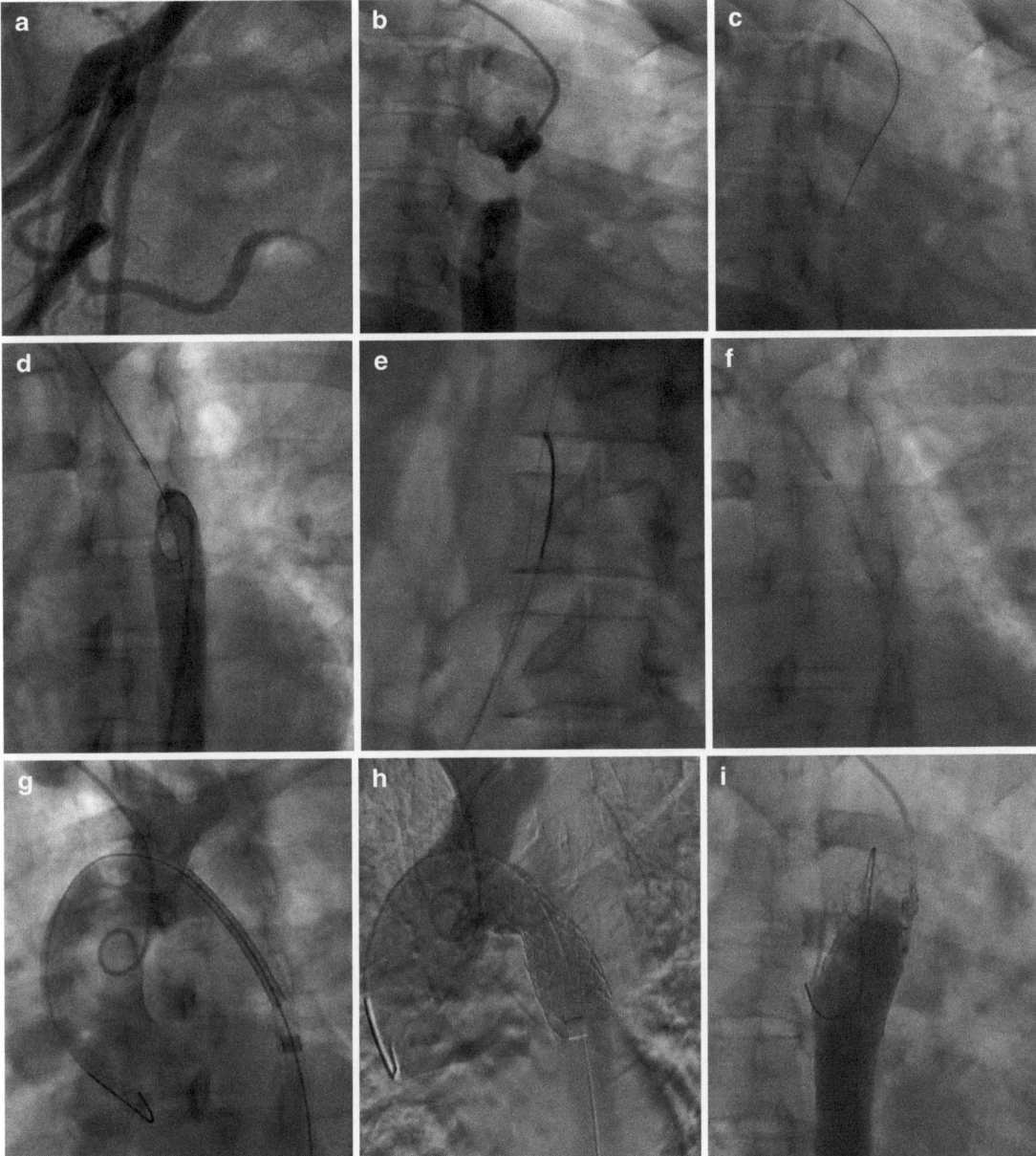

Fig. 8 (**a–i**) Right CFA angiography showed an acceptable diameter of the SFA, CFA, EIA, and CIA (**a**). Simultaneous antegrade and retrograde aortography at the level of the aortic isthmus and descending aorta with Pigtail catheter and Multipurpose catheter at working view projection depicted interrupted aorta just at the level of left subclavian artery. The interrupted segment length was discrete and both proximal and distal ends were tapered (**b**). Antegrade wiring was performed by CTO guidewire (Gaia 2nd) and after confirming of the position of the wire to be in the true lumen by aortography in several projections (**c, d**), the wire was snared in the CIA (**e**). Through the diagnostic Multipurpose catheter, the interrupted segment was dilated by coronary balloon (2.5*15) and by balloon swallow technique, the catheter was advanced toward the descending aorta (**f**). After manual crimping of the covered Optimus CoCor stent XL-48 mm on the table, it was passed through the sheath and by repetitive aortography by Pigtail catheter, it's appropriate position was confirmed (**g**). Final angiography demonstrated appropriate position of the stent without any complications (**h, i**). The final gradient was zero

(Fig. 8c, d), the wire was snared in the CIA (Fig. 8e). After that, through the diagnostic Multipurpose catheter, the interrupted segment was dilated by coronary balloon (2.5*15) and by balloon swallow technique, the catheter was advanced toward the descending aorta (Fig. 8f). After insertion a super-stiff guidewire 260 cm (Amplatzer), a long delivery sheath (Cook-14F) was advanced with it's tip positioned in the aortic arch and the dilator was removed and the sheath was de-aired. Based on the size of the transverse aorta, BIB 20*40 was selected. After manual crimping of the covered Optimus CoCor stent XL-48 mm on the table, it was passed through the sheath and by repetitive aortography by Pigtail catheter, it's appropriate position was confirmed (Fig. 8g). After retracting the sheath, first, the inner balloon was inflated to stabilize the stent and then the outer balloon was inflated. Finally, after deflating the balloon, the sheath was advanced over that, and the balloon was removed. Final angiography demonstrated appropriate position of the stent without any complications (Fig. 8h, i). The final gradient was zero.

Post-procedure Aortic CT Angiography

Aortic CTA, 1 month later illustrated: Patent stent at the proximal and distal portion of descending aorta, no evidence of recoarctation, no sign of complication at the site of stenting (Fig. 9a and b).

Complications

During the procedure, major complications occur in approximately 15% of cases: Intimal tearing, dissection, perforation, stent migration, CVA (<3%), tamponade, and the most important one, vascular complications (<1%). As the chance of delayed complications such as: aneurysm and pseudoaneurysm formation at the site of the stenting, re-coarctation, restenosis, stent fracture, and progressive aortic dilatation and dissection especially in those with BAV appears to be increased with more extended follow-up periods, all patients need careful periodic surveillance (Fig. 10).

Another issue in these patients is persistent, recurrent, and resistant systemic hypertension and disproportionate systolic hypertension with exercise.

- Hypertension is more common in patients whose repair was performed after 20 years of age compared with those who were corrected in early childhood [17]. So, close observation and treatment of hypertension by beta-blockers, angiotensin converting enzyme (ACE) inhibitors, or angiotensin receptor blockers (ARB) is mandatory.

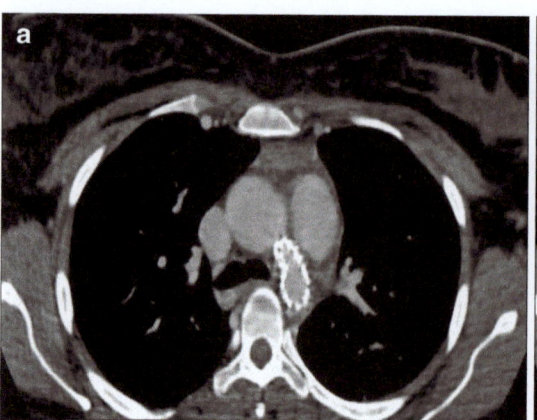 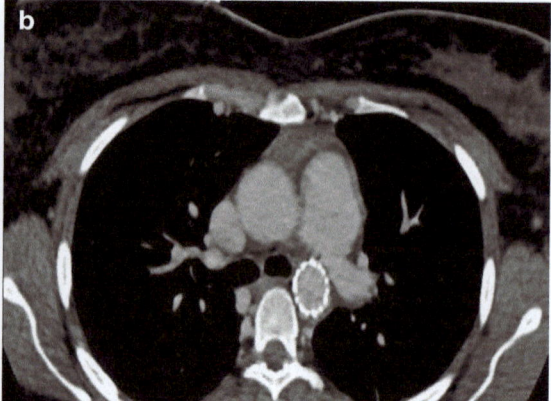

Fig. 9 (**a** and **b**) Follow-up aortic CTA 1 month later confirmed patent stent at proximal and distal portions of descending aorta, without evidence of recoarctation or any complications at the site of stenting (**a** and **b**)

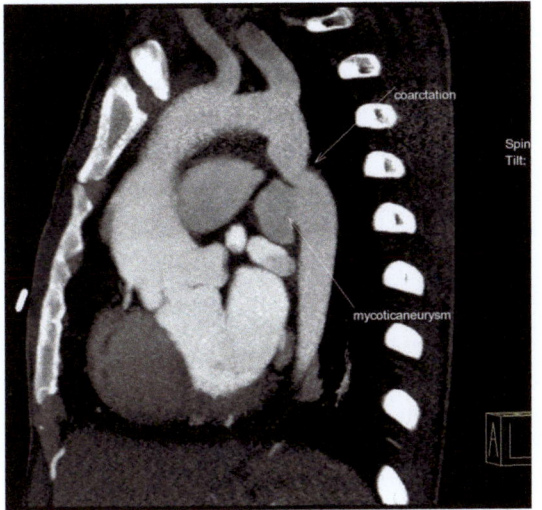

Fig. 10 CT angiogram sagittal plane showing Coarctation of Aorta complicated by mycotic aneurysm formation and infective endocarditis

Clinical Controversies and Pearls

- While balloon angioplasty effectively relieves vascular obstructions, it has some limitations, including elastic recoil of the vessel wall and intimal dissection.
- Stent insertion after balloon angioplasty or surgery reduces the complications, improves luminal diameter, results in minimal residual gradient, and sustains hemodynamic benefit [11, 12].
- The choice of stent depends on the coarctation anatomy, patient size and operator's preference. The imaging findings (the type and location of the COA or IAAs, the residual lumen width, the length of the stenosis or interruption, collateral vessels, and the size of the thoracoabdominal aorta at different levels and finding the optimal fluoroscopic angles especially in those with IAAs), assist in selecting the appropriate trans-catheter approach (either antegrade or retrograde approach) and selecting the proper balloon and stent size and type.
- Final stent diameter is based on the proximal arch diameter (transverse or distal arch), with the diameter not exceeding the size of the aorta at the diaphragm level. Furthermore, the ratio of stent diameter to pre-intervention narrowest coarctation segment should be <3.5 [13].
- There are several types of balloons and stents (either balloon-expandable or self-expandable, bare metal or covered types) at marketing. Each of them has its singular designs which have been improved during recent years regarding their materials (from stainless steel to platinum-iridium alloy, and chromium-cobalt alloy), expansion diameters, cell types and sizes (open or close cell design), wall thickness, foreshortening percentage, flexibility, profile, and the delivery sheath sizes.
- Both balloon-expandable and self-expandable stents have been used for the endovascular treatment of CoA. A randomized trial by Sadeghipour et al. [14] revealed that both balloon-expandable CP stents and self-expandable nitinol stents are safe and effective in treating native coarctation.
- Also, Firouzi et al [15] showed that both stent types were safe and effective in the treatment of non-interrupted COA during 1-year follow-up by CTA. A comparison between covered and non-covered stents in the non-interrupted aorta was made in a randomized controlled trial by Sohrabi et al. [16], who confirmed no significant superiority for covered stents.
- Regarding the potential risk of aortic dissection or perforation during the wiring and initial ballooning, most experts have recommended covered stents in the treatment of IAAs. Covered stents have been used by our group in these patients with the following conditions: (1) critical or sub-atretic obstructions, defined by a minimum diameter at the COA site of 2–3 mm on angiography (2) COA associated with the atresia of the aortic lumen (interrupted) [11].

Key Points
Coarctation of aorta (COA) is a congenital juxta ductal localized aortic narrowing (usually post-ductal in adults) that mainly remains undiagnosed in adulthood and

detected incidentally in a hypertensive patient with Radial-Femoral pulse delay.

An Interrupted aortic arch (IAA) is an anatomical and luminal disruption between the ascending and descending aorta that can be considered the most severe form of CoA.

The most common causes of death are congestive heart failure, aortic dissection, rupture of the aorta, infective endocarditis, premature coronary artery disease, and intra-cranial hemorrhage. In adults, the most common presentation is systemic hypertension, accounting for 0.2% of all hypertension cases in adults.

The systolic blood pressure gradient ≥20 mmHg between upper (right arm) and lower extremities suggests significant CoA that requires therapeutic intervention.

TTE showing suprasternal window provides the best view for visualizing the narrowing of the aorta and accelerated flow proximal to the narrowing with a characteristic Doppler pattern of "Sawtooth" appearance. Abdominal aorta Doppler study shows delayed and low velocity systolic and diastole forward flow associated with absent early diastolic flow reversal

Cardiac magnetic resonance (CMR) imaging and computed tomography (CT) angiography are recommended imaging modalities for evaluating CoA site, entire aorta and planing surgical vs trans-catheter approach.

Surgery is the standard management of native coarctation in infants and young children and TC approach is the preferred method in older children, adolescents, and adults.

Both balloon-expandable and self-expandable stents have been shown to be safe and effective for the endovascular treatment of CoA.

Interval surveillance by physical examination and imaging modalities (Echocardiography, CTA, and MRA), seems to be crucial as the chance of delayed complications such as: aneurysm and pseudoaneurysm formation at site of the stenting or surgical repair, re-coarctation, restenosis, stent fracture, and progressive aortic dilatation and dissection especially in those with BAV appears to increase during longer follow-up periods.

Patients need close monitoring and optimal treatment for their systemic hypertension.

CTA and preferably MRA are suggested imaging modalities to assess the postinterventional anatomy and possible complications every 3–5 years (Table 1).

Table 1 Imaging modalities

Imaging study	Benefits	Disadvantages
Echocardiogram	– The proper initial imaging modality for detecting the COA in suspicious cases. Also, assess biventricular function, the aortic valve (eg, bicuspid aortic valves, aortic stenosis, and aortic insufficiency), as well as detects other concomitant anomalies. – No radiation	– Limited value to define the detailed thoracoabdominal aorta anatomy in CoA and IAA
CT	The gold-standard tool to characterize the types and site of the COA or IAAs, the residual lumen width, the length of the stenosis or interruption, collateral vessels, and the size of the aorta at the level of sinus of valsalva, ascending, proximal arch, transverse arch, descending aorta at the level of the diaphragm by 3D volume-rendered and define any other anomalies. Further, assist to sort out the most appropriate treatment options (surgical or trans-catheter approach [TC]) in the pre-procedural planning and appropriate device selection before invasive angiography, and finding the optimal fluoroscopic views especially in those with IAAs	– Radiation exposure during follow-up – Risk of iodinated contrast nephropathy
MRI	– Additional information about ventricular size and function – No radiation – Preferred modality during follow-up	– Needs patient's cooperation
Angiogram	– The gold-standard tool to confirm the diagnosis and hemodynamic assessment of CoA, to characterize the types and site of the COA or IAAs, the residual lumen width, the length of the stenosis or interruption, collateral vessels, and the size of the aorta define the suitability for the trans-catheter approach and the device type	– Invasive – Radiation exposure – Risk of iodinated contrast nephropathy

Disclosures There are no conflicts of interest to disclose.

Chapter Review Questions

1. Which of the following Doppler study is NOT compatible with significant CoA of aorta?
   A. High-velocity systolic turbulent flow in the thoracic aorta detected in the suprasternal window
   B. Diastolic antegrade flow (diastolic tail) in the thoracic aorta detected in the suprasternal window
   C. The delayed and low-velocity systolic flow of the abdominal Aorta by pulse wave Doppler study
   D. Early diastolic flow reversal of the abdominal Aorta by pulse wave Doppler study

   Answer: D

   Explanation: In patients with significant CoA of aorta, abdominal pulse wave Doppler study shows slow and low-velocity systolic flow extending to the diastole with absent early diastolic flow reverse. More importantly, in post-CoA evaluation, the presence of the early diastolic flow reverse of the abdominal Aorta suggests no significant stenosis.

2. In an 18-year-old man with a history of severe hypertension and possible diagnosis of CoA, which of the following is NOT correct:
   A. Weak or absent pulses in the lower extremities are seen in all CoA patients
   B. Figure 3 configuration and rib notching can be seen in the Chest X Ray
   C. Continuous murmurs in inter-scapular might be heard on cardiac auscultation
   D. Radial-Femoral pulse delay is a common finding

   Answer: A

   Explanation: Radial-Femoral pulse delay and weak or absent pulses in the lower extremities are common findings except in the presence of the significant AR

3. A 25 years old woman with uncontrolled hypertension was referred to the ACHD clinic for further evaluation of coarctation (CoA) of aorta. Which of the following findings are NOT consistent with significant CoA:
   A. Mean Doppler systolic gradient at CoA site >20 mmHg

B. Mean Doppler gradient at CoA site >10 mmHg associated with significant AR or decreased LV systolic function
C. Mean Doppler gradient at CoA site >10 mmHg with collateral flow
D. Mean Doppler gradient at CoA site >10 mmHg with less than 50% narrowing of aorta relative to the aortic diameter at the level of the diaphragm

Answer: D

Explanation: In the significant CoA, more than 50% narrowing of aorta is seen relative to the aortic diameter at the level of the diaphragm

4. The preferred method of management of adults with significant coarctation of aorta is:
   A. End to end surgical repair
   B. CoA balloon aortoplasty
   C. CoA balloon aortoplasty with stenting
   D. Medical treatment and blood pressure control

Answer: C

Explanation: Trans catheter approach is the preferred method in older children, adolescents, and adults.

5. What is the recommended imaging interval follow-up in patients without associated anomaly after coarctation of aorta interventional treatment?
   A. CMR or CTA every 1–2 years
   B. CMR or CTA every 2-3 years
   C. CMR or CTA every 3–5 years
   D. Usually, TTE is the recommended follow up imaging modality

Answer: C

Explanation: CTA and preferably MRA are suggested imaging modalities to assess the postinterventional anatomy and possible complications every 3–5 years.

References

1. Topol EJ, Teirstein PS, editors. Textbook of interventional cardiology. 8th ed. Amsterdam, Netherlands: Elsevier; 2019. p. 959–62.
2. Rao PS. Coarctation of the aorta. Curr Cardiol Rep. 2005;7:425–32.
3. Campbell M. Natural history of coarctation of the aorta. Br Heart J. 1970;32:633–40.
4. Backer CL, Mavroudis C. Congenital heart surgery nomenclature and database project: patent ductus arteriosus, coarctation of the aorta, interrupted aortic arch. Ann Thorac Surg. 2000;69(4 Suppl):S298–307.
5. Hoffman JI, Kaplan S. The incidence of congenital heart disease. J Am Coll Cardiol. 2002;39(12):1890–900.
6. Ramirez Alcantara J, Mendez MD. Interrupted aortic arch. In: StatPearls. Treasure Island, FL: StatPearls Publishing; 2020.
7. Celoria GC, Patton RB. Congenital absence of the aortic arch. Am Heart J. 1959;58:407–13.
8. Sudhir Chandra Sinha. Transcatheter intervention for Coarctation of aorta: current status. Indian J Clin Cardiol. 2021;2(1):44–50.
9. Baumgartner H, Backer JD, Babu-Narayan SV, et al. 2020 ESC guidelines for the management of adult congenital heart disease: the task force for the management of adult congenital heart disease of the European Society of Cardiology (ESC). Eur Heart J. 2020;42(6):563–645. https://doi.org/10.1093/eurheartj/ehaa554.
10. Stout KK, Daniels CJ, Aboulhosn JA, Bozkurt B, Broberg CS, Colman JM, et al. 2018 AHA/ACC guideline for the management of adults with congenital heart disease: a report of the American College of Cardiology/American Heart Association Task Force on clinical practice guidelines. Circulation. 2019;139(14):e698–800.
11. Firouzi A, Hosseini Z, et al. Paradigm shift in management of interrupted aortic arch in adulthood. Curr Probl Cardiol. 2021;46(3):100717.
12. Chessa M, Carrozza M, Butera G, Piazza L, Negura DG, Bussadori C, et al. Results and mid-long-term follow-up of stent implantation for native and recurrent coarctation of the aorta. Eur Heart J. 2005;26(24):2728–32.
13. Forbes TJ, Moore P, et al. Intermediate follow-up following intravascular stenting for treatment of coarctation of the aorta. Catheter Cardiovasc Interv. 2007;70:569–77.
14. Sadeghipour P, Mohebbi B, Firouzi A, et al. Balloon-expandable Cheatham-platinum stents versus self-expandable nitinol stents in Coarctation of aorta. JACC Cardiov Interv. 2022;15:308–17.
15. Firoozi A, Mohebbi B, Noohi F, Bassiri H, Mohebbi A, Abdi S, et al. Self-expanding versus balloon-expandable stents in patients with isthmic Coarctation of the aorta. Am J Cardiol. 2018;122(6):1062–7.
16. Sohrabi B, Jamshidi P, Yaghoubi A, Habibzadeh A, Hashemi-Aghdam Y, Moin A, et al. Comparison between covered and bare Cheatham-platinum stents for endovascular treatment of patients with native post-ductal aortic coarctation: immediate and intermediate-term results. JACC Cardiovasc Interv. 2014;7(4):416–23.
17. Fawzy ME, Fathala A, Osman A, Badr A, Mostafa MA, Mohamed G, et al. Twenty-two years of follow-up results of balloon angioplasty for discreet native coarctation of the aorta in adolescents and adults. Am Heart J. 2008;156(5):910–7. Epub 2008/12/09

Percutaneous Closure of Patent Ductus Arteriosus

Lourdes Prieto and Daniel Duarte

Abstract

A patent ductus arteriosus (PDA) is a connection between the aorta and the pulmonary artery typically the proximal LPA. It is reported in 1 in 2000 full-term births, and accounts for 10% of all congenital heart defects. Although most of these are detected early in life, some of them are picked up in the adult population. Most patients are asymptomatic; however, some present with heart failure or with pulmonary hypertension and Eisenmenger syndrome. Percutaneous closure is now considered the standard of care. This section will discuss the physiology, as well as the role of different imaging modalities in the diagnosis of a PDA, indications for closure and periprocedural assessment.

Keywords

Patent ductus arteriosus · Percutaneous closure · Congenital heart disease · Transcatheter closure · Cardiac imaging in PDA

Supplementary Information The online version contains supplementary material available at https://doi.org/10.1007/978-3-031-50740-3_15.

L. Prieto (✉) · D. Duarte
Pediatric and Congenital Interventional Cardiology, Heart Institute, Nicklaus Children's Hospital, Miami, FL, USA
e-mail: lourdes.prieto@nicklaushealth.org; daniel.duarte-caceres@nicklaushealth.org

Abbreviations

CT	Computed tomography
LA	Left atrial
LPA	Left pulmonary artery
LV	Left ventricle
MRI	Magnetic resonance imaging
PA	Pulmonary artery
PDA	Patent ductus arteriosus
PVR	Pulmonary vascular resistance
RV	Right ventricle
SVR	Systemic vascular resistance
TTE	Transthoracic echocardiography

Test your learning and check your understanding of this book's contents: use the "Springer Nature Flashcards" app to access questions using ▶ https://sn.pub/ambACS. To use the app, please follow the instructions in the chapter "Transcatheter Aortic Valve Replacement."

Learning Objectives

1. Understand the pathophysiology and natural history of a PDA.
2. Know the most common clinical presentations and choose the most adequate imaging modality.

3. Understand the indications and contraindications for PDA closure, as well as potential complications.
4. Know how to evaluate the patient pre and post procedure, and when to follow up.

> **Case Study**
> A 20-year-old patient presented for murmur evaluation noticed by the primary care physician during an office visit. He had no significant past medical history. He recently immigrated from Central America for college and according to him, he had no symptoms referable to the cardiovascular system such as activity intolerance, chest pain or palpitations.

Background and Definitions

Introduction

The ductus arteriosus is a vascular connection of the proximal left pulmonary artery with the aorta. In-utero, this connection is maintained in fetal life by prostaglandins and low oxygen levels and diverts the blood from the pulmonary circulation into the systemic circulation. After birth, blood oxygen concentration increases inducing contraction of the smooth muscle resulting in physiologic closure within the first 72 h. Then, the endothelium necroses, and anatomical closure is finally achieved after 2–4 weeks. However, in some cases it can remain patent. The incidence of a patent ductus arteriosus (PDA) is reported as 1 in 2000 (0.3–0.8%) live births accounting for 5–10% of all congenital heart disease, yet this number can be underestimated in silent cases [1–3].

High altitudes, congenital rubella syndrome, prematurity and some gene mutations, such as TFAP2B, have been identified as risk factors for PDA [2]. Although it is commonly associated with more complex congenital heart defects the scope of this chapter is the isolated PDA.

Pathophysiology

The diameter of the PDA, and to a lesser degree the length, are the major determinant factors for the flow resistance. In large PDAs, the resistance is minimal and therefore, the flow will depend on the difference between the systemic and the pulmonary vascular resistance. Normally the pulmonary vascular resistance is lower than the systemic vascular resistance, and the shunt is left to right causing pulmonary overcirculation. To maintain adequate cardiac output, the left ventricle increases the stroke volume by increasing the end diastolic volume, or preload, and over time the end diastolic pressure increases. Different than ventricular septal defects, the shunting across the PDA occurs throughout the cardiac cycle, and in large PDAs the "run-off" of flow during diastole decreases the diastolic pressure. Occasionally, the combination of decreased diastolic pressure and increased ventricular end diastolic pressure can compromise the perfusion pressure of the coronary circulation [2, 4].

Clinical Assessment

The clinical presentation mostly depends on the size of the PDA, and it varies from asymptomatic patients with no signs of volume overload, to patients with heart failure or Eisenmenger physiology if left untreated. Frequently, large PDAs induce symptoms early in life that are noticed by the parents. However, it is not unusual for some of these patients to deny symptoms but avoid any physical activity. When symptoms are present, dyspnea and palpitations are the most frequent symptoms at the time of diagnosis [3, 5]. Left atrial dilatation can result in arrhythmias and sometimes it is the initial presentation. Wu et al. showed the incidence of tachyarrhythmias in adult patients with a PDA can be as high as 30% by age 59 [6].

Physical Examination
The typical murmur is a continuous "machinery" murmur throughout systole and diastole heard in the left upper parasternal border [2, 7].

Occasionally, there can be a diastolic rumble at the apex and the point of maximal impulse is deviated to the left. In a large PDA, the diastolic pressure is low increasing the pulse pressure resulting in bounding peripheral pulses. It is necessary to measure upper and lower extremities saturations to look for differential cyanosis that could indicate Eisenmenger syndrome, in which case the shunting is right to left. In these cases, the lower extremities saturation is lower than the upper, and can eventually manifest as lower extremity clubbing. In Eisenmenger syndrome, the typical murmur of the PDA is absent but the S2 component can be accentuated [2].

Cardiac Imaging

Echocardiogram: Echocardiogram is crucial to establish the diagnosis. The main objectives of the echocardiogram are:

- Visualizing the PDA by 2D, Doppler and Color Doppler study. Figure 1a, Movie 1 showing the typical location of PDA in parasternal short axis view by Doppler and color Doppler study
- Define anatomy: Defining the arch anatomy is essential especially before transcatheter closure is pursued. In patients with a right aortic arch the origin of the left subclavian artery may be aberrant coursing behind the esophagus. In these cases, most of the time, the PDA originates from the left subclavian artery constituting a vascular ring which can result in airway compression. Percutaneous closure of the defect can result in exacerbation of airway compression.
- Determine the directionality and velocity of the shunt by color and spectral Doppler. The velocity across the PDA is an indirect way to estimate the PA pressures (measure simultaneous systemic BP). A large, unrestrictive PDA

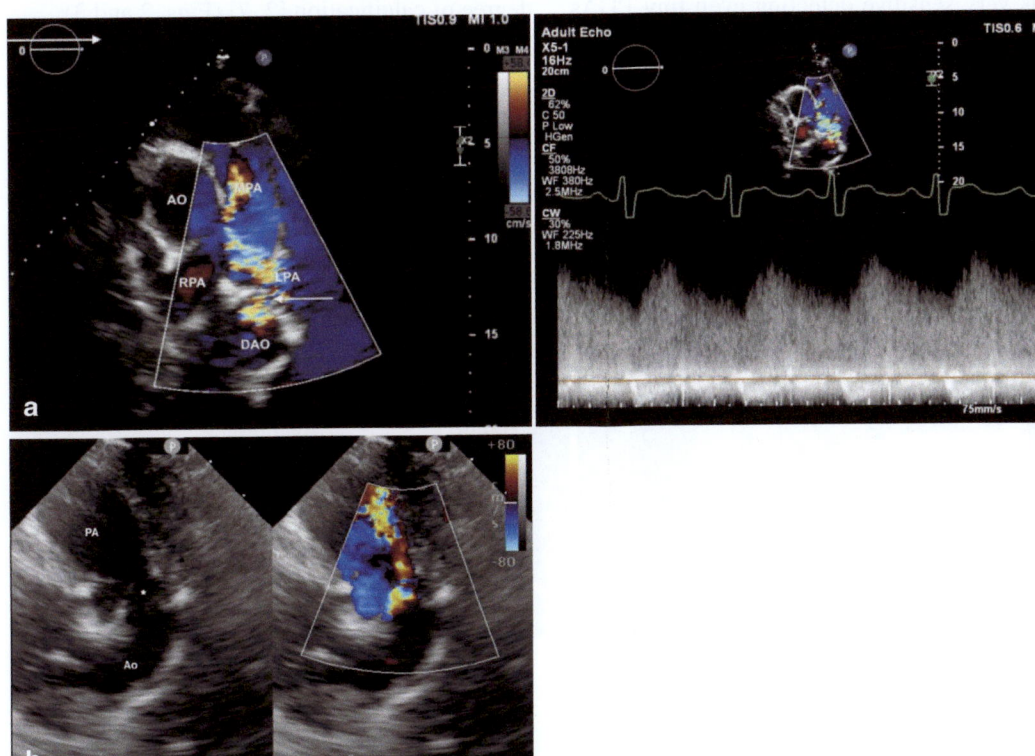

Fig. 1 Transthoracic echocardiogram (**a**) Parasternal short axis view, color Doppler imaging shows PDA flow (**b**) Continuous flow by Doppler study (**c**) 2D and color images demonstrating a PDA (star) with left to right shunting. *Ao* aorta; *PA* pulmonary artery; *RPA* right pulmonary artery; *LPA* left pulmonary artery; *DAO* descending aorta

has laminar flow and no turbulence in color Doppler indicating equal systolic pressure in the PA and aorta.
- Evaluate for volume overload. Enlargement of the left sided heart structures, left atrium and left ventricle, indicate volume overload. However, in patients with a large PDA who have developed Eisenmenger physiology, the left sided structures may be of normal size.
- Assess for other intra and extracardiac associated lesions such as coarctation of the aorta or LPA stenosis. As previously mentioned, a PDA can be associated with other congenital heart defects.

Acoustic windows in adults are generally limited, and the best view often is obtained from the suprasternal long axis view, angling the probe posteriorly to visualize the aorta and parasternal short axis view. Although 2D imaging can be useful to show the anatomy, color Doppler interrogation is very sensitive detecting even tiny PDAs, and estimates the degree of ductal shunting (Fig. 1). In patients with Eisenmenger and unrestrictive PDA, the ductal flow can be difficult to discern from flow in the LPA [7, 8].

Computed Tomography and Cardiac MRI

In younger patients transthoracic echocardiogram is often adequate to establish the diagnosis. However, in adult patients echocardiography may not be sufficient to make a definitive diagnosis, or to visualize other important anatomic features. In such cases, either cardiac CT or MRI should be performed to delineate the anatomy and size of the PDA. Additionally, 3D imaging can be helpful when the arch branching is questionable such as in vascular rings or cervical arches. It can also rule out a ductal aneurysm, although this is a very rare finding in the adult population. When performed, the MRI can help provide the Qp:Qs. In cases when surgical ligation is needed, the CT can help establish the degree of calcification [2, 7] (Figs. 2 and 3).

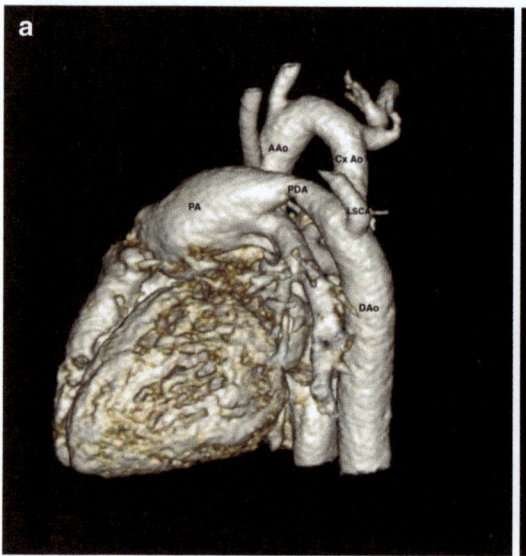
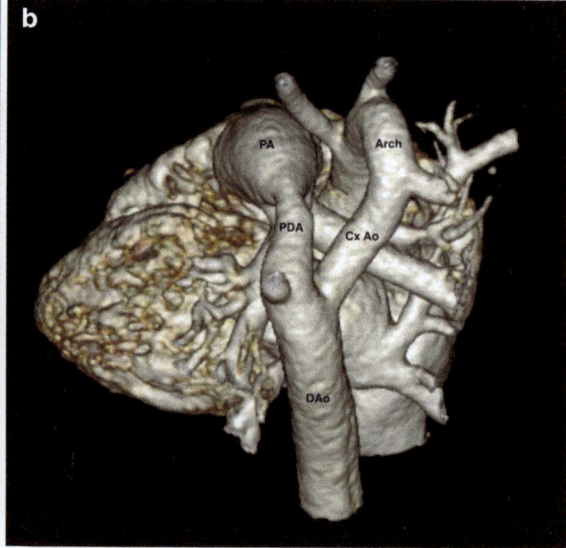

Fig. 2 (**a** and **b**) Three-dimensional render of a CT showing a patient with a large PDA in the setting of a vascular ring: right aortic arch with circumflex retroesophageal aorta, left descending aorta (DAo), aberrant left subclavian artery and left-sided PDA. *AAo* ascending aorta; *DAo* descending aorta; *PA* pulmonary artery; *PDA* patent ductus arteriosus; *Cx Ao* circumflex aorta

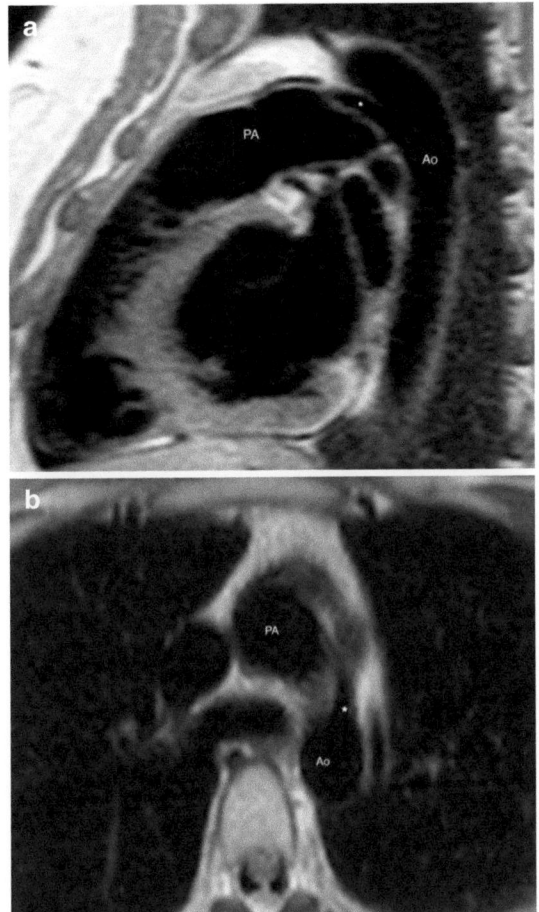

Fig. 3 (**a** and **b**) Sagital and transverse MRI "black blood" images of a PDA (star). *Ao* aorta; *PA* pulmonary artery

Cardiac Catheterization

Cardiac catheterization affords the opportunity to evaluate the anatomy by angiography, measure hemodynamics, and provide treatment during the same intervention. It is important to obtain hemodynamics prior to angiography as contrast can falsely increase the filling pressures. If PVR is elevated, pulmonary vasodilation testing should be performed with oxygen and nitric oxide to assess reversibility and determine whether the PDA can be closed [1, 9]. In patients with Eisenmenger syndrome the systemic saturation in the descending aorta will be lower than normal, thus the saturation must be obtained in the ascending aorta, and should be equal to the left atrial saturation.

Angiography is performed in the descending aorta just above the ductal ampulla to evaluate the ductal anatomy. A straight lateral projection shows the PDA anatomy best, including the narrowest diameter, length, and size of the ampulla. The anterior projection can be in straight AP or RAO [10]. Morphologic classification was established by Krichenko et al. based on the location of the narrowest diameter and the shape of the PDA (Fig. 4) (Table 1).

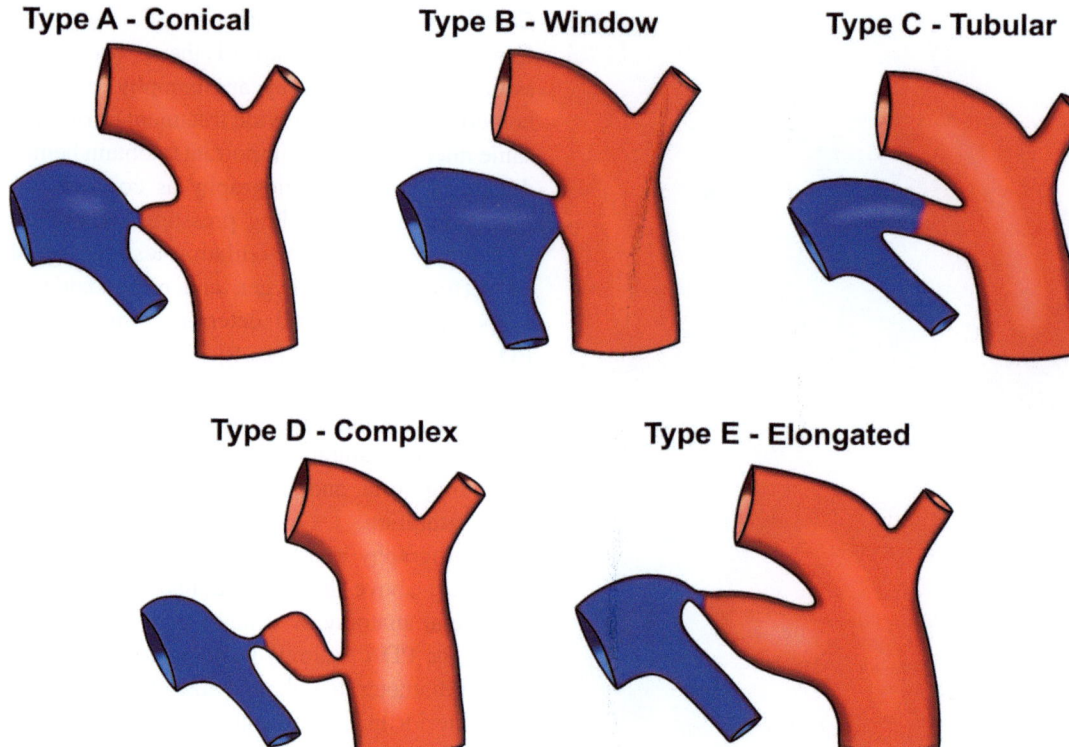

Fig. 4 PDA Krichenko classification

Table 1 PDA classification by size

PDA size	Physiology	Clinical findings	Management
Silent	Highly pressure restrictive and not hemodynamically significant	Silent on auscultation. Usually, an incidental finding	Observation
Small but audible	Highly pressure restrictive and not hemodynamically significant—no volume overload	No symptoms. Systolic grade I-II/VI in the left parasternal border. Normal LV and LA size. Possible risk of infectious endocarditis (see later discussion)	Percutaneous closure vs. observation (see controversies)
Moderate	Hemodynamically significant. Pulmonary overcirculation. Pressure restriction between Ao and PA	Symptomatic: – Dyspnea on exertion – Chest pain – Palpitations – Dizziness Continuous "machinery" on left upper parasternal border. Echocardiogram with enlargement of LA and LV	Cardiac catheterization and percutaneous closure indicated
Large	No or little pressure restriction between Ao and PA. +/− pulmonary vascular disease +/− Eisenmenger physiology	Symptomatic: – Possible arrhythmias due to chronic LA dilation – Differential cyanosis suggests Eisenmenger physiology	Cardiac catheterization for hemodynamic assessment. Percutaneous closure contraindicated in Eisenmenger physiology

Diagnosis and Pre-procedural Assessment

This patient had recently emigrated from Central America. Neither he nor his parents had ever been told he had a murmur before. Although he denied physical activity intolerance, he preferred more "quiet" activities and had voluntarily avoided physical education at school for the last 15 years because according to him, he "was not as fast as the other students". He denied palpitations.

His physical examination showed a PMI displaced to the left. There was a thrill on palpation over his chest. Auscultation revealed a grade III/VI continuous "machinery type" murmur in the left parasternal border. Pulses were 3+ in all extremities with no radiofemoral delay. The saturation in the upper and lower extremities was 96%.

Based on this, a PDA was suspected. A TTE was obtained demonstrating a moderate-size PDA with left-to-right shunting with LA and LV enlargement. Diastolic flow reversal in the descending aorta was seen. Spectral Doppler showed a peak velocity close to 4 m/s (Fig. 5). The arch was left-sided and the branching pattern was normal.

Since transthoracic echocardiography defined the arch branching pattern and ruled out other structural abnormalities no further imaging was obtained, and he underwent catheterization for hemodynamic assessment and possible device closure (Table 2).

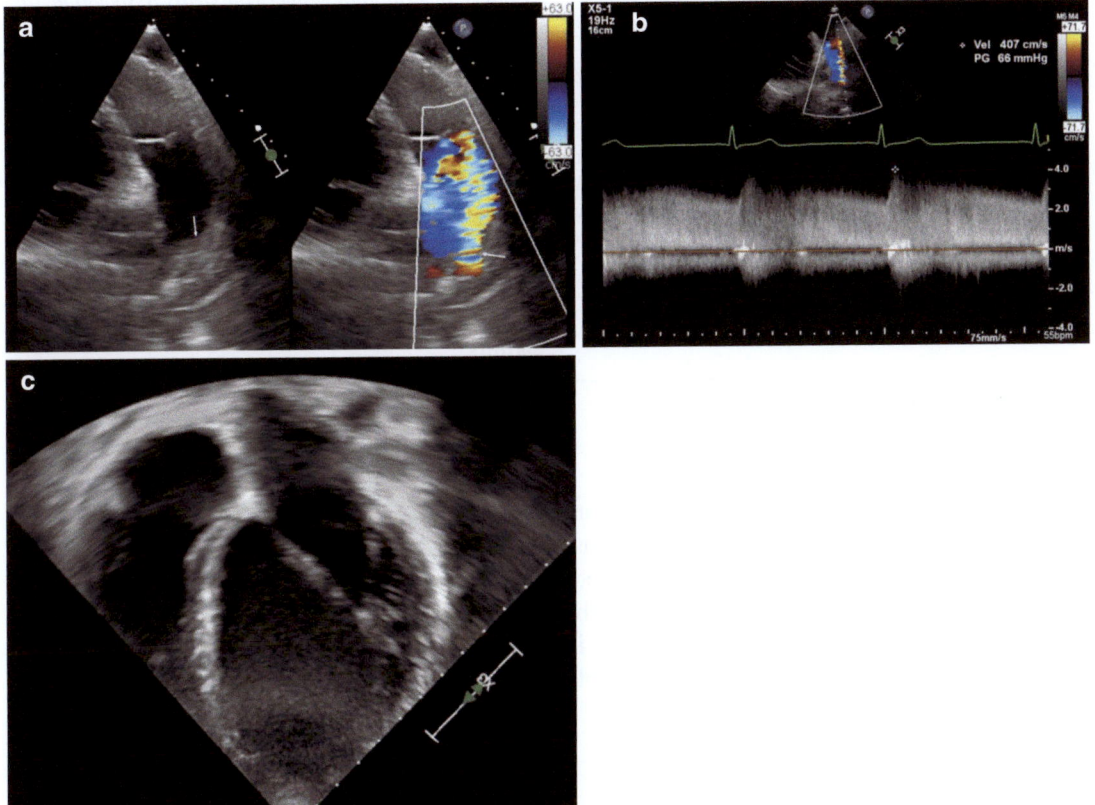

Fig. 5 (**a–c**) Transthoracic echocardiography shows a moderate sized PDA (white arrow) with continuous restrictive left to right shunting. The LV is dilated

Table 2 Patient hemodynamics

	Saturation	Pressure
SVC	74%	–
RA	74%	a = 10, v = 9, m = 9
RV	74%	44/10
PA	86%	44/25, mean = 35
LPA	82%	44/25, mean = 35
LPCWp		18
RPA	89%	44/25, mean = 35
RPCWp		18
LA	–	–
LV	–	98/18
AAo	96%	98/52, mean = 71
Dao	96%	98/52, mean = 71

Hemoglobin	14.5 g/dL
VO2	130 mL/kg/min
Qs	5.1 L/min (3.3 L/min/m^2)
Qp	11.35 L/min (7.3 L/min/m^2)
PVR	1.5 Wu (2.3 Wu * m^2)
SVR	12 Wu (18.8 Wu * m^2)
Qp/Qs	2.2
PVR/SVR	0.1

SVC superior vena cava; *RA* right atrium; *RV* right ventricle; *PA* pulmonary artery; *LPA* left pulmonary artery; *LPCWp* left pulmonary capillary wedge pressure; *RPA* right pulmonary artery; *RPCWp* right pulmonary capillary wedge pressure; *LA* left atrium; *LV* left ventricle; *AAo* ascending aorta; *Dao* descending aorta; *VO2* peak oxygen uptake; *Qs* systemic flow indexed to body surface area; *Qp* pulmonary flow indexed to body surface area; *PVR* pulmonary vascular resistance; *SVR* systemic vascular resistance

Heart Team Approach and Discussion

Although his mean pulmonary arterial pressures are elevated, the calculated pulmonary vascular resistance was within normal limits and thus, no pulmonary vasodilation testing was needed. Leaving the PDA open for a longer time would likely result in pulmonary vascular disease and possibly Eisenmenger. Therefore, closure was indicated.

Indications for PDA Closure

Closure of the PDA is indicated when there are symptoms of congestive heart failure, and/or signs of volume overload such as LA or LV enlargement. In patients with pulmonary hypertension without Eisenmenger physiology, PDA closure may be considered depending on careful hemodynamic evaluation. Table 3 summarizes the guideline recommendations of the American Heart Association/American College of Cardiology (AHA/ACC) for PDA closure in adults.

Table 3 Guideline recommendations

AHA/ACC 2019		
Recommendation	Class	LOE
PDA closure in adults recommended if LA or LV enlargement is present with net left to right shunt, PA systolic pressure <50% systemic and PVR <1/3 systemic	I	C-LD
PDA closure in adults may be considered in the presence of a net left to right shunt if PA systolic pressure is >50% systemic and the PVR >1/3 systemic	IIb	B-NR
PDA closure should not be performed in adults with a net right to left shunt and PA systolic pressure >2/3 systemic or PVR >2/3 systemic	III	C-LD

Obtained with permission from: *Stout KK, Daniels CJ, Aboulhosn JA, Bozkurt B, Broberg CS, Colman JM*, et al. *2018 AHA/ACC Guideline for the Management of Adults With Congenital Heart Disease: A Report of the American College of Cardiology/American Heart Association Task Force on Clinical Practice Guidelines. Circulation. 2019;139(14):e698–e800*

Heart Team Decision

Surgery

In contrast to the pediatric population, surgical ligation of the ductus in the adult carries a significant degree of morbidity. Calcification, ductal aneurysm or coexisting coronary artery disease require anterior sternotomy approach on cardiopulmonary bypass. Nowadays, surgery is reserved only for cases where transcatheter device closure is not possible or is contraindicated, as is the case in right aortic arch with aberrant left subclavian artery and left-sided PDA with airway compression, very large PDAs, or large ductal aneurysms [7, 11].

Percutaneous Closure

Percutaneous closure is currently the method of choice to address a PDA. The success rate is close to 100% and the rate of complications is minimal [1–3, 7, 9, 10, 12]. The largest reported series in 141 adults showed a success rate of 99% with no major complications [3]. The procedure can be performed under local anesthesia, and for most cases, it requires less than 24 h of observation.

Once the anatomy is defined, the ductus can be closed either by a prograde approach advancing a catheter from the venous side into the pulmonary artery and crossing the ductus to the descending aorta; or for symmetric devices retrograde from the aortic side crossing to the pulmonary artery. Nowadays, coils are rarely used as they have been replaced by newer occluding devices (i.e.: Amplatzer Duct Occluder I) (Fig. 6). If crossing from the PA is not possible, as sometimes happens in adult patients, a wire can be snared after the crossing from the aortic side to form an arterio-venous rail, allowing closure with an Amplatzer Duct Occluder I.

Intraprocedural Imaging Modalities and Measurements

Angiography was obtained in the descending aorta just above the ductal ampulla in RAO/caudal and straight lateral projections showing a moderate sized PDA. It is important to obtain adequate measurements with especial attention to the narrowest diameter. These will determine the size and type of device. In contrast to the pediatric population, it is rare for the devices to result in compression of the LPA or the descending aorta. Once the device is placed, angiography should be obtained in the aorta to evaluate for device position and residual shunting (Fig. 7).

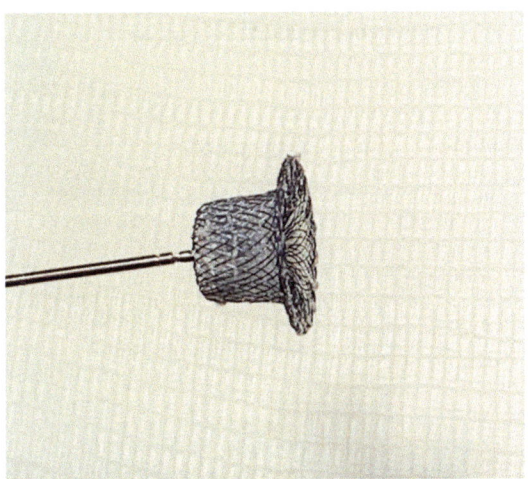

Fig. 6 Amplatzer Duct Occluder attached to the delivery wire. (Photo by the author)

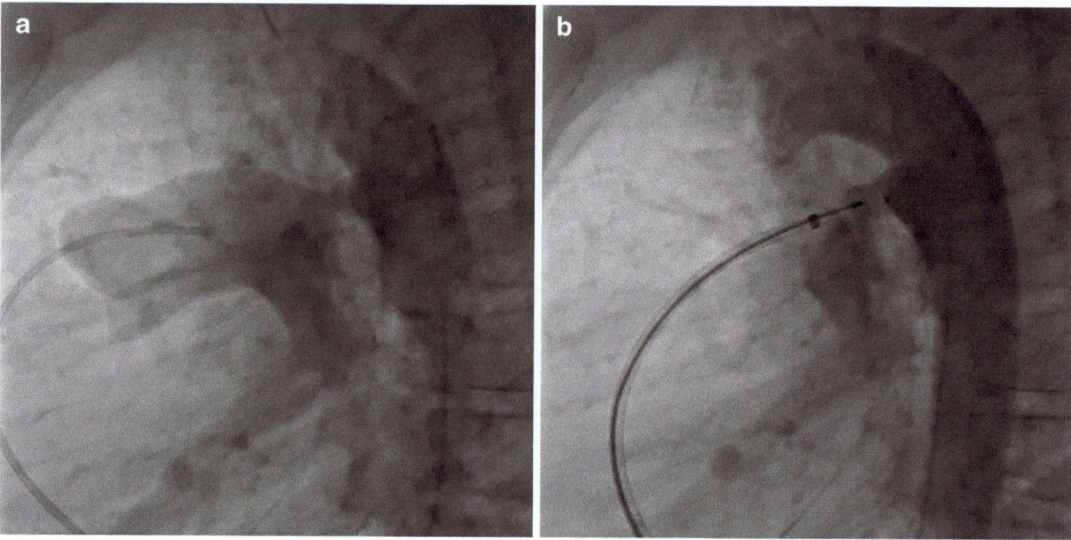

Fig. 7 (**a** and **b**) Angiogram in the descending aorta in the lateral projection demonstrating a moderate size PDA (Krichenko type A) pre and post-device closure

Post Procedural Assessment

Immediate postoperative evaluation should include transthoracic echocardiogram and CXR. Occasionally, left ventricular dysfunction can be seen following PDA closure especially when the PDA is large and pulmonary vascular resistance is still low. This is secondary to a sudden increase in afterload when the PDA is closed.

In this case, transthoracic echocardiogram performed after the procedure showed no residual flow through the ductus, no obstruction of the LPA or descending aortic flow, and normal LV function.

Follow Up

- First 24 h: Transthoracic echocardiogram and CXR to verify stable position of the device and evaluate residual shunting.
- Six months: outpatient visit with echocardiogram. If no residual shunting, normal PA pressures, and normal LV size and function, patient can be discharged.
- If elevated PVR or abnormal LV function—follow up every 1–3 years [9].

Multimodality imaging comparison

Imaging study	Benefits	Disadvantages
Echocardiogram	– More accessible. – Provides physiological data such as directionality of shunting, signs of volume overload, RV and PA pressures, LV function. – Rules out other anatomical lesions. – No radiation	– Acoustic windows in adults are limited and may not offer adequate anatomic information
CT	– Detailed anatomic evaluation. – Evaluates degree of calcification. – Can help evaluate the ventricular function	– No physiological information. – Radiation exposure

Imaging study	Benefits	Disadvantages
MRI	– Provides flow evaluation (Qp:Qs) as well as detailed anatomic evaluation and ventricular function. – No radiation	– Not adequate to evaluate for calcification
Cath and angiogram	– Anatomic and detailed physiologic information. – Opportunity to treat	– Invasive

Clinical Controversies and Clinical Pearls

- Bacterial endocarditis in small PDAs has been reported in a few cases, and closing a small, hemodynamically insignificant PDA for prevention is a matter of controversy [12].
- The rate of significant complications of transcatheter closure is quite low and thus, some argue the lifetime risk of endarteritis is higher than the procedural risks.
- PDA closure is indicated in patients with congestive heart failure symptoms and/or with evidence of LV volume overload and most agree to the closure a small, hemodynamically insignificant PDA as long as it is audible.
- PDA diagnosis is established by transthoracic echocardiogram in most cases, but 3D imaging, or other cardiac imaging may be necessary in adult patients.

Key Points
- A patent ductus arteriosus (PDA) is a vascular connection between the LPA and the aorta, and it comprises 10% of congenital heart disease cases.
- Moderate and large PDAs result in volume overload and eventually pulmonary arterial hypertension with vascular changes, and if uncorrected can result in Eisenmenger physiology.
- Transthoracic echocardiogram is the imaging modality of choice for diagnosis and evaluation of the anatomy, flow directionality and pressure restriction across the PDA.
- CT or MRI should be obtained when echocardiographic windows are not adequate and further anatomical detail is necessary, and/or if a ductal aneurysm is suspected by echocardiography.
- When indicated, transcatheter PDA device closure is the method of choice with high success rates and minimal complications.

Chapter Review Questions

1. What is the main determinant of the shunt direction in a PDA?
   A. Length and diameter of the PDA
   B. Difference between SVR and PVR
   C. Left ventricular end diastolic pressure
   D. A and C
   Answer: B
   Explanation: Although the restriction of the flow is mostly determined by the narrowest segment of the PDA, the direction of the shunt (right to left or left to right) is determined by the difference between the SVR and PVR. Normally the SVR is higher than the PVR, and thus the shunt is left to right. However, for untreated large, unrestrictive PDAs, once the PVR is greater than the SVR the shunt flow reverses, and patients develop Eisenmenger physiology.

2. Which of the following is NOT an indication for PDA closure?
   A. Signs of volume overload by echocardiography.
   B. Signs and symptoms of heart failure.
   C. Small non-audible "silent" PDA.
   D. Moderate PDA with mildly elevated PA pressures.

Answer: C

Explanation: Small non-audible PDA is frequently an incidental finding. They are hemodynamically insignificant and the risk of endocarditis is felt to be negligible to non-existent. Therefore, closure is not indicated.

3. A 20-year-old male patient presents for evaluation of a murmur. The echocardiogram showed moderate sized PDA with left to right shunt. The spectral Doppler showed restrictive PDA with peak gradient of 3.8 m/s and a simultaneous blood pressure of 100/70. The LV and LA are dilated. The arch is left-sided, and the branching pattern is normal. What is the best next step?
   A. Start diuretics and re-evaluate in 3 months.
   B. Computed tomography of the chest with contrast.
   C. Cardiac magnetic resonance.
   D. Transcatheter closure.

Answer: D

Explanation: The echocardiogram provided all the necessary information, and transcatheter closure is indicated. There is no need for further imaging.

4. (Questions 4 and 5) A 55-year-old female presents with lower extremity clubbing. Echocardiographic windows are very limited but shows a large PDA with possible bidirectional shunting. Spectral Doppler showed no significant restriction. What is the next step in evaluation of this patient?
   A. Cardiac catheterization.
   B. Cardiac MRI.
   C. Transesophageal echocardiogram.
   D. Surgical closure.

5. After evaluation, the patient undergoes cardiac catheterization for hemodynamic evaluation. Hemodynamics showed severe pulmonary hypertension with calculated PVR of 15 WU and Qp:Qs of 0.7. Pulmonary vasodilatory testing shows partial response to oxygen and nitric oxide with improvement of the PVR to 12. Angiography shows a large PDA with significant calcification. Based on the above:
   A. PDA should be closed in the catheterization laboratory.
   B. Surgical closure is indicated.
   C. Closure is contraindicated.
   D. None of the above

Answer to Question 4: A

Answer to Question 5: C

Explanation: The patient has clubbing of the lower extremities, and this is caused by chronic lower oxygen saturation in the descending aorta due to right to left shunting at the ductal level. It is necessary to obtain hemodynamics in the catheterization laboratory and test for reversibility. In this case hemodynamics showed the PVR is greater than the SVR and the Qp:Qs is lower than 1, indicating she has Eisenmenger physiology. Therefore, closure is contraindicated. Surgery is reserved for cases where device closure is contraindicated by the anatomy such as vascular rings with compression of the airway, or large ductal aneurysms.

References

1. Stout KK, Daniels CJ, Aboulhosn JA, Bozkurt B, Broberg CS, Colman JM, et al. 2018 AHA/ACC guideline for the management of adults with congenital heart disease: a report of the American College of Cardiology/American Heart Association Task Force on Clinical Practice guidelines. Circulation. 2019;139(14):e698–800.
2. Taggart NW, Mohammed YQ. Patent ductus arteriosus and aortopulmonary window. In: Allen HD, Shaddy RE, Penny DJ, Feltes TF, Cetta F, editors. Moss and Adams' heart disease in infants, children, and adolescents: including the fetus and young adults, vol. 1. 9th ed. Philadelphia, PA: Lippincott Williams & Wilkins; 2016.
3. Wilson WM, Shah A, Osten MD, Benson LN, Abraha N, Breitner D, et al. Clinical outcomes after percutaneous patent ductus arteriosus closure in adults. Can J Cardiol. 2020;36(6):837–43.
4. Sommer RJ, Hijazi ZM, Rhodes JF Jr. Pathophysiology of congenital heart disease in the adult: part I: shunt lesions. Circulation. 2008;117(8):1090–9.
5. Sudhakar P, Jose J, George OK. Contemporary outcomes of percutaneous closure of patent ductus arteriosus in adolescents and adults. Indian Heart J. 2018;70(2):308–15.
6. Wu MH, Lu CW, Chen HC, Kao FY, Huang SK. Adult congenital heart disease in a nationwide population 2000–2014: epidemiological trends, arrhythmia,

and standardized mortality ratio. J Am Heart Assoc. 2018;7(4):e007907.
7. Schneider DJ, Moore JW. Patent ductus arteriosus. Circulation. 2006;114(17):1873–82.
8. Arya B, Sable CA. Abnormalities of the ductus arteriosus and pulmonary arteries. In: Lai WW, Mertens LL, Cohen MS, Geva T, editors. Echocardiography in pediatric and congenital heart disease. 2nd ed. Chichester, UK: Wiley; 2016. p. 317–35.
9. Baumgartner H, De Backer J, Babu-Narayan SV, Budts W, Chessa M, Diller GP, et al. 2020 ESC guidelines for the management of adult congenital heart disease. Eur Heart J. 2021;42(6):563–645.
10. Bentham J, Wilson N. Patent ductus arteriosus (PDA): background and indications for closure. In: Interventions in structural, valvular, and congenital heart disease. 2nd ed. Boca Raton, FL: Taylor & Francis Group; 2015. p. 611–6.
11. Kouchoukos NT, Blackstone EH, Hanley FL, Kirklin JK. Congenital heart disease in the adult. In: Kouchoukos NT, Blackstone EH, Hanley FL, Kirklin JK, editors. Kirklin/Barratt-Boyes cardiac surgery: morphology, diagnostic criteria, natural history, techniques, results, and indications. 4th ed. Philadelphia, PA: Elsevier; 2013. p. 1061–147.
12. Fortescue EB, Lock JE, Galvin T, McElhinney DB. To close or not to close: the very small patent ductus arteriosus. Congenit Heart Dis. 2010;5(4):354–65.

Index

A
Alcohol septal ablation (ASA), 107, 108, 115, 195–205, 209, 212–217, 222–224
Amulet, 179, 181, 184–186, 188
Aortic regurgitation, 10, 20, 21, 34, 36–43, 46, 50, 54, 57, 61, 63, 156, 167, 170, 206, 288, 290, 292, 310, 311, 314, 316–318, 320, 321, 330
Aortic stenosis, 4–26, 28, 31, 38, 51, 52, 63, 139, 152, 167, 199, 329, 341
Atrial fibrillation (AF), 26, 58, 74, 88, 120, 121, 126, 127, 130, 135, 138, 156, 169, 178, 230, 246, 256–257, 265, 267, 270, 272, 311
Atrial septal defect (ASD), 113, 181, 189, 247, 264–266, 268–273, 275, 276, 280, 281, 297

B
Balloon valvuloplasty, 47, 51–54, 56, 57, 61–64
Bicuspid aortic valve, 28–37, 54, 63, 264, 288, 310, 329, 330, 334, 341

C
Cardiac computer tomography angiography (CCTA), 179, 189
Cardiac imaging, 37, 77, 122, 140, 284–294, 345–349, 353
Coarctation of aorta (COA), 328–334, 338–342
Complications of myocardial infarction, 233
Congenital heart disease, 138, 141, 144, 153, 168, 298, 328, 344, 346, 350, 353
Continuous murmur, 296, 297, 307, 310, 311, 322, 329, 341
Coronary artery fistulas (CAFs), 296, 306, 307
Coronary-cameral fistulas (CCFs), 296, 304, 306
Coronary obstruction, 13, 16, 19, 20, 28, 31, 33, 36, 38, 45–49, 51, 52, 54, 162

D
Device closure, 165, 178, 186, 233, 265, 266, 270–273, 285, 286, 289, 294, 298, 304, 320, 349, 350, 354
Diastolic dysfunction, 4, 121, 147, 250, 298

E
Echocardiography, 5–10, 20, 21, 24–26, 28, 34, 35, 40, 44, 47, 49, 59, 76, 97, 115, 122, 124, 126, 128, 133, 140, 144, 152, 158, 160–162, 164, 165, 168, 180, 197, 200, 201, 203, 205–209, 213, 216, 223, 224, 231, 233, 240, 269, 284, 297, 299, 306, 319, 320, 322, 330, 340, 346, 349, 353
Elevated gradients, 22–26, 47, 49–51, 112

H
Heart failure with mild range ejection fraction (HFmrEF) treatment, 246, 247
Heart failure with preserved ejection fraction (HFpEF) treatment, 120, 246, 247, 250, 252–254, 257
Hypertension, 28, 52, 71, 77, 87, 88, 98, 99, 104, 135, 178, 196, 246, 313, 321, 328, 329, 331, 333, 338, 340, 341, 350, 354
Hypertrophic cardiomyopathy (HCM), 196, 197, 203, 204, 212–214
Hypoattenuating leaflet thickening (HALT), 22

I
Interatrial shunt device, 246–248, 250, 254, 255, 257, 259
Inter-atrial shunting, 264, 280, 281
Intra-procedural guidance, 87, 94, 97, 115, 134, 191, 268
Interrupted aortic arch (IAA), 328–342

L
Left atrial appendage closure (LAAC), 177–181, 183–186, 188, 189, 191, 192
Left atrial hypertension, 246, 250
Luminal disruption, 340

M
Mitral balloon valvuloplasty, 88
Mitral regurgitation, 5, 20, 26, 28, 33, 57, 70, 73, 86, 91, 97, 102, 103, 116, 170, 197, 204, 206, 223, 231, 268, 312

Mitral stenosis, 73, 80, 88, 97, 98, 102–104, 116, 180, 191
Mitral valve disease, 26, 31, 73, 102, 115, 116, 199, 223, 269
Mitral valve in valve, 98–101, 104, 114
Mitral valve replacement, 71, 98, 102, 169, 199
Multimodality imaging, 25, 35, 42, 43, 49, 70, 86, 87, 97, 110, 134, 144, 158, 161, 189, 205, 240, 312, 315, 321–322, 352–353
Multimodality imaging for tricuspid intervention, 119–134
Muscular, 284, 286, 288, 293, 294, 316, 318, 320
Myocardial infarction, 57, 124, 196, 216, 231, 233, 240, 296, 304, 305, 307, 312, 320

P

Paravalvular leak, 13, 19, 21, 34, 39, 41–43, 48, 51, 111, 156, 157, 160–162, 164, 168, 169, 171
Paravalvular regurgitation, 8, 21, 33–35, 39, 42, 45, 49, 54, 61, 63, 110, 113, 156, 157, 159, 165–168, 170, 171
Patent ductus arteriosus (PDA), 139, 297, 300, 301, 329, 344, 346, 353
Patent foramen ovale (PFO), 264–266, 269–273, 275, 276, 280, 281
Percutaneous, 5, 43, 57, 61, 88, 89, 127, 162–164, 167, 168, 170, 171, 186, 189, 191, 192, 196, 203–205, 222, 230, 231, 233, 235, 237, 239–241, 266, 269–273, 275, 284–286, 288–290, 292, 293, 298, 312, 314, 320, 345, 348, 351
Percutaneous closure, 19, 157, 160, 162–168, 185, 230, 231, 233, 235, 237, 239–241, 266, 269–271, 273, 275, 284, 286, 288–290, 292, 293, 305, 314, 320, 345, 348, 351
Perimembranous, 284, 288, 289, 292
Post-myocardial infarction ventricular septal defect, 230
Pre-procedural planning, 38, 77, 87, 97, 115, 126, 165, 185, 297, 306, 307
Prosthetic stenosis, 99
Pulmonic valve, 138, 139, 147, 148, 151–153

R

Right heart disease, 122, 128
Right ventricle, 34, 76, 109, 122, 123, 125, 126, 130, 133, 135, 138, 139, 151, 200, 201, 286, 289, 298, 300, 301, 306, 307, 311, 312, 314, 318, 321, 350
Right ventricular outflow tract (RVOT), 138, 165, 289, 311–313, 318
Ruptured, 74, 297, 301, 310–322

S

Septal reduction therapy (SRT), 196, 198, 203, 204, 213, 214, 216

Sinuses of Valsalva (SOVA), 8, 12, 26, 30, 31, 46, 48, 56, 57, 59, 300, 310–322, 329, 341
Structural heart, 126, 186, 204, 284–294, 298, 321
Surgical myectomy, 196, 197, 199, 203, 206, 212, 214–216, 222
Surgical repair, 80, 87, 128, 138, 139, 232, 233, 286, 290, 293, 296, 312, 317–320, 329, 340

T

Transcatheter aortic paravalvular leak closure, 165–167
Transcatheter aortic valve replacement, 3–64, 102, 126
Transcatheter closure, 157, 158, 162, 163, 165, 169, 231, 233, 234, 292, 297, 305, 306, 310–322, 345
Transcatheter coarctoplasty, 328, 331
Transcatheter edge-to-edge repair (TEER), 71, 127, 132
Transcatheter heart valves, 21, 33, 45, 50, 102
Transcatheter intervention, 13, 70, 126, 128, 132, 135, 138, 152, 157, 158
Transcatheter mitral paravalvular leak closure, 156, 163
Transcatheter mitral valve replacement (TMVR), 102, 104, 107
Transcatheter pulmonic valve replacement, 153
Transcatheter tricuspid paravalvular leak closure, 168
Transcatheter tricuspid valve intervention, 130
Transesophageal, 5, 71, 76, 86, 97, 102, 115, 140, 151, 152, 156, 158, 161–163, 165–167, 169, 170, 180, 208, 230, 231, 240, 266–268, 273, 284, 285, 289, 299, 300, 307, 311, 322
Transesophageal echocardiography (TEE), 5, 12, 19–21, 24, 25, 30, 31, 35, 37, 38, 40, 41, 43, 45, 47–50, 52, 53, 61, 76, 82, 85, 86, 91–93, 95, 97, 102–106, 109, 110, 115, 125, 127, 161, 164, 165, 167, 168, 181, 182, 206, 234, 236, 266, 285, 286, 291, 292, 307, 312, 314, 315, 318, 320
Transthoracic, 5, 21, 37, 49, 61, 73, 86, 88, 91, 97, 115, 122–123, 140, 151, 152, 156, 158, 161–163, 166–170, 179, 180, 197, 198, 200, 203, 212, 223, 224, 230, 231, 239, 240, 246, 265, 279, 284, 292, 297, 304, 307, 311, 329, 345, 346, 349, 352, 353
Tricuspid regurgitation, 120–122, 124–126, 128, 130, 131, 134, 135, 156, 238, 254, 312

V

Valve-in-valve, 42–52, 115, 164, 171
Valvular disease, 38, 88, 180, 247
Ventricular septal defect (VSD), 138, 160, 284, 288, 291, 297, 310, 315, 321, 329, 344

W

Watchman, 178, 179, 181, 183–186, 191

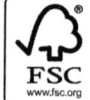

MIX
Papier aus verantwortungsvollen Quellen
Paper from responsible sources
FSC® C105338

If you have any concerns about our products,
you can contact us on
ProductSafety@springernature.com

In case Publisher is established outside the EU,
the EU authorized representative is:
Springer Nature Customer Service Center GmbH
Europaplatz 3, 69115 Heidelberg, Germany

Printed by Libri Plureos GmbH
in Hamburg, Germany